METHODS IN MOLECULAR BIOLOGY™

Series Editor
John M. Walker
School of Life Sciences
University of Hertfordshire
Hatfield, Hertfordshire, AL10 9AB, UK

For other titles published in this series, go to
www.springer.com/series/7651

Cystic Fibrosis

Diagnosis and Protocols, Volume I: Approaches to Study and Correct CFTR Defects

Edited by

Margarida D. Amaral

Centre for Biodiversity and Functional and Integrative Genomics,
Faculty of Sciences, University of Lisboa,
Lisboa, Portugal

Karl Kunzelmann

Department of Physiology, University of Regensburg,
Regensburg, Germany

Humana Press

Editors
Margarida D. Amaral
Centre for Biodiversity & Functional
and Integrative Genomics
University of Lisboa
Lisboa 1749-016, Portugal
mdamaral@fc.ul.pt

Karl Kunzelmann
Department of Physiology
University of Regensburg
Regensburg 93053, Germany
karl.kunzelmann@vkl.uni-regensburg.de

ISSN 1064-3745 e-ISSN 1940-6029
ISBN 978-1-4939-5787-3 ISBN 978-1-61779-117-8 (eBook)
DOI 10.1007/978-1-61779-117-8
Springer New York Dordrecht Heidelberg London

Printed on acid-free paper

Humana Press is part of Springer Science+Business Media (www.springer.com)

Foreword

This book represents a milestone in the worldwide cystic fibrosis (CF) community's efforts to continue to pave the way toward the development of new and innovative therapies that address the basic defect in CF. But no book on this subject would be possible without the invaluable contributions of the many patients, families, and disease-related organizations that played a key role in creating the science outlined in these chapters. As an orphan disease, CF does not receive sufficient funding from traditional supporting agencies but depends instead on a vast network of people who selflessly give their time and energy to raise the dollars to support the research that will lead to new treatments and a cure. Much of the science described in the pages that follow is the result of funds raised by the CF community, as well as the willingness of patients to provide tissue specimens, share their data in patient registries, and participate in clinical studies. These contributions have been critical to the success that CF research is experiencing worldwide.

The global cystic fibrosis community is clearly unique and has often been described as a "culture of research." Shared among the many patient groups that represent about 70,000 people with CF worldwide is the belief that we will ultimately cure this disease through research. The constancy of this shared mission to cure CF by focusing on research is part of what sets the CF community apart from other rare diseases. The clear promise of small molecules and the excitement over gene therapy have kindled a sense of optimism that is critical to sustaining the momentum toward finding a cure.

In addition to the consistent focus on research, there are a number of other unique traits that the CF community around the world possesses that make it one of a kind. Some of the distinguishing qualities include the following:

- *Willingness to share*: Because of the insidious nature of CF, there is a rare sense of cooperative spirit among scientists, physicians, caregivers, patients, and families all over the world who are dedicated to a cure. CF research data know no borders, and waiting until data are published is not part of the CF research culture. The advancement of science is an open book, and the rapid exchange of new ideas and approaches is a mainstay of CF conferences and workshops in North America and overseas.
- *Willingness to take risks*: The search for the gene in the 1980s is an example of the risks and rewards of the pioneering work of the global CF populace. In the early 1980s, CF communities began to collect blood and tissue samples from families with multiply-affected individuals with CF. With newly evolved technologies (such as chromosome jumping), which could be quickly applied to these samples, and the rapid exchange of information, numerous efforts to find the gene were launched. The discovery of the CF gene in 1989 was the result of an intricate and highly successful international collaboration and is hailed today as one of the major milestones in modern medical research. Because of the involvement of CF families, patients, and the US Cystic Fibrosis Foundation, this groundbreaking discovery occurred over 14 years prior to the publication of the human genome. Importantly, it gave scientists an opportunity to explore the relationship of the genetic defect with the pathogenesis associated with CF. This discovery was a prelude to the effort to move from a knowledge acquisition

mode of research to the current CF research efforts, whereby scientists are using acquired knowledge about CF to develop new approaches to treat the disease.

- *Willingness to take responsibility for its own destiny*: Because there are only 70,000 CF patients throughout the world, there has been reluctance in the biopharmaceutical arena to enter the field of CF. Without their involvement, the ability to develop novel therapeutics is limited. In the late 1990s, frustrated by this fact, the US CF Foundation dramatically changed its business model and created a program to reduce risk of industry involvement in CF research by providing early funding and access to scientific and clinical expertise. This successful array of alliances with industry has led to an exciting clinical pipeline of products, including small molecules that are now being tested in centers worldwide, any of which could have a profound impact on individuals with CF.

Similarly, upon realizing industry's dwindling interest in gene therapy for CF, the British Trust launched a Gene Therapy Consortium that has painstakingly worked through some of the critical issues and problems associated with applying this pioneering mode of therapy for CF. As a result, and with a significant financial investment by the British Trust, the most comprehensive gene therapy clinical trial process is underway in the British Isles.

More recently, clinical trial networks have been established throughout North America and Europe to facilitate the evaluation of new clinical entities in order to hasten the regulatory process leading to drug approval. These clinical trial networks are linked through the sharing of data, expertise, and experience to contribute to the worldwide clinical trial efforts.

These are just a few examples of the willingness of the CF community to make strategic investments, some of which, in the case of other diseases, would be taken by industry or the government to bring us closer to accomplishing our mission.

- *Willingness to accept responsibility for the coordinating role in the areas of care, teaching, and research*: In many countries, scientists and clinicians look to the government for funding – agencies like the US National Institutes of Health and other equivalent organizations. However, not only is the science of CF frequently funded by CF organizations, but its direction is often defined by these entities as well. Similarly, the outstanding care that is provided all over the world is driven by the standards and guidelines set by these universal CF organizations. These guidelines are commonly established in international forums sponsored by CF groups. Once again, the community looks to CF organizations for leadership.

These volumes are the result of a distinct and worldwide undertaking. The environment, funding, and culture that have been put in place by patient organizations, coupled with the ability to bring the best minds to the field of CF, have made the science described in this book possible. This publication will be a useful tool as we continue to translate the knowledge acquired during decades of basic research to the development of new therapies that will modify and change the course of the disease in CF patients in the years ahead. *Cystic Fibrosis: Diagnosis and Protocols* is the fulfillment of decades of hard work by the volunteers and staff of the patient groups and organizations that have helped to pave the way toward our ultimate goal: a cure and control for cystic fibrosis.

President and Chief Executive Officer
Cystic Fibrosis Foundation

Robert J. Beall

Preface

More than 20 years have passed since the identification of the gene responsible for cystic fibrosis (CF) and undoubtedly many milestones have highlighted this area of research. But we have to admit it, progress towards finding a way of curing the disease has been slower than we initially expected and wished.

Apparently, this is not due to a lack of research efforts in the field, since in recent years the CF research community has been producing on average ~1,500 papers annually. So, probably we still need to dig deeper and with better tools to understand further the basic biological mechanisms underlying this complex disease. Nevertheless, it is increasingly difficult to grasp and use the already wide and still growing range of diverse methods currently employed to study CF so as to understand it in its multidisciplinary nature.

The aim of these *Cystic Fibrosis: Diagnosis and Protocols* volumes is thus to provide the CF research community (and that in related fields) with a very wide range of high-quality experimental tools, as an easy way to grasp and use classical and novel methods applied to CF. Hence, it is expected that it will contribute to accelerate the advancement of knowledge in this area. The purpose is thus to offer selected "good practice protocols" with a level of technical detail which is rarely published in peer-reviewed journals. Moreover, it is expected that this information will also enable researchers to identify subtle differences regarding techniques in their own laboratories, which often account for apparently "contradictory" data in the literature. Co-authorship from both sides of the Atlantic was particularly encouraged.

In the 2002 edition of this volume and in another previous comprehensive compilation of *Methods for Cystic Fibrosis and CFTR Research*[1], a large set of classical techniques used for CF research were already covered. So, here the focus is placed on innovative methodologies (some revolutionizing our way of doing science) by describing in detail how to perform and exploit these emergent techniques applied to CF. Moreover, a complete section has been devoted to available resources such as useful software and databases, as well as cell lines and animal models, reviewed for their usefulness towards multiple purposes. Notwithstanding, the more "classical" methods can also undergo improvements and thus their most up-to-date and revised versions are also recapped here by the leading experts. All book sections are introduced by an overview discussing the applicability and practicality of the protocols with examples.

It is hoped that the methods presented and revised here will provide users with optimal working tools to address their pressing questions in the best technical way while helping all of us, as a research and clinical community, to move faster hand-in-hand towards unravelling the secrets of this (and possibly other) challenging disorder(s) and cure it.

Finally, we wish to thank all authors for their enthusiasm in joining us in this project by contributing with their best protocols to this book and also for their patience with

[1] Journal of Cystic Fibrosis (2004), volume 3 (Supplement 2), a special issue focused on "Methods for Cystic Fibrosis and CFTR Research" and The online "Virtual Repository of the Cystic Fibrosis European Network" at http://central.igc.gulbenkian.pt/cftr/vr/index.htm

our multiple requests. Special thanks to Renata Vincent for her help in dealing with the manuscripts. Moreover, we would like to express our gratitude to the whole CF community in general, researchers, clinicians and all caregivers and other professionals, not forgetting CF patients and their families, for their continuous efforts towards finding a way out of this still devastating disease. We believe that we will be there soon and we hope this book somehow contributes to getting there sooner. Then, when our goals are met, all efforts will have been worthwhile, or as the Portuguese poet Fernando Pessoa has put it, "All is worthwhile if the soul is not small".

Margarida D. Amaral
Karl Kunzelmann

Contents

Contributors

ERIC W.F.W. ALTON • *Department of Gene Therapy, Imperial College London, London, UK*

RODRIGO ALZAMORA • *Renal-Electrolyte Division, School of Medicine, University of Pittsburgh, Pittsburgh, PA, USA*

MARGARIDA D. AMARAL • *Faculty of Sciences, BioFiG-Centre for Biodiversity and Functional and Integrative Genomics, University of Lisboa, Lisbon, Portugal; Department of Genetics, National Institute of Health, Lisbon, Portugal; Centre of Human Genetics, National Institute of Health, Lisboa, Portugal; EMBL Heidelberg, Heidelberg, Germany*

P. ANDREW CHONG • *Molecular Structure and Function, Hospital for Sick Children, Toronto, ON, Canada*

PIRJO APAJA • *Department of Physiology, McGill University, Montréal, QC, Canada*

MELISSA ASHLOCK • *Cystic Fibrosis Foundation Therapeutics, Bethesda, MD, USA*

PASCAL BARBRY • *CNRS, Université de Nice Sophia Antipolis, IPMC, UMR6097, Sophia Antipolis, France*

HERVE BARRIÈRE • *Department of Physiology, McGill University, Montréal, QC, Canada*

YVES BERTHIAUME • *Centre de Recherche du Centre Hospitalier de l'Université de Montréal, Université de Montréal, Hôtel Dieu, Montréal, QC, Canada*

JAMES BIRTLEY • *Faculty of Life Sciences, Manchester Interdisciplinary Biocentre, The University of Manchester, Manchester, UK*

JENNIFER M. BOMBERGER • *Department of Microbiology and Immunology, Dartmouth Medical School, Hanover, NH, USA*

SILVIA G. BOMPADRE • *Department of Medical Pharmacology and Physiology, Dalton Cardiovascular Research Center, University of Missouri-Columbia, Columbia, MO, USA*

INEZ BRONSVELD • *Department of Pulmonology and Tuberculosis, University Medical Center Utrecht, Utrecht, The Netherlands*

BILL BURTON • *Vertex Pharmaceuticals Incorporated, San Diego, CA, USA*

ZHIWEI CAI • *Department of Physiology and Pharmacology, School of Medical Sciences, University of Bristol, Bristol, UK*

BRUNO CARDINAUD • *CNRS, Université de Nice Sophia Antipolis, IPMC, UMR6097, Sophia Antipolis, France*

JOHN PAUL CLANCY • *Departments of Medicine, Pediatrics, Physiology, Biophysics MCLM, University of Alabama, Birmingham, AL, USA*

JEAN PAUL CLANCY • *Department of Pediatrics, University of Alabama, Birmingham, AL, USA*

HEATHER CLARK • *Vertex Pharmaceuticals Incorporated, San Diego, CA, USA*

LUKA A. CLARKE • *Faculty of Sciences, BioFiG-Centre for Biodiversity and Functional and Integrative Genomics, University of Lisboa, Lisbon, Portugal*

LANE L. CLARKE • *Department of Biomedical Sciences, Dalton Cardiovascular Research Center, University of Missouri, Columbia, MO, USA*

DAVID M. CLARKE • *Departments of Medicine and Biochemistry, University of Toronto, Toronto, ON, Canada*
CHRISTELLE CORAUX • *INSERM UMRS 903, CHU Maison Blanche, Reims, France*
PIERRE J. COURTOY • *CELL Unit, de Duve Institute, Université Catholique de Louvain Medical School, Brussels, Belgium*
LÁSZLÓ CSANÁDY • *Department of Medical Biochemistry, Semmelweis University, Budapest, Hungary*
DOUGLAS M. CYR • *Department of Cell and Developmental Biology, School of Medicine, The UNC-Cystic Fibrosis Center, University of North Carolina, Chapel Hill, NC, USA*
JANE C. DAVIES • *Department of Gene Therapy, Imperial College London, London, UK*
KRIS DE BOECK • *Department of Pediatrics, University of Leuven, Leuven, Belgium*
NICO DERICHS • *Cystic Fibrosis Center, Pediatric Pulmonology and Neonatology, Medizinische Hochschule Hannover, Hannover, Germany; CFTR Biomarker Center, Christiane-Herzog-Zentrum für Mukoviszidose, Charité Universitätsmedizin Berlin, Berlin*
OLIVIER DEVUYST • *Division of Nephrology, Université Catholique de Louvain Medical School, Brussels, Belgium*
NIKOLAY V. DOKHOLYAN • *Department of Biochemistry and Biophysics, University of North Carolina, Chapel Hill, NC, USA*
EUGENIO FERNANDEZ-ALANIS • *Human Molecular Genetics, International Centre for Genetic Engineering and Biotechnology, Trieste, Italy*
ROBERT C. FORD • *Faculty of Life Sciences, Manchester Interdisciplinary Biocentre, The University of Manchester, Manchester, UK*
JULIE D. FORMAN-KAY • *Molecular Structure and Function, Hospital for Sick Children, Toronto, ON, Canada; Department of Biochemistry, University of Toronto, Toronto, ON, Canada*
DAVID C. GADSBY • *Laboratory of Cardiac/Membrane Physiology, The Rockefeller University, New York, NY, USA*
LUIS J.V. GALIETTA • *Laboratorio di Genetica Molecolare, Istituto Giannina Gaslini, Genova, Italy*
LISA GIOVANNINI-CHAMI • *CNRS, Université de Nice Sophia Antipolis, IPMC, UMR6097, Sophia Antipolis, France; Service de Pédiatrie, Unité de Pneumo-Allergologie, CHU de Nice, France*
ELISA GOINA • *Human Molecular Genetics, International Centre for Genetic Engineering and Biotechnology, Trieste, Italy*
NATHALIE GRANDVAUX • *Centre de Recherche du Centre Hospitalier de l'Université de Montréal, Université de Montréal, Hôpital Saint-Luc, PEA, Montréal, QC, Canada*
MICHAEL A. GRAY • *Epithelial Research Group, Institute for Cell and Molecular Biosciences, Newcastle University, Newcastle Upon Tyne, UK*
DIANE E. GROVE • *Department of Cell and Developmental Biology, School of Medicine, The UNC-Cystic Fibrosis Center, University of North Carolina, Chapel Hill, NC*
WILLIAM B. GUGGINO • *Department of Physiology, Johns Hopkins University School of Medicine, Baltimore, MD, USA*
ATTILA GULYÁS-KOVÁCS • *Laboratory of Cardiac/Membrane Physiology, The Rockefeller University, New York, NY, USA*
KENNETH R. HALLOWS • *Renal-Electrolyte Division, School of Medicine, University of Pittsburgh, Pittsburgh, PA, USA*

ANN HARRIS • *Human Molecular Genetics Program, Children's Memorial Research Center, Northwestern University Feinberg School of Medicine, Chicago, IL; Department of Pediatrics, Northwestern University Feinberg School of Medicine, Chicago, IL, USA*
MARTIN J. HUG • *Pharmacy, University Medical Center Freiburg, Freiburg, Germany*
TZYH-CHANG HWANG • *Department of Medical Pharmacology and Physiology, Dalton Cardiovascular Research Center, University of Missouri-Columbia, Columbia, MO, USA*
FRANÇOIS JOURET • *Division of Nephrology, Université Catholique de Louvain Medical School, Brussels, Belgium*
VOULA KANELIS • *Department of Chemical and Physical Sciences, University of Toronto Mississauga, Mississauga, ON, Canada*
BATSHEVA KEREM • *Department of Genetics, The Life Sciences Institute, The Hebrew University, Jerusalem, Israel*
J DARWIN KING • *Renal-Electrolyte Division, School of Medicine, University of Pittsburgh, Pittsburgh, PA, USA*
KARL KUNZELMANN • *Department of Physiology, University of Regensburg, Regensburg, Germany*
CHUNYING LI • *Department of Biochemistry and Molecular Biology, Wayne State University School of Medicine, Detroit, MI, USA*
LIAT LINDE • *Department of Genetics, The Life Sciences Institute, The Hebrew University, Jerusalem, Israel*
TIP W. LOO • *Departments of Medicine and Biochemistry, University of Toronto, Toronto, ON, Canada*
GERGELY L. LUKACS • *Department of Physiology, McGill University, Montréal, QC, Canada*
BRICE MARCET • *CNRS, Université de Nice Sophia Antipolis, IPMC, UMR6097, Sophia Antipolis, France*
BERNARD MARI • *CNRS, Université de Nice Sophia Antipolis, IPMC, UMR6097, Sophia Antipolis, France*
YOSHIHIRO MATSUMURA • *Department of Biochemistry and Molecular Biology, Oregon Health and Science University, Portland, OR, USA*
JUAN L. MENDOZA • *Department of Physiology, University of Texas Southwestern Medical Center, Dallas, TX, USA*
ANJAPARAVANDA P. NAREN • *Department of Physiology, University of Tennessee Health Science Center, Memphis, TN, USA*
TIMOTHY NEUBERGER • *Vertex Pharmaceuticals Incorporated, San Diego, CA, USA*
TSUKASA OKIYONEDA • *Department of Physiology, McGill University, Montréal, QC, Canada*
CHRISTOPHER J. OTT • *Human Molecular Genetics Program, Children's Memorial Research Center, Northwestern University Feinberg School of Medicine, Chicago, IL, USA; Department of Pediatrics, Northwestern University Feinberg School of Medicine, Chicago, IL, USA*
FRANCO PAGANI • *Human Molecular Genetics, International Centre for Genetic Engineering and Biotechnology, Trieste, Italy*
NICOLETTA PEDEMONTE • *Laboratorio di Genetica Molecolare, Istituto Giannina Gaslini, Genova, Italy*

ANABELA S. RAMALHO • *Faculty of Sciences, BioFiG-Centre for Biodiversity and Functional and Integrative Genomics, University of Lisboa, Lisbon, Portugal; Department of Genetics, National Institute of Health, Lisbon, Portugal*
KARINE ROBBE-SERMESANT • *CNRS, Université de Nice Sophia Antipolis, IPMC, UMR6097, Sophia Antipolis, France*
LEEANN ROONEY • *Department of Biochemistry and Molecular Biology, Oregon Health and Science University, Portland, OR, USA*
MARK F. ROSENBERG • *Faculty of Life Sciences, Manchester Interdisciplinary Biocentre, The University of Manchester, Manchester, UK*
MEREDITH F.N. ROSSER • *Department of Cell and Developmental Biology, School of Medicine, The UNC-Cystic Fibrosis Center, University of North Carolina, Chapel Hill, NC, USA*
STEVEN M. ROWE • *Departments of Medicine, Pediatrics, and Physiology and Biophysics MCLM, University of Alabama, Birmingham, AL, USA*
ANDRÉ SCHMIDT • *Department of Physiology, University of Texas Southwestern Medical Center, Dallas, TX, USA*
ADRIAN W.R. SEROHIJOS • *Department of Physics and Astronomy, Program in Molecular and Cellular Biophysics, University of North Carolina, Chapel Hill, NC, USA; Department of Chemistry and Chemical Biology, Harvard University, Cambridge, MA, USA*
DAVID N. SHEPPARD • *Department of Physiology and Pharmacology, School of Medical Sciences, University of Bristol, Bristol, UK*
WILLIAM R. SKACH • *Department of Biochemistry and Molecular Biology, Oregon Health and Science University, Portland, OR, USA*
YOSHIRO SOHMA • *Department of Pharmacology and Neuroscience, Keio University School of Medicine, Tokyo, Japan*
BRUCE A. STANTON • *Department of Microbiology and Immunology, Dartmouth Medical School, Hanover, NH, USA*
PATRICK H. THIBODEAU • *Department of Cell Biology and Physiology, University of Pittsburgh School of Medicine, Pittsburgh, PA, USA*
PHILIP J. THOMAS • *Department of Physiology, University of Texas Southwestern Medical Center, Dallas, TX, USA*
FREDRICK VAN GOOR • *Vertex Pharmaceuticals Incorporated, San Diego, CA, USA*
PAOLA VERGANI • *Department of Neuroscience, Physiology and Pharmacology, University College London, London, UK*
RAINER WALDMANN • *CNRS, Université de Nice Sophia Antipolis, IPMC, UMR6097, Sophia Antipolis, France*
RICHARD L. WATKINS • *Department of Cell and Developmental Biology, School of Medicine, The UNC-Cystic Fibrosis Center, University of North Carolina, Chapel Hill, NC, USA*
MICHAEL WILSCHANSKI • *Pediatric Gastroenterology, Hadassah University Hospitals, Jerusalem, Israel*
LAURE-EMMANUELLE ZARAGOSI • *CNRS, Université de Nice Sophia Antipolis, IPMC, UMR6097, Sophia Antipolis, France*
OLGA ZEGARRA-MORAN • *Laboratorio di Genetica Molecolare, Istituto Giannina Gaslini, Genova, Italy*
LIANG ZHANG • *Department of Cell Biology and Physiology, University of Pittsburgh, Pittsburgh, PA, USA*

Section I

Strategies to Correct the Basic Defect in CF and Assess Efficacy in Human Clinical Trials

Chapter 1

Introduction to Section I: The Relevance of CF Diagnostic Tools for Measuring Restoration of CFTR Function After Therapeutic Interventions in Human Clinical Trials

Kris De Boeck and Melissa Ashlock

Abstract

The pilocarpine sweat test, and in vivo assessment of CFTR function via nasal potential difference or intestinal current measurement are important tools to confirm the diagnosis of CF in subjects with suggestive symptoms. Since these tests reflect CFTR function and thus relate to the basic disease process in CF, changes in these parameters are also being used to assess the pharmacologic effect of compounds aimed at restoring CFTR function. However, longitudinal data proving that changes in these measurements are associated with meaningful clinical improvements in the course of disease in CF patients are needed. Consequently, many CF clinical investigators need to be facile with these existing methods to measure CFTR-related outcomes. This introduction sets the stage for more in-depth discussion of existing strategies to measure changes in CFTR function generated by gene therapy or small molecule modulators of CFTR function such as correctors and potentiators. It is hoped that lessons learned through the use of these measures will inform the future development of other robust methods to assess novel therapeutic strategies uncovered by basic scientists.

Key words: Cystic fibrosis, diagnostic tests, outcome parameters, new therapies.

1. Clinical Aspects of Cystic Fibrosis

Cystic fibrosis (CF) is an autosomal recessive multisystem disease affecting thousands of subjects around the world, with the highest incidence in individuals of northern European descent. As awareness of the disease increases, CF appears less rare than originally thought (1). Over the last 50 years, intensive follow up and treatment have improved the outcome to a median survival of more

M.D. Amaral, K. Kunzelmann (eds.), *Cystic Fibrosis*, Methods in Molecular Biology 741,
DOI 10.1007/978-1-61779-117-8_1, © Springer Science+Business Media, LLC 2011

than 37 years (2–4) so that in many countries nearly 50% of individuals with CF are 18 years of age or older (3, 5). National programs for CF newborn screening are instituted in several countries. If resultant CF diagnoses are linked to specialized treatment programs early in life, further improvements in clinical outcomes are expected (6). However, CF remains a burdensome and eventually devastating life-shortening disease. Thus, effective therapies aimed at changing the pathogenesis are necessary to change the face of this disease.

Cystic fibrosis is caused by mutations in the cystic fibrosis transmembrane regulator (*CFTR*) gene, whose protein product (CFTR) functions in unaffected individuals as a cAMP-regulated chloride channel. The normal CFTR protein is present in the apical membrane of epithelial cells in the various organs that can become involved in CF, including respiratory, pancreatic, intestinal, sweat gland and reproductive tissues. Consequently, a CF diagnosis consists of at least one of the following: a phenotypic symptom known to be associated with CFTR dysfunction, a positive newborn screening result (based on elevated immunoreactive trypsinogen or IRT in the blood), a positive history of CF in a sibling plus some evidence of CFTR dysfunction in the form of an abnormal sweat chloride or nasal potential difference (NPD) test, or the presence of disease-causing mutations in both *CFTR* alleles (7, 8).

The main cause of mortality in CF is respiratory failure secondary to chronic lung infection and inflammation. There is a poorly understood propensity towards lung infection with *Staphylococcus aureus, Pseudomonas aeruginosa, Burkholderia cepacia* and *Xanthomonas maltophilia*. Among these pathogens, the link between chronic *P. aeruginosa* infection and accelerated lung function decline is the most obvious and has been known for many years (9). Also at present, nearly 80% of adult patients with CF are chronically infected with *P. aeruginosa* (10). Intensive "microbial" surveillance of the airway and aggressive antibiotic treatment of initial lung infections have delayed the mean age at which *P. aeruginosa* infection becomes chronic (5, 11, 12).

Ninety percent of individuals with CF suffer from severe maldigestion because of pancreatic insufficiency secondary to CFTR dysfunction. The intestinal manifestations of CF can include meconium ileus at birth, distal intestinal obstruction syndrome, rectal prolapse, intussusception and possibly inclination towards intestinal malignancies in later life (13). Ten to 20% of individuals with CF also suffer from progressive liver disease (14).

Male infertility secondary to bilateral absence of the vas deference and decreased fertility in females because of altered viscosity of cervical secretions become apparent in most individuals with CF in adulthood.

Salt loss syndromes, manifest in individuals with CF by abnormally high levels of chloride in sweat, may lead to acute dehydration during hot summer days or to chronic salt depletion and electrolyte imbalance especially in infants. The acute salt loss syndrome led to the discovery of a chloride transport defect in the sweat duct in CF and was followed by characterization of that defect and its link to the basic defect in CFTR function (15).

2. Diagnostic Tools for CF

One of the easiest, cheapest, most sensitive and specific diagnostic tests for CF in individuals suspected to harbour the disease continues to be the "sweat test" – determination of the chloride concentration in a sweat collection obtained after stimulation of the sweat gland by pilocarpine (7, 8, 16–18). When the *CFTR* gene was discovered through linkage analysis, it came with little surprise that chloride conductance was a major function of this protein channel (19). One single type of mutation, resulting in a deletion of the amino acid phenylalanine at position 508 in the NBD1 domain of the protein (F508del), accounts for 50–80% of mutations found in individuals with CF. But numerous other mutations (>1,800), the majority of which are extremely rare, have been reported. Basic laboratory research into the cellular phenotype associated with some of the most common mutations has led to a mutation classification system that is described in more detail in **Section III**. The study of CFTR modulators as potential therapies for CF (described below and in **Chapters 2**, **3** and **4**) has highlighted the importance of further refining this classification system.

A search for mutations in the *CFTR* gene is a useful diagnostic test, but determining which of the numerous mutations to include in a diagnostic panel is difficult and varies upon the ethnic origin of the subject tested. In northern European countries, the situation is relatively simple with up to 90% of mutations being detected when using a panel of about 30 mutations (1). Increasingly, people with mild or partial disease manifestations linked to mutations in the *CFTR* gene are also being recognized; clinicians at times differ in their opinions on whether to classify these subjects as suffering from CF or not (16, 20).

Normal activity of the CFTR chloride channel is associated with inhibition of the epithelial sodium channel (ENaC), decreasing absorption of sodium by these cells. Consequently in CF, CFTR dysfunction results in hyperabsorption of sodium through the ENaC channel in addition to impaired chloride channel activity. In vivo tests such as the NPD test have been developed to measure the electric charge reflecting the chloride and sodium movement at the mucosal surface (21, 22). A limited number of centres are currently equipped to perform the test routinely. But because of the potential of this measure as a diagnostic tool and as a biomarker of CFTR function in CF clinical trials, efforts are underway to increase the availability of this test as described in **Chapter 6**. A similar assessment of CFTR and ENaC functions can be performed ex vivo on rectal tissue after biopsy (intestinal current measurement or ICM) but this technique is even less widely available (23). Worldwide, standardization of this procedure as a diagnostic tool and as an exploratory biomarker for CF clinical trials is under development and discussed in **Chapter 7**.

Many other tools are available to monitor lung disease severity in general and have been applied in CF clinical care. These include pulmonary function tests such as the forced expiratory volume in 1 s (FEV_1) and lung clearance index, imaging techniques, microbial profiling of airway fluids to establish the type and degree of airway infection, monitoring the frequency of pulmonary exacerbations and various patient-reported outcomes. Many of these tools are used extensively in clinical studies and their value as clinical outcome measures will be discussed in subsequent chapters (e.g. **Chapter 5**).

3. Using CF Diagnostic Tools to Detect CFTR Function After Therapeutic Interventions

When considering the use of diagnostic tests for CF as measures of restoration of CFTR function, it is important to consider how the diagnostic tests relate to the basic disease process and whether the test is validated and standardized for use in CF clinical trials (24). The sweat chloride test has a long history of use by clinicians to discriminate CF subjects from non-CF subjects. Some subjects with milder or mono-symptomatic disease (e.g. only pancreatic or intestinal disease) have been found to have sweat chloride values in the borderline range (30–60 mmol/l) or even in the normal range (below 30 mmol/l) (6, 25). When studying subjects with various degrees of organ system involvement from the most severe CF with pancreatic insufficiency, through CF with pancreatic sufficiency, patients with atypical disease, carriers of a *CFTR* mutation and finally unaffected individuals, mean sweat chloride values show the same gradient from definitely abnormal (>60 mmol/l) to intermediate (30–60 mmol/l) to normal (26).

On the whole, disease severity is milder in groups of subjects with lower sweat chloride values (20) and mean sweat chloride values are lower in subjects with pancreatic sufficiency compared with those with pancreatic insufficiency (27). Thus, since sweat chloride values seem to reflect the amount of CFTR activity present, using the sweat chloride value to monitor restoration of CFTR activity seems logical. There are however many caveats to using sweat chloride value alone to reflect changes in CFTR function as there are other ways besides modulation of CFTR function to mediate changes in this chloride concentration such as modifying salt intake and/or exercise-induced sweating (28). Some anti-epileptics are also known to change sweat chloride values but have no proven effect on CFTR function (29). It is important to acknowledge that while simple to measure and perhaps relatively easy to interpret, sweat chloride value alone will not suffice as an outcome measure unless it is associated with improvements in the respiratory manifestations of the disease. Although sweat chloride values are abnormal in subjects with CF, there is as yet no proof that lowering or normalizing sweat chloride values without demonstrating improvement in CFTR function in the other involved organ systems, specifically the lung, will be associated with slowing, stopping or reversing of the disease or its progression.

In contrast to sweat chloride test, NPD measurements are thought to reflect disease in the CF airway and to discriminate between unaffected individuals and those with CF (21, 22). But just as noted for sweat chloride values above, some individuals with mild CF phenotypes have intermediate NPD values. The ratio of the response of the airway epithelium to zero chloride plus isoproterenol response/amiloride is the most reliable parameter to distinguish between CF and non CF (30). This measure has been used effectively over nearly two decades to assess restoration of CFTR function during clinical trials of gene therapy agents (31). But again, just as with sweat chloride values, longitudinal data proving that changes in NPD measurement are associated with or serve as markers for correction of the entire disease course are lacking. It is also unclear as to what degree of improvement in CFTR function will be necessary to have an impact on disease course. Thus, at present, any measure of CFTR activity is considered as an exploratory biomarker in a clinical trial rather than as a surrogate outcome measure that reflects disease course. To qualify as a surrogate outcome measure, a biomarker needs to be shown to reflect both the positive and negative effects of the therapy on a clinically meaningful outcome in the disease. In CF therapeutics, since the majority of individuals succumb to respiratory failure, the most commonly used clinically meaningful outcomes relate to respiratory status (32).

4. What Therapies Are on the Horizon to Restore CFTR Function and What Role Do CF Diagnostic Measures Play in the Evaluation of These Therapies?

Several small molecule therapeutic approaches such as mutation class-specific therapies are currently undergoing clinical evaluation. For example, stop codon read-through compounds are under study in individuals with class 1 mutations and CFTR correctors and potentiators are under study in individuals with class 2 and 3 mutations. In these studies, as with prior gene therapy trials, measures of CFTR activity have been explored as biomarkers of the effectiveness of the therapeutic approach. For example, changes in the zero chloride plus isoproterenol response have been used in phase 2 trials with CFTR "modulators" (compounds that induce changes in CFTR function). One such modulator, Ataluren, has been studied in subjects with class 1 mutations (33, 34). A small but statistically significant improvement in NPD was seen, suggesting that this drug may have the potential to improve CFTR function. Statistically significant improvements in the zero chloride plus isoproterenol response on NPD were seen in individuals with CF who harbour the G551D class 3 mutation treated with another CFTR modulator under study, the CFTR potentiator compound VX-770 (35). In addition to improvements in NPD measures, sweat chloride values improved and a marked positive effect was seen on lung function in this phase 2 trial. Follow-up studies in larger numbers of individuals for longer periods of time are underway with both categories of compounds since effects on clinically meaningful disease outcomes and hence disease outcome have yet to be confirmed. The results of similar outcome measures from the early phase study of corrector compounds in individuals with the much more common class 2 mutation, F508del, are not yet available. The current diagnostic measures used in these trials are reviewed in more detail in **Chapters 6** and **7**. Given the promise of modulating CFTR as a therapeutic strategy, significant effort is underway worldwide to discover more CFTR modulators. High-throughput screening as a method to find additional CFTR modulators is discussed in **Chapter 2**. Pre-clinical evaluation of CFTR correctors and potentiators in human cells and animal studies is reviewed in **Chapters 3** and **4**.

Large-scale gene therapy studies in the UK also offer an opportunity to further define appropriate outcome measures of CFTR activity in pre-clinical animal models as well as in human subjects (31). These measures are similar to those described above but also include methods to quantify the presence of CFTR mRNA and CFTR protein.

In addition to the biomarkers of CFTR activity and the frequently used clinical outcome measures described above, other measures such as those used to assess the airway surface liquid height and mucociliary clearance may prove to be of value in clinical studies. Measuring the effects of new therapies on airway infection and inflammatory markers in sputum through exhaled breath and bronchoalveolar lavage fluid is also being considered. In **Chapter 5**, investigators from the UK gene consortium share their vast experience with these types of assessments.

The therapeutic approaches to improve CFTR activity are being studied at a time when the course of CF disease is changing in a positive way because of the awareness regarding the need for regular symptomatic treatment soon after diagnosis (36). This exciting era of better clinical outcomes has brought on new difficulties when assessing promising therapeutic options. Since the disease progression may be slower and variable between subjects, large groups of patients in longer multicenter, multinational trials are needed to evaluate the potential clinical benefit from new drugs in these individuals. Large research networks such as CFF-Therapeutics Development Network (TDN) and the recently established European Cystic Fibrosis Society-Clinical Trial Network (ECFS-CTN) (37) aim to evaluate candidate therapeutics and subsequently bring safe and effective new drugs to patients as quickly as possible. Reaching consensus on standardized and optimal methods to perform all of the relevant outcome measures will be very beneficial to the advancement of CF research. Coordinated efforts regarding outcome measure interpretation should improve the efficiency with which the clinical research community comes to consensus on the utility of potential new therapies as well. The following chapters written by eminent basic and clinical researchers address the many issues inherent to developing strategies to improve the lives of individuals with this complex disease.

References

1. WHO (2004) The molecular genetic epidemiology of cystic fibrosis. Report of a joint meeting of WHO/ECFTN/ICF(M)A/ECFS http://www.who.int/genomics/publications/en/ and WHO Geneva, Human Genetics Programme WHO/HGN/CF/WG/04.02.
2. Buzzetti, R., Salvatore, D., Baldo, E., Forneris, M. P., Lucidi, V., Manunza, D., et al. (2009) An overview of international literature from cystic fibrosis registries: 1. Mortality and survival studies in cystic fibrosis. *J. Cyst. Fibros.* **8**, 229–237.
3. CFF (2007) *CFF patient Registry annual data report 2007.* Available from: http://www.cff.org/UploadedFiles/research/ClinicalResearch/2007-Patient-Registry-Report.pdf
4. Dodge, J. A., Lewis, P.A., Stanton, M., and Wilsher, J., (2007) Cystic fibrosis mortality and survival in the UK: 1947–2003. *Eur. Respir. J.* **29**, 522–526.
5. ECFS. (2009) *European Registry for Cystic Fibrosis, Report 2006.* http://www.ecfs.eu/files/webfm/webfiles/File/ecfs_registry/ECFRreport2006.pdf
6. Lebecque, P., Leal, T., De Boeck, C., Jaspers, M., Cuppens, H., and Cassiman, J. J. (2002) Mutations of the cystic fibrosis gene and intermediate sweat chloride levels in

children. *Am. J. Resp. Crit. Care Med.* **165**, 757–761.
7. De Boeck, K., Wilschanski, M., Castellani, C., Taylor, C., Cuppens, H., Dodge, J., et al. (2006) Cystic fibrosis: Terminology and diagnostic algorithms. *Thorax* **61**, 627–635.
8. Rosenstein, B. J., and Cutting, G. R. (1998) The diagnosis of cystic fibrosis: A consensus statement. Cystic fibrosis foundation consensus panel. *J. Pediatr.* **132**, 589–595.
9. Henry, R. L., Mellis, C. M., and Petrovic, L. (1992) Mucoid Pseudomonas aeruginosa is a marker of poor survival in cystic fibrosis. *Pediatr. Pulmonol.* **12**, 158–161.
10. Ashlock, M. A., Beall, R. J., Hamblett, N. M., Konstan, M. W., Penland, C. M., Ramsey, B. W., et al. (2009) A pipeline of therapies for cystic fibrosis. *Semin. Respir. Crit. Care Med.* **30**, 611–626.
11. Frederiksen, B., Koch, C., and Hoiby, N. (1997) Antibiotic treatment of initial colonization with Pseudomonas aeruginosa postpones chronic infection and prevents deterioration of pulmonary function in cystic fibrosis. *Pediatr. Pulmonol.* **23**, 330–335.
12. Proesmans, M., Balinska-Miskiewicz, W., Dupont, L., Bossuyt, X., Verhaegen, J., Høiby, N., et al. (2006) Evaluating the "Leeds criteria" for Pseudomonas aeruginosa infection in a cystic fibrosis centre. *Eur. Respir. J.* **27**, 937–943.
13. Borowitz, D., Durie, P. R., Clarke, L. L., Werlin, S. L, Taylor, C. J., Semler, J., et al. (2005) Gastrointestinal outcomes and confounders in cystic fibrosis. *J. Pediatr. Gastroenterol. Nutr.* **41**, 273–285.
14. Colombo, C. (2007) Liver disease in cystic fibrosis. *Curr. Opin. Pulm. Med.* **13**, 529–536.
15. Quinton, P. M. (2007) Cystic fibrosis: Lessons from the sweat gland. *Physiology (Bethesda)* **22**, 212–225.
16. Farrell, P. M., Rosenstein, B. J., White, T. B., Accurso, F. J., Castellani, C., Cutting, G. R., et al. (2008) Guidelines for diagnosis of cystic fibrosis in newborns through older adults: Cystic fibrosis foundation consensus report. *J. Pediatr.* **153**, S4–S14.
17. Bush, A. (2008) Editorial overview: Newborn screening for cystic fibrosis – Benefit or bane? *Paediatr. Resp. Rev.* **9**, 301–302.
18. LeGrys, V. A., Yankaskas, J. R., Quittell, L. M., Marshall, B. C., and Mogayzel, P. J. Jr. (2007) Diagnostic sweat testing: The Cystic Fibrosis Foundation guidelines. *J. Pediatr.* **151**, 85–89.
19. Collins, F. S. (1992) Cystic fibrosis: Molecular biology and therapeutic implications. *Science* **256**, 774–779.
20. Goubau, C., Wilschanski, M., Skalicka, V., Lebecque, P., Southern, K. W., Sermet, I., et al. (2009) Phenotypic characterisation of patients with intermediate sweat chloride values: Towards validation of the European diagnostic algorithm for cystic fibrosis. *Thorax* **64**, 683–691.
21. Knowles, M. R., Paradiso, A. M., and Boucher, R. C. (1995) In vivo nasal potential difference: Techniques and protocols for assessing efficacy of gene transfer in cystic fibrosis. *Hum. Gene Ther.* **6**, 445–455.
22. Middleton, P. G., Geddes, D. M., and Alton, E.W. (1994) Protocols for in vivo measurement of the ion transport defects in cystic fibrosis nasal epithelium. *Eur. Respir. J.* **7**, 2050–2056.
23. De Boeck, C., Derichs, N., Fajac, I., et al. (2011) New clinical diagnostic procedures for cystic fibrosis in Europe. *J. Cyst. Fibros.* **10 Suppl 1**, S53–S66.
24. Rowe, S. M., Accurso, F., and Clancy, J. P. (2007) Detection of cystic fibrosis transmembrane conductance regulator activity in early-phase clinical trials. *Proc. Am. Thorac. Soc.* **4**, 387–398.
25. Highsmith, W. E., Burch, L. H., Zhou, Z., et al. (1994) A novel mutation in the cystic fibrosis gene in patients with pulmonary disease but normal sweat chloride concentrations. *N. Engl. J. Med.* **331**, 974–980.
26. Wilschanski, M., Dupuis, A., Ellis, L., Jarvi, K., Zielenski, J., Tullis E., et al. (2006) Mutations in the cystic fibrosis transmembrane regulator gene and in vivo transepithelial potentials. *Am. J. Respir. Crit. Care Med.* **174**, 787–794.
27. Corey, M., Edwards, L., Levison, H., and Knowles, M. (1997) Longitudinal analysis of pulmonary function decline in patients with cystic fibrosis. *J. Pediatr.* **131**, 809–814.
28. Morgan, R. M., Patterson, M. J., and Nimmo, M.A. (2004) Acute effects of dehydration on sweat composition in men during prolonged exercise in the heat. *Acta Physiol. Scand.* **182**, 37–43.
29. Yilmaz, K., Tatli, B., Yaramis, A., Aydinli, N., Caliskan, M., and Ozmen, M. (2005) Symptomatic and asymptomatic hypohidrosis in children under topiramate treatment. *Turk. J. Pediatr.* **47**, 359–363.
30. Wilschanski, M., Famini, H., Strauss-Liviatan, N., Rivlin, J., Blau, H., Bibi, H., et al. (2001) Nasal potential difference

measurements in patients with atypical cystic fibrosis. *Eur. Respir. J.* **17**, 1208–1215.

31. Griesenbach, U., and Boyd, A. C. (2005) Pre-clinical and clinical endpoint assays for cystic fibrosis gene therapy. *J. Cyst. Fibros.* **4**, 89–100.
32. Rosenfeld, M. (2007) An overview of endpoints for cystic fibrosis clinical trials: One size does not fit all. *Proc. Am. Thorac. Soc.* **4**, 299–301.
33. Kerem, E., Hirawat, S., Armoni, S., Yaakov, Y., Shoseyov, D., Cohen, M., et al. (2008) Effectiveness of PTC124 treatment of cystic fibrosis caused by nonsense mutations: A prospective phase II trial. *Lancet* **372**, 719–727.
34. Sermet-Gaudelus, I., Boeck, K. D., Casimir, G. J., et al. (2010) Ataluren (PTC124) induces cystic fibrosis transmembrane conductance regulator protein expression and activity in children with nonsense mutation cystic fibrosis. *Am. J. Respir. Crit. Care Med.* **182**, 1262–1272.
35. Accurso, F. J., Rowe, S. M., Clancy, J. P., et al. (2010) Effect of VX-770 in persons with cystic fibrosis and the G551D-CFTR mutation. *N. Engl. J. Med.* **363**, 1991–2003.
36. Ashlock, M., and Olson, E. R. (2011) Therapeutics development for cystic fibrosis: a successful model for a multisystemic genetic disease. *Annu. Rev. Med.* **62**, 107–125.
37. De Boeck, C., Bulteel, V., Tiddens, H., et al. (2011) Guideline on the design and conduct of CF clinical trials: the ECFS Clinical Trials Network (ECFS-CTN). *J. Cyst. Fibros.* **10 Suppl 1**, S67–S74.

Chapter 2

High-Throughput Screening of Libraries of Compounds to Identify CFTR Modulators

Nicoletta Pedemonte, Olga Zegarra-Moran, and Luis J.V. Galietta

Abstract

Small molecules acting as selective activators (potentiators), inhibitors, or "correctors" of the CFTR chloride channel represent candidate drugs for various pathological conditions including cystic fibrosis and secretory diarrhea. The identification of CFTR pharmacological modulators may be achieved by screening highly diverse synthetic or natural compound libraries using high-throughput methods. A convenient assay for CFTR function is based on the halide sensitivity of the yellow fluorescent protein (YFP). CFTR activity can be simply assessed by measuring the rate of YFP signal decrease caused by iodide influx. This assay can be automated to test thousands of compounds per day.

Key words: Cystic fibrosis, CFTR, fluorescent protein, high-throughput screening, drug discovery.

1. Introduction

The CFTR chloride channel is an important pharmacological target to treat various genetic and nongenetic diseases (1). In cystic fibrosis (CF), mutations affecting the *CFTR* gene cause a large variety of defects including altered CFTR channel gating (class III mutations such as G551D and G1349D) or impaired CFTR protein maturation (class II mutations such as F508del). Therefore, compounds increasing CFTR-dependent chloride transport are potentially useful as drugs to treat CF patients. In particular, pharmacological activators of CFTR, called potentiators, are useful to overcome the gating defect caused by class III CF mutations. Conversely, other compounds, called correctors, may help the F508del-CFTR protein to escape the endoplasmic reticulum and reach the plasma membrane. Potentiators are also useful

M.D. Amaral, K. Kunzelmann (eds.), *Cystic Fibrosis*, Methods in Molecular Biology 741,
DOI 10.1007/978-1-61779-117-8_2, © Springer Science+Business Media, LLC 2011

for F508del. Indeed, this mutation causes also a gating defect, although less severe than that of classical class III mutations. On the other hand, CFTR inhibitors are potentially useful to treat secretory diarrhea and polycystic kidney disease, two pathological conditions characterized by increased CFTR activity (1).

The identification of novel pharmacological modulators (potentiators, correctors, and inhibitors) of the CFTR chloride channel may be achieved by performing high-throughput screenings of large chemical libraries using a functional assay. This assay has to measure the main function of the CFTR protein, i.e., the transmembrane transport of chloride and other small anions. CFTR function may be determined directly with electrophysiological techniques. However, these methods are time consuming and expensive. Usually, high-throughput screenings are better performed using fluorescence-based techniques. For CFTR, a convenient fluorescent probe is the halide-sensitive yellow fluorescent protein (HS-YFP).

YFP is a derivative of the green fluorescent protein (GFP). Its fluorescence is quenched in the presence of chloride at high concentrations. Its sensitivity to anions has been further improved by mutagenesis. The replacement of histidine by glutamine at position 148 (H148Q) was initially found to enhance the affinity of the YFP protein to iodide and chloride, the corresponding K_i values being 20 and 100 mM, respectively (2). Subsequently, a second isoleucine to leucine mutation at position 152 (I152L) further increased the affinity for halides ($K_i \sim 2$ mM for iodide and 20 mM for chloride) (3).

The different sensitivity of the HS-YFP toward iodide and chloride allows to perform assays measuring the transport of anions through the plasma membrane as changes in cell fluorescence. For this assay, the cells expressing HS-YFP are equilibrated in a physiological chloride-rich saline solution (e.g., Dulbecco's PBS). During fluorescence reading, cells are exposed to a high concentration of iodide. Iodide influx quenches the cell fluorescence with a rate that depends on the halide permeability of cell membrane, and therefore, on the activity of anion channels or transporters (**Fig. 2.1**).

The YFP assay has been applied to CFTR (4–7), pendrin (8), and the Ca^{2+}-activated Cl^- channel (9). Because of its simplicity and sensitivity, it can be automated. Therefore, it has been applied to perform high-throughput screenings of large chemical libraries in order to identify pharmacological modulators of CFTR.

Here we present a schematic description of procedures used to evaluate CFTR function in high-throughput format with HS-YFP. We also describe an adaptation of the HS-YFP assay for transiently transfected cells (HEK-293). Although this method has a significantly lower throughput, it is useful for initial evaluation of novel CFTR mutants or activity of a limited number of compounds.

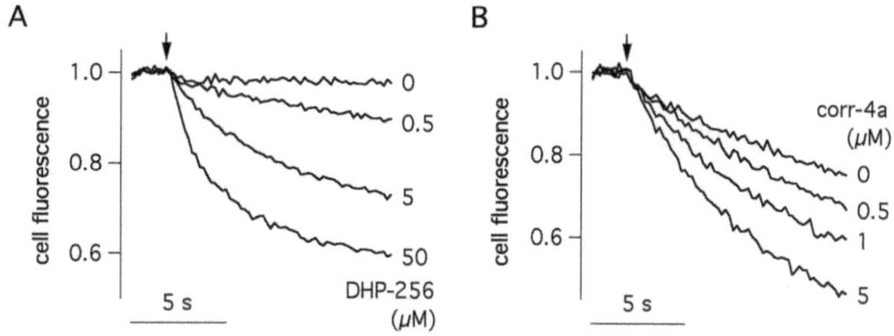

Fig. 2.1. Evaluation of CFTR correctors and potentiators with the HS-YFP assay. The figure shows representative cell fluorescence recordings acquired with a microplate reader. (**a**) Potentiator assay: FRT cells expressing G551D-CFTR. Cells were acutely stimulated with forskolin (20 μM) plus the potentiator DHP-256 at the indicated concentrations. (**b**) Corrector assay: FRT cells expressing F508del-CFTR. Cells were treated for 24 h with corr-4a at the indicated concentrations. After treatment, cells were acutely stimulated with forskolin (20 μM) and genistein (50 μM). In both panels, the *arrow* indicates iodide addition.

2. Materials

2.1. Cell Culture Media and Transfection Reagents

1. Cell culture medium for FRT cells: Coon's modification of F-12 (Sigma-Aldrich). This is a powder medium that requires addition of sodium bicarbonate as indicated by the supplier. After solubilization, the medium is supplemented with 2 mM glutamine, 100 U/ml penicillin, 100 μg/ml streptomycin, and 10% fetal bovine serum.
2. Cell culture medium for A549 and HEK-293 cells: Dulbecco's modified Eagle's medium–Ham's F-12 (DMEM/F-12 1:1) (Euroclone) supplemented with 2 mM glutamine, 100 U/ml penicillin, 100 μg/ml streptomycin, and 10% fetal bovine serum.
3. The selection agents zeocin, hygromycin B (Invitrogen), and geneticin (Calbiochem) are dissolved in tissue culture-grade water at 100 mg/ml, stored in aliquots at −20°C (zeocin) or at 4°C (hygromycin B and geneticin), and then added to cells as required.
4. PBS solution without Ca^{2+} and Mg^{2+} (Euroclone).
5. Trypsin solution (0.05%) and ethylenediaminetetraacetic acid (EDTA) (0.02%) (Euroclone).
6. Transfection reagent: Lipofectamine 2000 (Invitrogen).
7. Synthetic medium to use for DNA–Lipofectamine 2000 complex formation: Opti-MEM (Invitrogen).

2.2. CFTR and YFP Plasmids

Common plasmids or other vectors carrying the CFTR coding sequence and suitable for stable transfections can be used. Plasmids for the YFP-H148Q or YFP-H148Q/I152L can be obtained from our laboratory or from Dr. A.S. Verkman (verkman@ucsf.edu).

2.3. Saline Solutions

1. Standard Dulbecco's PBS: 137 mM NaCl, 2.7 mM KCl, 8.1 mM Na_2HPO_4, 1.5 mM KH_2PO_4, 1 mM $CaCl_2$, and 0.5 mM $MgCl_2$ (pH 7.4).
2. Iodide-rich Dulbecco's PBS: 137 mM NaI, 2.7 mM KCl, 8.1 mM Na_2HPO_4, 1.5 mM KH_2PO_4, 1 mM $CaCl_2$, and 0.5 mM $MgCl_2$ (pH 7.4).

2.4. Equipment

1. For automated testing on stable transfected cells: a microplate reader equipped with one or two syringe pumps, temperature control, and high-quality excitation (HQ500/20X: 500 ± 10 nm) and emission (HQ535/30 M: 535 ± 15 nm) filters for EYFP (Chroma Technology Corp., Brattleboro, VT).
2. For manual testing on transiently transfected cells: an inverted fluorescence microscope equipped with optical filters for EYFP (excitation: 505 nm; emission: 535 nm; dichroic: 515 nm). Optical filters for EGFP or similar probes (485 for excitation and 520 for emission) are also acceptable. The microscope needs one of the following acquisition systems: (1) photomultiplier tube (PMT, Hamamatsu) connected to an analog-to-digital converter (e.g., PowerLab 2/25; ADInstruments) or a camera (e.g., CoolSNAP cf; Photometrics) with relatively fast acquisition rate (at least four images per second).

2.5. Compounds

Compounds are dissolved as 10 mM stock solutions in dimethyl sulfoxide (DMSO) and arrayed in 96-well master plates. Daughter plates are made at 1–2 mM concentration in DMSO. Plates are stored at -80°C. Compounds are added to cells dissolved in saline solution (potentiators and inhibitors) or in the culture medium (correctors). Final DMSO concentration should not exceed 0.5–1.0%. Appropriate controls to evaluate effect of DMSO alone should be included throughout the screening.

Screenings are usually performed by testing a single compound per well. However, screenings of small compound pools (four per well) have also been carried out.

3. Methods

3.1. Generation and Use of Stable Transfectants for CFTR Functional Assays

Clones of Fischer rat thyroid (FRT) or A549 cells stably co-expressing human CFTR and the halide-sensing YFP (9) are generated with the following scheme:

1. Cells are first transfected with the plasmid carrying the coding sequence of wild-type or mutant CFTR using Lipofectamine 2000 (Invitrogen).
2. Twenty-four hours after transfection, cells are treated with the appropriate selection agent (e.g., 0.6 mg/ml zeocin or 0.75 mg/ml geneticin).
3. After 3–6 days, surviving cells are plated in 96-well microplates at clonal density (0.5–1 cell per well) for further selection.
4. Positive clones are identified by immunofluorescence or with functional assays (e.g., short-circuit current measurements for FRT cells).
5. Cells with stable CFTR expression are retransfected with the plasmid carrying the coding sequence for the halide-sensitive YFP and treated with a second selection agent to isolate pure fluorescent clones (*see* **Note 1**).
6. Stable clones co-expressing CFTR and the fluorescent protein are evaluated with functional assays. If needed, the cells can be re-cloned again to isolate cells with homogeneous expression of both proteins. After expansion of the best clone(s), the cells are frozen in several aliquots to keep a large stock for future screenings.

FRT and A549 cells expressing CFTR and YFP are cultured in the continuous presence of the corresponding selection agents. When needed for screenings, the cells are plated (50,000 cells/well) on clear-bottomed 96-well black microplates (Corning Life Sciences, Acton, MA) (*see* **Note 2**).

3.2. Generation of Transiently Transfected Cells for CFTR Functional Assays

This method is suitable for transient transfection in cells like HEK-293:

1. Cells are plated in 96-well microplates (25,000 cells/well) in 100 μl of DMEM/F-12 medium supplemented with 10% serum *without antibiotics*.
2. After 6 h, the cells are co-transfected with the plasmids coding for CFTR and the halide-sensitive YFP.
3. The transfection complex solution contains 0.2 μg total plasmidic DNA and 0.5 μl of Lipofectamine 2000 (Invitrogen) in 50 μl of Opti-MEM (Invitrogen) per well.
4. The mixture is incubated for 1 h at room temperature to allow formation of DNA/Lipofectamine 2000 complexes before addition to the cells (final volume in the well is therefore 150 μl).
5. After 24 h, the complexes are removed by replacement with fresh medium (*see* **Note 3**).

3.3. CFTR Assay by Microplate Reader

This method has been successfully used for high-throughput screening of large compound libraries to find CFTR inhibitors (4), potentiators (5, 6), and correctors (7):

1. At the time of the assay (24–48 h after cell plating in 96-well microplates), the cell culture medium is removed and the cells are washed and incubated for 30–45 min with 60 μl of Dulbecco's PBS containing compounds for CFTR stimulation/inhibition (e.g., forskolin, CPT-cAMP, and potentiators).
2. Microplates are transferred to a microplate reader for CFTR activity determination.
3. The assay in each well consists of a continuous 14 s fluorescence reading with 2 s before and 12 s after injection of 165 μl of the iodide-rich Dulbecco's PBS. This step ensures that the cells are exposed to a final iodide concentration of 100 mM. Injection flow rate is set at 100–160 μl/s. Cell incubation and assay are carried out at 37°C.

3.4. CFTR Assay by Fluorescence Microscope

This method has been successfully used to study the effect of CFTR inhibitors (10) and potentiators (11) after transient transfection in cells like HEK-293:

1. At the time of assay (48 h after transfection in 96-well microplates), cells are washed twice with standard Dulbecco's PBS.
2. After washing, the cells are incubated for 30–45 min with 60 μl PBS with and without compounds for CFTR stimulation/inhibition (e.g., forskolin, CPT-cAMP, and potentiators).
3. After this step, the microplates carrying the cells are transferred to the microscope to perform the assay, one well at a time.
4. Cell fluorescence is continuously recorded (with a PMT or a camera) before and after addition of 165 μl of iodide-containing Dulbecco's PBS.

3.5. Conditions for Screening (Potentiators, Inhibitors, and Correctors)

3.5.1. Conditions for the Screening of Correctors on F508del-CFTR Cells

1. Eighteen to twenty-four hours before the assay, the cells are treated with test compounds at the desired concentration in the culture medium. Each microplate is used to test 80 compounds with the rest of wells available for positive controls (known correctors) and negative controls (DMSO vehicle alone). Additional microplates can be incubated at 27°C (in a 5% CO_2–95% air atmosphere) as another positive control.
2. At the time of assay, cells are washed with standard Dulbecco's PBS and stimulated for 30–45 min with forskolin (20 μM) plus genistein (50 μM) in a final volume of 60 μl of the same saline solution.

3.5.2. Conditions for the Screening of Potentiators on F508del-CFTR Cells

1. Eighteen to twenty-four hours before the assay, the cells are incubated at 27°C (in a 5% CO_2–95% air atmosphere) to allow rescue of the mutant protein to the plasma membrane.
2. At the time of assay, cells are washed with standard Dulbecco's PBS and stimulated for 30–45 min with forskolin (20 μM) and test compounds (at the desired concentration) in a final volume of 60 μl of the same saline solution. Positive controls include genistein and/or other known potentiators at maximally effective concentrations.

3.5.3. Conditions for the Screening of Potentiators on G551D- and G1349D-CFTR Cells

The conditions are identical to those used to test potentiators on F508del-CFTR cells except that the step of incubation at low temperature is omitted. Furthermore, higher concentrations of potentiators are required for G551D cells since this mutant is more refractory to pharmacological stimulation (e.g., genistein needs to be tested at 100–200 μM instead of 50 μM).

3.5.4. Conditions for the Screening of Inhibitors on Wild-Type CFTR Cells

1. Twenty-four to forty-eight hours after plating in 96-well microplates, cells with stable expression of wild-type CFTR and the halide-sensitive YFP are washed with Dulbecco's PBS.
2. Cells are treated for 30–45 min with a stimulating cocktail containing forskolin (20 μM) and IBMX (100 μM) plus test compounds (at the desired concentration) in a final volume of 60 μl Dulbecco's PBS.

3.6. Data Analysis

Data analysis is usually performed as follows:

1. Subtracting the background fluorescence (i.e., well with saline solution but no cells);
2. Normalizing each trace by the initial fluorescence;
3. Fitting of the fluorescence decay (skipping the first few points to avoid the injection artifact) with a single exponential function (**Fig. 2.2a**);
4. Determination of maximal slope by differentiation of the fit (*see* **Note 4**).

Fluorescence subtraction and normalization can be done with Excel. Fitting needs a program such as Igor (Wavemetrics). The entire calculation, or part of it, can be done using automated procedures.

An alternative method to quantify fluorescence quenching is based on the determination of the decrease in signal at a fixed time point (**Fig. 2.2a**). This approach is simpler and may be more adequate for cells with a complex shape of the cell fluorescence decrease that does not follow a single exponential decay.

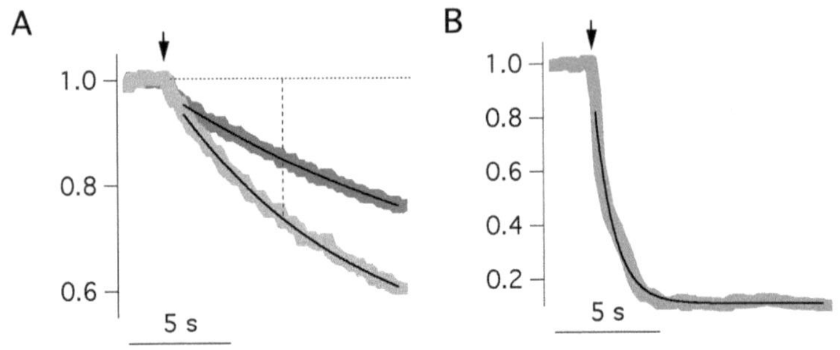

Fig. 2.2. Analysis of HS-YFP assay data. (**a**) Representative traces from FRT cells showing two different levels of F508del-CFTR activity (*light gray* and *dark gray lines*). The fluorescence decay was fitted with exponential functions (*smooth black curves*) to calculate initial maximal slope. As an alternative method, decay was also measured as the fraction of initial fluorescence at a fixed time point (*dashed vertical line*). (**b**) Example of artifact generated by incubation with a toxic compound. Presence of toxic compounds during corrector screenings causes cell detachment at the time of iodide solution injection during the HS-YFP assay. This results in a sharp fluorescence drop that may appear as a "high CFTR activity."

A software to analyze cell fluorescence intensity (e.g., MetaMorph; Molecular Devices) needs to be utilized if fluorescence changes are acquired as a series of images (microscope equipped with a fast acquisition camera). This method is time consuming compared to acquisition of an integrated signal from a cell population, as done with a microplate reader or with a microscope equipped with a PMT. However, it gives the advantage to determine CFTR activity in single cells.

4. Notes

1. In theory, transfection of cells with the HS-YFP in first place and then with the CFTR plasmid should be more practical. Indeed, after the second transfection, the HS-YFP assay can be used to rapidly screen hundreds of clones to identify the ones that express CFTR. However, for unknown reasons, this procedure is associated in our hands with a very low probability of positive clones, at least in FRT cells.
2. Besides FRT and A549 cells, other cell lines can also be used to perform the HS-YFP assay. One of the requirements is that the cell line has no endogenous activity of other anion channels and transporters that could interfere with the CFTR activity. Another important requirement is that the chosen cell line must be strongly attached to the plastic of the microplate to resist washings and iodide solution

injection. Cell plating density needs to be determined for each cell line.

3. Percentage of HEK-293 cells expressing HS-YFP is in the 30–50% range using the indicated conditions.

4. The initial points after iodide injection are an important source of artifacts. Solution addition causes a fast drop in fluorescence that is usually smaller than 5% of total signal. If not skipped during the fitting step, it could erroneously generate a large value of fluorescence decay rate. The extent of the artifact caused by solution injection should be monitored each time by running wells in which the cells are not stimulated. During screenings and automatic analysis of data, the presence of toxic compounds may generate false positives (**Fig. 2.2b**) because of large decreases in cell fluorescence upon iodide injection (due to cell detachment). These artifacts can be easily detected by visual inspection of traces (they appear as sharp drops in cell fluorescence) and cells (there will be a visible detachment at the center of the well).

References

1. Verkman, A. S., and Galietta, L. J. (2009) Chloride channels as drug targets. *Nat. Rev. Drug Discov.* **8**, 153–171.
2. Jayaraman, S., Haggie, P., Wachter, R. M., Remington, S. J., and Verkman, A. S. (2000) Mechanism and cellular applications of a green fluorescent protein-based halide sensor. *J. Biol. Chem.* **275**, 6047–6050.
3. Galietta, L. J., Haggie, P. M., and Verkman, A. S. (2001) Green fluorescent protein-based halide indicators with improved chloride and iodide affinities. *FEBS Lett.* **499**, 220–224.
4. Ma, T., Thiagarajah, J. R., Yang, H., Sonawane, N. D., Folli, C., Galietta, L. J., et al. (2002) Thiazolidinone CFTR inhibitor identified by high-throughput screening blocks cholera toxin-induced intestinal fluid secretion. *J. Clin. Invest.* **110**, 1651–1658.
5. Yang, H., Shelat, A. A., Guy, R. K., Gopinath, V. S., Ma, T., Du, K., et al. (2003) Nanomolar affinity small molecule correctors of defective Delta F508-CFTR chloride channel gating. *J. Biol. Chem.* **278**, 35079–35085.
6. Pedemonte, N., Sonawane, N. D., Taddei, A., Hu, J., Zegarra-Moran, O., Suen, Y. F. et al. (2005) Phenylglycine and sulfonamide correctors of defective deltaF508 and G551D cystic fibrosis transmembrane conductance regulator chloride-channel gating. *Mol. Pharmacol.* **67**, 1797–1807.
7. Pedemonte, N., Lukacs, G. L., Du, K., Caci, E., Zegarra-Moran, O., Galietta, L. J. et al. (2005) Small-molecule correctors of defective DeltaF508-CFTR cellular processing identified by high-throughput screening. *J. Clin. Invest.* **115**, 2564–2571.
8. Pedemonte, N., Caci, E., Sondo, E., Caputo, A., Rhoden, K., Pfeffer, U. et al. (2007) Thiocyanate transport in resting and IL-4-stimulated human bronchial epithelial cells: Role of pendrin and anion channels. *J. Immunol.* **178**, 5144–5153.
9. Caputo, A., Caci, E., Ferrera, L., Pedemonte, N., Barsanti, C., Sondo, E. et al. (2008) TMEM16A, a membrane protein associated with calcium-dependent chloride channel activity. *Science.* **322**, 590–594.
10. Caci, E., Caputo, A., Hinzpeter, A., Arous, N., Fanen, P., Sonawane, N. et al. (2008) Evidence for direct CFTR inhibition by CFTR(inh)-172 based on Arg347 mutagenesis. *Biochem. J.* **413**, 135–142.
11. Caputo, A., Hinzpeter, A., Caci, E., Pedemonte, N., Arous, N., Di Duca, M. et al. (2009) Mutation-specific potency and efficacy of cystic fibrosis transmembrane conductance regulator chloride channel potentiators. *J. Pharmacol. Exp. Ther.* **330**, 783–791.

Chapter 3

Repair of CFTR Folding Defects with Correctors that Function as Pharmacological Chaperones

Tip W. Loo and David M. Clarke

Abstract

The major cause of cystic fibrosis is the presence of processing mutations in CFTR (such as deletion of Phe-508 (F508del-CFTR)) that disrupt folding of the protein and trafficking to the cell surface. Processing mutations appear to inhibit folding of CFTR so that it accumulates in the endoplasmic reticulum as a partially folded protein. Expressing the proteins in the presence of small molecules called correctors can repair CFTR folding defects. Some correctors appear to function as pharmacological chaperones that specifically bind to the CFTR processing mutants and induce them to complete the folding process. In this chapter, we describe techniques to examine the effects of correctors on folding of CFTR processing mutants.

Key words: F508del-CFTR, corrector, processing mutant, protein folding, glycosylation, disulfide cross-linking, protein maturation.

1. Introduction

The cystic fibrosis transmembrane conductance regulator (CFTR) chloride channel is located at the apical surface of epithelial cells of many organs where it plays an important role in salt and fluid homeostasis (1). Genetic mutations that inhibit expression, activity, or trafficking of CFTR to the cell surface (2) cause cystic fibrosis (CF). The primary cause of CF (over 90% of CF patients express at least one copy) is deletion of Phe508 (F508del-CFTR) in the first nucleotide-binding domain (NBD). Repair of F508del-CFTR would prevent CF in most patients. F508del-CFTR has three major defects. The mutant is defective

M.D. Amaral, K. Kunzelmann (eds.), *Cystic Fibrosis*, Methods in Molecular Biology 741,
DOI 10.1007/978-1-61779-117-8_3,

in folding and trafficking to the cell surface, has low channel activity relative to the wild-type protein, and is unstable at the cell surface. In previous studies on the structurally similar P-glycoprotein drug pump, we found that defects in folding and activity could be specifically and efficiently repaired when the protein was expressed in the presence of compounds that bound directly to the protein (3). Subsequent screening of chemical libraries showed that expression, delivery to the cell surface, and activity of F508del-CFTR could be enhanced by carrying out expression in the presence of small molecules called correctors (4–7). Correctors have also been shown to repair folding defects in other CFTR processing mutants (8). The term "processing mutation" is used to describe a mutation that inhibits folding of CFTR such that it accumulates in the endoplasmic reticulum as a core-glycosylated immature protein. Processing mutations appear to act as thermodynamic hurdles for CFTR folding, so the mutants accumulate in the endoplasmic reticulum as proteins that resemble partially folded wild-type CFTR (9, 10). The immature processing mutants appear to be in a loosely folded conformation as they are more sensitive to proteases than the mature protein (9). They show incomplete domain–domain interactions (11) and packing of the transmembrane (TM) segments (12). A goal is to use correctors to induce CFTR processing mutants to complete the folding process to yield functional protein at the cell surface.

The ideal corrector would act as a pharmacological chaperone that is targeted directly and specifically toward CFTR mutants. Specific rescue would reduce potential side effects because they would be less likely to alter the expression or the activity of other proteins. The bioavailability of oral medications would also be increased if they were not substrates for the drug pumps that block entry in the intestine or catalyze excretion in the kidney and liver.

This chapter describes the techniques involved in "rescuing" CFTR processing mutants with correctors and examining corrector-induced structural changes in the protein. The most versatile expression system for studying CFTR mutants is transient expression in human embryonic kidney (HEK 293) cells. Expression is very rapid in these cells and the mutant proteins can be characterized 1–3 days after transfection. Several commercial sources have expression vectors for transient transfection (e.g., pcDNA3 from Invitrogen, San Diego, CA). The pcDNA3 vector can also be used to generate stable cell lines since it contains the neomycin resistance gene. Stable cell lines are needed for procedures such as iodide efflux measurement because of the large number of washing steps that must be performed.

2. Materials

2.1. Transient Transfection

1. HEK 293 cells (ATCC, American Type and Culture Collection (*see* **Note 1**)).
2. Media: Dulbecco's modified Eagle's medium (DMEM) with high glucose and supplemented with non-essential amino acids, 4 mM L-glutamine, 10 IU/ml penicillin, 0.1 mg/ml streptomycin, and 10% (v/v) fetal bovine serum.
3. cDNA in the appropriate expression vector purified using a Qiagen (Qiagen, Inc.) Maxi-Prep column and suspended in sterile TE buffer (10 mM Tris–HCl (pH 8.0) and 1 mM EDTA).
4. 2.5 M $CaCl_2$ stock in sterile water (Tissue culture grade $CaCl_2$; Sigma, Cat. # C-7902).
5. 2× BES: 50 mM BES [*N,N*-bis(2-hydroxyethyl)-2-aminoethanesulfonic acid; Sigma, Cat #: B-4554], 280 mM NaCl, and 1.5 mM $Na_2HPO_4{\cdot}7H_2O$. Adjust pH to 6.96 with NaOH (*see* **Note 2**).
6. Endoglycosidase H_f and 10× Endo H_f buffer (New England Biolabs).

2.2. Pulse Labeling

1. S-minus media: Dulbecco's modified Eagle's medium with high glucose, without L-methionine or L-cystine (Invitrogen, Inc.). To this, add non-essential amino acids and 10% (v/v) fetal bovine serum.
2. [^{35}S]Translabel (specific activity: 1180 Ci/ml; MP Biomedicals, USA).
3. Buffer I: 25 mM Tris–HCl, pH 7.5, 150 mM NaCl, 1% (w/v) Triton X-100, 0.5% (w/v) sodium deoxycholate, and 1 mM EDTA.
4. Protein A Sepharose CL-4B (GE Healthcare, Quebec).

2.3. Cell Surface Labeling

1. Biotin hydrazide (Pierce).
2. Horseradish peroxidase conjugated to streptavidin (Kirkegaard and Perry Laboratories).
3. PBSCM: PBS buffer (pH 7.4) with 1 mM $MgCl_2$ and 0.1 mM $CaCl_2$.
4. Acetate buffer: 100 mM sodium acetate, pH 5.5, 1 mM $MgCl_2$, and 0.1 mM $CaCl_2$.

2.4. Cross-linking Analysis

1. LIS buffer: 10 mM Tris–HCl, pH 7.5, 0.5 mM $MgCl_2$.
2. Solution A: 10 mM Tris–HCl, pH 7.5, 0.5 M sucrose, and 0.3 M KCl.

3. Copper phenanthroline: 25 mM copper sulfate and 75 mM 1, 10-phenanthroline.
4. TBS: 10 mM Tris–HCl, pH 7.4, 150 mM NaCl.

2.5. Measurement of Iodide Efflux Activity

1. CHO Flp-In cells, vectors, and hygromycin are available from Invitrogen.
2. G418 sulfate: potency greater than 0.65 mg/g.
3. Loading buffer: 136 mM NaI, 4 mM KNO_3, 2 mM $Ca(NO_3)$, 2 mM $Mg(NO_3)$, 11 mM glucose, 20 mM HEPES, pH 7.4.
4. Efflux buffer: 136 mM $NaNO_3$, 4 mM KNO_3, 2 mM $Ca(NO_3)$, 2 mM $Mg(NO_3)$, 11 mM glucose, and 20 mM HEPES, pH 7.4.
5. Stimulation buffer: Efflux buffer plus 0.01 mM forskolin, 200 nM IBMX, 500 nM chlorophenylthio-cAMP (CPT-cAMP), and 0.01 mM VX-532.

3. Methods

3.1. Small-Scale Expression of CFTR Processing Mutants and Rescue with Correctors

Maturation of CFTR processing mutants can be monitored by glycosylation of the protein. CFTR is glycosylated at two sites in the extracellular loop that connects transmembrane segments 7 and 8. The protein is core glycosylated in the endoplasmic reticulum. When the protein folds into a native state, it leaves the endoplasmic reticulum and enters the Golgi where complex carbohydrate is added. The immature core-glycosylated form of CFTR (in the endoplasmic reticulum) migrates in SDS gels with an apparent mass of about 160 kDa, while the mature form of CFTR migrates with an apparent mass of about 180 kDa. Therefore, the glycosylation pattern of CFTR in SDS gels serves as an important preliminary tool for indicating whether a mutant protein has been processed after rescue with a corrector. Subsequent biochemical tests with endoglycosidases will indicate whether the CFTR protein has been fully processed. As the protein moves from the ER to the Golgi, their carbohydrates are modified and they become resistant to endoglycosidase H_f, but not to endoglycosidase F.

To identify the concentration of chemical chaperone required, the cells are first transfected with the mutant cDNA (in six-well plates) and then incubated with different concentrations of the corrector. Different concentrations are tested to determine optimum rescue and determine the levels that are toxic to the cells. Transfection using the calcium phosphate co-precipitation method (13) is relatively inexpensive and works well. There are two approaches to carry out the transfections. In the first method, cells are suspended, mixed with the transfection mix, and the cells are then added to plates. In the second method, cells are plated the day before transfection. The next day, transfection mixes are added to the plated cells:

1. All procedures are done in a tissue culture hood. The following protocol is sufficient to transfect a six-well plate. In a 50-ml sterile polypropylene conical tube, mix 0.01 mg cDNA (CFTR processing mutant in the chosen expression vector) and sterile water to give a volume of 0.45 ml. Then add 0.05 ml of 2.5 M $CaCl_2$ and mix. Then slowly add 0.5 ml of 2× BES solution (dropwise and with constant mixing) and let the mixture incubate at room temperature (21°C) for 10 min. During this interval, prepare the cells.
2. Remove the media from a 75-cm^2 flask of HEK 293 cells (grown to about 50–75% confluency). Give the flask a hard tap. This will dislodge the cells from the bottom of the flask. Add 5 ml of media (*see* **Note 3**). Pipette the cells up and down 3–4 times to break any clumps of cells and add another 55 ml of media. Take 12 ml of this cell suspension and add to the DNA/$CaPO_4$ mixture above. Mix gently and immediately pipette 1.5 ml of this suspension into each well of a six-well plate (*see* **Notes 4** and **5**).
3. The alternative approach would be to plate the cells a day before transfection. Remove the media from a 75-cm^2 flask of HEK 293 cells (grown to about 50–75% confluency). Give the flask a hard tap. This will dislodge the cells from the bottom of the flask. Add 5 ml of media. Pipette the cells up and down 3–4 times to break any clumps of cells and add about another 145 ml of media. Add 1.5 ml per well of six-well plates and let incubate overnight. The next day transfect the cells. For one six-well plate, mix 0.01 mg cDNA (in the chosen expression vector) and sterile water to give a volume of 0.45 ml in a 50-ml sterile polypropylene conical tube. Then add 0.05 ml of 2.5 M $CaCl_2$ and mix. Then add slowly 0.5 ml of 2× BES solution (dropwise and with constant mixing) and let the mixture incubate at room temperature (21°C) for 10 min. Add 10 ml of media. Aspirate the media from the cells and add 1.5 ml of the transfection mix to each well.
4. After transfection by either approach, incubate the plate overnight at 37°C in 2.5% CO_2 (*see* **Note 6**).
5. Next day, prepare fivefold serial dilutions of a corrector to test. A concentration of 0.05 mM as the highest concentration is a useful starting point in our experience (prepare a drug stock of 50 mM in DMSO). Remove the six-well plate from the incubator and gently aspirate the media. Then add

1.5 ml of the diluted drug/media mixture to each well. Plain media is added to one well. Incubate for 24–48 h at 37°C in 5% CO_2. Repeat this step on a plate of transfected cells but with no corrector (these are the mock-treated samples that will serve as controls). Another plate of cells that was transfected with cDNA for wild-type CFTR should also be treated with and without different concentrations of corrector (these samples will indicate whether the corrector had an effect on the wild-type protein) (*see* **Note 7**).

6. Harvest the transfected cells by pipetting the media up and down several times to dislodge the cells and then transfer to a 1.5-ml microcentrifuge tube (*see* **Note 8**). Pellet cells by centrifugation at 2,000×*g* for 3 min at room temperature. Remove the supernatant and resuspend cells in 1 ml PBS. Pellet the cells again by centrifugation. Resuspend pellet in 0.025 ml of PBS, then add 0.2 ml of 2× SDS sample buffer (125 mM Tris–HCl, pH 6.8, 4% (w/v) SDS, 4% (v/v) 2-mercaptoethanol, 20% (v/v) glycerol and 50 mM EDTA (*see* **Note 9**)).
7. Load 0.01 ml on 5.5% SDS gels (Minigel; 1.5 mm spacers and 15 wells). Electroblot the gel onto a piece of nitrocellulose (Western blot) and do immunoblot analysis with anti-CFTR antibody (available commercially) followed by enhanced chemiluminescence (14). If the corrector promoted maturation of the CFTR processing mutant, then the ratio of mature to immature protein will increase. Although the level of glycosylation can vary in different cell lines, immature CFTR migrates as a 160-kDa protein when expressed in HEK 293 cells, whereas mature CFTR migrates as a 180-kDa protein (*see* **Note 10**) (*see* **Fig. 3.1**).
8. Immature and mature CFTRs can also be distinguished by testing their sensitivity to digestion by endoglycosidase H.

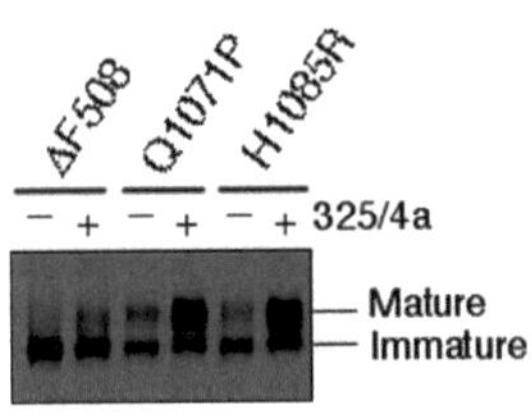

Fig. 3.1. Example of rescue of CFTR processing mutants by correctors. HEK 293 cells expressing the CFTR processing mutants, F508del, Q1071P, or H1085R, were incubated with media containing no corrector (–) or 0.05 mM VX-325 plus 0.015 mM corr-4a (+). After 18 h at 37°C, the cells were harvested and solubilized with SDS sample buffer containing 50 mM EDTA, and subjected to immunoblot analysis with a polyclonal anti-CFTR antibody. In the absence of corrector, the major CFTR product is the 160-kDa immature protein. Expression in the presence of correctors promoted maturation (180 kDa protein) of each of the processing mutants.

Take 0.45 ml of the whole-cell extract and add 0.05 ml 10× Endo H buffer (500 mM sodium citrate, pH 5.5, 5% (w/v) SDS, 100 mM EDTA and 10% (v/v) 2-mercaptoethanol) and 0.001 ml of Endo H_f (1,000 U/ml; New England Biolabs). Mix gently and incubate at 37°C for 15 min. Add 1 vol. of 2× SDS sample buffer and load 0.01 ml onto 5.5% SDS gels. Do Western blot analysis.

3.2. Pulse Labeling to Monitor Time Course of Maturation

The time course of maturation of a CFTR processing mutant in the presence or the absence of a corrector can be determined by pulse-chase experiments using radiolabeled [^{35}S]methionine and cystine. The steps described below involve the use of the correctors VX-325 plus corr-4a. The use of VX-325 plus corr-4a is the most efficient method to promote maturation of CFTR processing mutants (11):

1. HEK 293 cells are plated on day 1. Media is aspirated from a subconfluent T-75 flask of HEK 293 cells. Rap the flask on the edge of the hood to dislodge the cells. Add 10 ml of media to the flask and pipet up and down three times to break up any clumps of cells. Add about 120 ml of media and then add to 12 numbered 10-cm plates. Six of the plates will be used to monitor maturation in the absence of correctors and six plates will be used to monitor maturation in the presence of VX-325 plus corr-4a.
2. The next day transfect the cells. Add 0.1 mg of cDNA for a CFTR processing mutant to sterile water to give a total volume of 4.5 ml. Add 0.5 ml of 2.5 M $CaCl_2$. Add 5 ml of 2× BES dropwise. After 10 min, add the transfection mix to 100 ml of media in a T-75 flask. Aspirate the media from the cells plated the day before. Add 9 ml of this mixture to the 10-cm-diameter culture dishes (total of 12 dishes). Incubate the cells for overnight at 37°C in a 2.5% CO_2 incubator.
3. Next day gently aspirate off the media from each plate and gently add 9 ml of S-minus media (no L-methionine or L-cystine) and again remove media (*see* **Note 11**). Then add 9 ml of S-minus media and incubate cells for 30 min at 37°C. While cells are incubating, prepare the radioactive label.
4. In one 50-ml conical tube, add 0.04 mCi/ml [^{35}S]Translabel (contains [^{35}S]L-methionine and [^{35}S]cystine) to 50 ml S-minus media with no correctors (control). In another 50-ml conical tube, add 0.04 mCi/ml [^{35}S]Translabel (contains [^{35}S]L-methionine and [^{35}S]cystine) to 50 ml S-minus media with 0.05 mM VX-325 plus 0.015 mM corr-4a (+ corr). To start labeling, remove media from cells and add 8 ml of the radioactive media. Incubate the cells for 30 min at 37°C.

5. Remove radioactive media and add 8 ml of regular media containing no correctors or 0.05 mM VX-325 plus 0.015 mM corr-4a. (This is Time = 0 min, and the start of the chase part of the experiment.)
6. At times 0, 1, 2, 4, 8, and 24 h, remove the media. Add 1.5 ml PBS and collect the cells in a 2-ml microfuge tube.
7. Collect cells by centrifugation at 2,000×*g* for 3 min and wash the pelleted cells four times with 1.5 ml PBS.
8. Suspend the cells in 0.1 ml PBS containing 5 mM EDTA. Add 1.5 ml of buffer I, mix, and let incubate on ice for 10 min. Centrifuge at 14,000×*g* for 10 min at 4°C. Transfer the supernatant to a fresh microfuge tube and then add 2 μg of anti-CFTR monoclonal antibody (such as M3A7). Incubate for 2 h overnight at 4°C and then add 0.05 ml of Protein A Sepharose CL-4B beads (the Protein A Sepharose CL-4B beads are prepared as a 50% (v/v) slurry in buffer I).
9. Incubate for 1 h at 4°C on a rotator or a platform shaker. Centrifuge at 4,000×*g* for 1 min to pellet the beads. Resuspend the beads in 1 ml of buffer I, then centrifuge to pellet the beads. Wash the bead another four times with 1 ml buffer I. Add 0.05 ml of 2× SDS sample buffer to the final pelleted beads (*see* **Note 12**). Load 0.015 ml of the supernatant onto a 5.5% Minigel (1.5 mm thick). After gel electrophoresis, soak the gels in 10% (v/v) acetic acid for 15 min at room temperature. Rinse the gel twice with distilled water and soak the gel in Amplify (GE Healthcare) for 30–60 min at room temperature. Place the gel onto a piece of 3-mm filter paper and dry at 60–70°C for 1 h in a vacuum dryer (*see* **Note 13**).
10. Place the dried gel in a film cassette and expose to film for various times at –80°C (*see* **Note 14**).

3.3. Cell Surface Labeling

There are several ways to determine if a fully glycosylated (mature) CFTR protein has been transported from the Golgi to the cell surface. A biochemical method is cell surface labeling of the carbohydrate group in the protein. When CFTR is at the cell surface, its carbohydrate groups are exposed to the outside of the cell and can be modified and labeled (*see* **Note 15**):

1. Transfect HEK 293 cells with wild-type, misprocessed CFTR mutant or with expression vector (mock-transfected) in 10-cm^2 culture plates (two plates each). Incubate overnight at 37°C in 2.5% CO_2 incubator.
2. Remove media from each pair of plates. Add fresh plain media to one plate and fresh media containing 0.05 mM VX-325 plus 0.015 mM corr-4a to the other plate. Incubate for another 24–48 h at 37°C in a 5% CO_2 incubator.

3. The remaining steps are done at 4°C. Gently wash the cells four times with 3 ml PBSCM buffer (*see* **Note 16**).
4. Add 2 ml of 10 mM $NaIO_4$ in PBSCM buffer and leave the plates in the dark for 30 min.
5. Wash the cells three times with 3 ml PBSCM buffer and once with 3 ml acetate buffer.
6. Add 2 ml of 2 mM biotin hydrazide in acetate buffer and incubate for 30 min in the dark.
7. Wash cells four times with PBSCM. Collect cells in 1 ml PBS and transfer to a 1.5-ml microfuge tube. Pellet cells by centrifugation and suspend in 0.1 ml PBS and then add 1 ml of buffer I.
8. Centrifuge at 14,000×*g* for 10 min. Transfer supernatant to a fresh microfuge tube and do immunoprecipitation as described above.
9. Run immunoprecipitates on SDS gels, transfer onto nitrocellulose, and develop with HRP conjugated to streptavidin. It will be observed that expression in the presence of corrector will enhance expression of CFTR at the cell surface.

3.4. Disulfide Cross-linking of CFTR in Whole Cells to Monitor Effects of Correctors on CFTR Folding

A convenient method for testing whether the corrector has promoted folding of a CFTR processing mutant into a native conformation is to monitor disulfide cross-linking between cysteines introduced into different domains of the protein. It has previously been demonstrated that CFTR processing mutations trap CFTR as a partially folded protein in the endoplasmic reticulum (15). Correctors promote folding into a native structure. Disulfide cross-linking between cysteines introduced into various domains can be used to distinguish between native and immature forms of CFTR. An initial problem with cross-linking studies on CFTR was the fact that the protein contained 18 endogenous cysteines. The presence of endogenous cysteines would make cross-linking studies difficult because it would not be known if cross-linking would involve introduced cysteines or native cysteines. Therefore, a cysteine-less CFTR was made. All of the native cysteines were mutated to alanines. A problem with the initial cysteine-less CFTR was that the protein failed to mature (12). To improve the maturation efficiency of Cys-less CFTR, cysteines 590 and 592 were replaced with leucines (16) and valine 510 was changed to alanine (17). To monitor folding of CFTR processing mutants, cysteines were introduced at various domain interfaces of the protein. Examples of reporter cysteines that showed differences in the immature and mature forms of CFTR were cysteines introduced into transmembrane segments 6 and 12 of transmembrane domains 1 (TMD1) and 2 (TMD2), respectively (15), and between cysteines introduced into the first nucleotide-binding domain (NBD1) and an intracellular loop in TMD2 (11).

In both cases the presence of processing mutations inhibited maturation of CFTR and inhibited cross-linking between cysteines in different domains (15, 18). Carrying out expression in the presence of correctors could restore maturation and cross-linking. The following protocols describe disulfide cross-linking between cysteines introduced into NBD1 (V510C) and the fourth intracellular loop in TMD2 (A1067C) of a F508del-CFTR processing mutant expressed in the presence or the absence of correctors. These cysteines can be used to monitor folding of CFTR. Immature CFTR shows little cross-linking (18). Cross-linking was observed, however, when maturation of the mutant was promoted by carrying out expression in the presence of correctors (11). Since these cysteines are located in cytoplasmic regions of CFTR, cross-linking must be carried out on membranes prepared from the transfected cells:

1. Remove media from two subconfluent T-75 flasks of HEK 293 cells by aspiration. Rap the flasks to dislodge cells. Add 5 ml of media to each flask, pipet up and down three times, and pool the cells into a total volume of about 200 ml. Add 9 ml of cells to 10-cm^2 plates to yield two sets of 10 plates – one set will be treated with correctors and the other set will serve as a control. Incubate the cells overnight.

2. The next day, add 0.17 mg of (V510C)/(A1067C)/F508del-CFTR cDNA to sterile water to give a total volume of 7.65 ml. Add 0.85 ml of 2.5 M $CaCl_2$ and then add dropwise 8.5 ml 2× BES solution. Let mixture sit at room temperature for 10 min. Add the transfection mix to 170 ml of media. Aspirate media from the transfected cells and add 9 ml of media containing the transfection mix. Incubate the cells overnight.

3. Next day, remove the media and replace with fresh media containing 0.05 mM VX-325 plus 0.015 mM corr-4a to 10 plates and plain media to the second set of plates (control). Incubate at 37°C in a 5% CO_2 incubator overnight.

4. The next day, harvest cells and use immediately or suspend in 3 ml of media containing 10% (v/v) DMSO and store in a –80°C freezer.

5. To prepare membranes, wash the cells three times with 6 ml of PBS. All steps are performed on ice or at 4°C. We use 13-ml polypropylene tubes and centrifuge at 3,000×*g* for 3 min each time. Suspend the cells in 3 ml of LIS buffer. Transfer into a 7-ml Dounce homogenizer and break cells using 40 strokes with a glass "loose" homogenizer. Add 3 ml of solution A followed by 15 additional strokes. Transfer the broken cells back to the 13-ml tube and centrifuge at 6,000×*g* for 5 min. Transfer the supernatant to a 30-ml polycarbonate tube containing 20 ml of TBS. Centrifuge at

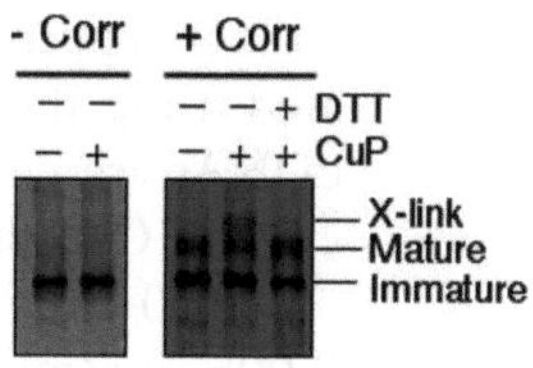

Fig. 3.2. Effect of correctors on cross-linking of CFTR mutant F508del/V510C (NBD1)/A1067C(TMD2). HEK 293 cells were transfected with mutant F508del/V510C(NBD1)/A1067C(TMD2) cDNA and grown in the presence (+ Corr) or the absence (– Corr) of 0.05 mM VX-325 plus 0.015 mM corr–4a for 18 h. Membranes were prepared from the transfected cells and samples were treated with (+) or without (–) 1 mM copper phenanthroline (CuP) for 15 min at 0°C. The reactions were stopped by addition of SDS sample buffer without (– DTT) or with 40 mM dithiothreitol (+ DTT). Samples were subjected to immunoblot analysis. The positions of immature, mature, and cross-linked (X-link) forms of CFTR are indicated. The results show that only mature CFTR is cross-linked.

40,000×*g* for 45 min and discard the supernatant. Suspend the crude membrane pellet in about 0.4 ml of TBS.

6. Cross-linking is performed on ice. Put 0.002 ml of water (blank) or 20 mM copper phenanthroline in tubes on ice. Add 0.018 ml of membranes and let incubate on ice for 15 min. Add 0.1 ml of 2× SDS sample buffer (containing no thiol-reducing agents) with 50 mM EDTA to stop the reactions. Load 0.01 ml on 6.5% acrylamide gels. Then perform immunoblot analysis with an anti-CFTR antibody. Cross-linking of the mature protein is observed after expression in the presence of correctors (*see* **Note 17**) (*see* **Fig. 3.2**).

3.5. Measurement of CFTR Activity by Iodide Efflux

It is important to test if rescue of CFTR processing mutants with correctors yields functional mutants. One approach is to measure iodide efflux in whole cells. CFTR can mediate protein kinase A-dependent efflux of anions such as chloride or iodide with linear conductance. Since CFTR is one of the few channels that can conduct iodide current, measurement of iodide efflux in cells loaded with iodide can be used to assay for activity. A disadvantage of the assay is that iodide efflux is much lower than chloride efflux due to the larger size of the iodide ion. The first step is to generate a cell line expressing a CFTR processing mutant. Since the assay requires many washing steps of cells attached to the plates, a more adherent cell line than HEK 293 cells is required. We describe an approach to measure iodide efflux in stable Chinese hamster ovary (CHO) cells or baby hamster kidney (BHK) cells. Transfections are carried out using the calcium phosphate precipitation method as described above for HEK 293 cells. The main differences are that cells must be released from the plates using tissue culture grade trypsin in PBS and cytotoxic drugs are used to select transfected cells:

1. In one approach, stable CHO cell lines can be generated using the Flp-In system. Wild-type or F508del-CFTR cDNAs are cloned into pcDNA5-FRT vectors. Subconfluent CHO cells (maintained on F-12 media (Invitrogen)) on a 10-cm^2 tissue culture plate are co-transfected with 0.005 mg/ml of the plasmid containing CFTR cDNA with POGO DNA at a 1:9 ratio. The next day, the media is replaced with fresh F-12 media. After 2 days, the cells are trypsinized and transferred to five 10-cm^2 tissue culture plates in media containing 0.6 mg/ml hygromycin. The media is changed every 2–3 days to remove dead cells. Colonies will appear after about a week. The colonies should be large enough to isolate (about 2 weeks) after transfection. Aspirate the media and then pick the colonies using about 0.02 ml of media in a pipettor. Transfer about half the cells to one well of a 24-well plate and the remainder to a second well of another 24-well plate. Cells are maintained in the presence of 0.6 mg/ml hygromycin in F-12 media. One 24-well plate will be used to check for expression of CFTR using immunoblot analysis of whole-cell extracts. A similar approach can be used to prepare stable cell lines of BHK cells expressing CFTR. For BHK cells, the vector and media are the same as described for HEK 293 cells. BHK cells are co-transfected with the CFTR plasmid and vector containing the neomycin resistance gene (such as pWL-neo) at a 1:9 ratio (*see* **Note 18**). The next day, media is changed to plain media. The following day, media is added that contains 1 mg/ml G418. Colonies are selected after 7–10 days and CFTR-expressing clones identified and expanded as described above.
2. For iodide efflux measurements, stable lines expressing wild-type CFTR, F508del-CFTR, or control cells that do not express CFTR are used. Each stable line is plated in duplicate on six-well plates to allow measurements to be carried out in triplicate. One set of plates will be treated with plain media and the other set treated with correctors. In our hands, the most efficient correctors are a combination of 0.05 mM VX-325 plus 0.015 mM corr-4a. Cells are grown to about 75% confluency, correctors are added, and iodide efflux measurements are performed 24–48 h later.
3. Media is aspirated from the cells. The cells are then washed three times with loading buffer.
4. Cells are then loaded with NaI by incubation at room temperature with 2 ml of loading buffer for 1 h in the dark.
5. Cells are then washed 13 times at 1 min intervals with 0.5 ml of efflux buffer. Solutions from the first 10 washes

are discarded. The last three washes are collected and used to create a pre-stimulation baseline.

6. Stimulation buffer is then added to the cells and removed at 1 min intervals for 12 min. The removed solutions are collected and stored in the dark until all samples have been collected.
7. When all samples have been collected, the relative voltages are measured using an iodide-specific electrode. Standard iodide curves are generated using different concentrations of NaI in efflux buffer.

4. Notes

1. The proper name for the cells is 293 cells. Although many laboratories use these cells for transfection studies, all are not morphologically similar. The reason is unknown. It may be that with prolonged passage, the cells may have altered characteristics because of their embryonic nature. Therefore, it is important to grow and freeze many vials of cells as stock from the initial cell stock. Usually after about a year of continuous passage, transfection efficiency decreases. Then one will need to start a fresh vial of cells for transfection.
2. It is important that the pH is exact. Even the smallest deviation from this will adversely affect the level of expression.
3. Some lots of serum contain considerable levels of precipitate. The precipitate will reduce the transfection efficiency, so it should be removed by filtering the media used for transfection.
4. Expression is best if the cells are actively growing and very poor if the cells are 100% confluent.
5. HEK 293 cells are unlike other cells (e.g., COS-1 cells) because they do not attach very well to the bottom of the flask. Therefore, one has to be gentle when moving the cells from the incubator to the culture hood. An advantage is that trypsin is not required to dislodge the cells from the bottom of the flask.
6. A 5% CO_2 incubator can also be used if a 2.5% CO_2 incubator is unavailable.
7. At the higher concentrations, some hydrophobic correctors will precipitate when mixed with the media. It is still worthwhile to add these mixtures to the cells. Alternatively,

one could titrate the drug concentration that will remain in solution.

8. Many compounds are cytotoxic and will cause some cells to detach from the bottom of the plate. These floating cells should be harvested because they may contain mutant CFTR that has been rescued by correctors.
9. Metal-dependent proteases seem to be present in HEK 293 cells that are resistant to SDS (Loo and Clarke, unpublished observations). The presence of EDTA protects CFTR from degradation after solubilization of whole cells.
10. The whole-cell SDS extract is often too viscous to load onto the SDS gels because of the presence of genomic DNA. If this is the case, then pass the entire sample through a Qiagen miniprep plasmid DNA isolation column. Load the extract onto the spin column and centrifuge at 14,000 × *g* for 1 min at room temperature. Load the pass-through material onto the gel.
11. This step is essential as it removes residual media containing cold methionine and cystine that if left will interfere with the efficiency of labeling.
12. Do not boil the sample! Membrane proteins, unlike the soluble proteins, will irreversibly aggregate upon heating. Once aggregation has occurred, nothing can be done to repair the damage. The whole experiment will have to be repeated.
13. Do not break the vacuum until the gel is dry. SDS gels will crack into many pieces if drying is interrupted.
14. Develop the film after 12–16 h exposure. In a good labeling experiment, a strong signal is easily present and you can decide whether to get a more or less intense signal by varying the exposure time. If signal is barely visible, then be prepared to repeat the experiment. A poor transfection (low expression) will also affect the intensity of signal obtained.
15. An alternative method for labeling cell surface proteins is to use NHS–biotin (Pierce) that labels amino groups.
16. If HEK 293 cells detach too easily, then transfect COS-1 cells.
17. Cross-linking causes CFTR to migrate slower on SDS-PAGE gels.
18. The pcDNA3 vector already contains a neomycin resistance gene, so co-transfection is not necessary. Some of our CFTR cDNAs have been cloned into the pMT21 vector that does not contain a neomycin resistance gene, so co-transfection must be performed with PWL-neo.

Acknowledgments

This work was supported by funds from the Canadian Institutes for Health Research (Grant 62832) and the Cystic Fibrosis Foundation (Grant CLARKE08GO).

References

1. Riordan, J. R., Rommens, J. M., Kerem, B., Alon, N., Rozmahel, R., Grzelczak, Z. et al. (1989) Identification of the cystic fibrosis gene: cloning and characterization of complementary DNA. *Science* **245**, 1066–1073.
2. Welsh, M. J., and Smith, A. E. (1993) Molecular mechanisms of CFTR chloride channel dysfunction in cystic fibrosis. *Cell* **73**, 1251–1254.
3. Loo, T. W., and Clarke, D. M. (1997) Correction of defective protein kinesis of human P-glycoprotein mutants by substrates and modulators. *J. Biol. Chem.* **272**, 709–712.
4. Loo, T. W., Bartlett, M. C., and Clarke, D. M. (2005) Rescue of ΔF508 and other misprocessed CFTR mutants by a novel quinazoline compound. *Mol. Pharm.* **2**, 407–413.
5. Van Goor, F., Straley, K. S., Cao, D., Gonzalez, J., Hadida, S., Hazlewood, A., et al. (2006) Rescue of ΔF508 CFTR trafficking and gating in human cystic fibrosis airway primary cultures by small molecules. *Am. J. Physiol. Lung Cell Mol. Physiol.* **290**, L1117–L1130.
6. Pedemonte, N., Lukacs, G. L., Du, K., Caci, E., Zegarra-Moran, O., Galietta, L. J., et al. (2005) Small-molecule correctors of defective DeltaF508-CFTR cellular processing identified by high-throughput screening. *J. Clin. Invest.* **115**, 2564–2571.
7. Carlile, G. W., Robert, R., Zhang, D., Teske, K. A., Luo, Y., Hanrahan, J. W. et al. (2007) Correctors of protein trafficking defects identified by a novel high-throughput screening assay. *Chembiochem* **8**, 1012–1020.
8. Loo, T. W., and Clarke, D. M. (2005) Rescue of folding defects in ABC transporters using pharmacological chaperones. *J. Bioenerg. Biomembr.* **37**, 501–507.
9. Chen, E. Y., Bartlett, M. C., and Clarke, D. M. (2000) Cystic fibrosis transmembrane conductance regulator has an altered structure when its maturation is inhibited. *Biochemistry* **39**, 3797–3803.
10. Du, K., Sharma, M., and Lukacs, G. L. (2005) The ΔF508 cystic fibrosis mutation impairs domain-domain interactions and arrests post-translational folding of CFTR. *Nat. Struct. Mol. Biol.* **12**, 17–25.
11. Loo, T. W., Bartlett, M. C., and Clarke, D. M. (2009) Correctors enhance maturation of DeltaF508 CFTR by promoting interactions between the two halves of the molecule. *Biochemistry* **48**, 9882–9890.
12. Chen, E. Y., Bartlett, M. C., Loo, T. W., and Clarke, D. M. (2004) The ΔF508 mutation disrupts packing of the transmembrane segments of the cystic fibrosis transmembrane conductance regulator. *J. Biol. Chem.* **279**, 39620–39627.
13. Chen, C., and Okayama, H. (1987) High-efficiency transformation of mammalian cells by plasmid DNA. *Mol. Cell Biol.* **7**, 2745–2752.
14. Loo, T. W., and Clarke, D. M. (1994) Reconstitution of drug-stimulated ATPase activity following co-expression of each half of human P-glycoprotein as separate polypeptides. *J. Biol. Chem.* **269**, 7750–7755.
15. Loo, T. W., Bartlett, M. C., and Clarke, D. M. (2008) Correctors promote folding of the CFTR in the endoplasmic reticulum. *Biochem. J.* **413**, 29–36.
16. Mense, M., Vergani, P., White, D. M., Altberg, G., Nairn, A. C., and Gadsby, D. C. (2006) In vivo phosphorylation of CFTR promotes formation of a nucleotide-binding domain heterodimer. *EMBO. J.* **25**, 4728–4739.
17. Wang, Y., Loo, T. W., Bartlett, M. C., and Clarke, D. M. (2007) Correctors promote maturation of cystic fibrosis transmembrane conductance regulator (CFTR)-processing mutants by binding to the protein. *J. Biol. Chem.* **282**, 33247–33251.
18. Loo, T. W., Bartlett, M. C., and Clarke, D. M. (2008) Processing mutations disrupt interactions between the nucleotide binding and transmembrane domains of P-glycoprotein and the cystic fibrosis transmembrane conductance regulator (CFTR). *J. Biol. Chem.* **283**, 28190–28197.

Chapter 4

Use of Primary Cultures of Human Bronchial Epithelial Cells Isolated from Cystic Fibrosis Patients for the Pre-clinical Testing of CFTR Modulators

Timothy Neuberger, Bill Burton, Heather Clark, and Fredrick Van Goor

Abstract

The use of human bronchial epithelial (HBE) cell cultures derived from the bronchi of CF patients offers the opportunity to study the effects of CFTR correctors and potentiators on CFTR function and epithelial cell biology in the native pathological environment. Cultured HBE cells derived from CF patients exhibit many of the morphological and functional characteristics believed to be associated with CF airway disease in vivo, including abnormal ion and fluid transport leading to dehydration of the airway surface and the loss of cilia beating. In addition, they can be generated in sufficient quantities to support routine lab testing of compound potency and efficacy and retain reproducible levels of CFTR function over time. Here we describe the development and validation of the CF HBE pharmacology model and its use to characterize, optimize, and select clinical candidates. It is expected that the pre-clinical testing of CFTR potentiators and correctors using epithelial cell cultures derived from CF patients will help to increase their likelihood of clinical efficacy.

Key words: Cystic fibrosis transmembrane conductance regulator, CFTR potentiators, CFTR correctors, Transepithelia current, Airway surface liquid, Cilia beat frequency.

1. Introduction

Cystic fibrosis (CF) is a fatal genetic disease caused by mutations on both alleles in the gene encoding the CF transmembrane conductance regulator (CFTR) (1, 2), a PKA-activated epithelial Cl^- channel involved in salt and fluid transport in multiple organs (3–6). Disease-causing *CFTR* mutations result in a loss of CFTR-mediated Cl^- secretion by causing a reduction in the number of CFTR channels at the cell surface or by impairing the ability of the

M.D. Amaral, K. Kunzelmann (eds.), *Cystic Fibrosis*, Methods in Molecular Biology 741,
DOI 10.1007/978-1-61779-117-8_4, © Springer Science+Business Media, LLC 2011

channel to open or conduct anions (7). A therapeutic strategy to treat CF is to develop drugs that target these underlying defects in CFTR protein function, resulting in enhanced ion transport (8–11). Such drugs are known as CFTR modulators and can be grouped into two classes based on their mode of action. CFTR modulators that increase the cellular processing and delivery of CFTR proteins, such as F508del-CFTR, to the cell surface are called CFTR correctors (9–11). The second class of CFTR modulators increase the flow of ions through activated CFTR that is present at the cell surface and are called CFTR potentiators (8).

Drug discovery efforts to identify CFTR modulators have been aided by high-throughput screening (HTS) campaigns that allow for the testing of several hundred thousand compounds (8, 10, 11). To profile compound activity on CFTR-mediated Cl^- transport and epithelial cell function in a physiologically relevant disease model, we developed methods to isolate and culture human bronchial epithelial (HBE) cells derived from CF patients. The goal was to develop methods that result in the large-scale production of isolated HBE cells and fully differentiated cultures that exhibit several of the morphological and functional defects in airway epithelia believed to contribute to the development of CF lung disease. These include the loss of CFTR-mediated Cl^- and fluid secretion, excessive epithelial Na^+ channel (ENaC)-mediated Na^+ and fluid absorption, and decreased cilia beating secondary to decreased surface fluid (2, 4, 6, 12, 13). To support lead optimization efforts over several years and because of the limited availability of CF lung tissue, it was also necessary that the methods allowed for the large-scale isolation and production of cells from a single lung. Key to achieving this goal was the development of cell expansion and dissociation methods that allowed for the freezing and storage of a large number of cells that could be later thawed and differentiated with reproducible levels of CFTR function. The ability to obtain reproducible levels of CFTR function during each thaw/differentiation cycle was critical for evaluating the structure–activity relationship throughout the multi-year lead optimization effort needed to improve the potency (effective concentration) and efficacy (magnitude of the increase in CFTR function) of the HTS hits. Here, we describe the materials and methods for the isolation, expansion and storage, and differentiation of cultured HBE cells derived from CF lung tissue to support drug discovery efforts to identify CFTR modulators.

2. Materials

1. Rinse solution: Minimum essential medium (MEM), dithiothreitol (0.5 mg/ml), DNase I (25 U/ml; Roche, Catalog # 04 536 280 001).

2. Dissociation solution: MEM, DNase (2.5 U/ml), ceftazidime (100 μg/ml), tobramycin (80 μg/ml), amphotericin B (1.25 μg/ml), pronase (Sigma, Catalog # P-6911; 4.4 U/ml).
3. Accutase^{TM} (Innovative Cell Technologies, Catalog # AT104).
4. Growth media: Bronchial epithelial growth medium (BEGM) plus all components provided in the accompanying Bullet kit (Lonza, Catalog # CC 3170). To the media, add an additional 50 μl of 100 μM all-*trans*-retinoic acid, as well as ceftazidime (100 μg/ml), tobramycin (80 μg/ml), and amphotericin B (1.25 μg/ml).
5. Differentiation media: Dulbecco's MEM (DMEM)/F12, Ultroser-G (2.0%; Pall, Catalog # 15950-017), fetal clone II (2%), insulin (2.5 μg/ml), bovine brain extract (0.25%; Lonza, Kit #CC-4133, component # CC-4092C), hydrocortisone (20 nM), triiodothyronine (500 nM), transferrin (2.5 μg/ml: Invitrogen, Catalog # 0030124SA), ethanolamine (250 nM), epinephrine (1.5 μM), phosphoethanolamine (250 nM), and retinoic acid (10 nM).
6. NIH-3T3 conditioning media: DMEM, fetal bovine serum (10%), penicillin (100 U/ml), streptomycin (100 μg/ml), non-essential amino acids (0.1 mM), Na^+ pyruvate (1 mM), and HEPES (10 mM).
7. Ussing chamber solution: 135 mM NaCl, 1.2 mM $CaCl_2$, 1.2 mM $MgCl_2$, 2.4 mM K_2HPO_4, 0.6 mM $KHPO_4$, 10 mM *N*-2-hydroxyethylpiperazine-*N'*-2-ethanesulfonic acid (HEPES), and 10 mM dextrose (pH 7.4; NaOH).
8. Low Cl^- Ussing chamber solution: 145 mM Na gluconate, 1.2 mM $CaCl_2$, 1.2 mM $MgCl_2$, 2.4 mM K_2HPO_4, 0.6 mM $KHPO_4$, 10 mM HEPES, and 10 mM dextrose (pH 7.4; NaOH).

3. Methods

3.1. Isolation of Bronchial Tube Sections from the Lung

1. Whole lungs were obtained from non-CF and CF subjects following autopsy or lung transplantation. After removal, the lung was packed in Dulbecco's phosphate buffered saline (DPBS) maintained at 4°C and processed within 24 h. All procedures were performed in a class II, biological safety cabinet and universal precautions were followed.
2. Place lungs in a tray containing DPBS (~4°C), remove the primary and secondary bronchial tubes, and clean of connective tissue by blunt dissection.

3. Cut the bronchial tubes into ~5 cm lengths and place 1–2 pieces in a 50-ml conical tube containing MEM (~4°C) until the lung dissection is complete.
4. To clean the mucus from the bronchial tubes, replace the MEM with rinse solution and place the conical tubes on a rocker plate (~40 cycles/min) in a 37°C incubator for 20 min. Repeat this step until all the mucus is removed.
5. After the last rinse cycle, replace the rinse solution with dissociation solution and rock the conical tubes (~40 cycles/min) for 36 h at 4°C.
6. Place the bronchial tubes in a 150-mm Petri dish containing MEM (~4°C). Under a dissecting microscope, cut each bronchial tube along its entire length, open, and lay flat.
7. To separate the epithelial cell layer from the underlying connective tissue, gently place a number 21 Feather scalpel above the epithelial cell layer and then draw the scalpel along the length of the tube without making contact with the epithelial cell layer (*see* **Note 1**).
8. Transfer the epithelial sheets into 15-ml conical tubes containing MEM (~4°C).

3.2. Preparation and Expansion of Dissociated Epithelial Cells

1. To disperse the epithelial sheets, replace the MEM with 14 ml of Accutase™ and incubate at 37°C for 20 min (*see* **Note 2**). To keep the sheets in suspension, invert the conical tubes at 5 min intervals.
2. Spin the conical tubes for 5 min at 500×*g* to pack the epithelial sheets. Before removing the Accutase™, note the volume of packed epithelial sheets in each 15-ml conical tube to determine the number of T75 flasks to be seeded, as described in step 4. Remove the Accutase™.
3. Resuspend and dissociate the epithelial sheets by adding 1 ml of growth medium and gently triturate ~10 times using a 1-ml pipette tip.
4. Based on the amount of packed epithelia noted in step 2, equally divide the 1 ml of dispersed cells into NIH-3T3 conditioned media coated T75 flasks (20 μl of compact epithelia/T75 flask). For example, if ~60 μl of packed epithelial sheets was noted in step 2, equally divide the 1 ml of dispersed cell solution into three T75-flasks.
5. To expand the cells, incubate the T75 flasks at 37°C (5% CO_2, 90% humidity) until the cells reach 90% confluence, replacing the growth media every 24 h (*see* **Note 3**).
6. When the cell density reaches 90% confluence, harvest the dispersed HBE cells for further expansion or cryoprotect and bank for future use (*see* **Note 4**).

3.3. Cell Harvesting for Cell Expansion or Banking of Undifferentiated HBE Cells

1. To harvest the cells, remove the growth media and add a sufficient volume of warm (~37°C) Accutase™ solution to cover the bottom of the T flask, gently swirl, and let the flasks sit at room temperature for ~4 min. The cells should remain attached to the flask.
2. Replace with fresh Accutase™ solution and incubate for 10 min at 37°C (5% CO_2; 95% humidity). The majority of cells should be detached after the 10-min incubation.
3. Collect the cells by adding an equal volume of growth media to the flask containing Accutase™ and gently swirl the flasks to dislodge any remaining attached cells.
4. Transfer the dissociated HBE cells to a 15-ml conical tube and pellet the cells by spinning at 500×*g* for 5 min. Remove the Accutase™ solution and resuspend the cell pellet in 1 ml of warm growth media by gentle trituration using a 1-ml pipette.
5. Add approximately 3 ml of BEGM to 1 ml of cell suspension and transfer the cells through a 30-μm filter into a 50-ml conical tube.
6. Count the cells to determine the cell yield using a hemocytometer. The expected cell yields for T25, T75, and T225 flasks are ~3, 6, and 12 million cells, respectively.
7. For further cell expansion, seed the HBE cells into NIH-3T3 conditioned media coated T flasks at a density of 6,667 cells/cm^2. The cells can be passed up to five times to expand the number of HBE cells available for functional studies (*see* **Note 5**). During the expansion, split the cells into new flasks when the cell density reaches 90% confluence.
8. Change the growth media every 24 h during the cell expansion (*see* **Note 6**).
9. For cryoprotection, pellet the cells by spinning at 500×*g* for 5 min and resuspend in CryoStor™ CS-10 (Biolife Solutions, Catalog # 640222) at a density of 1 million cells/ml. Place 1 ml of dispersed HBE cells into each cryovial and freeze using a cryofreezing machine before transferring to a liquid nitrogen tank for long-term storage.
10. To thaw the frozen HBE cells, place a vial in a 37°C water bath for ~2 min and then transfer the cells to NIH-3T3 conditioned media coated T flasks (6,667 cells/cm^2) and expand as described above.

3.4. Generation of Differentiated HBE Cultures

1. Coat Corning SnapWell™ inserts with NIH-3T3 conditioned media at least 24 h prior to seeding with HBE cells.
2. Harvest the cells as described above and resuspend in 3 ml of growth media.

3. Pass the cells through a 30-μm filter into a 50-ml conical tube and count using a hemocytometer. If needed, dilute with growth media to achieve a final cell density of ~1.43×10^6 cells/ml.
4. Add 350 μl of dispersed HBE cells into each six-well, 0.4-μm NIH-3T3 conditioned media coated SnapWell™ culture insert (~5×10^5 cells/insert). Add 2 ml of growth media to the bottom well and incubate for 24 h at 37°C (5% CO_2 and 90% humidity).
5. Replace the growth medium with differentiation medium on both the insert and the well and incubate at 37°C (5% CO_2, and 90% humidity) for an additional 72 h, replacing the differentiation media once at 48 h.
6. After 72 h, remove the differentiation media from the filter to establish an air–liquid interface. This will result in fully differentiated HBE cell cultures in ~14 days that exhibit the desired morphological (*see* **Note** 7), bioelectric (*see* **Note 8**), and fluid transport (*see* **Note 9**) characteristics of differentiated airway epithelia.
7. Change the media in the bottom well at least three times per week to prevent acidification, which reduces the ENaC- and CFTR-mediated currents and the response to CFTR modulators.

3.5. NIH-3T3 Conditioned T Flasks and SnapWell Culture Plates

1. NIH-3T3 cells were grown at 37°C (5% CO_2 and 95% humidity) in T225 flasks in NIH-3T3 growth medium until 100% confluence.
2. After reaching confluence, replace the medium with 50 ml of fresh NIH-3T3 growth media and incubate for 10 days at 37°C (5% CO_2 and 95% humidity). The conditioned media was collected, filtered through a 0.2-μm filter, and stored at 4°C for up to 1 month.
3. To condition the cultureware, cover the bottom of the T flasks or SnapWell™ filters with NIH-3T3 conditioned media for 12 h at 37°C. Remove the media and store at 4°C.

3.6. Ussing Chamber Recordings of Potential Difference and Transepithelial Current

1. All cells were grown on Costar® SnapWell™ cell culture inserts and maintained at 37°C.
2. Mount the cell culture inserts into an Ussing chamber (VCC MC8; Physiologic Instruments, Inc., San Diego, CA) to record transepithelial current (I_T) ($V_{hold} = 0$ mV) or the potential difference (PD) (PD = $V_{basolateral} - V_{apical}$) using Acquire and Analyze software (version 2; Physiologic Instruments, Inc., San Diego, CA).
3. For recordings of PD or fluid transport and cilia beat frequency (CBF), equimolar Cl^- solutions were added to the

basolateral and apical sides unless otherwise indicated. For recording the CFTR-mediated I_T, a basolateral-to-apical Cl^- gradient was established by replacing apical NaCl with equimolar Na^+ gluconate (*see* **Note 10**).

4. To calibrate the CFTR-mediated secretion in CF HBE cells to that observed in non-CF HBE cells, we normalized the peak forskolin-stimulated I_T in CF HBE cells to that in non-CF HBE cells and expressed it as percentage of non-CF (*see* **Note 11**).

3.7. Measurement of Fluid Transport and CBF in Cultured CF and Non-CF HBE Cells

1. All cells were grown on Costar® SnapWell™ cell culture inserts maintained at 37°C.
2. The apical surface of the HBE cells was washed two times with normal Cl^- apical solution followed by addition of 100 μL of normal Cl^- apical solution to the apical layer. To prevent evaporation, the cell plates were wrapped in a damp paper towel and placed in a modular incubation chamber (Billups-Rothenberg, Inc.; cat#MIC-101) filled with a gas mixture of 5% CO_2 and 95% air and maintained at 37°C.
3. To monitor the airway surface liquid (ASL), the fluid remaining after up to 72 h of incubation was collected from the apical surface and placed in pre-weighed 1.5-ml Eppendorf tubes.
4. The CBF was monitored as previously described (14). Briefly, the cilia beating was recorded at 43 fps using a phase-contrast AxioVert 200 microscope equipped with a 20× Zeiss Achroplan objective and a digital camera (Edmond Optics; EO-0413 Mono LE USB). Each frame was divided into six equal segments, in which three regions of interest (ROIs), measuring 3 × 3 pixels, were placed over a single beating cilium. If no cilia beating were visible, the ROI was placed next to the cell body. The mean grey level for each ROI was determined using Image-J (v.1.41o) and a Fourier transformation was used to measure the CBF.

4. Notes

1. Moving the scalpel along the length of the tube causes the fluid within the tube to swirl and is usually sufficient to dislodge the sheets of epithelial cells from the underlying connective tissue. The epithelial dissociation media contains pronase, which is a bacterial enzyme that digests extracellular matrix proteins without cleaving the intercellular adhesion proteins that hold the epithelial cells together. If done

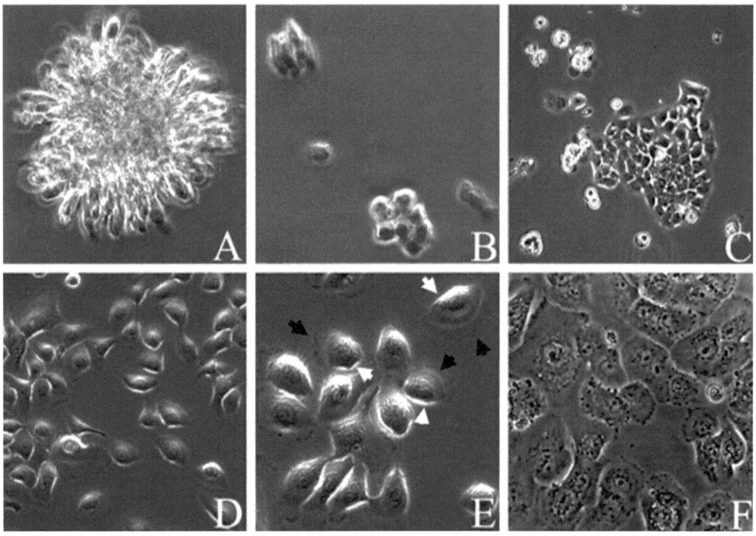

Fig. 4.1. Morphology of HBE cells at different stages during the isolation and culture. (**a**) Photomicrograph of an intact epithelial sheet separated from the bronchial tube by pronase digestion. (**b**) Morphology of the epithelial cells immediately after dispersion of the epithelial sheet and after 24 h (**c**) and 96 h (**d**) in culture as viewed using a phase-contrast microscope (20× magnification). (**e**) Higher magnification (×40 magnification) of cultured epithelial cells after 96 h in culture revealed a mature, undifferentiated morphology that is characterized by a smooth, phase bright edge (*white arrows*), and a ruffled edge (*black arrows*). (**f**) Granulated HBE cell morphology after 96 h in cell culture where the media was not replaced every 24 h.

properly, the epithelial cell layer can be dislodged from the underlying connective tissue as large intact sheets of cells (**Fig. 4.1a**). If the extracellular matrix is not sufficiently digested, it may be necessary to bring the scalpel in contact with the epithelial cell layer as it is drawn across the length of the tube. However, contact between the scalpel and the cell layer should be minimized so as not to dislodge the underlying connective tissue which contains fibroblasts. Viable epithelial sheets should contain columnar cells with beating cilia. If not, discard.

2. The proper combination of Accutase™ treatment and trituration will yield a mixture of single cells and small aggregates of cells (**Fig. 4.1b**). Immediately after dissociation, the majority of cells should appear to be phase bright and the columnar cells should still display rapidly beating cilia, indicating good cell viability. If these features are not observed, the incubation time in Accutase™ and/or the amount of trituration should be decreased. If the majority of the epithelial cells remain as large, multi-cell aggregates, the incubation time in Accutase™ and the amount of trituration should be increased.

3. Twenty-four hours after epithelial cell dissociation from the epithelial sheets, ~75% of the cells should be attached and a mixture of single cells and small islands of epithelial cells, some of which will have beating cilia, should be observed (**Fig. 4.1c**). The beating cilia, however, will disappear over the next several days. A small number of fibroblasts may also be present, but should die off during subsequent passing and expansion. After 96 h, monolayers of cells should be formed and the cells should acquire a mature, undifferentiated morphology characterized by a smooth, phase bright surface on one side and a ruffled surface on the other side (**Fig. 4.1d**, **e**).
4. If the cells during the initial isolation or subsequent expansion are allowed to grow beyond 90% confluence, we have observed that they do not provide differentiated HBE cell cultures with the desired morphology and functional properties.
5. Additional passages allow for the generation of large quantities of cells that can be banked or plated into six-well SnapWell™ plates for functional analysis. We have found that the desired morphological and functional characteristics are maintained for up to five passages.
6. We have found that exchanging the HBE cell growth media every 24 h is critical to maintain the desired epithelial cell morphology during cell expansion. As long as this feeding schedule is maintained, HBE cells remain as isolated cells. If the media is not exchanged every 24 h, the HBE cells become granulated and begin to migrate toward each other to form cell aggregates (**Fig. 4.1f**). Once this cell morphology has been obtained, we are unable to obtain differentiated cells with the desired morphology and function.
7. Differentiated HBE cells should appear as a uniform monolayer consisting of ciliated columnar epithelial cells and goblet cells (**Fig. 4.2a**). Transmission electron microscopy confirmed the presence of ciliated columnar cells throughout the differentiated non-CF HBE (**Fig. 4.2b**, **c**) and F508del-HBE (**Fig. 4.2d**) cultures. Unlike the non-CF HBE cultures, a thick electron-dense mucin layer that compressed the underlying cilia was observed in cultured F508del-HBE cells (**Fig. 4.2d** vs. **c**). This is consistent with the accumulation of the thick sticky mucus and reduced ciliary movement that is characteristic of the CF lung (12, 13, 15). Interspersed among the ciliated columnar cells were mucin-secreting goblet cells, identified by their secretory granules. Brush cells identified by microvilli-like projections extending into the apical space and numerous basal

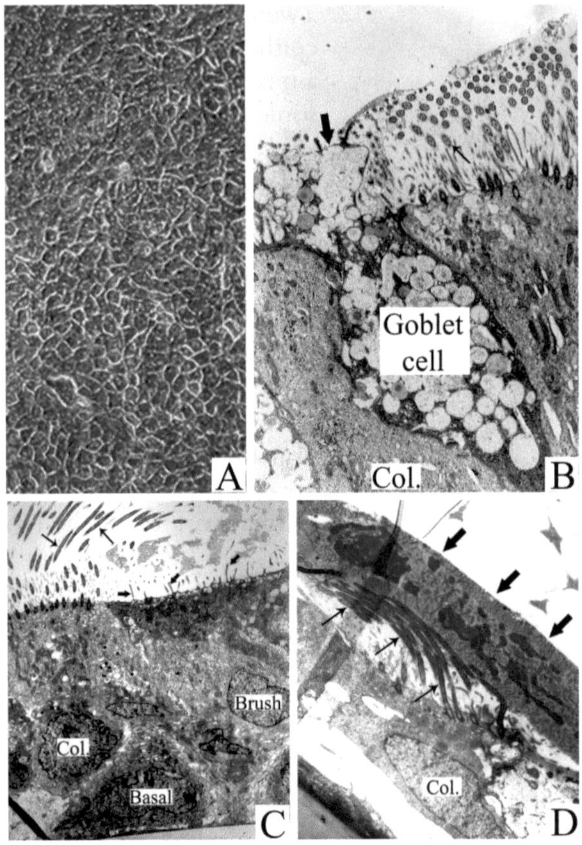

Fig. 4.2. Morphology of differentiated non-CF HBE and F508del-HBE cells. (**a**) Phase-contrast photomicrograph of differentiated non-CF HBE cells cultured for 14 days under an air–liquid interface. Transmission electron photomicrographs of differentiated non-CF HBE (**b, c**) and F508del-HBE cultures (**d**) fixed with Karnovsky's fixative and stained with osium tetroxide and uranyl acetate to increase electron density. (**b**) Goblet cells releasing mucin (*thick arrow*) onto the apical surface and columnar epithelial cells (*Col.*) with numerous cilia (*thin arrows*) projecting into the mucin layer. (**c**) Basal cells localized to the basal surface and brush cells with microvilli (*thick arrows*) were also observed. (**d**) Differentiated HBE cultures derived from F508del-HBE cells appeared similar to non-CF HBE cultures except for the thick electron-dense mucin layer (*thick arrows*) which compressed the cilia (*thin arrows*).

cells located on the basolateral surface were also present. These four cell types produced the characteristic pseudostratified columnar epithelium typical of human airway tissue (16).

8. The methods described herein produced cultured F508del-HBE cells that exhibit several of the ion transport defects in airway epithelia that are believed to contribute to the development of CF lung disease (4, 6, 17). As observed in in vivo recordings of the nasal potential difference in CF patients (17), the in vitro baseline potential difference (PD) was elevated and the amiloride response was

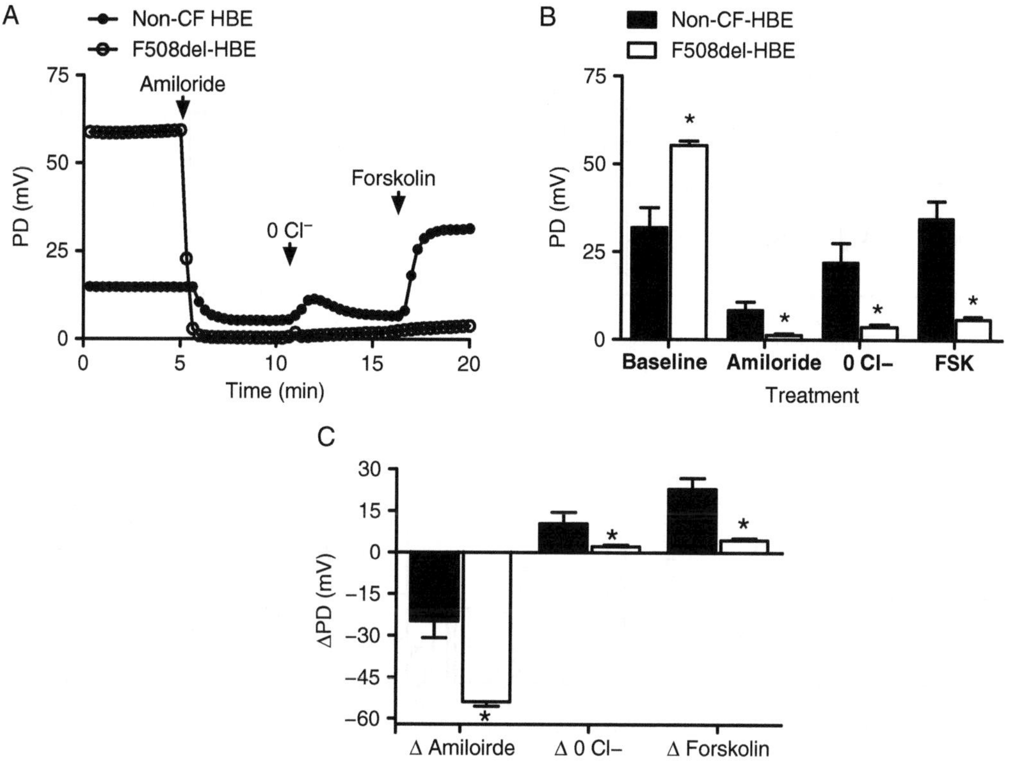

Fig. 4.3. Potential difference (PD) in cultured non-CF HBE and F508del-HBE cells recorded using Ussing chamber techniques. (**a**) Representative recording of the PD in non-CF HBE cells (*filled circles*) and F508del-HBE cells (*open circles*). (**b**) Quantification of the data shown in (**a**) (mean ± SEM; $n = 12$). (**c**) Net change in PD to amiloride, 0 Cl^-, and forskolin additions (mean ± SEM; $n = 12$). *Asterisks* indicate significant difference compared to non-CF HBE cells (two-way ANOVA followed by Bonferroni post test).

larger in cultured F508del-HBE cells compared to non-CF HBE cells (**Fig. 4.3**). In addition, the response to 0 Cl^- and the cAMP agonist, forskolin, was markedly reduced in F508del-HBE cells (**Fig. 4.3**). Similarly, transepithelial current (I_T) measurements showed that there is a marked reduction in the CFTR-mediated I_T in cultured F508del-HBE cells compared to non-CF HBE cells (**Fig. 4.4**). In non-CF HBE cells isolated from four separate individuals, the I_T response to a maximally effective forskolin concentration (10 μM; $EC_{50} = 13 \pm 1$ nM: $n = 3$) reached a peak amplitude of 56 ± 6 μA/cm^2 and then declined to a steady-state level of 35 ± 4 μA/cm^2 (**Fig. 4.4a–c**). In cultured F508del-HBE cells isolated from the bronchi of 10 F508del homozygous CF patients, addition of 10 μM forskolin resulted in small increase in the I_T compared to that measured in non-CF HBE cells (**Fig. 4.4d–f**). The forskolin-stimulated I_T was not blocked by prior addition of the Ca^{2+}-activated Cl^- channel blocker,

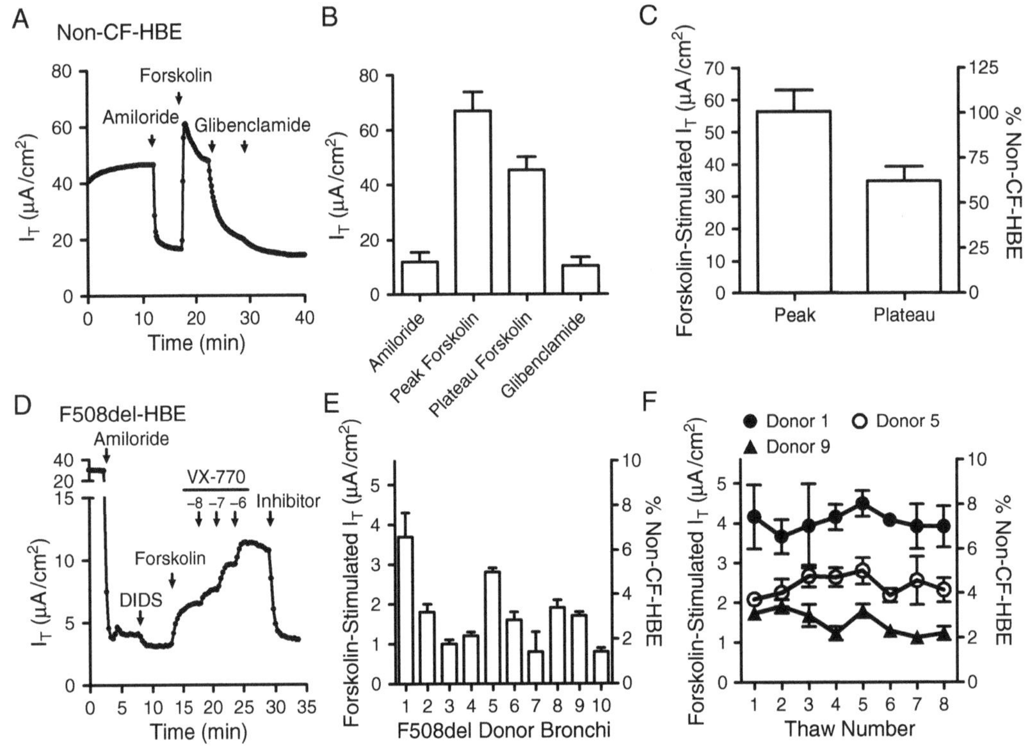

Fig. 4.4. CFTR-mediated I_T in cultured non-CF HBE and F508del-HBE cells recorded using Ussing chamber techniques. To isolate the CFTR-mediated I_T, 30 μM amiloride was added to the apical membrane to block ENaC, a basolateral-to-apical Cl^- gradient was established, and forskolin was added to activate CFTR. (**a**) Representative I_T trace from non-CF HBE cells. (**b**) Quantification of the data shown in A (mean ± SEM; $n = 20$; combined data from four donor lungs). (**c**) Change from the baseline I_T in the presence of amiloride to the peak or plateau level in the presence of forskolin (forskolin-stimulated I_T). (**d**) Representative I_T trace from F508del-HBE cells. (**e**) Forskolin-stimulated I_T in cultured F508del-HBE cells isolated from 10 CF patients maintained at 37°C prior to recording. (**f**) Forskolin-stimulated I_T in differentiated F508del-HBE cells prepared from different thaws of frozen cells isolated from three separate donor lungs. The *right* y-axis represents the forskolin-stimulated I_T normalized to peak forskolin-stimulated I_T in cultured non-CF HBE cells isolated from four individuals and expressed as percentage of non-CF HBE cells.

4,4′-diisothiocyanostilbene-2,2′-disulfonic acid (DIDS), was increased by acute addition of the investigational CFTR potentiator, VX-770 (8), and was abolished by the addition of glibenclamide (**Fig. 4.4d**). These data indicate that the forskolin-stimulated I_T is due to a small amount of F508del-CFTR that is able to exit the ER and traffic to cell surface. The level of residual F508del-CFTR function appeared to be different in HBE cells isolated from the different donor bronchi and remained stable after several thaw/culture cycles (**Fig. 4.4e, f**). This suggests that the methods outlined here led to stable and reproducible levels of CFTR activity in F508del-HBE cells from each individual donor.

9. In the CF lung, the decrease in CFTR-mediated Cl^- and fluid secretion and the associated increase in ENaC-mediated Na^+ and fluid absorption are believed to cause the dehydration of the airway surface (12). This likely contributes to the inability of the cilia to extend and beat normally, preventing them from supplying the motive force for mucus transport that is important in clearing infection-causing microbes from the airway. Compared to cultured non-CF HBE cells, the ASL volume was markedly reduced (**Fig. 4.5a**), consistent with a decrease in CFTR-driven fluid secretion and an increase in ENaC-driven fluid absorption (12). The dehydration of the ASL in the F508del-HBE cultures was accompanied by a decrease in the CBF compared to non-CF HBE cultures (**Fig. 4.5b, c**).

10. The use of Ultroser-G in the differentiation media significantly increased the amplitude of ENaC-mediated and CFTR-mediated I_T (**Fig. 4.6a–c**). The use of a basolateral-

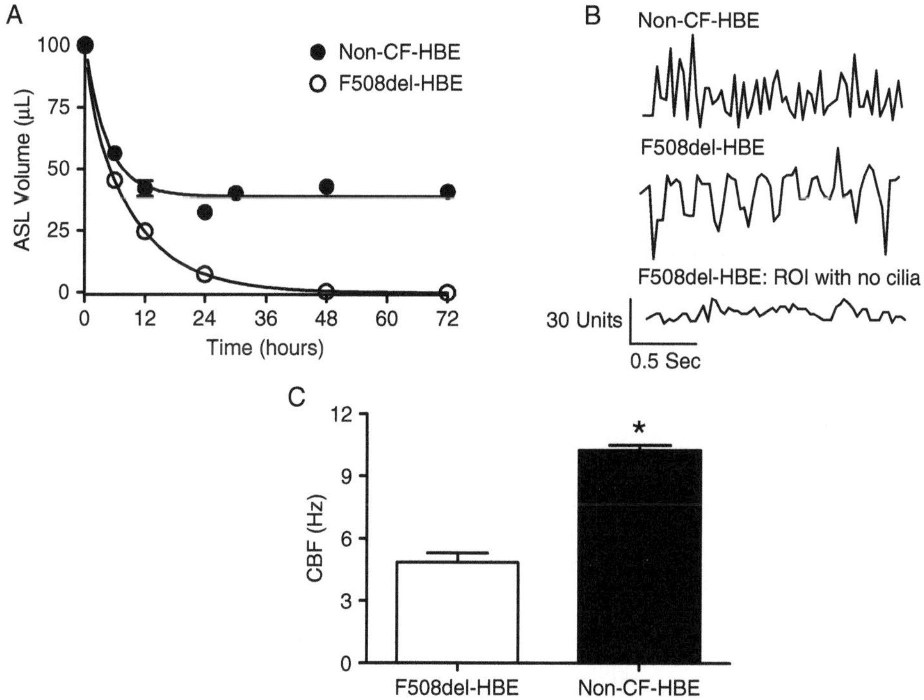

Fig. 4.5. Fluid transport and CBF in cultured non-CF HBE and F508del-HBE cells. (**a**) The ASL volume in cultured non-CF HBE (*filled circles*) and F508del-HBE cells (*open circles*) after up to 72 h incubation at 37°C in the presence of 30 nM VIP added to the basolateral surface. (**b**) Representative tracings of the light intensity (*y*-axis in relative units) derived from a single region of interest (ROI) containing cilia in cultured non-CF HBE and F508del-HBE cells monitored 72 h after adding 100 μl of fluid to the apical surface. An ROI in F508del-HBE cells without cilia is also shown. (**c**) Quantification of the data in B (mean ± SEM; $n = 4$). *Single asterisk* indicates significant difference ($p < 0.05$: paired *t*-test) compared to non-CF HBE cells.

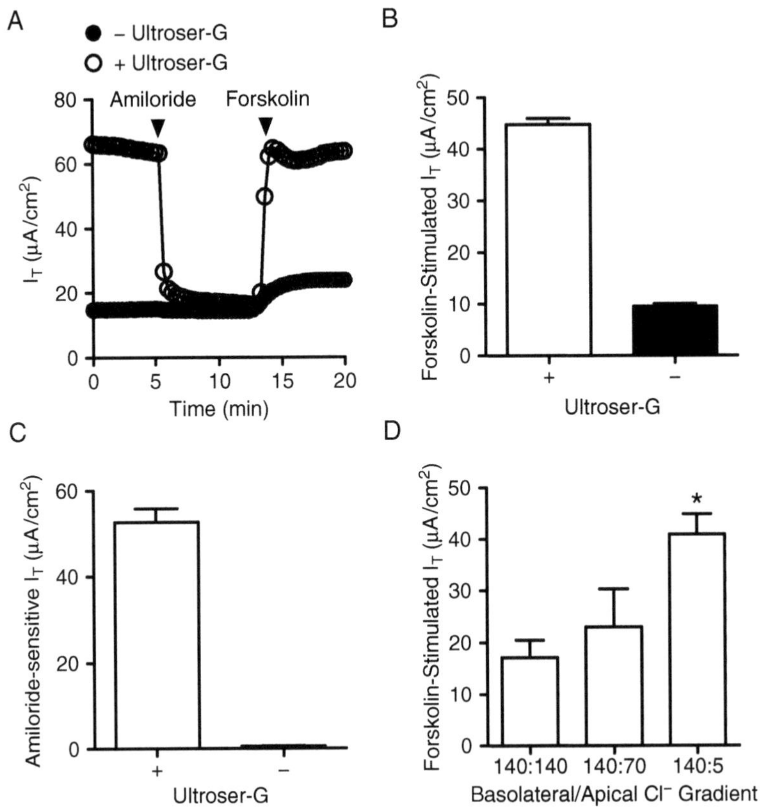

Fig. 4.6. Ultroser-G and a basolateral-to-apical Cl^- gradient increase the magnitude of the CFTR-mediated I_T. (**a**) Representative I_T trace in cultured non-CF HBE cells prepared with (*open circles*) or without (*Filled circles*) Ultroser-G in the differentiation media. Quantification (mean ± SEM; $n = 6$) of the data in (**a**) showing the forskolin-stimulated (**b**) and the amiloride-sensitive I_T (**c**). (**d**) Forskolin-stimulated I_T in non-CF HBE cells with 140 mM Cl^- on the basolateral surface and 140, 70, or 5 mM Cl^- on the apical surface. *Single asterisk* indicates significantly different ($p < 0.05$) equimolar Cl^- on both sides.

to-apical Cl^- gradient in the Ussing chamber recordings also increased the magnitude of the CFTR-mediated I_T (**Fig. 4.6d**). These conditions improved the assay window which in turn facilitated the assessment of the structure–activity relationship during lead optimization efforts.

11. To compare the level of cAMP/PKA-stimulated CFTR function in vivo with that observed in cultured CF HBE cells, the forskolin-stimulated I_T in cultured F508del-HBE cells was normalized to the peak forskolin-stimulated I_T in non-CF HBE cells isolated from four separate individuals (56 ± 6 μA/cm²). In cultured F508del-HBE cells isolated from 10 different donor bronchi, the level of residual CFTR function ranged from 0.8 to 3.7% μA/cm², or 1.4–6.6% of non-CF HBE cells with a mean of 3 ± 1% non-CF HBE cells. The low level of forskolin-stimulated CFTR

function in all 10 F508del-HBE cells is consistent with the low CFTR function and severe CF disease observed in F508del homozygous individuals (18). This method of normalization does not account for the low basal "cAMP tone" on CFTR-mediated Cl^- secretion, which can be quantified by the application of a CFTR inhibitor in the absence of forskolin. For example, in non-CF HBE cells, glibenclamide reduced the I_T in the absence of forskolin by 5 ± 2 μA/cm2, which is consistent with a low basal "cAMP tone" on CFTR-mediated Cl^- secretion (19).

References

1. Kerem, B., Rommens, J. M., Buchanan, J. A., Markiewicz, D., Cox, T. K., Chakravarti, A. et al. (1989) Identification of the cystic fibrosis gene: genetic analysis. *Science* **245**, 1073–1080.
2. Riordan, J. R., Rommens, J. M., Kerem, B., Alon, N., Rozmahel, R., Grzelczak, Z. et al. (1989) Identification of the cystic fibrosis gene: cloning and characterization of complementary DNA. *Science* **245**, 1066–1073.
3. Berger, H. A., Anderson, M. P., Gregory, R. J., Thompson, S., Howard, P. W., Maurer, R. A. et al. (1991) Identification and regulation of the cystic fibrosis transmembrane conductance regulator-generated chloride channel. *J. Clin. Invest.* **88**, 1422–1431.
4. Knowles, M., Gatzy, J., and Boucher, R. (1983) Relative ion permeability of normal and cystic fibrosis nasal epithelium. *J. Clin. Invest.* **71**, 1410–1417.
5. Li, C., Ramjeesingh, M., Wang, W., Garami, E., Hewryk, M., Lee, D. et al. (1996) ATPase activity of the cystic fibrosis transmembrane conductance regulator. *J. Biol. Chem.* **271**, 28463–28468.
6. Quinton, P. M. (1983) Chloride impermeability in cystic fibrosis. *Nature* **301**, 421–422.
7. Welsh, M. J., and Smith, A. E. (1993) Molecular mechanisms of CFTR chloride channel dysfunction in cystic fibrosis. *Cell* **73**, 1251–1254.
8. Van Goor, F., Hadida, S., Grootenhuis, P. D., Burton, B., Cao, D., Neuberger, T. et al. (2009) Rescue of CF airway epithelial cell function in vitro by a CFTR potentiator, VX-770. *Proc. Natl. Acad. Sci. USA* **106**, 18825–18830.
9. Van Goor, F., Hadida, S., and Grootenhuis, P. D. J. (2008) Pharmacological Rescue of mutant CFTR function for the treatment of cystic fibrosis. *Top. Medic. Chem.* **3**, 29.
10. Van Goor, F., Straley, K. S., Cao, D., Gonzalez, J., Hadida, S., Hazlewood, A. et al. (2006) Rescue of DeltaF508-CFTR trafficking and gating in human cystic fibrosis airway primary cultures by small molecules. *Am. J. Physiol. Lung Cell. Mol. Physiol.* **290**, L1117–1130.
11. Pedemonte, N., Lukacs, G. L., Du, K., Caci, E., Zegarra-Moran, O., Galietta, L. J. et al. (2005) Small-molecule correctors of defective DeltaF508-CFTR cellular processing identified by high-throughput screening. *J. Clin. Invest.* **115**, 2564–2571.
12. Boucher, R. C. (2007) Cystic fibrosis: a disease of vulnerability to airway surface dehydration. *Trends Mol. Med.* **13**, 231–240.
13. Jiang, C., Finkbeiner, W. E., Widdicombe, J. H., McCray, P. B., Jr., and Miller, S. S. (1993) Altered fluid transport across airway epithelium in cystic fibrosis. *Science* **262**, 424–427.
14. Sisson, J. H., Stoner, J. A., Ammons, B. A., and Wyatt, T. A. (2003) All-digital image capture and whole-field analysis of ciliary beat frequency. *J. Microsc.* **211**, 103–111.
15. Gibson, R. L., Burns, J. L., and Ramsey, B. W. (2003) Pathophysiology and management of pulmonary infections in cystic fibrosis. *Am. J. Respir. Crit. Care Med.* **168**, 918–951.
16. Souma, T. (1987) The distribution and surface ultrastructure of airway epithelial cells in the rat lung: a scanning electron microscopic study. *Arch. Histol. Jpn.* **50**, 419–436.
17. Knowles, M. R., Paradiso, A. M., and Boucher, R. C. (1995) In vivo nasal potential difference: techniques and protocols for assessing efficacy of gene transfer in cystic fibrosis. *Hum. Gene Ther.* **6**, 445–455.
18. Ahrens, R. C., Standaert, T. A., Launspach, J., Han, S. H., Teresi, M. E., Aitken, M. L. et al. (2002) Use of nasal potential difference and sweat chloride as outcome measures in

multicenter clinical trials in subjects with cystic fibrosis. *Pediatr. Pulmonol.* **33**, 142–150.

19. Blouquit, S., Sari, A., Lombet, A., D'Herbomez, M., Naline, E., Matran, R. et al. (2003) Effects of endothelin-1 on epithelial ion transport in human airways. *Am. J. Respir. Cell. Mol. Biol.* **29**, 245–251.

Chapter 5

Design of Gene Therapy Trials in CF Patients

Jane C. Davies and Eric W.F.W. Alton

Abstract

The report of the first CF patients to receive *CFTR* gene therapy appeared in 1993; since then, there have been over 20 clinical trials of both viral and non-viral gene transfer agents. These have largely been single dose to either nose or lower airway and have been designed around molecular or bioelectrical outcome measures. Both transgene mRNA and partial correction of chloride secretion have been reported, although sodium hyperabsorption has not been improved. The UK CF Gene Therapy Consortium is focussed on a clinical programme to establish whether these proof-of-principle measures translate into clinical benefit. Here, we discuss the considerations in designing such a programme, focusing in particular on our choice of the optimal, currently available delivery method and established and novel outcome measures. We highlight the logistic and regulatory complexities of such a clinical programme and finally, we look to the future and consider possible alternative strategies.

Key words: CFTR, clinical trial, gene delivery, gene transfer, outcome measures, vector.

1. Introduction

Gene therapy for CF has been a focus of research and clinical trial interest for the last two decades. Despite this, clinical benefit has not yet been demonstrated and emphasis has decreased worldwide of late, related, at least in part, to some of the major challenges encountered. Almost two-thirds of clinical trials have utilised viral vectors with the remainder using a variety of synthetic agents, most commonly lipid based. Most have been single dose, focussing on proof-of-principle outcome measures: both molecular evidence of gene expression and functional correction based on bioelectrical measures have been demonstrated but to variable levels. Side effects, where observed, have been generally mild.

M.D. Amaral, K. Kunzelmann (eds.), *Cystic Fibrosis*, Methods in Molecular Biology 741,
DOI 10.1007/978-1-61779-117-8_5,

Unlike many of the topics covered in this book, there are no agreed protocols for the design of such trials; indeed the design needs to be individually tailored to the gene transfer agent being studied and the phase of the study. In this chapter, we aim therefore to review the field, identify the outstanding questions relating to *CFTR* gene therapy, summarise the design and results of the clinical trials performed to date, and look to the future on the basis of our work within the UK CF Gene Therapy Consortium.

2. Outstanding Basic Questions

2.1. Which Cells to Transfect?

Maximal CFTR expression in non-CF airways appears to be in the submucosal glands (1, 2), and in the surface epithelium of the distal small airways. It is in this latter site that clinically detectable disease begins. Topical application, for example via inhalation, is likely to target the surface epithelium but is less likely to reach the deeper submucosal gland cells. Whether or not gene transfer to these cells will be necessary for clinical effect remains to be determined. Furthermore, the surface epithelium is terminally differentiated, although its lifespan may be significantly longer than originally thought (3). Although there is increasing understanding of the stem cell populations at various levels throughout the airway, methods to target these cells, which are usually not accessible directly on the airway surface, and to achieve long-term expression have yet to be identified.

2.2. What Degree of Correction Will Be Required for Clinical Benefit?

Different levels of expression are likely to be required to restore the various functions of CFTR. For example, at least in vitro lower numbers of cells (approximately 5%) need to be corrected to restore chloride transport than those required for normalisation of sodium absorption (4), and differences have also been observed with regard to the correction of glycoconjugate sulphation and ion transport (5). Which function(s) of CFTR are most important for respiratory health and whether all identified functions (and perhaps as yet unrecognised ones) need to be corrected to prevent disease initiation/progression are important questions, which remain to be resolved. Based on genetic studies, it would seem that as little as 5–10% of wild-type levels of CFTR in each cell may be sufficient for a normal disease-free phenotype (6). A recent study has demonstrated that restoration of mucus transport could be achieved when 25% of cells in a cultured monolayer were transfected with parainfluenza virus-mediated CFTR (7).

2.3. How to Achieve Long-Term Expression?

As a chronic, lifelong disease, CF will be best treated with a continuous level of CFTR expression; this could be achieved either by repeated application or with a long-duration expression system. As discussed further below, viral vectors appear difficult to administer repeatedly (8–11), in contrast to synthetic approaches (12). Novel approaches to target and transfect stem cells may be more attractive in this regard; although based on recent clinical data from the bone marrow field (13), concerns may exist over the long-term safety of integrating vectors.

3. Published Trials

3.1. Pros and Cons of Clinically Available Gene Transfer Agents

The first clinical trials of gene therapy in patients took place within a short time of the *CFTR* gene being identified in 1989 and were initially focussed on viral vectors (**Table 5.1**). To date, clinical trials have been conducted with engineered adeno (Ad) virus or adeno-associated virus (AAV). Limitations to this approach were soon identified which included (a) the absence of certain specific receptors on the apical surface of respiratory epithelia (14), (b) inflammatory responses, leading in some cases to unacceptable toxicity (15) (this has largely been overcome in more recent trials) and (c) the development of immune responses and the detrimental impact of these on expression after repeated application (8–11). Expression levels will need to be long lived to be therapeutic and in the context of a respiratory epithelium with a limited lifespan, this is most likely to require either repeated application or long duration of expression within a progenitor cell population. Non-viral agents include cationic lipids (12, 16–21), compacted DNA nanoparticles (22) and naked DNA (19). The major advantage of certain of these is that they can be repeatedly administered (12). However, they are not universally without side effects, as discussed below.

3.2. Routes and Methods of Delivery

The nasal mucosa, similar in composition and ion transport abnormalities to that of the lower airway, provided an attractive site for early phase, proof-of-principle studies. Dosing has been achieved by nasal nebulisation, spray or perfusion. One group used the maxillary sinus and instilled via an antrostomy (23). Delivery to the lower airways has been achieved via bronchoscopy or with conventional nebulisation. Of note, it appears that the toxicity profiles of administration to the two organs may differ significantly (20); as such, safety for lung dosing should not be extrapolated from nasal studies.

Table 5.1
Characteristics of gene therapy trials for CF

Reference	Vector	Organ	Placebo controlled?	Repeated dose?	Number	Safety concerns	Efficacy
Viral							
(42)	Ad	Nose	No	No	3	No	Nasal PD: decreases baseline toward normal values; mRNA: –ve; CFTR protein: –ve
(15)	Ad	Nose Lung	No	No	4	Yes, with highest lung dose	Nasal PD: inconclusive mRNA: some positive nose; lung –ve
(33)	Ad	Nose	No	No	12	Mild mucosal inflammation at highest dose	Nasal PD: no change *CFTR* mRNA: some +ve
(43)	Ad	Nose	No	No	9	No	Nasal PD: partial correction
(8)	Ad	Nose	No	Yes	6	No	Nasal PD: partial correction of Cl^- in some; effect reduced with subsequent doses
(44)	Ad	Nose Lung	No	No	6	No	mRNA: some positive in both organs
(9)	Ad	Lung	No	Yes	14	No	mRNA: some positive; decreased with subsequent doses
(23)	AAV	Sinus	No	No	10	No	Nasal PD: partial Cl^- correction in some; *CFTR* mRNA: –ve
(34)	Ad	Lung	No	No	11	Flu-like symptoms at high dose	Vector DNA: +ve on day 4, transient
(35, 36)	Ad	Lung	No	No	36	Mild, non-specific inflammatory response	mRNA: some +ve
(37)	AAV	Lung	No	No	12	±	*CFTR* mRNA: –ve
(32)	AAV	Sinus	Yes	No	23	No	No change: sinusitis, nasal PD, histology, IL-8 Increase in IL-10

Table 5.1 (continued)

Reference	Vector	Organ	Placebo controlled?	Repeated dose?	Number	Safety concerns	Efficacy
(38)	AAV	Nose Lung	No	No	25	±	Nasal PD: no change; DNA: some +ve Lung: DNA: some +ve
(10)	AAV	Lung	Yes	Yes	37	No	FEV1, IL-8 and IL-10: trends to improvement mRNA: –ve
(11)	AAV	Lung	Yes	Yes	102	No	FEV1, sputum markers, requirement for antibiotics: no significant improvement
Non-viral							
(16)	DC-Chol/DOPE	Nose	Yes	No	15	No	NPD: partial correction (20%) of Cl^- defect *CFTR* mRNA: –ve
(17)	DC-Chol/DOPE	Nose	Yes	No	12		Nasal PD: some correction of Cl^-
(18)	DOTAP	Nose	Yes	No	16	No	Nasal PD: partial Cl^- correction up to 4 weeks mRNA: some +ve
(19)	GL67 vs. naked pDNA	Nose	No	No	12	No	NPD: statistically significant correction of Cl^- with no difference between vectors *CFTR* mRNA: –ve, technical problems
(20)	GL67	Lung Nose	Yes	No	16	Flu-like symptoms	Bronchial PD: significant Cl^- correction to 25% of normal values Reduced IL-8 and inflammatory cells in sputum mRNA: –ve

Table 5.1 (continued)

Reference	Vector	Organ	Placebo controlled?	Repeated dose?	Number	Safety concerns	Efficacy
(12)	DC-Chol/DOPE	Nose	Yes	Yes	12	No	*CFTR* mRNA: some +ve; CFTR protein: some +ve Nasal PD: partial Cl^- correction in some No loss of efficacy with repeated dosing
(21)	GL67	Lung	No	No	8	Flu-like symptoms	*CFTR* mRNA: 4/8 +ve
(22)	DNA nanoparticles	Nose	Yes	No	12	No	NPD: partial to complete Cl^- correction 8/12 *CFTR* DNA: 12/12 +ve in active but cross-contamination in placebo

Ad, adenovirus; AAV, adeno-associated virus; PD, potential difference; mRNA, messenger RNA.

4. Methods

4.1. Molecular Assays

4.1.1. CFTR mRNA

Whereas quantification of transgene DNA will provide confirmation of delivery, only detection of mRNA provides proof of gene expression. The majority of clinical trials have included RT-PCR-based methods of quantifying mRNA, although results have been highly variable (**Table 5.1**). Endogenous levels of CFTR in airway epithelial cells are very low (2) and detection of levels adequate for clinical benefit poses technical challenges related to assay sensitivity. Further, the assay is most commonly performed on either airway brushings (or, less commonly, biopsies), both of which contain abundant cells of non-epithelial origin, including leucocytes and connective tissue cells. Gene transfer to such cells could lead to false-positive results, making either enrichment of the sample for epithelial cells or some method to render the assay epithelium-specific highly desirable. Finally, the complex post-translational biogenesis of CFTR means that mRNA levels may not necessarily correlate with CFTR protein levels or function and so this assay should not be relied upon in isolation (*see* also **Chapter 9, Section II**).

4.1.2. CFTR Protein

One of the major advantages of immunohistochemistry is the ability to visualise the localisation of the protein on the apical surface and to co-stain for proteins such as cytokeratin, confirming epithelial expression. However, the presence of detectable protein levels on the cells of many patients with CF (24) together with the technical challenges surrounding these techniques (25, 26) makes quantification difficult (*see* also **Chapter 2, Section I, Volume II**).

4.2. Assays of CFTR Function

4.2.1. Potential Difference

The passage of charged ions across an intact epithelial surface generates a measurable millivoltage potential difference (PD) across the epithelium, whereby the outside of the cell is negatively charged compared to the inside. CF subjects have a more negative nasal PD and a greater response to the sodium channel blocking agent amiloride (both reflecting increased sodium absorption) with reduced or absent chloride secretory responses (stimulated with low/zero chloride solutions and the cAMP agonist isoproterenol) (27). The US CF TDN has standardised SOPs for performing nPD in multicentre settings (28) and the European equivalents are shortly to be published. Many of the reported gene therapy trials (and trials of novel small molecule drugs (29)) have employed nasal PD as an outcome. However, there are several issues to be considered (*see* also **Chapter 6**, **Section I**):

- There is a high degree of intra-operator and intra-subject variability; the latter is particularly notable for measures of sodium transport (30).
- It is unknown what degree of change (and in which parameter(s)) might be relevant for clinical benefit.
- When changes have been observed in gene therapy trials, these have generally been related to Cl^- secretion with no correction of the sodium hyperabsorption.
- Baseline readings will also be reduced (mimicking correction towards wild-type) by epithelial damage or inflammation, which must be considered as a possible confounding factor.

More recently, the technique has been adapted for use in the lower airway via a bronchoscope, with similar CF/non-CF differences in chloride secretion being observed in as far out as seventh- or eighth-generation airways (31). Our group reported a significant increase in chloride secretion 2 days after a single dose of non-viral *CFTR* gene therapy (20), confirming its utility as an outcome measure and we are using it in a current single-dose study. However, this technique is best performed under general anaesthetic, making it unsuitable for studies requiring repeated measurements.

4.2.2. Inflammatory Markers

Few gene therapy trials have included inflammatory markers as efficacy outcomes. We reported decreased levels of sputum IL-8 and neutrophils after a single dose of liposome-mediated *CFTR* gene therapy (20) and the former was also found after the first (10), but not subsequent (11), dose of AAV-mediated *CFTR* gene therapy. Levels of the anti-inflammatory cytokine IL-10 increased in the maxillary sinus after administration of a single dose of AAV- mediated *CFTR* (32). Methodological issues may be major factors in both processing samples and measuring such inflammatory markers and need to be taken into consideration (*see* also **Chapter 4**, **Section I**, **Volume II**).

4.2.3. Spirometry

Two AAV trials performed by the same group have been designed with FEV_1 as an efficacy outcome measure. In the first and smaller of these (10), a significant improvement was observed after the first of three monthly doses, although not thereafter. In the second trial, which included 102 relatively mild subjects, such a beneficial effect was not observed (11).

4.2.3.1. Safety/Toxicity Measures

In general, safety has not been a major concern in studies limited to the upper airway, although nasal mucosal inflammation has been reported after viral administration (33). In contrast, both viral and non-viral agents administered to the lungs have reported flu-like symptoms and/or a rise in inflammatory markers (15, 20, 21, 34–38). Whilst with viral vectors this most likely reflects an inflammatory response to viral proteins, with non-viral vectors it is thought that this reflects a host response to the unmethylated CpG motifs present in plasmid DNA (39). Studies in which both upper and lower airways have been treated support the fact that safety in the lung cannot be extrapolated from nasal delivery (20). Whether this relates to organ-specific differences or is simply a reflection of delivery or dose issues remains unclear. Respiratory safety measures have included spirometry (which has in some cases shown acute, transient drop after delivery), transfer factor (ditto) and radiology including plain films and CT scans; in general, any changes observed in these have been unremarkable.

5. Looking to the Future: The UK CF Gene Therapy Consortium

The UKCFGTC (http://www.cfgenetherapy.org.uk/) was formed several years ago from the three centres in the UK with CF clinical trial experience: Oxford University, Edinburgh University and Imperial College London/Royal Brompton Hospital. The purpose of the collaboration was to streamline efforts, rationalise resources and hopefully thereby advance progress more rapidly. The clinical trials discussed above had largely already been reported, from which proof of principle had been confirmed for both viral and non-viral gene delivery methods. However, the key question of whether the demonstrated degree of molecular benefit is sufficient to produce clinical benefit when sustained over a long period had not been addressed.

The primary aim of the Consortium is to develop gene therapy to produce clinical benefit in CF. We focussed on two waves of research: Wave 1, a programme to determine whether such clinical benefit was achievable with the best, currently available gene transfer agent, and Wave 2, more futuristically, to explore novel approaches that were then not yet available for clinical use. We are currently midway through Wave 1, on which the remainder of this chapter will focus. The design of the programme has evolved from several premises:

- Repeated application will be required for clinical benefit; thus a non-viral GTA will be required and toxicity will need to be minimised to an acceptable level.
- Duration of expression should be maximised to allow a reasonable dosing interval.

- Benefit should be confirmed with clinically relevant outcome measures and therefore
  - large numbers treated for a prolonged duration are likely to be required;
  - sensitive, relevant outcome measures should be developed.

6. Rationale and Strategy

6.1. Choice of a Non-viral Gene Delivery Method

Based on published data and our own experience, we considered it unlikely that, within the time frame of Wave 1, a repeatable viral gene transfer agent would be available. This led to our assessing available non-viral vectors with the following criteria:

- Nebulisable
- Manufacturable to GMP in sufficient quantities
- Repeatable
- Reasonable preclinical toxicity profile

From a short list, the cationic lipid GL67 was identified and chosen as meeting these criteria.

6.2. Plasmid Modifications

In a previous clinical trial using GL67 (20), we had noted flu-like responses and observed a relatively short duration of gene expression. Modifications were therefore made to (a) remove the pro-inflammatory CpG motifs and (b) exchange the viral promoter for a mammalian promoter, capable in preclinical testing of sustaining prolonged gene expression (40).

6.3. Trial Design: How Might We Search for Clinical Benefit?

In this programme, we wish to design a trial to assess *clinical benefit* rather than simply changes in molecular or bioelectrical markers. Conventionally, lung function (most commonly FEV_1) is used as a primary outcome for CF clinical trials. However, this outcome is noisy, changes only very slowly over time in most clinics currently and is therefore difficult to power for (41). The Consortium is currently midway through a series of studies to address the feasibility and utility of other potential outcomes (Run-in study). These are being assessed longitudinally at periods of both stability and exacerbation and include a potentially more sensitive physiological technique (multiple breath washout); lung CT; mucociliary clearance assessed with radioisotope scans; inflammatory markers in sputum, serum, exhaled breath condensate and urine; sputum physical properties and quantitative culture; quality of life questionnaires and symptom scores; and exercise tests. From these studies, we hope to be able to choose primary outcome measure(s) on which we can power a trial over a period of up to 12 months.

6.4. Regulatory and Logistic Requirements

The UK requires permission to be obtained from the Medicines and Healthcare Regulatory Agency (MHRA), the Gene Therapy Advisory Committee (GTAC) and local Research & Development Offices before an interventional trial commences. This creates a huge burden of work for groups such as our own performing trials sponsored by the host institution rather than a commercial company, within which entire departments are devoted to producing the documentation required. Any amendment to protocols must also be approved by these same bodies, resulting often in significant time delays. There are also internal logistic hurdles, such as the provision of vented cubicles suitable for nebulisation of genetically modified material; the availability of a dedicated trial pharmacist for the lengthy formulation required on the day of dosing; the requirements for segregation of CF patients at all times to prevent cross-infection and the impact of this on throughput.

7. What Might the Future Hold?

Proof of the ability of *CFTR* gene transfer to achieve clinical improvement will pave the way for future strategies to improve efficacy further; these might include targeting stem/progenitor cells of the airway for longer term benefit, achieving either long-term expression or the ability to repeatedly deliver high-expressing viral vectors, and increasing safety such that it is ethical and feasible to delivering to the relatively clean, undamaged airway of the newly diagnosed newborn.

8. Conclusions

During 20 years of clinical research in CF gene therapy, we have proved the principle of gene delivery to the CF airway and correction of some of the basic functions of the CFTR protein. Our challenge now is to understand what these changes mean for patients with the disease and how they might correlate with measures of real clinical improvement. This will lead to our ability to refine further and improve current gene transfer approaches with the ultimate goal of providing a treatment that can halt the progression of CF lung disease.

References

1. Engelhardt, J. F., Yankaskas, J. R., Ernst, S. A., Yang, Y., Marino, C. R., Boucher, R. C., et al. (1992) Submucosal glands are the predominant site of CFTR expression in the human bronchus. *Nat. Genet.* **2**, 240–248.
2. Engelhardt, J. F., Zepeda, M., Cohn, J. A., Yankaskas, J. R., and Wilson, J. M. (1994) Expression of the cystic fibrosis gene in adult human lung. *J. Clin. Invest.* **93**, 737–749.
3. Rawlins, E. L., and Hogan, B. L. (2008) Ciliated epithelial cell lifespan in the mouse trachea and lung. *Am. J. Physiol. Lung Cell. Mol. Physiol.* **295**, L231–234.
4. Johnson, L. G., Boyles, S. E., Wilson, J., and Boucher, R. C. (1995) Normalization of raised sodium absorption and raised calcium-mediated chloride secretion by adenovirus-mediated expression of cystic fibrosis transmembrane conductance regulator in primary human cystic fibrosis airway epithelial cells. *J. Clin. Invest.* **95**, 1377–1382.
5. Zhang, Y., Jiang, Q., Dudus, L., Yankaskas, J. R., and Engelhardt, J. F. (1998) Vector-specific complementation profiles of two independent primary defects in cystic fibrosis airways. *Hum. Gene Ther.* **9**, 635–648.
6. Gan, K. H., Veeze, H. J., van den Ouweland, A. M., Halley, D. J., Scheffer, H., van der Hout, A., et al. (1995) A cystic fibrosis mutation associated with mild lung disease. *N. Engl. J. Med.* **333**, 95–99.
7. Zhang, L., Button, B., Gabriel, S. E., Burkett, S., Yan, Y., Skiadopoulos, M. H. et al. (2009) CFTR delivery to 25% of surface epithelial cells restores normal rates of mucus transport to human cystic fibrosis airway epithelium. *PLoS Biol.* 7, e1000155.
8. Zabner, J., Ramsey, B. W., Meeker, D. P., Aitken, M. L., Balfour, R. P., Gibson, R. L., et al. (1996) Repeat administration of an adenovirus vector encoding cystic fibrosis transmembrane conductance regulator to the nasal epithelium of patients with cystic fibrosis. *J. Clin. Invest.* **97**, 1504–1511.
9. Harvey, B. G., Leopold, P. L., Hackett, N. R., Grasso, T. M., Williams, P. M., Tucker, A. L., et al. (1999) Airway epithelial CFTR mRNA expression in cystic fibrosis patients after repetitive administration of a recombinant adenovirus. *J. Clin. Invest.* **104**, 1245–1255.
10. Moss, R. B., Rodman, D., Spencer, L. T., Aitken, M. L., Zeitlin, P. L., Waltz, D., et al. (2004) Repeated adeno-associated virus serotype 2 aerosol-mediated cystic fibrosis transmembrane regulator gene transfer to the lungs of patients with cystic fibrosis: a multicenter, double-blind, placebo-controlled trial. *Chest* **125**, 509–521.
11. Moss, R. B., Milla, C., Colombo, J., Accurso, F., Zeitlin, P. L., Clancy, J. P., et al. (2007) Repeated aerosolized AAV-CFTR for treatment of cystic fibrosis: a randomized placebo-controlled phase 2B trial. *Hum. Gene Ther.* **18**, 726–732.
12. Hyde, S. C., Southern, K. W., Gileadi, U., Fitzjohn, E. M., Mofford, K. A., Waddell, B. E., et al. (2000) Repeat administration of DNA/liposomes to the nasal epithelium of patients with cystic fibrosis. *Gene Ther.* 7, 1156–1165.
13. Thrasher, A. J., Gaspar, H. B., Baum, C., Modlich, U., Schambach, A., Candotti, F., et al. (2006) Gene therapy: X-SCID transgene leukaemogenicity. *Nature* **443**, E5–E7.
14. Walters, R. W., Grunst, T., Bergelson, J. M., Finberg, R. W., Welsh, M. J., and Zabner, J. (1999) Basolateral localization of fiber receptors limits adenovirus infection from the apical surface of airway epithelia. *J. Biol. Chem.* **274**, 10219–10226.
15. Crystal, R. G., McElvaney, N. G., Rosenfeld, M. A., Chu, C. S., Mastrangeli, A., Hay, J. G., et al. (1994) Administration of an adenovirus containing the human CFTR cDNA to the respiratory tract of individuals with cystic fibrosis. *Nat. Genet.* **8**, 42–51.
16. Caplen, N. J., Alton, E. W., Middleton, P. G., Dorin, J. R., Stevenson, B. J., Gao, X., et al. (1995) Liposome-mediated CFTR gene transfer to the nasal epithelium of patients with cystic fibrosis. *Nat. Med.* **1**, 39–46.
17. Gill, D. R., Southern, K. W., Mofford, K. A., Seddon, T., Huang, L., Sorgi, F., et al. (1997) A placebo-controlled study of liposome-mediated gene transfer to the nasal epithelium of patients with cystic fibrosis. *Gene Ther.* **4**, 199–209.
18. Porteous, D. J., Dorin, J. R., McLachlan, G., Davidson-Smith, H., Davidson, H., Stevenson, B. J., et al. (1997) Evidence for safety and efficacy of DOTAP cationic liposome mediated CFTR gene transfer to the nasal epithelium of patients with cystic fibrosis. *Gene Ther.* **4**, 210–218.
19. Zabner, J., Cheng, S. H., Meeker, D., Launspach, J., Balfour, R., Perricone, M. A., et al. (1997) Comparison of DNA-lipid complexes and DNA alone for gene transfer to cystic fibrosis airway epithelia in vivo. *J. Clin. Invest.* **100**, 1529–1537.
20. Alton, E. W., Stern, M., Farley, R., Jaffe, A., Chadwick, S. L., Phillips, J., et al. (1999) Cationic lipid-mediated CFTR gene transfer

to the lungs and nose of patients with cystic fibrosis: a double-blind placebo-controlled trial. *Lancet* **353**, 947–954.

21. Ruiz, F. E., Clancy, J. P., Perricone, M. A., Bebok, Z., Hong, J. S., Cheng, S. H., et al. (2001) A clinical inflammatory syndrome attributable to aerosolized lipid-DNA administration in cystic fibrosis. *Hum. Gene Ther.* **12**, 751–761.
22. Konstan, M. W., Davis, P. B., Wagener, J. S., Hilliard, K. A., Stern, R. C., Milgram, L. J., et al. (2004) Compacted DNA nanoparticles administered to the nasal mucosa of cystic fibrosis subjects are safe and demonstrate partial to complete cystic fibrosis transmembrane regulator reconstitution. *Hum. Gene Ther.* **15**, 1255–1269.
23. Wagner, J. A., Messner, A. H., Moran, M. L., Daifuku, R., Kouyama, K., Desch, J. K., et al. (1999) Safety and biological efficacy of an adeno-associated virus vector-cystic fibrosis transmembrane regulator (AAV-CFTR) in the cystic fibrosis maxillary sinus. *Laryngoscope* **109**, 266–274.
24. Kälin, N., Claass, A., Sommer, M., Puchelle, E., and Tümmler, B. (1999) DeltaF508 CFTR protein expression in tissues from patients with cystic fibrosis. *J. Clin. Invest.* **103**, 1379–1389.
25. Carvalho-Oliveira, I., Efthymiadou, A., Malhó, R., Nogueira, P., Tzetis, M., Kanavakis, E., et al. (2004) CFTR localization in native airway cells and cell lines expressing wild-type or F508del-CFTR by a panel of different antibodies. *J. Histochem. Cytochem.* **52**, 193–203.
26. Davidson, H., Wilson, A., Gray, R. D., Horsley, A., Pringle, I. A., McLachlan, G., et al. (2009) An immunocytochemical assay to detect human CFTR expression following gene transfer. *Mol. Cell Probes* **23**, 272–280.
27. Middleton, P. G., Geddes, D. M., and Alton, E. W. (1994) Protocols for in vivo measurement of the ion transport defects in cystic fibrosis nasal epithelium. *Eur. Respir. J.* **7**, 2050–2056.
28. Standaert, T. A., Boitano, L., Emerson, J., Milgram, L. J., Konstan, M. W., Hunter, J., et al. (2004) Standardized procedure for measurement of nasal potential difference: an outcome measure in multicenter cystic fibrosis clinical trials. *Pediatr. Pulmonol.* **37**, 385–392.
29. Clancy, J. P., Rowe, S. M., Bebok, Z., Aitken, M. L., Gibson, R., Zeitlin, P., et al. (2007) No detectable improvements in cystic fibrosis transmembrane conductance regulator by nasal aminoglycosides in patients with cystic fibrosis with stop mutations. *Am. J. Respir. Cell. Mol. Biol.* **37**, 57–66.
30. Yaakov, Y., Kerem, E., Yahav, Y., Rivlin, J., Blau, H., Bentur, L., et al. (2007) Reproducibility of nasal potential difference measurements in cystic fibrosis. *Chest* **132**, 1219–1226.
31. Davies, J. C., Davies, M., McShane, D., Smith, S., Chadwick, S., Jaffe, A., et al. (2005) Potential difference measurements in the lower airway of children with and without cystic fibrosis. *Am. J. Respir. Cell. Mol. Biol.* **171**, 1015–1019.
32. Wagner, J. A., Nepomuceno, I. B., Messner, A. H., Moran, M. L., Batson, E. P., Dimiceli, S., et al. (2002) A phase II, double-blind, randomized, placebo-controlled clinical trial of tgAAVCF using maxillary sinus delivery in patients with cystic fibrosis with antrostomies. *Hum. Gene Ther.* **13**, 1349–1359.
33. Knowles, M. R., Hohneker, K. W., Zhou, Z., Olsen, J. C., Noah, T. L., Hu, P. C., et al. (1995) A controlled study of adenoviral-vector-mediated gene transfer in the nasal epithelium of patients with cystic fibrosis. *N. Engl. J. Med.* **333**, 823–831.
34. Zuckerman, J. B., Robinson, C. B., McCoy, K. S., Shell, R., Sferra, T. J., Chirmule, N., et al. (1999) A phase I study of adenovirus-mediated transfer of the human cystic fibrosis transmembrane conductance regulator gene to a lung segment of individuals with cystic fibrosis. *Hum. Gene Ther.* **10**, 2973–2985.
35. Joseph, P. M., O'Sullivan, B. P., Lapey, A., Plog, M. S., O'Sullivan, B. P., Joseph, P. M., et al. (2001) Aerosol and lobar administration of a recombinant adenovirus to individuals with cystic fibrosis. I. Methods, safety, and clinical implications. *Hum. Gene Ther.* **12**, 1369–1382.
36. Perricone, M. A., Morris, J. E., Pavelka, K., Plog, M. S, O'Sullivan, B. P., Joseph, P. M., et al. (2001) Aerosol and lobar administration of a recombinant adenovirus to individuals with cystic fibrosis. II. Transfection efficiency in airway epithelium. *Hum. Gene Ther.* **12**, 1383–1394.
37. Aitken, M. L., Moss, R. B., Waltz, D. A., and Dovey, M. E. Tonelli, M. R., McNamara, S. C., et al. (2001) A phase I study of aerosolized administration of tgAAVCF to cystic fibrosis subjects with mild lung disease. *Hum. Gene Ther.* **12**, 1907–1916.
38. Flotte, T. R., Zeitlin, P. L., Reynolds, T. C., Heald, A. E., Pedersen, P., Beck, S., et al. (2003) Phase I trial of intranasal and endobronchial administration of a recombinant

adeno-associated virus serotype 2 (rAAV2)-CFTR vector in adult cystic fibrosis patients: a two-part clinical study. *Hum. Gene Ther.* **14**, 1079–1088.

39. Yew, N. S., and Cheng, S. H. (2004) Reducing the immunostimulatory activity of CpG-containing plasmid DNA vectors for non-viral gene therapy. *Expert Opin. Drug Deliv.* **1**, 115–125.
40. Hyde, S. C., Pringle, I. A., Abdullah, S., Lawton, A. E., Davies, L. A., Varathalingam, A., et al. (2008) CpG-free plasmids confer reduced inflammation and sustained pulmonary gene expression. *Nat. Biotechnol.* **26**, 549–551.
41. Davis, P. B., Byard, P. J., and Konstan, M. W. (1997) Identifying treatments that halt progression of pulmonary disease in cystic fibrosis. *Pediatr. Res.* **41**, 161–165.
42. Zabner, J., Couture, L. A., Gregory, R. J., Graham, S. M., Smith, A. E., and Welsh, M. J. (1993) Adenovirus-mediated gene transfer transiently corrects the chloride transport defect in nasal epithelia of patients with cystic fibrosis. *Cell* **75**, 207–216.
43. Hay, J. G., McElvaney, N. G., Herena, J., and Crystal, R. G. (1995) Modification of nasal epithelial potential differences of individuals with cystic fibrosis consequent to local administration of a normal CFTR cDNA adenovirus gene transfer vector. *Hum. Gene Ther.* **6**, 1487–1496.
44. Bellon, G., Michel-Calemard, L., Thouvenot, D., Jagneaux, V., Poitevin, F., Malcus, C., et al. (1997) Aerosol administration of a recombinant adenovirus expressing CFTR to cystic fibrosis patients: a phase I clinical trial. *Hum. Gene Ther.* **8**, 15–25.

Chapter 6

Nasal Potential Difference Measurements to Assess CFTR Ion Channel Activity

Steven M. Rowe, John Paul Clancy, and Michael Wilschanski

Abstract

The Nasal potential difference measurement is used to measure the voltage across the nasal epithelium, which results from transepithelial ion transport and reflects in part CFTR function. The electrophysiologic abnormality in cystic fibrosis was first described 30 years ago and correlates with features of the CF phenotype. NPD measurement is an important in vivo research and diagnostic tool, and is used to assess the efficacy of new treatments such as gene therapy and ion transport modulators. This chapter will elaborate on the electrophysiological principles behind the test, the equipment required, the methods, and the analysis of the data.

Key words: Nasal potential difference, CFTR, ENaC, amiloride, cAMP, isoproterenol, electrodes, ion transport.

1. Introduction

The measurement of nasal potential difference (NPD) provides a direct and sensitive evaluation of sodium and chloride transport in secretory epithelial cells via assessment of transepithelial bioelectric properties (1–3). This serves as a diagnostic aid in difficult cases where abnormal CFTR function is suspected (4, 5). As the only direct in vivo measure capable of separating sodium and chloride transport, NPD has been used as an important endpoint in clinical trials evaluating therapeutic agents intended to replace dysfunctional CFTR with wild-type CFTR cDNA (including viral and nonviral gene transfer (6–8)), restore mutant CFTR function (9–14), or address other abnormalities in CF ion transport such

M.D. Amaral, K. Kunzelmann (eds.), *Cystic Fibrosis*, Methods in Molecular Biology 741,
DOI 10.1007/978-1-61779-117-8_6, © Springer Science+Business Media, LLC 2011

as novel high-affinity ENaC blockers, channel-activating protease inhibitors, or activators of alternate Cl^- channels (15–18).

1.1. Principles Underlying Nasal Potential Difference Measurements

The premise behind NPD measurements is that the bioelectric abnormality of the CF nasal airway reflects transport abnormalities observed in the lower airways of CF patients. In non-CF patients, the potential is maintained by a balance of sodium absorption and chloride transport, resulting in the tight regulation of the airway surface liquid volume and ionic content, both of which are important for maintaining normal mucociliary clearance. The nasal cavity is accessible which makes it a good site to examine the ion transport characteristics of airway epithelia. Because respiratory epithelia form a tight monolayer harboring a stable and sufficient transepithelial resistance, the active secretion or absorption of charged salts such as sodium (Na^+) and chloride (Cl^-) ions induces a potential difference, measured as a voltage across the epithelial surface (19). The bioelectric potential can be measured by using a high-impedance voltmeter between two electrodes, with one in continuity with each side of the epithelial surface. The electrode on the airway surface (the exploring electrode) rests against the surface of the target epithelium. The internal electrode (the reference electrode) can theoretically be placed in any interstitial compartment of the body, although generally the subcutaneous tissue of the forearm is used. Due to the importance of appropriate placement within the nasal cavity, and the need for an electrically quiet environment, some training and experience are required to achieve accuracy and reproducibility with the method.

1.2. General Methodology

Less than a centimeter into the nose, the squamous ("skin type") epithelium becomes ciliated pseudocolumnar epithelium under the inferior turbinate, sharing many characteristics with the more distal airways (20–22). Under basal conditions, Na^+ absorption is the primary ion transport activity in normal airway epithelia (1). The resulting (or basal) PD is negative or polarized (viewed from the epithelial surface) and in normal subjects, it is usually between −15 and −25 mV. The measurement continues by the sequential perfusion of compounds that block inwardly directed sodium transport through inhibition of ENaC (amiloride), followed by augmentation of chloride transport through CFTR. During perfusion of amiloride, the potential difference depolarizes as ENaC transport is reduced, and the PD typically approaches a low polarizing value (typically between 0 and −10 mV). Perfusion of a chloride-free solution induces a chloride diffusion PD through CFTR channels, resulting in a rapid and often large hyperpolarization of the PD. CFTR-mediated Cl^- transport is further enhanced pharmacologically by the addition of agents known to activate CFTR, such as isoproterenol (which increases intracellular cyclic AMP as a β2 receptor agonist) (23, 24). It is not unusual to observe transient hyperpolarization that is believed to represent Cl^- transport through calcium-activated chloride channels (CaCCs) during chloride-free perfusion (with or without isoproterenol). These transient polarizations typically resolve within 1–2 min and are not CFTR dependent. Finally, ATP is perfused, which activates chloride secretion through alternative (non-CFTR) CaCCs and serves as a marker of epithelium integrity.

1.3. Healthy and CF Nasal PD Measurements

Example tracings in normal and CF subjects are shown in **Fig. 6.1**. In CF, this ion transport profile is abnormal and the nasal PD measurement has a number of features that distinguish the PD signature. At the beginning of the measurement with buffered Ringer's solution, the basal PD in CF is much more negative due to increased ENaC activity, thought to be due to the absence of regulation of ENaC function by CFTR. As expected, the depolarizing response to amiloride is also enhanced. Although the sodium abnormality is usually readily apparent, the most consistent abnormality in CF is the absence of hyperpolarization following perfusion with chloride-free solution and isoproterenol. In CF, the addition of ATP (or other purines) leads to a large hyperpolarization and occurs through non-CFTR-mediated chloride secretory pathways, including stimulation of P2Y2 receptors which activate CaCCs (an approach now being tested as a potential CF therapy through long-acting derivatives of UTP (25)). In aggregate, the differences in Na and Cl transport are sufficient to discriminate CF from non-CF subjects, and also detect individuals with intermediate phenotypes (**Table 6.1**) (26, 27).

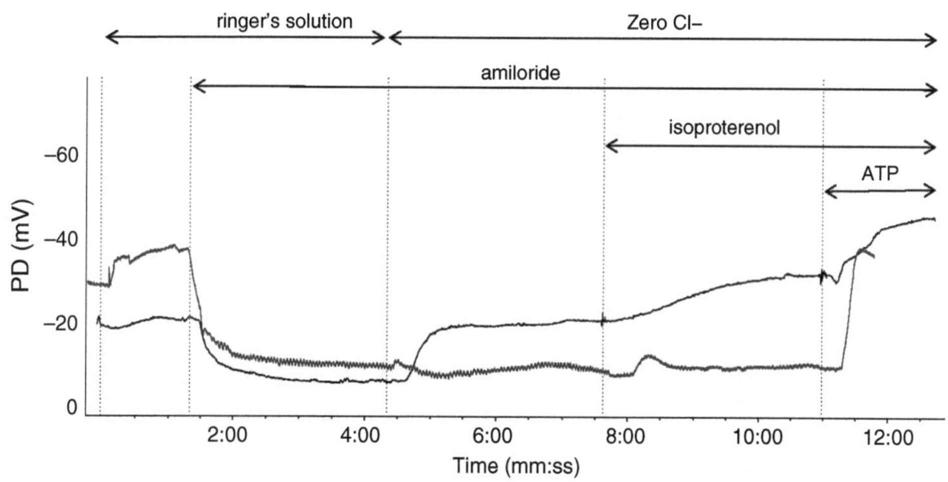

Fig. 6.1. Representative nasal potential difference tracings from a normal (*black*) and a CF (*gray*) subject. Contents and duration of each perfused solution is designated above.

Table 6.1
Relationship between NPD parameters, sweat chloride and CFTR genotype

				Nasal potential difference (mv)				
Group	n	Age (yr)	Sweat chloride (mmol/l)	Max PD	ΔAmil	ΔCl−free	ΔCl−free+Iso	ΔAmil+Cl−free+Iso
Control	25	30±6	20±11	−24±8	13±4	−15±9	−29±10	−16±12
Incidental heterozygote	6	24±2	34±16	−26±9	15±6	−12±4	−27±3	−12±5
CF heterozygote	21	37±10	26±13	−22±6	14±5	−11±10	−23±10	−9±9
CBAVD−0	6	33±3	22±9	−25±7	12±4	−8±6	−22±10	−9±8
CBAVD−1	18	37±6	44±23	−28±11	19±7	−5±5	−12±7	+7±10
CBAVD−2	36	34±5	54±23	−35±9	23±10	−2±3	−8±7	+15±11
CF−PS	24	32±10	73±21	−44±13	27±12	+3±5	+2±5	+28±13
CF−PI	26	20±9	102±14	−54±9	36±8	+3±4	+4±5	+40±7

Definition of abbreviations: Amil, amiloride; CBAVD, congenital bilateral absence of the vas deferens; CF, cystic fibrosis; CF-PI, pancreatic-insufficient cystic fibrosis; CF-PS, pancreatic-sufficient cystic fibrosis; Iso, isoproterenol; PD, potential difference.
Values are mean ± SD.
Reprinted with permission of the American Thoracic Society. Copyright © American Thoracic Society. Wilschanski M, Dupuis A, Ellis L, et al., (26).

2. Materials

There are numerous choices in regard to equipment and supplies that can be employed to successfully perform the NPD measurement and capture the data generated. There are advantages and disadvantages to various setup choices, and often the final choice at a given NPD site is a balance of the desire to standardize performance across sites, feasibility, and cost. The equipment described below is based upon experience developed through sites participating in clinical trials through the CFF-TDN. The use of the electronic data capture, sequence, solutions, and electrodes has been validated through comparative testing across a number of NPD sites in CF and non-CF subjects (28). Equipment that is felt to be highly important for standardization across study sites participating in therapeutic clinical trials is noted by an asterisk.

2.1. Electronic Data Capture (EDC) Equipment

Hardware and software employed for NPD measurements that have been standardized across study sites for use in therapeutic clinical trials have been based on pilot testing of performance, manufacturer support, and good laboratory practice (GLP) compatibility (21CFTR part11 compliance) (28). This equipment is available from ADInstruments (www.adinstruments.com):

- *PowerLab 4/30 data acquisition system.
- *BMA-200 AC/DC portable bioamplifier.
- *ISO-Z isolation headstage for BMA-200.
- *ADInstruments software: LabChart Pro (GLP Client V6 (win) or higher).

2.2. Perfusion Equipment and Supplies

Ensuring that the NPD perfusates are delivered at 5 ml/min typically requires the use of programmable syringe pumps (capable of holding 60-ml syringes) and relatively large diameter perfusion tubing. The larger bore also helps to ensure that target temperatures are achieved for perfusates (by passing the tubing through a water bath). Specific equipment (pumps and disposables) are listed below:

- Infusion pump for 60-ml syringes (Medfusion 3,500 Syringe Pump or equivalent).
- Isotemp 210 water bath (Fisher Scientific, Cat. # 15-462-10).
- *Electrodes – mini-calomel reference (Fisher Scientific, Cat. # 13-620-79).
- *PE50 tubing (0.023 in. i.d., 1 × 100 ft; Becton Dickenson, Cat # 427411).

- *PE90 tubing (0.034 in. i.d., 1 × 100 ft; Becton Dickenson, Cat. # 427421).
- *Silastic tubing (0.058 in. i.d., 0.077 in. o.d.; Dow Corning, Cat. # 508-006).
- IV extension tubing (30 in., 50/Box; International Limited, Cat. # IMN30).
- Three-way stopcock (50/Box; Medex, Cat # MX5311L).
- Intramedic luer stub adapter (20 G; Becton Dickenson, Cat. # 427564).
- Syringe 60 cm^3 w/o needle luer slip (30/Box; Becton Dickenson, Cat. # 309653).
- 23G.3/4 vacutainer needles (0.6 mm × 19 mm, 50 U/Box; Becton Dickenson, Cat. # 367283).
- Difco Laboratories agar (Fisher Scientific, Noble 100 g, Cat. # 0142-15-2; or equivalent).
- Welch Allyn rhinoscope 71000-C; 3.5 V convertible handle battery 72300; nasal illuminator 26530.

2.3. Solutions and Reagents

There are three isotonic base NPD solutions used in most NPD protocols:

Solution #1 = Ringer's solution + phosphates.
Solution #2 = Ringer's solution + phosphates + amiloride (100 μM).
Solution #3 = $0[Cl^-]$ + phosphates + amiloride.

Isoproterenol (final concentration = 10 μM) and ATP (final concentration = 100 μM) are added to solution #3 to make solutions #4 and #5, respectively. While there is uncertainty regarding the optimal salt concentrations to maximize detection of CFTR activity, the following recipes for base solutions (when stored in sterile, single-use glass bottles) have been tested for stability of osmolality, sodium, chloride, calcium, potassium, and amiloride concentrations. Repeated measurements indicate that these concentrations vary by ≤15% over 18 months (29). In efforts to reduce variability in NPD performance during multicenter trials, base solutions have been centrally produced through partnerships with academic or industry pharmacies. Since NPD solutions are not routinely available outside of sponsored clinical trials, it is often necessary for sites to have the capability to mix solutions on-site. The CFF-TDN recommends the use of USP-grade agents when available and storage at 4°C in single-use, 50–100-ml bottles or vials following sterile filtration at 4 °C. The instructions for mixing solutions and 3% agar dissolved in Ringer's solution (for bridges and nasal non-perfusion catheter probes) provided below are based on CFF-TDN Standard Operation Procedures (SOPs; 2009) and have been successfully used to discriminate between

CF and non-CF subjects, and to detect biologic activity of CFTR modulators (13):

- *Ringer's solution (solution #1)*: Commercial Ringer's solution injection (Baxter Healthcare) + phosphates (pH 5.5, 147.5 meq Na, 4 meq K, 4.5 meq Ca, 156 meq Cl, 309 mOsm)

	Salts	MW	mM/L	G/L
	NaCl	58	148	8.58
	$CaCl_2 \bullet 2H_2O$	147	2.25	0.33
	KCl	74	4.05	0.30
Add	*K_2HPO_4*	*174*	*2.4*	*0.42*
Add	*KH_2PO_4*	*136*	*0.4*	*0.05*
Add	*$MgCl_2 \bullet 6H_2O$*	*203*	*1.2*	*0.24*

- *Amiloride (solution #2)*: 30 mg/L of amiloride HCl (MW = 302) is added to the Ringer's solution + phosphates described above. Warming of the solution to 35–37°C and stirring can help to dissolve the amiloride. The base solution used is double distilled H_2O.
- *Zero Cl^- (solution #3)*: 0 [Cl^-] solution (to otherwise match Ringer's solution injection): (pH 5.5, 147.5 meq Na, 4 meq K, 4.5 meq Ca, 156 meq Cl, 309 mOsm). The base solution used is ddH_2O.

	Salts	MW	mM/L	G/L
Add	Na gluconate	218	148	32.26
Add	Ca gluconate	430	2.25	0.97
Add	K gluconate	234	4.05	0.95
Add	K_2HPO_4	174	2.4	0.42
Add	KH_2PO_4	136	0.4	0.05
Add	$MgSO_4 \bullet 7H_2O$	246	1.2	0.30

The pH of solutions is adjusted to 7.4 (1 N NaOH), followed by sterile filtering (0.22 μm) and storage in single-use, 50–100-ml bottles or polystyrene tubes. Solutions should be stored at 4°C and warmed immediately prior to use.

- *Isoproterenol (solution #4)*: It is made by adding sterile isoproterenol (e.g., Hospira, Inc., Lake Forest, IL; 0.2 mg/ml; MW = 248) to solution #3 to a final concentration of 10 μM. Isoproterenol should be added immediately prior to use and protected from light. It can be frequently ordered through the institutional pharmacy.

- *ATP (solution #5)*: It is made by adding ATP to solution #4 to a final concentration of 100 μM. A stock solution of concentrated ATP can be made by adding 55 mg to 2 ml of ddH_2O, sterile filtering, and storing as 0.10 ml aliquots at –20°C. About 0.10 ml is then added to 50 ml of solution #4.
- *3% agar in Ringer's solution* is used to make the skin bridge and the nasal non-perfusion probe catheter. To make stock, 6 g of agar (Difco or equivalent) is dissolved in 200 ml of solution #1 in a large-mouth, autoclave-tolerant bottle with a screw top. The sealed bottle is then autoclaved (160°C, 30 min) and allowed to cool. This process fully dissolves the agar and removes all bubbles, which helps to ensure that the single-use bridges and catheters are free from bubbles when made immediately prior to NPD performance.
- *3 M KCl* dissolved in H_2O is used to store the calomel electrodes. The glass end of the two calomels should be submerged in the 3 M KCl, and the two calomel solutions should be connected by a 3% agar bridge when not in use to ensure that no offsets develop between the calomels. Periodically check to ensure that the 3 M KCl solutions are full and the calomels are submerged. The internal chamber of the calomels is also filled with 3 M KCl and should be periodically checked to ensure that the solution has not been depleted/evaporated. Excess KCl crystals on the surfaces of the calomels and calomel solutions should be removed.

3. Methods

3.1. Preparation and Setup of the Potential Difference Apparatus

- Warm stock solutions #1, #2, and #3 prior to use. Make solution #4 by adding aliquoted isoproterenol to solution #3. Make solution #5 by adding aliquoted isoproterenol and ATP to solution #3.
- Place all solutions in syringes labeled #1, #2, #3, #4, and #5.
- Attach infusion tubing to syringes, and place three-way stopcocks on the free ends of the infusion sets as shown in **Fig. 6.2**. The stopcocks can then be connected and taped to the side of the warmer bath.
- Pass the infusion tubing through the warming water bath (typically set at approximately 40°C to achieve probe temperature of 32–37°C). Check the temperature of the solution exiting the probe catheter to ensure that it is in the appropriate range.

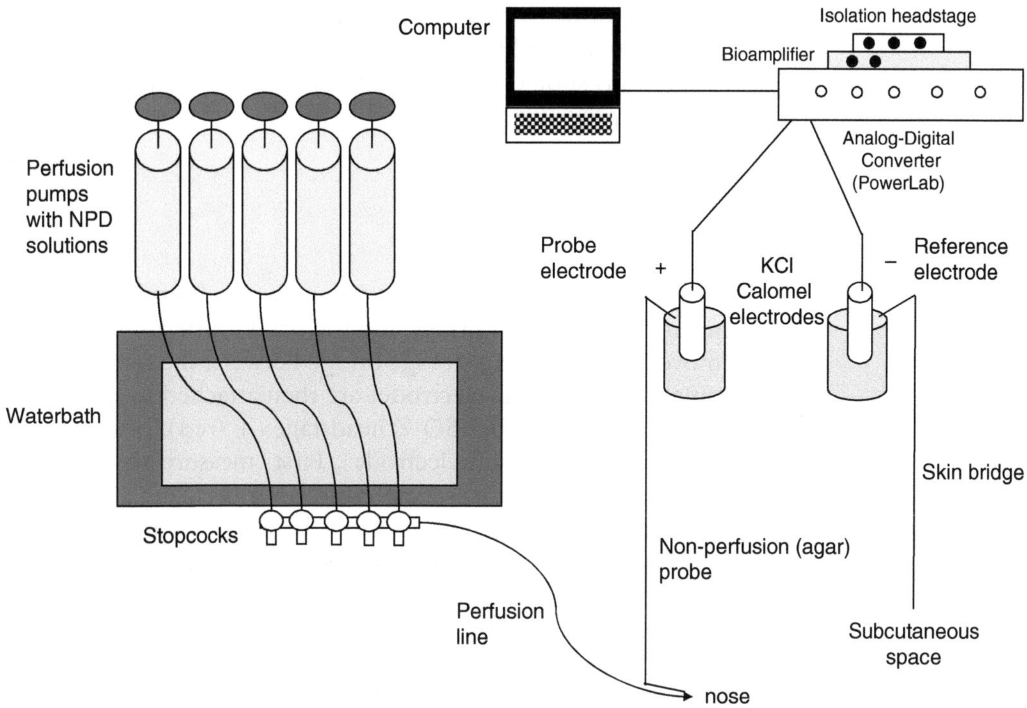

Fig. 6.2. Schematic diagram of the nasal potential difference apparatus.

- To make the skin bridge, loosen the lid of the agar bottle and warm the 3% agar for 10–30 s in a microwave. Carefully remove approximately 5 ml with a 10-ml sterile syringe and remove bubbles. Attach the syringe to a 23-gauge butterfly needle luer lock. Slowly inject the agar until the agar escapes from the needle end of the butterfly and backfill the luer lock to ensure that no bubbles are entrained. Allow the bridge to cool (~5 min).
- To make the non-perfusion nasal catheter probe, measure approximately 3 ft of PE90 and PE50 tubing. Bring the end of both tubes together and place a 1-cm silastic sleeve over the end of the tubes (helped by dipping the tip in 70% EtOH). Cut the end so that the sleeved end is flushed. Attach a 23-gauge needle to the free end of the PE50, and attach the luer lock end to the first stopcock. For the non-perfusion probe, place a 20-gauge luer stub adapter on the free end of the PE90 tube. Slowly inject the warmed 3% agar through the PE90 until the agar is seen exiting the sleeved end. Backfill the luer lock to ensure that no bubbles are entrained and allow it to cool (~5 min).
- Backflush the five perfusates through the probe electrode catheter, including perfusion of solutions #5, #4, #3, #2, and #1 for approximately 30 s each. Turn the stopcocks in

reverse order during this procedure to ensure that later solutions are cleared from the nasal probe. Solution #1 (Ringer's solution) should be the solution filling the tubing at the end of this procedure.

3.2. The Nasal Potential Difference Procedure

3.2.1. Offsets and Calibration

The next steps are to ensure that there are no offsets in the entire setup and that the skin bridge and the nasal probe are functional. Remove the connecting storage bridge between the two 3 M KCl calomel solutions. The electrodes are then attached to the appropriate connectors of the ISO-Z headstage (+ (red) for nasal electrode, – (black) for skin electrode). First, measure the potential between the two calomels by placing both in a single 3 M KCl calomel solution. Dial any offset out by adjusting the bioamplifier. Second, place the two calomels in their separate 3 M KCl baths and connect the two solutions with the skin bridge. The PD should be near zero and confirms that the skin bridge is functional. Third, remove the skin bridge and replace with the nasal probe electrode catheter. Again, the PD should be near zero. Fourth, place the luer end of the skin bridge in the skin 3 M KCl solution and the luer end of the probe catheter in the nasal 3 M KCl solution. Place the free ends of the skin bridge and the probe catheter (the needle end of the skin bridge and the sleeved end of the nasal probe) in a single 50-ml tube of Ringer's solution and measure the PD. This is the "closed-loop offset," and ensures that all components of the PD apparatus are functional. The PD should be near zero (±3 mV). Dial the bioamplifier to remove any remaining offsets. If the offset is larger or the circuit is open, either the probe catheter or the skin bridge is dysfunctional and should be replaced.

3.2.2. Skin, Anterior Tip, and Basal PDs

Using sterile technique, place the skin bridge needle in the subcutaneous space of the forearm of the study subject and gently pinch the probe catheter tip between their index finger and thumb. Dipping the end of the probe catheter in the Ringer's solution may be necessary to make a stable connection. The skin PD is typically between –35 and –75 mV. Record the "skin PD." Place the probe catheter in the right nares under direct visualization with the otoscope and nasal illuminator, and advance the probe catheter into the inferior meatus (under the inferior turbinate) to 3 cm to measure the PD. Record the PD at 3, 2, 1.5, 1.0, and 0.5 cm for approximately 5 s each. Place the catheter on the anterior tip of the inferior turbinate (AT) at the completion of the basal measurements at the anterior tip of the inferior turbinate. This is the AT measurement and it is generally between 0 and –15 mV. This value is similar in CF and non-CF subjects, as the AT surface is typically squamous epithelium (and not respiratory epithelium) and serves as a reference value (along with the skin PD) to be rechecked throughout the procedure. Record the AT measurement for 5 s. Remove the catheter and repeat the procedure for the left nostril. These steps complete the basal PD measurements.

3.2.3. Performing the NPD Tracings

Measure the PD of the right nostril AT and then remove the nasal illuminator. Place a small piece of water-resistant tape on the tip of the nose. Place the probe catheter in the right nares under the inferior turbinate. This can often be done "blind" based on knowledge of the values obtained during the "basal PDs" but can also be performed by directly visualizing with a otorhinoscope or a nasal dilator and illuminating headlamp. Attempt to locate the most polarized PD under the right inferior turbinate and secure the catheter in position with tape. Check that the catheter is in the inferior meatus using the otoscope and nasal illuminator, and note the distance within the inferior meatus (0.5–3 cm). Start perfusion with solution #1 (Ringer's solution) and have the subject assume a comfortable position (often with head slightly down so that the perfusate exits the nostril). Begin recording the "tracing PD" and indicate the start of perfusion with "Ringer's solution." Once Ringer's solution has been perfused for 1 min and a stable PD has been obtained (± 1 mV) for a minimum of 30 s, turn off the solution #1 pump, turn the first stopcock "off" to solution #1, and open the solution #2 perfusate. Turn on the solution #2 (Ringer's solution + amiloride) pump, mark the initiation of "amiloride" perfusion, and record for a minimum of 3 min (maximum of 5 min). When a stable PD has been obtained, turn off the solution #2 pump, turn the second stopcock "off" to solution #2, and begin perfusion with solution #3 (zero Cl + amiloride). Mark the initiation of "zero Cl" perfusion and record for a minimum of 3 min (maximum of 5 min). When a stable PD has been obtained, turn off the solution #3 pump, turn the third stopcock "off" to solution #3, and begin perfusion with solution #4 (zero Cl + amiloride + isoproterenol). Mark the initiation of "Iso" perfusion and record for a minimum of 3 min (maximum of 5 min). When a stable PD has been obtained, turn off the solution #4 pump, turn the fourth stopcock "off" to solution #4, and begin perfusion with solution #5 (zero Cl + amiloride + isoproterenol + ATP). Mark the initiation of "ATP" perfusion and record for a minimum of 1 min (maximum of 5 min) until a peak value is obtained. Once completed, turn off solution #5 and stop recording. Remove the tape and probe catheter, and backflush solutions #4, #3, #2, and #1 in reverse order (30–60 s each), turning the stopcocks in reverse order. Using the nasal illuminator and otoscope, re-measure the right AT PD and record. Measure the skin PD and then repeat the "tracing PD" steps for the left nostril, including the left AT before and after the tracing. Re-measure the skin PD at the completion of the left tracing PD and then remove the skin bridge. Repeat the "closed-loop offset" measurement at the end of the procedure to ensure that no offsets have developed during the procedure (the value should again be near zero). This completes the entire NPD procedure.

3.3. Analysis

Nasal potential difference tracings should be reviewed by an expert familiar with the technique, as care must be taken to discriminate between tracings reflecting an accurate result and tracings that are unstable and therefore may not reflect the true potential difference of the subject. In the setting of clinical research trials, blinded review is strongly recommended to prevent potential bias from affecting interpretation of the NPD or determination of the validity of particular tracings. Review by a single interpreter should also be considered, as the inter-reader agreement between blinded reviewers has not been evaluated in a rigorous fashion. The analysis discussed below is based upon experience during CFF-TDN studies.

3.3.1. Scoring the Potential Difference Tracing

The basal PD is measured at various distances within the inferior meatus in the right nostril (3.0, 2.0, 1.5, 1.0, and 0.5 cm), followed by the left nostril. For each of these measures, a plateau value is obtained for approximately 5 s, and the mean PD is determined during the stable plateau. A similar method is used for the finger, anterior tip of the inferior meatus, and offset measurements. Based on these results, both the maximally negative (most polarizing) value and the mean basal PD are calculated for each nostril. To score each NPD tracing, the PD for each superperfusion solution is measured once the PD reaches a stable value after the minimum perfusion time (*see* **Section 3.2.3** above). The mean PD for the final 10 s of perfusion solution is calculated using the LabChart software and should represent a stable area of the tracing (**Fig. 6.3**). For solution #5 (ATP), the peak (most polarizing) value is calculated as the mean value over 2 s at the peak (most negative) value. From the values measured above, derived within tracing changes in PD can be calculated. These include alternative measures of sodium transport (change in PD following amiloride and percentage change in PD following amiloride), measures of CFTR-dependent chloride transport (change in PD following zero-chloride perfusion, change in PD following isoproterenol perfusion, and the sum of these changes), and measures of CFTR-independent chloride transport (change in PD following ATP perfusion). In CF, the Ringer's solution PD, the derived parameter of sodium transport, and the derived measures of CFTR-dependent Cl^- transport each correlates with the severity of the CF genotype (Table **6.1**). The change following zero chloride + isoproterenol is widely considered the

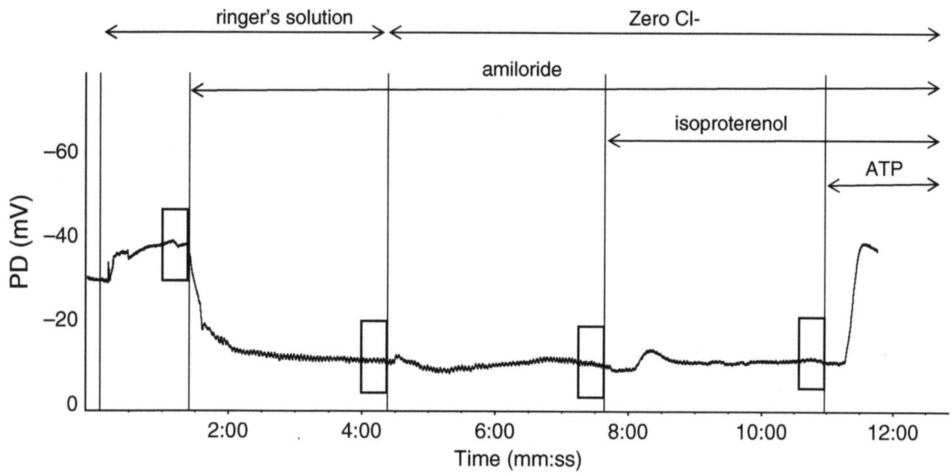

Fig. 6.3. Representative potential difference tracing from a CF subject demonstrating methodology used to calculate PD and quantify tracing stability. *Open boxes* represent the 10 s scoring interval used to quantify the PD and tracing stability.

most sensitive and specific indicator of CFTR-dependent anion transport, is included in diagnostic algorithms for CF, and is a frequent outcome measure in CF clinical trials of CFTR modulators. The total change in PD (end Cl-free isoproterenol – end Ringer's solution perfusion (26)) and the Wilschanski index [$e^{(\text{response to chloride-free isoproterenol/response to amiloride})}$, with a cut-off >0.70 to predict a CF diagnosis (30)] are alternative derived endpoints that incorporate both sodium and chloride transport and have also demonstrated reasonable diagnostic accuracy.

4. Notes

4.1. Alternative Methods

A number of alternative methods to measure the NPD have been developed since its first description, as the relative lack of standardization of the measure (until recently) encouraged a number of innovations to be developed at individual centers. While this section does not capture all of these alternative methods, a number of these are highlighted here.

4.1.1. Perfusion Catheter

Rather than using an exploring probe filled with agar gel, the exploring probe can be filled with Ringer's solution that continuously perfuses at a slow rate (12 ml/h) so that continuity with the nasal surface is maintained. This method was utilized in the original description by Knowles et al. and in previous standard operating procedures adopted by the CFF-TDN (2). A disadvantage with this method is that bubbles can form in the continuous perfusion line (a process predicted to occur by Bernoulli's principle when pumping solution with dissolved gas through a narrow caliber line), which results in artifact and breaks in the tracing, and can also induce an electrical resistance in the probe electrode. This method also detects greater electrical interference from the ambient environment which can include electrical noise from the continuous perfusion pumps used in the NPD setup.

4.1.2. Single Lumen Catheter

To reduce the size of the nasal probe, the perfusing line and the exploring probe can be united by a T connector (or equivalent device) proximal to the nasal interface (2). This has the advantage of allowing placement in infants and young children, or individuals with a small inferior meatus. The principal disadvantage is that the method is prone to artifacts from bubbles within the perfusion line, similar to the perfusion catheter. The perfusion line is the distal portion of the exploring probe and can transmit microbubbles and electrical noise into the NPD signal.

4.1.3. Nasal Floor Placement

Instead of placement within the inferior meatus, the nasal catheter can be placed in the floor of the medial nasal cavity (3). This is facilitated by the use of a larger diameter catheter (such as a pediatric Foley catheter) and one that utilizes a side port to allow directional orientation to the exploring interface. Placement of the catheter with this method allows blinded placement, but may be more uncomfortable for some patients (as perfusion is more likely to run into the pharyngeal space rather than out of the nostril), and is a limitation in individuals with small nasal orifices.

4.1.4. Ag–AgCl Electrodes

Ag–AgCl electrodes are frequently used for medical applications and have been successfully employed for NPD measurements in lieu of KCl calomel electrodes. Care must be taken to maintain the working surface of the Ag–AgCl electrode and offsets measured between paired electrodes on a regular basis. Interface with the metal surface of the electrode is typically made through Ringer's solution or a mixture of Ringer's solution and ECG cream (2, 3). Common Ag–AgCl electrodes used for this purpose include AgCl microelectrode holder half cell (Item No. Ref-2L, 64-1302; Warner Instruments) or pellet-type electrodes (Cat. # E-22X, 10-02060; CWE, Inc.).

4.1.5. Abrasion Subcutaneous Bridge

The reference bridge can connect with the subcutaneous space using a small needle placed and secured into position as described above, or by inducing a small dermal abrasion with a sterile rotary tool, permitting access to the subcutaneous compartment. The dermal abrasion interface is typically made by placing ECG conducting gel and a Ag–AgCl electrode over the abrasion, and securing with an adherent dressing (3, 31, 32). This method is particularly advantageous for individuals with needle anxiety but necessitates use of Ag–AgCl electrodes and ECG conducting gel to maintain symmetry between electrodes. The method also requires careful attention to maintain the sterility of the rotary tool between subjects.

4.1.6. Strip-chart Recorder

Strip-chart recorder can be used instead of the electronic data capture device to obtain NPD results (12). While providing the essential information, analog capture and low-pass filters intrinsic to strip-chart recorders do not allow monitoring of ambient electrical noise. Moreover, handwritten notes that accompany the strip-chart tracings may need special handling to ensure blinding. A typical strip chart utilized for NPD measurement include flatbed recorders (Item No. BD11E; Kipp and Zoe).

4.2. Interpretation of Potential Difference Results

Internal consistency of the tracing can be judged by repeated measures of the electrical offset, finger, and anterior tip of the inferior turbinate performed throughout the session. Tracings with frequent or sustained breaks in the tracing often indicate poor interface with the study subject, which can occur due to problems with the nasal catheter, reference bridge, or monitoring equipment. The most frequent cause is development of a bubble in the nasal probe or poor contact with the nasal mucosa, and is particularly problematic with nasal probes based on the continuous perfusion of Ringer's solution.

4.3. Tracing Interpretability and Quality

It is helpful to provide objective criteria regarding the quality of NPD tracings, a process facilitated by central review. The CFF-TDN Center for CFTR Detection at the University of Alabama at Birmingham assigns a "confidence score" to each tracing reviewed in a blinded fashion for research studies. Criteria that can contribute to a low confidence score include sustained breaks in the tracing (>30 s), abrupt changes in the PD (>5 mV over 1 s or less that do not rapidly return to baseline), or tracings that do not have a significant response (>3 mV change) to both amiloride and ATP (often due to disruptions in the nasal membrane) (13). Additional criteria that indicate accurate NPD results include tracing stability assessed by the variance of the PD plateau voltage and the frequency of tracing artifacts (defined as PD values that shift >5 mV and are not sustained or otherwise considered reliable), which likely represent transient breaks in the PD circuit (28).

4.4. Reproducibility

NPD measurement is a reproducible procedure within subject, but care must be taken to optimize results, particularly when used in the context of clinical trials (12, 33). Yaakov et al. (34) examined the within-patient repeatability of NPD measurements at a single center. They examined on at least two occasions 68 CF patients, 25 with classic disease and 43 with non-classic disease (defined as patients with a CF phenotype in at least one organ system but normal or borderline sweat chloride measurements, two

CF-causing mutations, and abnormal NPD). Using the paired *t*-test and Wilcoxon test, the repeated NPD measures were reproducible. In part to improve the reproducibility of NPD measurement in the context of multicenter trials, the standard operating procedure of the Cystic Fibrosis Therapeutics Development Network was devised. This has included several factors to improve between-center and between-operator variability, including use of warmed centrally produced perfusion solutions, standardized equipment, and technical training of NPD operators. Avoiding changes in nasal medication known to alter NPD, including nasal steroids in particular, is another caveat to consider.

Acknowledgments

The authors are grateful to Michael Knowles for providing a critical review of the material presented and also to Peter Durie for helpful critiques in devising current methods proposed here. Support for this work was provided by the US National Institute of Health grants 1K23DK075788-01 and 1R03DK084110-01 (to S.M.R.), 1P30DK072482-01A1 (to Eric J. Sorscher for infrastructural support) and Cystic Fibrosis Foundation grants CLANCY05Y2 (S.M.R. and J.P.C.). This project was supported in part by grants from the National Institute of Diabetes and Digestive and Kidney Diseases and the National Heart, Lung, and Blood Institute. The content is solely the responsibility of the authors and does not necessarily represent the official views of the National Institute of Diabetes and Digestive and Kidney Diseases; National Heart, Lung, and Blood Institute; or the National Institutes of Health.

References

1. Knowles, M., Gatzy, J., and Boucher, R. (1981) Increased bioelectric potential difference across respiratory epithelia in cystic fibrosis. *N. Engl. J. Med.* **305**, 1489–1495.
2. Knowles, M. R., Paradiso, A. M., and Boucher, R. C. (1995) In vivo nasal potential difference: Techniques and protocols for assessing efficacy of gene transfer in cystic fibrosis. *Hum. Gene Ther.* **6**, 445–455.
3. Middleton, P. G., Geddes, D. M., and Alton, E. W. (1994) Protocols for in vivo measurement of the ion transport defects in cystic fibrosis nasal epithelium. *Eur. Respir. J.* **7**, 2050–2056.
4. Farrell, P. M., Rosenstein, B. J., White, T. B., Accurso, F. J., Castellani, C., Cutting, G. R. et al. (2008) Guidelines for diagnosis of cystic fibrosis in newborns through older adults: Cystic fibrosis foundation consensus report. *J. Pediatr.* **153**, S4–S14.
5. De Boeck, K., Wilschanski, M., Castellani, C., Taylor, C., Cuppens, H., Dodge, J. et al. (2006) Cystic fibrosis: Terminology and diagnostic algorithms. *Thorax* **61**, 627–635.
6. Knowles, M. R., Hohneker, K. W., Zhou, Z., Olsen, J. C., Noah, T. L., Hu, P. C. et al. (1995) A controlled study of adenoviral-vector-mediated gene transfer in the nasal

epithelium of patients with cystic fibrosis. *N. Engl. J. Med.* **333**, 823–831.
7. Noone, P. G., Hohneker, K. W., Zhou, Z., Johnson, L. G., Foy, C., Gipson, C. et al. (2000) Safety and biological efficacy of a lipid-CFTR complex for gene transfer in the nasal epithelium of adult patients with cystic fibrosis. *Mol. Ther.* **1**, 105–114.
8. Middleton, P. G., Caplen, N. J., Gao, X., Huang, L., Gaya, H., Geddes, D. M. et al. (1994) Nasal application of the cationic liposome DC-Chol: DOPE does not alter ion transport, lung function or bacterial growth. *Eur. Respir. J.* 7, 442–445.
9. McCarty, N. A., Standaert, T. A., Teresi, M., Tuthill, C., Launspach, J., Kelley, T. J. et al. (2002) A phase I randomized, multicenter trial of CPX in adult subjects with mild cystic fibrosis. *Pediatr. Pulmonol.* **33**, 90–98.
10. Wilschanski, M., Yahav, Y., Yaacov, Y., Blau, H., Bentur, L., Rivlin, J. et al. (2003) Gentamicin-induced correction of CFTR function in patients with cystic fibrosis and CFTR stop mutations. *N. Engl. J. Med.* **349**, 1433–1441.
11. Kerem, E., Yaacov, Y., Armoni, S. et al. (2008) PTC124 induces time-dependent improvements in chloride conductance and clinical parameters in patients with nonsense-mutation-mediated cystic fibrosis. *Pediatr. Pulmonol. Suppl.* **31**, 294.
12. Clancy, J. P., Rowe, S. M., Bebok, Z., Aitken, M. L., Gibson, R., Zeitlin, P. et al. (2007) No detectable improvements in cystic fibrosis transmembrane conductance regulator by nasal aminoglycosides in patients with cystic fibrosis with stop mutations. *Am. J. Respir. Cell. Mol. Biol.* **37**, 57–66.
13. Accurso, F. J., Rowe, S. M., Clancy, J. P., Boyle, M. P., Dunitz, J. M., Durie, P. R., Sagel, S. D., Hornick, D. B., Konstan, M. W., Donaldson, S. H., Moss, R. B., Pilewski, J. M., Rubenstein, R. C., Uluer, A. Z., Aitken, M. L., Freedman, S. D., Rose, L. M., Mayer-Hamblett, N., Dong, Q., Zha, J., Stone, A.J., Olson, E. R., Ordonez, C. L., Campbell, P. W., Ashlock, M. A., and Ramsey, B. W. (2010) Effect of VX-770 in persons with cystic fibrosis and the G551D-CFTR mutation. *N. Engl. J. Med.* **363**, 1991–2003.
14. Konstan, M. W., Davis, P. B., Wagener, J. S., Hilliard, K. A., Stern, R. C., Milgram, L. J. et al. (2004) Compacted DNA nanoparticles administered to the nasal mucosa of cystic fibrosis subjects are safe and demonstrate partial to complete cystic fibrosis transmembrane regulator reconstitution. *Hum. Gene Ther.* **15**, 1255–1269.
15. Zeitlin, P. L., Boyle, M. P., Guggino, W. B., and Molina, L. (2004) A phase I trial of intranasal Moli1901 for cystic fibrosis. *Chest* **125**, 143–149.
16. Rowe, S. M., Accurso, F., and Clancy, J. P. (2007) Detection of cystic fibrosis transmembrane conductance regulator activity in early-phase clinical trials. *Proc. Am. Thorac. Soc.* **4**, 387–398.
17. Rowe, S. M., Reeves, G., Young, H. et al. (2008) Correction of sodium transport with nasal administration of the prostasin inhibitor QAU145 in CF subjects. *Pediatr. Pulmonol. Suppl.* **31**, A268.
18. Rowe, S. M., Miller, S., and Sorscher, E. J. (2005) Cystic fibrosis. *N. Engl. J. Med.* **352**, 1992–2001.
19. Gatzy, J. T. (1967) Bioelectric properties of the isolated amphibian lung. *Am. J. Physiol.* **213**, 425–431.
20. Knowles, M. R., Carson, J. L., Collier, A. M., Gatzy, J. T., and Boucher, R. C. (1981) Measurements of nasal transepithelial electric potential differences in normal human subjects in vivo. *Am. Rev. Respir. Dis.* **124**, 484–490.
21. Knowles, M. R., Buntin, W. H., Bromberg, P. A., Gatzy, J. T., and Boucher, R. C. (1982) Measurements of transepithelial electric potential differences in the trachea and bronchi of human subjects in vivo. *Am. Rev. Respir. Dis.* **126**, 108–112.
22. Davies, J. C., Davies, M., McShane, D., Smith, S., Chadwick, S., Jaffe, A. et al. (2005) Potential difference measurements in the lower airway of children with and without cystic fibrosis. *Am. J. Respir. Crit. Care Med.* **171**, 1015–1019.
23. Anderson, M. P., Gregory, R. J., Thompson, S., Souza, D. W., Paul, S., Mulligan, R. C. et al. (1991) Demonstration that CFTR is a chloride channel by alteration of its anion selectivity. *Science* **253**, 202–205.
24. Li, C., and Naren, A. P. (2005) Macromolecular complexes of cystic fibrosis transmembrane conductance regulator and its interacting partners. *Pharmacol. Ther.* **108**, 208–223.
25. Olivier, K. N., Bennett, W. D., Hohneker, K. W., Zeman, K. L., Edwards, L. J., Boucher, R. C. et al. (1996) Acute safety and effects on mucociliary clearance of aerosolized uridine 5′-triphosphate ± amiloride in normal human adults. *Am. J. Respir. Crit. Care Med.* **154**, 217–223.
26. Wilschanski, M., Dupuis, A., Ellis, L., Jarvi, K., Zielenski, J., Tullis, E. et al. (2006) Mutations in the cystic fibrosis transmembrane regulator gene and in vivo transepithe-

lial potentials. *Am. J. Respir. Crit. Care Med.* **174**, 787–794.
27. Fajac, I., Hubert, D., Guillemot, D., Honoré, I., Bienvenu, T., Volter, F. et al. (2004) Nasal airway ion transport is linked to the cystic fibrosis phenotype in adult patients. *Thorax* **59**, 971–976.
28. Solomon, G. M., Konstan, M. W., Wilschanski, M., Billings, J., Sermet-Gaudelus, I., Accurso, F., Vermeulen, F., Levin, E., Hathorne, H., Reeves, G., Sabbatini, G., Hill, A., Mayer-Hamblett, N., Ashlock, M., Clancy, J. P., and Rowe, S. M. (2010) An international randomized multicenter comparison of nasal potential difference techniques. *Chest* **138**, 919–928.
29. Cohen, M., Beamer, J. R., Clancy, J. P. et al. (2008) Centralized production and long term stability of electrolytes and amiloride in solutions for nasal potential difference testing. *Pediatr. Pulmonol. Suppl.* **31**, A275.
30. Wilschanski, M., Famini, H., Strauss-Liviatan, N., Rivlin, J., Blau, H., Bibi, H. et al. (2001) Nasal potential difference measurements in patients with atypical cystic fibrosis. *Eur. Respir. J.* **17**, 1208–1215.
31. Sermet-Gaudelus, I., Renouil, M., Fajac, A., Bidou, L., Parbaille, B., Pierrot, S. et al. (2007) In vitro prediction of stop-codon suppression by intravenous gentamicin in patients with cystic fibrosis: A pilot study. *BMC Med.* **5**, 5.
32. Leal, T., Lebacq, J., Lebecque, P., Cumps, J., and Wallemacq, P. (2003) Modified method to measure nasal potential difference. *Clin. Chem. Lab. Med.* **41**, 61–67.
33. Ahrens, R. C., Standaert, T. A., Launspach, J., Han, S. H., Teresi, M. E., Aitken, M. L. et al. (2002) Use of nasal potential difference and sweat chloride as outcome measures in multicenter clinical trials in subjects with cystic fibrosis. *Pediatr. Pulmonol.* **33**, 142–150.
34. Yaakov, Y., Kerem, E., Yahav, Y., Rivlin, J., Blau, H., Bentur, L. et al. (2007) Reproducibility of nasal potential difference measurements in cystic fibrosis. *Chest* **132**, 1219–1226.

Chapter 7

Measurement of Ion Transport Function in Rectal Biopsies

Martin J. Hug, Nico Derichs, Inez Bronsveld, and Jean Paul Clancy

Abstract

Cystic fibrosis (CF) is caused by mutations in the gene encoding for the cystic fibrosis transmembrane conductance regulator (CFTR). CFTR functions as an anion channel and is known to interact with a number of other cellular proteins involved in ion transport. To date more than 1,800 mutations are known, most of which result in various degrees of impaired transport function of the gene product. Due to the high inter-individual variability of disease onset and progression, CF still is a diagnostic challenge. Implemented almost 20 years ago, the measurement of electrolyte transport function of rectal biopsies is a useful ex vivo tool to diagnose CF. In this chapter we will review the different approaches to perform ion transport measurements and try to highlight the advantages and limitations of these techniques.

Key words: Epithelial cells, cystic fibrosis, CFTR, Ussing chamber, electrolyte transport.

1. Introduction

1.1. Epithelia – Structure and Function

Epithelia can be found wherever our body faces the environment such as in the airways, the gastrointestinal tract, part of the skin, and the urogenital tract.

Epithelial tissues serve two functions: they separate the body from and exchange substances with the environment. They are exposed to a constantly changing environment and have to adapt to the surrounding conditions. In order to fulfill these functions epithelial cells require two distinct features: a tight cell-to-cell connection and polarized expression of membrane proteins. These properties also determine whether a certain tissue may be categorized as a 'leaky' or a 'tight' epithelium, respectively. Generally these terms refer to the ratio between para- and transcellular transport of a given tissue.

M.D. Amaral, K. Kunzelmann (eds.), *Cystic Fibrosis*, Methods in Molecular Biology 741,
DOI 10.1007/978-1-61779-117-8_7, © Springer Science+Business Media, LLC 2011

To estimate the contribution of either pathway to the net transport of an epithelium we have to understand how one can measure this process. Let us therefore start by giving a brief overview about the many studies on electrolyte transport by epithelia.

1.2. Studies on Epithelial Transport

Studies on epithelial transport began in the year 1889 when the Scottish scientist Edward Waymouth Reid published one of the first reports about epithelial solute transport. He submitted a manuscript describing an apparatus that could be described as an early forerunner of what we now call an Ussing chamber (1). Reid mounted frog skin between two half-chambers that were filled with normal saline. Two cylinders connected to each side were used to monitor the volume of liquid filled in each chamber. Provided the tissue in the middle was viable, a decrease in the volume of the chamber facing the outside of the frog skin and an increase in the opposite chamber was observed over time. Due to the fact that the amount of volume shifted from one side to the other of the frog skin was also inversely correlated with the time the tissue was removed from its proprietor, Reid concluded that this phenomenon could only be explained by some energy-driven mechanism. Later he extended his studies to other epithelia such as the rabbit ileum where he noticed that under some conditions the direction of the transport could even be reversed (2).

The history of transepithelial ion transport measurements cannot be written without the Danish scientist Hans Henrikson Ussing. Born in 1911, Ussing followed the footsteps of his teacher, the Nobel Prize winner Schack August Steenberg Krogh, and started by studying transport processes in living cells. Similar to Reid, Ussing also chose the isolated frog skin to work with. Impressed by the observation that the frog skin has a negative voltage outside when compared to the inside, he wondered whether this voltage difference is the cause for or the result of the transport processes across that tissue. Ussing's studies were aided by the introduction of radioactive tracers to experimental physiology during the mid-1940s. His first approach was to mount a piece of frog skin between two half-chambers similar to the apparatus Reid had built almost 100 years earlier. But instead of studying the transport of liquid volume, Hans Ussing filled one chamber with Ringer's solution that contained the isotope $^{24}Na^{+}$ while the opposite chamber was supplemented with $^{22}Na^{+}$. Much to his surprise the transport of the labeled cations was almost unidirectional from the mucosal (apical, outside) to the serosal (basolateral, blood) side (3). In a further series of experiments Ussing could demonstrate that the Cl^{-} ions move in a passive fashion (4). It was apparent to him that a negative voltage on the outside cannot promote the flux of Na^{+} to the inside. Therefore Ussing concluded that the transepithelial voltage difference must be the

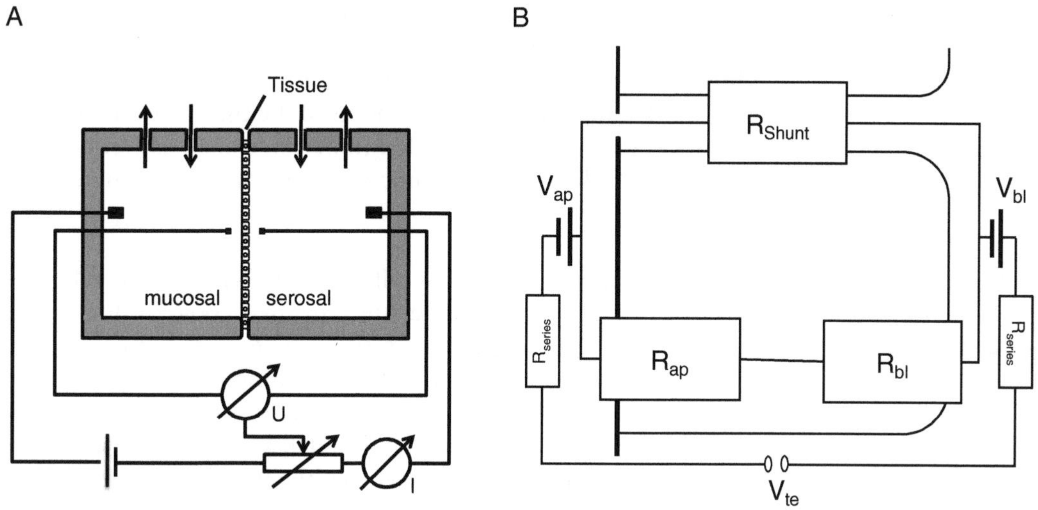

Fig. 7.1. (**a**) Schematic drawing of an Ussing chamber for the measurement of I_{SC}. (**b**) Equivalent circuit of a tissue consisting of a single monolayer of cells.

consequence and not the cause of the unidirectional transport of Na^+ ions. To test his hypothesis he modified his apparatus by adding a pair of electrodes connected to a voltmeter and another pair of electrodes wired to a battery in order to pass an external current through the epithelium (*see* **Fig. 7.1a**). Ussing's idea was that when he adjusted the external current loop so that the voltage across the epithelium became 0 he would essentially remove any driving force for ion transport via a diffusional pathway. This approach is generally referred to as short circuiting. A short circuit flows when you, for instance, connect the two poles of a battery thereby decreasing the resistance to nominally 0. Obviously, Ussing did not just connect the two sides of the frog skin with a piece of wire but used the external voltage source in order to overcome the limited capacity of the 'battery' epithelium. The current that was necessary to voltage clamp the epithelium to 0 was almost identical to the net transport of $^{24}Na^+$ and was named short circuit current (I_{SC}) from then on (5). With this tool in hand Ussing was able to perform I_{SC} measurements and use the current reading as a surrogate parameter for any transepithelial ion transport.

The apparatus designed by Hans Ussing has soon been adapted by many scientists worldwide and was named after its inventor 'Ussing chamber.' While the mechanical design has been customized to fit the various tissues studied, very little change has been done to the basic setup using two voltage and two current electrodes. Technical advances have been made over the years: the feedback loop through a simple voltage divider has been replaced by operational amplifiers built into integrated circuits and the shape and duration of the clamp voltage have been modified to meet the respective requirements. Modulating the clamp voltage at a spectrum of different frequencies and high-resolution sampling of the resulting current have made it possible to mathematically model the electrical components of the tissue mounted in the chamber (6). A technique called impedance analysis can be used to electronically dissect the mucosal from the serosal membrane (7, 8).

1.3. Electrolyte Transport by the Distal Colon

The distal colon is sometimes called a 'tight' epithelium. Whether this description is appropriate still remains a topic of discussion. Reports on the transepithelial resistance, R_{te}, of the colon vary from roughly 100 to 500 $\Omega{\cdot}cm^2$ depending on the species and cell type studied (9, 10). The ratio between para- and transepithelial transport can be as high as 1:10, which would suffice to classify the distal colon as a tight epithelium (10). The colonic mucosa is structurally divided into two morphologically and functionally distinct parts: the surface epithelial cells and the crypts. It is believed that the surface epithelial cells are responsible for the predominant function of the colon, the absorption of fluid and electrolytes (11). The model in **Fig. 7.2a** depicts the ion transporters in an absorbing colonic epithelial cell (CEC). The mechanism by which Na^+ is taken up by colonocytes is similar to what Ussing has demonstrated for the frog skin. Na^+ enters the CEC by selective ion channels. We now know that the molecular

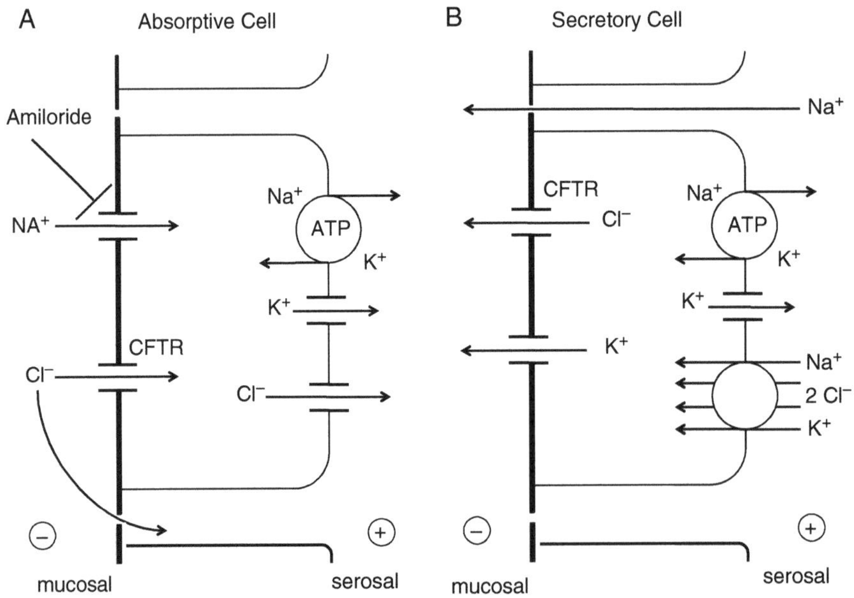

Fig. 7.2. Simplified models showing the ion channels and transport proteins of (**a**) an absorptive cell and (**b**) a secretory colonic epithelial cell.

correlate for this conductance is the epithelial Na^+ channel (eNaC, SCNN1) (12). The driving force for the entry through eNaC is the concentration gradient built up by the basolateral Na^+/K^+ ATPase, which is responsible for the bulk of Na^+ export out of the colonic epithelial cell. In order to keep this process running, K^+ recirculates across the basolateral membrane. A great deal of work has been done to elucidate the molecular entity of the basolateral K^+ conductance of the colonocyte (13). For all we know there are at least two types of K^+ channels, one of which is voltage dependent (KvLQT1, KCNQ1) (14) and the other regulated by the intracellular concentration of free Ca^{2+} (sK4) (15) that contributes to the K^+ homeostasis across the basolateral membrane of the colonic epithelial cell. There is a bulk of evidence that K^+ ions can also be secreted through the apical membrane of the colonocyte (16, 17). Experiments performed on BK channel-deficient mice have demonstrated that at least in rodents large conductance Ca^{2+} activated or 'Big' K^+ channels are responsible for K^+ secretion in the distal colon (18).

The anion movement across the colonic epithelium is not as well understood as the transport of cations. The most widely accepted hypothesis is that Cl^- ions move passively through the paracellular shunt – driven by V_{te}. Transcellular Cl^- absorption through apical anion channels as demonstrated for the sweat duct might be an alternative (19). The only anion channel that has thus far been shown to play a major role in the apical membrane of colonocytes is the cystic fibrosis transmembrane conductance regulator (CFTR) (20). Defective CFTR can lead to hypoabsorption of Na^+ and Cl^- in the jejunum of CF patients (21). Whether the same pathophysiological behavior applies to the colon of CF patients is yet unclear. To this end no plausible explanation for Cl^- exit across the basolateral membrane of the colonic epithelial cell has been given. Basolateral ClC channels (22) or electro-neutral transporters such as the Cl^-/HCO_3^- exchanger are implicated to play a role in this process (23).

But the colon does not only absorb electrolytes; it is also capable of Cl^- secretion. The base cells of the colonic crypts, which have the highest degree of CFTR expression in the distal colon, carry out this task (24). **Figure 7.2b** shows the principal components of a Cl^- secretory cell. It is easy to anticipate that the differences between absorptive and secretory cells are not so obvious. The main differences between the two cell types consist of the presence of a basolateral NKCC-1 co-transporter and the absence of apical Na^+ channels. The co-transporter is energized by the gradient for Na^+, which is in turn maintained by the Na^+/K^+ ATPase. Recirculation of K^+ ions occurs via the same channels as proposed for the surface cells. Due to the activity of the co-transporter the Cl^- concentration inside the crypt base cell can reach values up to 40 mmol/l. This concentration is sufficient to permit Cl^- exit through an apical anion conductance. Activation of CFTR by hormones that increase the intracellular concentration of cAMP leads to depolarization of V_{ap} and thereby generates a lumen-negative V_{te} provided by the concomitant activity of a basolateral K^+ conductance. These K^+ channels can either be activated by cAMP-mediated phosphorylation through PKA or by an increase in the intracellular Ca^{2+} concentration ($[Ca^{2+}]_i$). The predominant stimulus in the distal colon is the muscarinergic agonist acetylcholine, which is known to increase $[Ca^{2+}]$. The increase in V_{te} is sufficient to drive Na^+ ions through the paracellular shunt. Activation of the basolateral K^+ conductance provides the main driving force for Cl^- secretion by epithelial cells. Little is known about the exact composition of the fluid secreted by the crypt base. It is possible though that paracellular Na^+ transport plays only a minor role in this process and the predominant cation secreted is K^+. To this end we have to admit that the mechanisms of colonic absorption and secretion are far from being completely understood (25). The models proposed so far, however, are sufficient to explain the electric properties of the colonic mucosa under resting and stimulated conditions. They can also be applied to explain some of the pathophysiological properties of colonocytes obtained from CF patients.

1.4. Basic Principles of Short Circuit Current (I_{SC}/ICM) and Transepithelial Voltage (V_{te}) Measurements – Understanding Transepithelial Ion Transport from an Electrophysiologist's Point of View

When ions are transported across an epithelium this flux must not necessarily be unidirectional. The net amount of charges moving through the tissue is defined as follows:

$$J_{net} = J_{ap \to bl} - J_{bl \to ap} \quad [1]$$

This flux corresponds to the charges per time moving through the tissue. A flow of charges per time (J_X) is called an electric current (I). If we assume a configuration similar to what Hans Ussing was using in his lab we can write

$$J_X = \frac{I_{SC}}{zF} \quad [2a]$$

or

$$I_{SC} = J_X \cdot zF \quad [2b]$$

where z refers to the charge of the respective ion and F is the Faraday's constant.

From the lumped model in **Fig. 7.2** we can assume that I flows through a complex array of resistors in parallel and in series. Using Ohm's law we can write

$$I_{SC} = \frac{V_{te}}{R_{te}} \quad [3a]$$

or resolved for

$$V_{te} = R_{te} \cdot I_{SC} \quad [3b]$$

where V_{te} is the transepithelial voltage difference that is generated by the voltage of the apical membrane (V_{ap}) and the basolateral membrane (V_{bl}):

$$V_{te} = V_{ap} + V_{bl} \quad (4)$$

The total resistance of the epithelium (R_{te}) can be calculated according to Kirchhoff's law as

$$R_{te} = \frac{R_{shunt} \cdot (R_{ap} + R_{bl})}{R_{stunt} + R_{ap} + R_{bl}} \quad (5)$$

where R_{shunt} refers to the resistance of the shunt/paracellular pathway and R_{ap} and R_{bl} refer to the resistance of the mucosal and serosal membranes, respectively. It is worth noting that R_{shunt} is determined not only by the paracellular conductivity but to a much larger extent by the leak caused at the edges of the tissue mounted between the two sets of electrodes of the Ussing chamber. When we study a mostly planar tissue we also have to bear in mind that the current across the epithelium will depend on the total surface area. The most common unit for I_{SC} is $\mu A/cm^2$. It is evident that R_{te} is also a function of the area and has the unit $\Omega \cdot cm^2$.

In an experimental setup we may not forget that resistances in series can introduce errors. The series resistance is the sum of the resistance of the electrodes ($R_{electrodes}$) and the solution ($R_{solution}$), respectively:

$$R_{series} = R_{electrodes} + R_{solution} \quad [6]$$

With this we can determine the total resistance of our circuit as

$$R_{total} = R_{te} + R_{series} \quad [7]$$

It is evident from Eqs. (2a) and (2b) that I_{SC} and V_{te} can be converted into each other once R_{te} is known. An approach to assess R_{te} is to apply short current (ΔI) or voltage pulses (ΔV) across the epithelium and measure the resulting voltage or current responses, respectively. R_{te} can then be calculated using Ohm's law:

$$R_{te} = \frac{\Delta V_{te}}{\Delta I_{sc}}$$

1.5. Discussion and Summary: Impact of Functional Measurements of Ion Transport on Diagnosis, Prognosis, and Treatment of CF

1.5.1. Diagnosis and Prognosis

ICM is both a viable and valuable method to assess CFTR function in subjects with questionable or intermediate CF diagnostic information (e.g., clinical history and physical exam features, sweat chloride testing, nasal potential difference measurements). Detailed methodology has been developed at independent research laboratories that define CF and non-CF ion transport characteristics in human rectal biopsies, and these have been used to demonstrate that the measurement can be a valuable tool to aid in the diagnostic evaluation (9, 26–31). Meaningful ICM data can be obtained in biopsies procured by either suction biopsy apparatus or forceps through an endoscope, and center-specific diagnostic criteria can be applied based on ICM methodology in place. Advantages of ICM testing relative to other in vivo testing (sweat Cl^-, NPD) include the rapid and painless biopsy process (typically <5 min), the capacity to measure several ion transport features ex vivo (e.g., CFTR-dependent Cl^- transport, ENaC-mediated Na^+ transport, K^+ channel activity), the ability to use reagents that are not suitable for use in vivo (e.g., ion transport blockers, CFTR modulators), and tissue viability that allows biopsies to be restudied several times when maintained appropriately in ex vivo conditions (30). Disadvantages include the technical expertise necessary to mount and study the tissue in Ussing chambers, the cost and space needed for laboratory supplies and equipment, and potential patient unease regarding rectal biopsy performance.

Similar to other CFTR outcome measures, patients with partial function CFTR mutations often provide ICM results that are intermediate between pancreatic-insufficient CF and non-CF subjects (31). The flexibility in reagents and conditions that can be used in ICM protocols, however, provides great potential to better characterize the nature of CFTR dysfunction in a given CF patient. For example, use of ICM in subjects possessing rare and poorly characterized CFTR mutations may be very beneficial to their global assessment and future care planning, providing ex vivo data to determine if their mutation(s) retain localization to the plasma membrane and/or partial function to novel activating maneuvers (29, 32). This information will be of increasing importance as CFTR modulators move from clinical trials to clinical care, potentially identifying appropriate candidates for emerging treatments. Furthermore, rectal biopsies can serve as a logical means to monitor responsiveness to treatment plans, providing detailed information about CFTR biogenesis, maturation, and function on a patient-by-patient basis (further discussed below).

1.5.2. Treatment of CF Based on ICM Results – Development of GI Outcome Measures for Clinical Trials and Clinical Management

ICM and other GI outcome measures are relatively unexplored biomarkers of CFTR maturation, cell localization and activity for use in therapeutic trials of CFTR modulators, and potentially to guide treatment choices. Evidence indicates that ICM can segregate CF patients with two non-functional CFTR mutations from subjects with partial function mutations (most with pancreatic sufficiency), non-CF heterozygotes, and non-CF patients possessing two copies of the normal CF gene (31). Thus, ICM appears to be capable of detecting a hierarchy of CFTR function ranging from absent to full activity, correlating with predicted clinical outcomes across these patient populations. These measures can in principle serve as 'benchmarks' of ex vivo activity to predict clinical outcomes.

There are a number of potential advantages for their application in clinical trials to detect activity of CFTR modulators relative to other CFTR biomarkers that are more established for use in clinical trials (e.g., sweat Cl^- and NPD). First, a number of unique CFTR outcome measures can be explored in biopsied rectal tissue that cannot be tested in vivo, including ICM, to quantify CFTR-dependent ion transport, biochemical detection of immature and mature CFTR by Western blot or immunoprecipitation, immunohistochemical detection and localization of CFTR protein in epithelia, and monitoring of CFTR expression by real-time RT-PCR. Some of these principles have been demonstrated by Du and colleagues in CF animal models, measuring CFTR activity by ICM and by immunofluorescence in GI tissues of *hG542X CFTR* transgenic mice treated with suppressors of premature termination codons (PTCs) (33–36). Due to the high level of CFTR expression in rectal tissue compared with surface airway epithelia, small rectal biopsy samples are typically sufficient for sensitive detection by these methods. In contrast, nasal brushing may not provide adequate amounts of cells to detect CFTR protein biochemically, and immunofluorescent detection of CFTR in nasal cells has been difficult to standardize across research laboratories (37–40).

There are a large number of emerging reagents available to modulate CFTR expression and activity that could be applied to tissue that is studied ex vivo (41–46). First, a number of recently developed reagents to activate, block, or otherwise detect CFTR have become available over recent years that may demonstrate enhanced sensitivity to detect biologic effects of modulators relative to currently used CFTR biomarkers. For example, a large number of CFTR potentiators and inhibitors have been developed through high-throughput screening efforts (41, 45), many of which are available through Cystic Fibrosis Foundation Therapeutics-supported distribution programs. Small molecule potentiators and inhibitors of CFTR lack the necessary human GMP production, safety, and pharmacokinetic experience to adopt for use in nasal perfusion protocols, thus limiting their use for in vivo applications. In contrast, all of these reagents are potentially available for study in biopsied tissue studied ex vivo. Use of CFTR potentiators to detect and quantify mutant CFTR at the colonocyte cell membrane has many theoretic advantages, such as enhancing sensitivity to detect biologic effects of modulators. This principle may be of particular importance to support the development of drugs designed to increase the amount of mutant CFTR at the cell membrane (e.g., suppressors of PTCs or correctors of F508del-CFTR processing), as the mutant protein may not retain normal activation by standard CFTR stimuli (such as agonists to raise cAMP and phosphorylate CFTR). If the mutant CFTR delivered to the cell membrane in response to a small molecule modulator lacks normal gating characteristics (which has been described for F508del-CFTR following corrective maneuvers), it is possible that standard CFTR biomarkers may fail to identify primary biologic effects (47–50). This may be of even greater significance for suppressors of PTCs, since there are a large number of relatively rare, disease-causing PTC mutations that are relatively poorly characterized. If mutant CFTR proteins that result from PTC suppression lack normal regulation at the plasma membrane, biologic activity of suppressive agents may not be appreciated in select CF patients possessing these rare mutations. Specificity of modulator effects could also be enhanced by demonstrating blockade of Cl^- currents by novel CFTR blockers (that are not appropriate for in vivo use). Use of GI outcome measures could also improve the monitoring of response to small molecule treatment strategies, characterizing effects of CFTR modulators at both the biochemical and functional level. It is not difficult to imagine that GI outcome measures could also be used to test novel single and combination modulator strategies to enhance CFTR activity, testing relative effects of modulators in a controlled, patient-specific manner. GI outcome measures could thus serve as a flexible means to identify candidate subjects for novel treatment strategies. Finally, as CFTR modulator studies extend into younger and younger CF children, new biomarkers that are readily applicable to infant and toddler populations become more important, particularly since biomarkers such as the NPD may not be feasible for use in young children. Rectal biopsies may be an appropriate means to examine these biologic effects in this difficult to study population.

To bring GI outcome measures to human trials, a number of important steps are necessary. First, standardization of techniques is needed across study sites to ensure that results are comparable and interpretable in multicenter clinical trials. There are a number of technical variables that need to be considered and evaluated to optimize the available assays that can be utilized in ex vivo studies of rectal biopsies. For ICM, the choice of biopsy method (suction vs forceps), dissection (to remove the muscularis mucosa and enhance detection of epithelial ion transport), mounting equipment, buffer content, chamber temperature, Ussing chamber design (recirculating vs continuous exchange perfusion), reagents and sequence, electrophysiologic monitoring methods (voltage clamp vs open circuit), data capture, data over-read, and development of genotype-specific databases require clarification and standardization in preparation for use as a clinical trial outcome measure. While this list represents a potentially daunting number of hurdles to overcome, the need for standardization has been appreciated by the CF research community, and efforts are well underway to develop standard methodology across research sites, in both Europe and North America. In Europe the ECFS Clinical Trial Network standardization committee and the ECFS Diagnostic Network Working Group are working toward a SOP for ICM, both for diagnostic purposes and for use as endpoint in clinical trials. As an example of standardization testing in progress, investigative teams across three sites in the United States (The University of Alabama at Birmingham, The University of North Carolina in Chapel Hill, and the University of Iowa) have begun to develop standard operating procedures for rectal biopsy and ICM performance in human subjects. Standardize a number of aspects, including

- electrophysiologic equipment (voltage clamp amplifiers, tissue mounts, Ussing chambers, and software),
- gassed Ringer's bicarbonate buffers at 37°C,
- recirculating buffers in Ussing chambers,
- common reagent concentrations and sequences (10 μM indomethacin, 100 μM amiloride, 10 μM forskolin/100 μM IBMX, 100 μM carbachol, and 100 μM bumetanide), and
- centralized data interpretation.

Data from six to eight sequential non-CF subjects studied at each site indicate that similar CFTR-dependent currents can be obtained across sites with similar variability. These results suggest that standardized methodology is feasible and can produce similar results across several study sites and provide support for further efforts to optimize and standardize GI outcome measure performance.

Following the development of basic methodological SOPs, studies to examine potentiator and inhibitor dose/response relationships in human rectal biopsies, to address assay precision (including repeatability within human subjects), and to validate sensitivity of the assay to detect biologic activity of CFTR modulators in treated human subjects will be needed to establish ICM as a meaningful CFTR biomarker for clinical trials. Similar processes will be needed to develop other potential GI outcome measures (e.g., Western blot, immunoprecipitation, immunofluorescence, and/or real-time RT-PCR) and could benefit significantly by establishing centralized centers to process and measure these endpoints in clinical samples derived across study sites. In parallel to these studies to develop GI outcome measures, similar methodology could be incorporated into SOPs to develop rectal biopsied tissue as a preclinical model system for testing modulator strategies (30). Together, these steps could establish assays performed in rectal biopsies as extremely powerful tools to accelerate bringing novel CFTR modulators to CF patients.

2. Materials

2.1. Intestinal Current vs Voltage Measurements

CF is characterized by severe defects in electrolyte transport. This fact has been utilized for decades to diagnose the disease using the sweat test (51). It took until the early 1980s to supplement the sweat test with a different diagnostic tool, the measurement of the nasal potential difference (52). Some 10 years later, Henk Veeze and coworkers introduced a technique at the Sophia Children's Hospital, Rotterdam, that quickly became named intestinal current measurement (ICM) to the public (53). Veeze mounted small suction biopsies taken from the rectum of CF patients and healthy volunteers in an Ussing chamber that was customized for the size of the samples. He then treated the tissue with various inhibitors and stimuli while recording the I_{SC} generated by the epithelium. One remarkable finding was that the electrical response to stimuli of intestinal biopsies taken from CF patients greatly differed from that taken from healthy volunteers. The publication raised the attention of many scientists interested in epithelial transport. The laboratory of Rainer Greger in Freiburg quickly adopted the technique published by Veeze but modified it in several ways (27). In the following section we will discuss the differences and similarities between the measurement of ICM as established by the Rotterdam group and the measurement of V_{te} by the laboratory in Freiburg.

2.1.1. Intestinal Current Measurement

For the current measurements, specialized equipment and a well-trained technician are required (26). The rectal biopsy is taken with a suction biopsy device (Trewavis Surgical, Australia).

Micro-Ussing chambers are used with two half-chambers consisting of recirculating baths with a volume of 1.5 ml each. Between the half-chambers two mounting plates are compressed, positioned on guiding pins, between which the biopsy is fixed. These plates have an aperture of 1.2 mm in the middle and the exposed biopsy area is 1.13 mm^2. There are two calomel voltage electrodes (K401 Radiometer, Copenhagen, Denmark) connected to the bath solutions by 3 M KCl agar bridges located on the front side of the halves. The two platinum current electrodes are connected at the back of the half-chambers. Buffer temperature is kept at 37°C by water jackets around the baths connected to a water bath. The bath is continuously gassed with carbogen gas (95% O_2/5% CO_2). Phosphate-buffered saline (PBS: 1.5 mM KH_2PO_4, 3.2 mM Na_2HPO_4, 0.5 mM $MgCl_2$, 0.9 mM $CaCl_2$, 2.7 mM KCl, 137 mM NaCl) is used to transport the biopsies. The composition of the bath solutions (Meyler buffer) is 105 mM NaCl, 4.7 mM KCl, 1.3 mM $CaCl_2$, 1.0 mM $MgCl_2$, 20.2 mM $NaHCO_3$, 0.3 mM Na_2HPO_4, 0.4 mM NaH_2PO_4, 10 mM glucose, 10 mM HEPES; pH 7.4.

The voltage/current clamp is a DVC-1000 two-channel device with a DAM-50 differential amplifier (World Precision Instruments, Berlin, Germany). Data acquisition is digitally by PowerLab (AD Instruments, Colorado Springs, CO, USA) or by a strip chart recorder. All chemicals used are from Sigma (St. Louis, MO, USA).

2.1.2. Intestinal Voltage Measurement

The approach established in Freiburg differs from the aforementioned protocol in a couple of aspects. The tissue obtained by forceps (Karl Storz GmbH, Germany) biopsy is mounted on a slider with a pinhole area of 0.95 mm^2 that can be inserted between two half-chambers mounted on a heated manifold. Slider, chambers, and manifold are built by the machine shop of the Institute of Physiology in Freiburg. The most striking difference is, however, that both sides of the epithelium are continuously perfused by a gravity-driven system. The perfusate has the following composition (in mmol/l): NaCl 145, KH_2PO_4 0.4, $K_2HPO_4 \cdot 3H_2O$ 1.6, glucose 5, $MgCl_2 \cdot 6H_2O$ 1, Ca-gluconate $\cdot$ $1H_2O$ 1.3. The chambers and the perfusate are heated to 37°C by a water-jacked equipped system. Current electrodes are custom-made of Ag/AgCl wire directly inserted through channels on the sides of the half-chambers. For the recording of the voltage commercially available Ag/AgCl pellet electrodes (IVM E-207, Science Products, Hofheim, Germany) are coupled through Agar/KCl bridges that are placed in close proximity to the tissue surfaces. Both current and voltage electrodes are connected to an amplifier customized for this kind of measurements (UPG 3, AD-Elektronik, Buchenbach, Germany). Data are recorded on strip chart and on the hard disk of a computer using a custom-made software.

3. Methods

3.1. Measurement of ICM Using the 'Rotterdam /Hannover' Protocol

The ICM methodology and a standardized evaluation protocol have been used by the CF centers in Rotterdam and Hannover approximately since 15 years. After risk minimization by determination of capillary bleeding time and exclusion of a history of hemorrhoids, superficial rectal suction biopsies (3 mm in diameter) are taken with the suction biopsy tool without sedation or special preparation in a standardized procedure and defined suction pressure of 5 mmHg. Biopsies are preserved in ice-cold PBS, mounted in the recirculating Ussing chambers immediately, and incubated at 37°C with Meyler buffer. Voltage and current electrodes are connected to the chamber solution. Basal potential difference (PD_{basal}), short circuit current ($I_{SC\ basal}$), and transepithelial resistance ($R_{te\ basal}$) are determined, taking fluid resistance into account. Subsequently, the tissue is short circuited using voltage clamps and the I_{SC} as a direct measure for the net movement of ions across the epithelium. After equilibration of I_{SC} for at least 20 min, the ICM protocol presented here includes the following substances, added cumulatively to the luminal (L) and/or basolateral (BL) bathing solutions in a standardized sequence: amiloride (100 μM, L), indomethacin (10 μM, L+BL), carbachol (100 μM, BL), 8-bromo-cAMP (1 mM, L+BL), forskolin (10 μM, BL), 4,4′-diisothiocyanostilbene-2, 2′-disulfonic acid (DIDS) (200 μM, L), and histamine (500 μM, BL). The changes in I_{SC} are recorded subsequently, with next substance being added after stabilization of each I_{SC} response in general.

ICM recordings on rectal biopsies differ significantly between CF patients and healthy control. In pancreatic-insufficient CF (PI-CF), CFTR-mediated chloride secretion is absent or minimally preserved, whereas rectal tissue from patients with pancreatic-sufficient CF (PS-CF) is known to exhibit a variable amount of residual CFTR chloride secretion, which can be differentiated from the normal CFTR function in heterozygotes and healthy control (32, 53–55). Although sometimes presenting with a more variable I_{SC} baseline, short circuit ICM recordings have been proven to sensitively detect small amounts of residual CFTR chloride secretion (**Fig. 7.3**), which were missed by insignificant changes in the baseline of open circuit V_{te} recordings when directly compared to I_{SC} in a subset of diagnostic individuals (Derichs, unpublished data).

Recently, the diagnostic reliability of a standardized ICM protocol (31) was investigated in a large cohort of PS-CF and PI-CF, healthy control, and individuals with questionable CF, presenting with mild symptoms and equivocal results in the standard

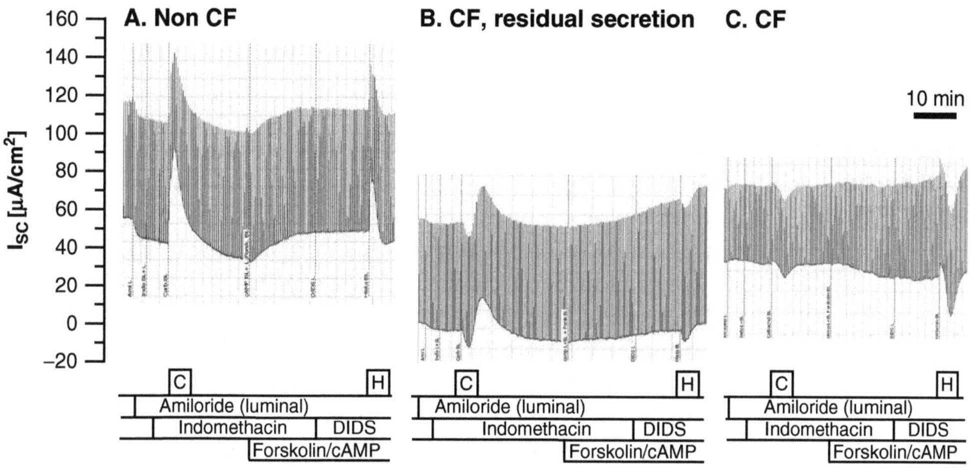

Fig. 7.3. Short circuit current (I_{SC}, baseline) ICM recordings and periodical transepithelial resistance recordings (ΔI_{SC} upon short 1 mV voltage impulses) on rectal biopsies in recirculating Ussing chamber (buffer volume ~1.5 ml/side, gassed 95% O_2/5% CO_2, rectal biopsy mounted between two discs with exposed tissue area of 1.13 mm^2). (**a**) CF, absent chloride secretion, (**b**) CF, residual chloride secretion, and (**c**) healthy control. ΔI_{SC} (µA/cm^2) after additive stimulation of CFTR chloride secretion with carbachol (100 µM BL), 8-Br-cAMP (1 mM L+BL)/forskolin (10 µM L), and histamine (500 µM BL) in the presence of DIDS (200 µM L) is registered; data are obtained in the presence of amiloride (100 µM L) and indomethacin (10 µM BL). Side of bathing solution: BL, basolateral; L, luminal.

diagnostic test (Derichs, unpublished data). For additional validation, extensive *CFTR* genotype analysis was performed in all subjects with questionable CF. This study first described the cumulative value of the Cl^- secretory responses $\Delta I_{SC\ carbachol}$, $\Delta I_{SC\ cAMP/forskolin}$, and $\Delta I_{SC\ histamine}$ ($I_{SC\ carb+cAMP+hista}$) as best diagnostic ICM marker with a clear cutoff value of 34 µA/cm^2 between PS-CF and control and summarizes I_{SC} reference values from previous studies obtained by the CF centers in Rotterdam and Hannover.

Besides the use of I_{SC} measurements on rectal biopsies for diagnostic purposes, a potential advantage of the ICM method has been recognized for the preclinical ex vivo analysis of novel small molecule compounds identified to rescue the CFTR basic defect (30). These CFTR potentiators and correctors mostly are identified by high-throughput screening programs and further evaluated and optimized on in vitro systems (animal models and cell cultures) (56–58). However, they might have different efficacy on native human epithelia, and a prediction on the clinical effect of compounds in CF patients is rather difficult by in vitro models. For a possible translation into early-phase in vivo clinical trials (59), a prioritization of most promising drugs by preclinical ex vivo analysis on human native tissue by ICM therefore seems to be a reasonable approach. Moreover, the ICM method is currently further standardized by committees of the CFF Therapeutics Development Network and the ECFS Clinical Trial Network, in order to develop and provide a standard operating procedure for monitoring CFTR function in future multicenter clinical trials.

3.2. Measurement of V_{te} Using the 'Freiburg' Protocol

Most recordings using the Freiburg protocol have been performed in 'open circuit' mode where V_{te} has been measured while short current pulses are applied to calculate R_{te}. Nevertheless it is also possible to directly measure I_{SC} using the same setup. Comparison between the two approaches revealed no significant differences. Due to the possibility of a constant perfusion the sequence of solutions applied to either side of the epithelium is different in the Freiburg protocol when compared to the Rotterdam/Hannover protocol. Representative recordings performed by this protocol are depicted in **Fig. 7.4**. After insertion into the chamber the tissue is perfused for about 20 min with a bicarbonate-free solution. Once a stable baseline of V_{te} is reached, amiloride (10 μmol/l) is added to the mucosal side. After 10 min carbachol (CCH, 100 μmol/l) is applied to the serosal side. CCH leads to a transient lumen-negative voltage deflection in non-CF while the opposite change is observed in CF. Next indomethacin is added to the serosal side to assess the amount of residual stimulation of the tissue by prostaglandins. While this maneuver has

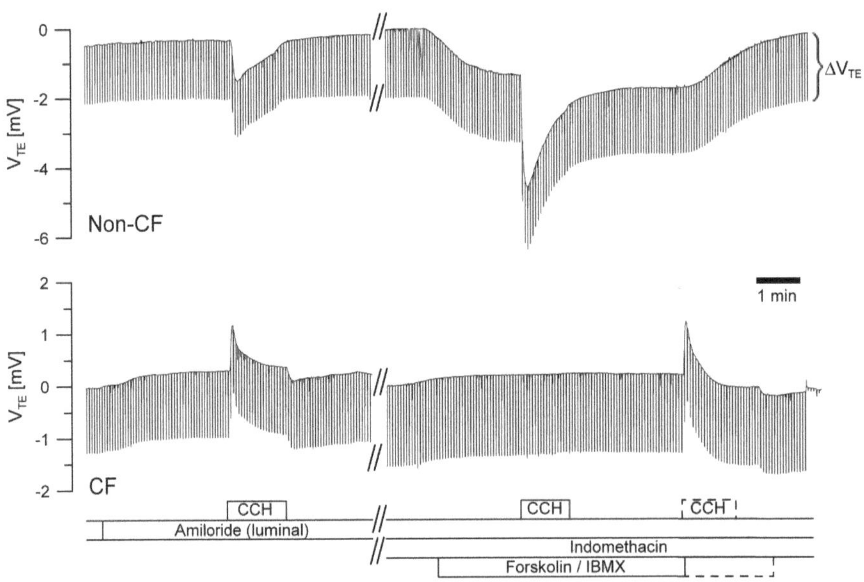

Fig. 7.4. Representative recording of V_{te} against time using rectal biopsies taken from non-CF (*top panel*) or CF patients (*bottom panel*). Downward deflections of V_{te} (ΔV_{TE}) are caused by short current pulses of 0.5 μA amplitude. ΔV_{TE} is proportional to R_{TE} which can be calculated using Ohm's law. Addition of carbachol (CCH, 100 μM BL) to the perfusate results in a lumen-negative change in V_{te} in non-CF whereas the opposite response can be observed in CF. Stimulation with forskolin + isobutylmethylxanthine (FSK 5 μM, IBMX 100 μM) leads to a slow change of V_{te} to more negative values in non-CF whereas a lumen-positive change can be observed in CF. The effect of CCH is augmented in the presence of FSK/IBMX.

hardly any effect in CF tissue, a change of V_{te} to more positive values is often but not always observed in normals. Addition of CCH in the presence of indomethacin often results in a CF-like response of the tissue. To this end the most likely explanation for this phenomenon is an inhibition of residual activity of CFTR by indomethacin, thereby preventing the bulk of transepithelial Cl^- secretion. Next the tissue is stimulated with a combination of forskolin (FSK, 5 μmol/l) and IBMX (100 μmol/l). This results in a change of V_{te} to more negative values in non-CF tissue while no effect or a slight change into the positive direction is observed in CF. Finally, CCH is applied in the presence of FSK + IBMX which leads to a pronounced decrease in V_{te} in non-CF, whereas a change to a positive V_{te} is seen in tissue from CF patients. The advantage of a perfused chamber is the ability to repetitively apply agonists and/or inhibitors to either side of the epithelium.

4. Notes

Both the ICM and the measurement of V_{te} with the perfused chamber are complex and time-consuming techniques, which need an expert technician and specialized personnel for guiding and interpretation of results. There are a few technical difficulties that might occur during the measurements. The biopsy can be reversely mounted which results in a mucosa in the opposite bathing solution. As a consequence, amiloride and carbachol will not evoke responses. To find out whether the orientation of the biopsy is reversed, the amiloride and/or carbachol can be added to the contralateral side which should give responses, however, in the opposite direction because also the current is opposite to the standardized protocol. When the reversed orientation is diagnosed, the experiment can continue with the addition of the secretagogues to the opposite sides compared to the protocol. To avoid wrongly mounted biopsies we use a microscope to mount the biopsy on the plate.

Sometimes the tissue is folded. This can not only result in non-responsiveness to the secretagogues but also give biphasic responses that are non-interpretable. When biopsies are folded it is very difficult to use the results since responses are usually a lot smaller and not reliable.

Minor pitfalls are air bubbles stuck in front of the biopsy against the chamber walls or in agar bridges. Delicate movement of the fluid with a Pasteur pipette and replacement of agar bridges are to be performed.

For the interpretation of the results there is the complication that when secretagogues like carbachol or histamine are added, the Cl^- and K^+ channels are both activated. The net current response that occurs is the summation of these individual currents (26). Therefore, the absence of a chloride secretory response upon carbachol does not automatically imply a complete absence of CFTR, but states that the K^+ secretory response overrides the Cl^- current.

Acknowledgments

MJH acknowledges the generous support from Mukoviszidose e.V. (N03/07), Innovative Medizinische Förderung Münster (HU 1 1 01 03), and EuroCare CF (LSHM-CT-2005-018932). The expert technical help of Tatjana v. Massenbach is highly appreciated.

ND acknowledges the financial support from Christiane Herzog Stiftung and Mukoviszidose e.V. ND and IB acknowledge the cooperation within the ECFS Diagnostic Network Working Group and IB acknowledges R.A. de Nooijer for technical assistance with NPD.

References

1. Reid, E. W. (1889) Report on experiments upon "absorption without osmosis". *Brit. Med. J.* **1**, 323–326.
2. Reid, E. W. (1901) Transport of fluid by certain epithelia. *J. Physiol.* **26(6)**, 436–444.
3. Levi, H., and Ussing, H. H. (1949) Resting potential and ion movements in the frog skin. *Nature* **164**, 928.
4. Koefoed-Johnsen, V., and Ussing, H. H. (1958) The nature of the frog skin potential. *Acta Physiol. Scand.* **42**, 298–308.
5. Ussing, H. H., and Zerahn, K. (1951) Active transport of sodium as the source of electric current in the short-circuited isolated frog skin. *Acta Physiol. Scand.* **23**, 110–127.
6. Kottra, G., Weber, G., and Frömter, E. (1989) A method to quantify and correct for edge leaks in Ussing chambers. *Pflügers Archiv. Eur. J. Physiol.* **415**, 235–240.
7. Gitter, A. H., Schulzke, J. D., Sorgenfrei, D., and Fromm, M. (1997) Ussing chamber for high-frequency transmural impedance analysis of epithelial tissues. *J. Biochem. Biophys. Methods* **35**, 81–88.
8. Singh, A. K., Singh, S., Devor, D. C., Frizzell, R. A., Driessche, W. V., Bridges, R. J. (2002) Transepithelial impedance analysis of chloride secretion, in (William R. S., ed.), *Cystic fibrosis methods and protocols*, Vol. 70, pp. 129–142. Humana Press Inc., Totowa, NJ, USA.
9. Kunzelmann, K., and Mall, M. (2002) Electrolyte transport in the mammalian colon: Mechanisms and implications for disease. *Physiol. Rev.* **82**, 245–289.
10. Gitter, A. H., Bendfeldt, K., Schulzke, J. D., and Fromm, M. (2000) Trans/paracellular, surface/crypt, and epithelial/subepithelial resistances of mammalian colonic epithelia. *Pflügers Arch.* **439**, 477–482.
11. Debongnie, J. C., and Phillips, S. F. (1978) Capacity of the human colon to absorb fluid. *Gastroenterology* **74**, 698–703.
12. Canessa, C. M., Schild, L., Buell, G., Thorens, B., Gautschi, I., Horisberger, J. D., et al. (1994) Amiloride-sensitive epithelial Na^+ channel is made of three homologous subunits. *Nature* **367**, 463–467.

13. Heitzmann, D., and Warth, R. (2008) Physiology and pathophysiology of potassium channels in gastrointestinal epithelia. *Physiol. Rev.* **88**, 1119–1182.
14. Schroeder, B. C., Waldegger, S., Fehr, S., Bleich, M., Warth, R., Greger, R., et al. (2000) A constitutively open potassium channel formed by KCNQ1 and KCNE3. *Nature* **403**, 196–199.
15. Joiner, W. J., Basavappa, S., Vidyasagar, S., et al. (2003) Active K^+ secretion through multiple KCa-type channels and regulation by IKCa channels in rat proximal colon. *Am. J. Physiol. Gastrointest. Liver Physiol.* **285**, G185–196.
16. Butterfield, I., Warhurst, G., Jones, M. N., and Sandle, G. I. (1997) Characterization of apical potassium channels induced in rat distal colon during potassium adaptation. *J. Physiol.* **501**, 537–547.
17. Matos, J. E., Sausbier, M., Beranek, G., Sausbier, U., Ruth, P., and Leipziger, J. (2007) Role of cholinergic-activated KCa1.1 (BK), KCa3.1 (SK4) and KV7.1 (KCNQ1) channels in mouse colonic Cl^- secretion. *Acta Physiol.* **189**, 251–258.
18. Sausbier, M., Matos, J. E., Sausbier, U., Beranek, G., Arntz, C., Neuhuber, W., et al. (2006) Distal colonic K(+) secretion occurs via BK channels. *J. Am. Soc. Nephrol.* **17**, 1275–1282.
19. Quinton, P., and Bijman, J. (1983) Higher bioelectric potentials due to decreased chloride absorption in the sweat glands of patients with cystic fibrosis. *N. Engl. J. Med.* **308**, 1185–1189.
20. Greger, R. (2000) Role of CFTR in the colon. *Annu. Rev. Physiol.* **62**, 467–491.
21. Russo, M. A., Hogenauer, C., Coates, S. W., Santa Ana, C. A., Porter, J. L., Rosenblatt, R. L., et al. (2003) Abnormal passive chloride absorption in cystic fibrosis jejunum functionally opposes the classic chloride secretory defect. *J. Clin. Invest.* **112**, 118–125.
22. Catalán, M., Niemeyer, M. I., Cid, L. P., and Sepúlveda, F. V. (2004) Basolateral ClC-2 chloride channels in surface colon epithelium: Regulation by a direct effect of intracellular chloride. *Gastroenterology* **126**, 1104–1114.
23. Traynor, T. R., and O'Grady, S. M. (1992) Mechanisms of Na and Cl absorption across the distal colon epithelium of the pig. *J. Comp. Physiol. B* **162**, 47–53.
24. Umar, S., Scott, J., Sellin, J. H., Dubinsky, W. P., and Morris, A. P. (2000) Murine colonic mucosa hyperproliferation. I. Elevated CFTR expression and enhanced cAMP-dependent Cl^- secretion. *Am. J. Physiol. Gastrointest. Liver Physiol.* **278**, G753–764.
25. Lucas, M. L. (2008) Enterocyte chloride and water secretion into the small intestine after enterotoxin challenge: Unifying hypothesis or intellectual dead end? *J. Physiol. Biochem.* **64**, 69–88.
26. Veeze, H. J., Sinaasappel, M., Bijman, J., Bouquet, J., and de Jonge, H. R. (1991) Ion transport abnormalities in rectal suction biopsies from children with cystic fibrosis. *Gastroenterology* **101**, 398–403.
27. Mall, M., Bleich, M., Schürlein, M., Kühr, J., Seydewitz, H. H., Brandis, M., Greger, R., and Kunzelmann, K. (1998) Cholinergic ion secretion in human colon requires coactivation by cAMP. *Am. J. Physiol. Gastrointest. Liver Physiol.* **275**, G1274–1281.
28. Mall, M., Hirtz, S., Gonska, T., and Kunzelmann, K. (2004) Assessment of CFTR function in rectal biopsies for the diagnosis of cystic fibrosis. *J. Cyst. Fibros.* **3**, 165–169.
29. Hirtz, S., Gonska, T., Seydewitz, H. H., Thomas, J., Greiner, P., Kuehr, J., et al. (2004) CFTR Cl^- channel function in native human colon correlates with the genotype and phenotype in cystic fibrosis. *Gastroenterology* **127**, 1085–1095.
30. Derichs, N., Knoll, J., Hyde, R., Pedemonte, N., Galietta, L. V., and Ballmann, M. (2009) Preclinical evaluation of CFTR modulators in ex vivo human rectal tissue. *Pediatr. Pulmonol.* **44**, 292.
31. de Jonge, H. R., Ballmann, M., Veeze, H. J., Bronsveld, I., Stanke, F., Tümmler, B., et al. (2004) Ex vivo CF diagnosis by intestinal current measurements (ICM) in small aperture, circulating Ussing chambers. *J. Cyst. Fibros.* **3**, 159–163.
32. Stanke, F., Ballmann, M., Bronsveld, I., Dörk, T., Gallati, S., Laabs, U., et al. (2008) Diversity of the basic defect of homozygous CFTR mutation genotypes in humans. *J. Med. Genet.* **45**, 47–54.
33. Du, M., Jones, J. R., Lanier, J., Keeling, K. M., Lindsey, J. R., Tousson, A., et al. (2002) Aminoglycoside suppression of a premature stop mutation in a Cftr–/– mouse carrying a human CFTR-G542X transgene. *J. Mol. Med.* **80**, 595–604.
34. Du, M., Keeling, K. M., and Fan, L. (2006) Clinical doses of amikacin provide more effective suppression of the human CFTR-G542X stop mutation than gentamicin in a transgenic CF mouse model. *J. Mol. Med.* **84**, 573–582.
35. Du, M., Liu, X., Welch, E. M., Hirawat, S., Peltz, S. W., and Bedwell, D. M. (2008) PTC124 is an orally bioavailable compound

that promotes suppression of the human CFTR-G542X nonsense allele in a CF mouse model. *Proc. Natl. Acad. Sci. USA* **105**, 2064–2069.

36. Du, M., Keeling, K. M., Fan, L., Liu, X., and Bedwell, D. M. (2009) Poly-L-aspartic acid enhances and prolongs gentamicin-mediated suppression of the CFTR-G542X mutation in a cystic fibrosis mouse model. *J. Biol. Chem.* **284**, 6885–6892.
37. Clancy, J. P., Rowe, S. M., Bebok, Z., Aitken, M. L., Gibson, R., Zeitlin, P., et al. (2007) No detectable improvements in cystic fibrosis transmembrane conductance regulator by nasal aminoglycosides in patients with cystic fibrosis with stop mutations. *Am. J. Respir. Cell Mol. Biol.* **37**, 57–66.
38. Davidson, H., Wilson, A., Gray, R. D., Horsley, A., Pringle, I. A., McLachlan, G., et al. (2009) An immunocytochemical assay to detect human CFTR expression following gene transfer. *Mol. Cell. Probes* **23**, 272–280.
39. Harris, C. M., Mendes, F., Dragomir, A., Doull, I. J., Carvalho-Oliveira, I., Bebok, Z., et al. (2004) Assessment of CFTR localisation in native airway epithelial cells obtained by nasal brushing. *J. Cyst. Fibros.* **3**, 43–48.
40. Wilschanski, M., Yahav, Y., Yaacov, Y., Blau, H., Bentur, L., Rivlin, J., et al. (2003) Gentamicin-induced correction of CFTR function in patients with cystic fibrosis and CFTR stop mutations. *N. Engl. J. Med.* **349**, 1433–1441.
41. Ma, T., Vetrivel, L., Yang, H., Pedemonte, N., Zegarra-Moran, O., Galietta, L. J., et al. (2002) High-affinity activators of cystic fibrosis transmembrane conductance regulator (CFTR) chloride conductance identified by high-throughput screening. *J. Biol. Chem.* **277**, 37235–37241.
42. Yang, H., Shelat, A. A., Guy, R. K., Gopinath, V. S., Ma, T., Du, K., et al. (2003) Nanomolar affinity small molecule correctors of defective Delta F508-CFTR chloride channel gating. *J. Biol. Chem.* **278**, 35079–35085.
43. Welch, E. M., Barton, E. R., Zhuo, J., Tomizawa, Y., Friesen, W. J., Trifillis, P., et al. (2007) PTC124 targets genetic disorders caused by nonsense mutations. *Nature* **447**, 87–91.
44. Robert, R., Carlile, G. W., Pavel, C., Liu, N., Anjos, S. M., Liao, J., et al. (2008) Structural analog of sildenafil identified as a novel corrector of the F508del-CFTR trafficking defect. *Mol. Pharmacol.* **73**, 478–489.
45. Van Goor, F., Straley, K. S., Cao, D., González, J., Hadida, S., Hazlewood, A., et al. (2006) Rescue of DeltaF508-CFTR trafficking and gating in human cystic fibrosis airway primary cultures by small molecules. *Am. J. Physiol. Lung Cell. Mol. Physiol.* **290**, L1117–1130.
46. Van Goor, F., Hadida, S., Grootenhuis, P. D., Burton, B., Cao, D., Neuberger, T., et al. (2009) Rescue of CF airway epithelial cell function in vitro by a CFTR potentiator, VX-770. *Proc. Natl. Acad. Sci. USA* **106**, 18825–18830.
47. Al-Nakkash, L., and Hwang, T. C. (1999) Activation of wild-type and deltaF508-CFTR by phosphodiesterase inhibitors through cAMP-dependent and -independent mechanisms. *Pflugers Arch.* **437**, 553–561.
48. Hwang, T. C., Wang, F., Yang, I. C., and Reenstra, W. W. (1997) Genistein potentiates wild-type and delta F508-CFTR channel activity. *Am. J. Physiol.* **273**, C988–998.
49. Wang, W., Bernard, K., Li, G., and Kirk, K. L. (2007) Curcumin opens cystic fibrosis transmembrane conductance regulator channels by a novel mechanism that requires neither ATP binding nor dimerization of the nucleotide-binding domains. *J. Biol. Chem.* **282**, 4533–4544.
50. Wang, W., Li, G., Clancy, J. P., and Kirk, K. L. (2005) Activating cystic fibrosis transmembrane conductance regulator channels with pore blocker analogs. *J. Biol. Chem.* **280**, 23622–23630.
51. Gibson, L. E., and Cooke, R. E. (1959) A test for concentration of electrolytes in sweat in cystic fibrosis of the pancreas utilizing pilocarpine by iontophoresis. *Pediatrics* **23**, 545–549.
52. Knowles, M., Gatzy, J., and Boucher, R. (1981) Increased bioelectric potential difference across respiratory epithelia in cystic fibrosis. *N. Engl. J. Med.* **305**, 1489–1495.
53. Veeze, H. J., Halley, D. J. J., Bijman, J., de Jongste, J. C., de Jonge, H. R., and Sinaasappel, M. (1994) Determinants of mild clinical symptoms in cystic fibrosis patients – Residual chloride secretion measured in rectal biopsies in relation to the genotype. *J. Clin. Invest.* **93**, 461–466.
54. Bronsveld, I., Mekus, F., Bijman, J., Ballmann, M., Greipel, J., Hundrieser, J., et al (2000) Residual chloride secretion in intestinal tissue of DF508 homozygous twins and siblings with cystic fibrosis. *Gastroenterology* **119**, 32–40.
55. Derichs, N., Mekus, F., Bronsveld, I., Bijman, J., Veeze, H. J., von der Hardt, H.,

et al. (2004) Cystic fibrosis transmembrane conductance regulator (CFTR)-mediated residual chloride secretion does not protect against early chronic Pseudomonas aeruginosa infection in F508del homozygous cystic fibrosis patients. *Pediatr. Res.* **55**, 69–75.

56 Pedemonte, N., Lukacs, G. L., Du, K., Caci, E., Zegarra-Moran, O., Galietta, L. J., et al. (2005) Small-molecule correctors of defective DeltaF508-CFTR cellular processing identified by high-throughput screening. *J. Clin. Invest.* **115**, 2564–2571.

57. Amaral, M. D., and Kunzelmann, K. (2007) Molecular targeting of CFTR as a therapeutic approach to cystic fibrosis. *Trends Pharmacol. Sci.* **28**, 334–341.

58. Verkman, A. S., and Galietta, L. J. (2009) Chloride channels as drug targets. *Nat. Rev. Drug Discov.* **8**, 153–171.

59. Rowe, S. M., Accurso, F., and Clancy, J. P. (2007) Detection of cystic fibrosis transmembrane conductance regulator activity in early-phase clinical trials. *Proc. Am. Thorac. Soc.* **4**, 387–398.

Section II

RNA Methods to Approach CFTR Expression

Chapter 8

Introduction to Section II: RNA Methods to Approach *CFTR* Expression

Ann Harris

Abstract

In this section, we review methods for the analysis of the *CFTR* gene and its transcript. First, we discuss techniques to accurately measure levels of CFTR mRNA in primary human cells; next, protocols for measuring *CFTR* transcripts that contain premature termination codons and for evaluating the role of nonsense-mediated decay which targets these transcripts; a further chapter considers methodology to investigate pre-mRNA splicing. The penultimate chapter concentrates on methods for evaluating microRNA regulation of gene expression in the context of airway disease. The final chapter considers methods to evaluate the chromatin structure of the active *CFTR* locus and to analyse the *cis*-acting regulatory elements that control it

Key words: *CFTR* gene, mRNA levels, pre-mRNA splicing, nonsense-mediated decay, microRNA, chromatin structure, regulatory elements.

Analysis of the *CFTR* transcript has made a major contribution to our understanding of the molecular basis of CF over the past 20 years. The complexity of the transcriptional mechanisms governing *CFTR* expression and the processing of CFTR mRNA remain topics of intensive investigation. Recent developments in the molecular techniques that can be applied to investigating the *CFTR* locus have significantly advanced the field.

The cystic fibrosis transmembrane conductance regulator (*CFTR*) gene encompasses 189 kb at chromosome 7q31.2. The full-length 6.2 kb transcript contains 27 exons and has a relatively long (1.5 kb) 3′-UTR. Many alternatively spliced forms of the CFTR mRNA have been identified in non-CF individuals though most, if not all, of these are non-functional. More than 15% of disease-associated mutations in the *CFTR* gene modulate pre-mRNA splicing, either through the disruption or creation of

M.D. Amaral, K. Kunzelmann (eds.), *Cystic Fibrosis*, Methods in Molecular Biology 741,
DOI 10.1007/978-1-61779-117-8_8, © Springer Science+Business Media, LLC 2011

intronic splicing motifs or by altering exonic splice sites. Some of these splicing mutations completely abolish the normally spliced transcript and are usually associated with a severe phenotype. Other splice site mutations generate a variable mixture of mis-spliced and correctly spliced transcripts. In these cases, the relative amount of normally spliced transcript is positively correlated with the mildness of the associated disease.

The frequency of splicing mutations together with their potentially variable clinical outcomes generates a need for robust methodology to evaluate and quantify the *CFTR* transcript. Moreover, some of the potential therapeutic avenues for CF that are currently being explored require endpoint measurement of *CFTR* transgene expression. Possible future therapies may also require measurement of the abundance of endogenous *CFTR* transcript as one gauge of efficacy. In **Chapter 9**, Ramalho et al. present methods to accurately measure *CFTR* transcript levels in several primary tissues/cell types. These techniques are based on RT-PCR technology, either using traditional quantitative and semi-quantitative methodology or quantitative real-time PCR. The mechanisms whereby mutations in a number of different splicing regulatory elements influence the efficiency of CFTR pre-mRNA splicing are examined in-depth by Goina et al. in **Chapter 11**. In this case the methodologies are based on evaluating the transcripts arising from hybrid minigenes, rather than endogenous *CFTR* expression.

Another clinically relevant aspect of CFTR mRNA processing relates to the class of mutations that generate premature termination codons (PTCs) in the transcript. PTCs can arise through several mechanisms, including deletions or insertions causing frame-shifts, from aberrant splicing or most frequently in *CFTR* by nonsense mutations. The *CFTR* PTCs result in non-functional proteins and have thus become the target of pharmacological approaches to promote translational read-through, for example, by the use of aminoglycoside antibiotics. The efficacy of read-through treatments such as gentamicin is influenced by the abundance of the PTC-bearing mRNA, which is controlled by both transcriptional and post-transcriptional mechanisms. The most important post-transcriptional mechanism in this context is nonsense-mediated decay (NMD), which specifically targets PTC-containing transcripts. In **Chapter 10**, Linde and Kerem describe protocols for measuring *CFTR* PTC-containing transcripts and evaluating the role of NMD in the context of read-through therapies.

The final two chapters in this section address relatively novel technologies that have broad ranging applications: In **Chapter 12** Giovannini-Chami et al. provide an overview of methods for evaluating microRNA regulation of gene expression in the context of airway disease. MicroRNAs (miRNAs) provide an additional mechanism of post-transcriptional control of gene expression. miRNAs are short (~22nt), endogenously expressed, non-coding RNAs that generally suppress gene expression by binding to the 3′-untranslated region (UTR) of mammalian transcripts (or in some cases, the coding sequence or 5′-UTR). Once bound, they may block translation or promote the degradation of the transcript. Each miRNA can bind to many targets and individual transcripts may be regulated by multiple miRNAs, thus greatly increasing the level of complexity of transcriptional networks.

Chapter 13 describes two of the new generation of genomic techniques developed to identify and characterize the regulatory elements of the genome, which are often hidden in non-coding regions. Expression of *CFTR* is strikingly different from that of its neighbours (*ASZ1* 5′ and *CTTNBP2* 3′) and is tightly regulated, exhibiting a complex pattern of tissue specificity. Despite this, the *CFTR* promoter appears to be a general ("housekeeping") promoter, and apparently to lack the key tissue-specific elements that control *CFTR* expression. A number of regulatory elements both within the gene and flanking it have now been identified and the mechanism of action of some of them has been elucidated. In **Chapter 13**, Ott and Harris provide details of two methods that have recently been used to identify and elucidate the function of key regulatory elements in the *CFTR* locus: (1) DNase chip, which utilizes DNase I-digested chromatin hybridized to tiled microarrays in order to locate regions of the *CFTR* locus that are "open" and thus likely regions of transcription factor binding; (2) quantitative chromosome conformation capture (q3C), which uses quantitative PCR analysis of digested and ligated, crosslinked chromosomes to measure physical interactions between distal genomic regions. When used together, these methods provide a powerful avenue to discover transcriptional regulatory elements within large genomic regions.

Chapter 9

Quantification of CFTR Transcripts

Anabela S. Ramalho, Luka A. Clarke, and Margarida D. Amaral

Abstract

Quantification and analysis of CFTR transcripts is of crucial importance not only for cystic fibrosis (CF) diagnosis and prognosis, but also in evaluating the efficiency of various therapeutic approaches to CF, including gene therapy. Reverse transcription (RT) followed by quantitative polymerase chain reaction (qPCR) is at present the most sensitive method for transcript abundance measurement. Classical RNA-based methods require significant expression levels in target samples for appropriate analysis, thus PCR-based methods have evolved towards reliable quantification. In this chapter we describe and discuss several protocols for the quantitative analysis of CFTR transcripts, including those variants that result from alternative splicing.

Key words: Cystic fibrosis, CFTR, quantification, transcripts, RT-PCR, primers, internal standards, real-time PCR, mRNA, splicing variants.

1. Introduction

Cystic fibrosis (CF) is a life-threatening disease caused by mutations in the cystic fibrosis transmembrane conductance regulator (CFTR) gene. Twenty years after the discovery of the CFTR gene (1) there are still many questions to be answered in the CF research field. The analysis and quantification of CFTR transcripts can provide valuable answers to the recurring question: "How much CFTR expression is needed to eliminate CF?" In fact, transcript analysis and quantification can also be a powerful tool for disease diagnosis and monitoring. Using different mRNA analyses and quantification techniques it is possible to quantify *CFTR* transcripts in different tissues and assess the effect of mutations on CFTR mRNA processing. The information thus obtainable

M.D. Amaral, K. Kunzelmann (eds.), *Cystic Fibrosis*, Methods in Molecular Biology 741,
DOI 10.1007/978-1-61779-117-8_9, © Springer Science+Business Media, LLC 2011

can allow (1) the identification of relevant target tissues/cells for therapy; (2) the determination of residual levels of normal, full-length *CFTR* transcripts that may either have prognostic significance; or (3) the evaluation of responses to gene therapy, or "corrective " therapies, i.e., pharmacological agents aimed at increasing the levels of *CFTR* gene expression (e.g., phenyl butyrate) or correcting defective splicing.

Ordinarily, mRNA makes up less than 6% of the total RNA content of a human/mammalian cell or tissue. In the respiratory tract, the abundance of CFTR mRNA is very low, with perhaps just 1–2 copies present per cell (2), so accurate CFTR transcript quantification may be problematic. The classic method of Northern blot allowing reliable quantification of unamplified RNA requires the target molecule to be present at a high-copy number in samples, making them unsuitable for CFTR. In contrast, polymerase chain reaction (PCR)-based techniques allow quantification by specific amplification of nucleic acid sequences starting with a very low copy number and/or limited amounts of sample. Reverse transcriptase (RT)-PCR, therefore, represents a sensitive and powerful tool for analyzing CFTR mRNA transcript abundance and quantitative (q) RT-PCR has tremendous potential, although a comprehensive knowledge of its technical aspects is required.

The scope of this chapter is to outline some of the basic methods for good quality RNA preparation from mammalian tissues and cells (including epithelial cells). Additionally, we give an outline of common techniques of measuring CFTR gene expression such as semi-quantitative RT-PCR and quantitative real-time (qRT)-PCR. These methods are designed to detect low abundance transcripts, which applies to CFTR mRNA in most cell types and tissues.

Quantitative real-time PCR (qRT-PCR) allows us to monitor the progress of a PCR reaction as it occurs in real time, and this combination of amplification and detection not only increases the accuracy of PCR product quantification but also eliminates the need for post-PCR manipulations. Two main experimental procedures can be followed, based on the use of either fluorescently labelled gene-specific probes (e.g., Taqman) or dyes that intercalate double-stranded DNA during product extension (e.g., SYBR Green). Furthermore, there are several experimental designs available for both relative and absolute quantification of CFTR transcripts. In this section we will describe one method for relative quantification of CFTR transcripts from a group of experimental vs. control samples, using a housekeeping gene as an internal control. This technique can be used to measure changes in CFTR mRNA abundance following experimental manipulations in cell cultures or to confirm altered expression of other genes in native tissues from patients vs. controls for validation of microarray data.

2. Materials

2.1. General Requirements

1. RNase-free water
2. Unpowdered gloves
3. RNaseout wipes
4. RNase-free 1.5 and 2.0 ml microcentrifuge tubes
5. Ice
6. 20 and –80°C freezers
7. Bench microcentrifuge (refrigerated)
8. Vortex
9. Micropipettes dedicated to RNA work
10. Sterile micropipette tips with filter
11. RNA*later* (Qiagen)

2.2. RNA Extraction and Native Nasal Cell Sampling

1. Interdental brushes (3 mm ref. 91016 or 2.5 mm ref. 91014 from Paro-Isola)
2. RNeasy® mini kit (cat no.74104 from Qiagen)
3. QIAshredder (cat no. 76654 from Qiagen) to homogenize cell lysates
4. Ethanol 100–96% and 70%
5. 14.5 M β-mercaptoethanol
6. TRIzol reagent (Invitrogen)
7. 1× PBS
8. Rubber cell scrapers
9. Chloroform
10. Isopropyl alcohol
11. Eye protection
12. Chemical fume hood

2.3. RT-PCR and Real-Time PCR Quantification

1. Thermal cycler (Biometra Tpersonal)
2. dNTP Set 100 mM Solutions (Amersham Biosciences, cat no. 27-2035-02)
3. Taq polymerase (Applied Biosystems, cat no. N808-0152)
4. Eppendorf tubes 0.2 and 0.5 ml
5. Automated sequencer (3,100 genetic Analyser, Applied Biosystems)
6. GeneScan® software (Applied Biosystems)
7. Real-time PCR device (e.g., ABI 7000 Sequence Detection System, Bio-Rad Cx96)

8. 96-Well plates (e.g., MicroAmp Optical 96-Well Reaction Plates, Applied Biosystems, or Hard Shell 96-Well PCR Plates, Bio-Rad) and sealing film (e.g., Microseal "B" film, Bio-Rad)

3. Methods

3.1. Sample Collection

All these procedures should be done using gloves and the appropriate clothing, and all instruments should be RNase free.

3.1.1. Collection of Nasal Epithelial Cells

1. Before collecting cells, prepare one 1.5 ml microcentrifuge tube per sample with 350 μl extraction buffer (RTL) supplemented with 1% (v/v) β-mercaptoethanol.
2. Nasal epithelial cells are collected from the nasal epithelium by gently brushing the inferior turbinate of both nostrils (**3**) using 2.5 or 3 mm interdental brushes.
3. After collecting cells, introduce the brush into the 1.5 ml microcentrifuge tube prepared in step 1 (*see* **Note 1**). By leaving the brush inside the tube covered by the extraction buffer (the cap may be closed leaving the end of the brush out – *see* **Fig. 9.1a**) greater yields are obtained. Before starting the extraction protocol, if the sample is frozen, thaw by incubation at 37°C for 10 min to ensure that all salt has dissolved and pass the brush several times through a P200 tip (previously cut in order to allow the brush to pass through it) to ensure all the cells are removed.
4. Additionally, to remove all fluid from the brush, immobilize the brush some millimetres from the bottom of the tube by closing the lid over the handle and spin down

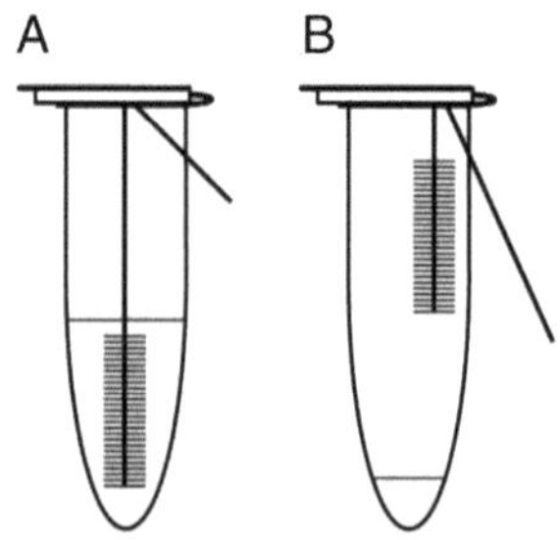

Fig. 9.1. (**a**) Image demonstrating how the brush should be introduced in the Eppendorf tube. It has to be completely immersed in the lysis buffer to avoid RNA degradation. (**b**) Illustration of how the brush should be placed in the Eppendorf tube to allow complete extraction of the samples from the brush by centrifugation.

(*see* **Fig. 9.1b**). Remove the brush from the tube and add the lysate obtained from this spin to the previous one on the same Qiashredder column.

3.1.2. Lung and Bronchial Tissue

Normally, human lung tissues are obtained following lung transplant. For the usage of human tissues in research, prior approval from the relevant institutional ethical review board and often also informed consent from the donor patients (or their legal representatives) are required. Small pieces are cut from the lung (3 mm diameter) and immediately frozen in liquid nitrogen and stored at –80°C, or each small piece is introduced into a 1.5 ml microcentrifuge tube containing 350 μl RTL buffer (Qiagen RNeasy kit) supplemented with 1% (v/v) β-mercaptoethanol and stored at –80°C. Alternatively the tissue fragments can be stored in RNA*later* (Qiagen: use according to manufacturer's instructions).

3.1.3. Colonic Tissues

Colonic tissues are usually obtained by rectal biopsies (suction or forceps) from patients undergoing this procedure for CF diagnosis/prognosis. Again, prior requirements for sample collection are approval from the relevant ethical review board and informed consent from patients (or their legal representatives). These samples are usually small pieces that can either be immediately frozen in liquid nitrogen and transferred to –80°C or can be stored at –80°C immersed in RTL buffer supplemented with 1% (v/v) β-mercaptoethanol. RNA*later* can also be used to protect the RNA from these tissues before RNA extraction.

3.1.4. Cultured Cells

Two methods can be used to prepare cells growing in a monolayer for RNA extraction, namely "direct lysis" or "trypsinization".

3.1.4.1. Direct Lysis

1. Remove all the medium from the culture flask.
2. Wash with PBS and then add the appropriate amount of lysis buffer (this depends on the number of cells in the culture flask) directly onto cells.
3. Collect the cell lysate with a rubber scraper.
4. Homogenize the mixture by pipetting up and down to ensure that all cell clumps are broken down.
5. Proceed with RNA extraction or store the sample at –80°C.

3.1.4.2. Trypsinization

1. Remove all growth medium from the culture flask.
2. Wash well with PBS and add trypsin to allow cells to detach.
3. Add medium to deactivate the trypsin, resuspend the cells and transfer them to a polypropylene centrifuge tube.
4. Centrifuge for pelleting at 300×*g* for 5 min.
5. Remove all medium and lyse the cells in the appropriate amount of lysis buffer, followed by homogenization of the sample by pipetting.

6. To collect cells that are grown in suspension, transfer the required number of cells to a polypropylene tube and pellet by centrifugation as above. Remove the medium completely and add the appropriate amount of lysis buffer, taking care to homogenize the sample by pipetting.

3.2. RNA Extraction

3.2.1. RNeasy Kit Method (Qiagen)

Unless otherwise stated, all procedures are carried out at room temperature.

1. If frozen lysates are used it is necessary to thaw them by incubation at 37°C for 10 min to ensure that all salt has dissolved.
2. Pipette the lysate onto a QIAshredder column sitting on a 2 ml collection tube (previously labelled).
3. Centrifuge the QIAshredder column for 2 min at full speed to homogenize.
4. Add 1 vol. (usually 350 μl) of 70% ethanol to column eluate and mix well by pipetting. Do not centrifuge.
5. Apply the whole volume of the sample (up to 700 μl) to one RNeasy mini spin column sitting on a 2 ml collection tube and centrifuge for 15 s at 12,000×*g*.
6. Pipette 700 μl of buffer RW1 onto the RNeasy column and centrifuge for 15 s at 12,000×*g*.
7. Transfer the RNeasy column into a new 2 ml collection tube. Pipette 500 μl of RPE buffer onto RNeasy column and centrifuge under the same conditions to wash.
8. Repeat step 7.
9. Transfer RNeasy column into a new 2 ml collection tube. Centrifuge for 2 min at 12,000×*g* as above (to ensure that all the ethanol is washed out from column membrane).
10. Transfer RNeasy column into a 1.5 ml collection tube and pipette 50 μl of RNase-free water directly onto the middle of the RNeasy membrane without touching it with the tip. Incubate at room temperature for 1 min and then centrifuge for 1 min at 12,000×*g* as above.
11. After centrifugation transfer the tubes to ice and use the samples immediately or store them at –80°C.

3.2.2. RNA Extraction Using TRIzol Solution Method

As TRIzol reagent contains phenol, contact with skin or breathing of vapour should be avoided, so gloves and eye protection should be used. The procedure should be carried out in a chemical fume hood.

For the homogenization of the sample, two different procedures can be used depending on the nature of the sample, namely whether tissue samples or cell monolayers.

3.2.2.1. Tissue Samples

Tissue samples should be homogenized in 1 ml of TRIzol reagent per 50–100 mg of tissue using a glass or power homogenizer. Sample volume should not exceed 10% of TRIzol reagent volume, and homogenizers should be washed in double-distilled water, 100% ethanol, 75% ethanol, double-distilled water and RNase-free water between uses if used for more than one sample. Once the tissue sample has been homogenized, it can be incubated 5 min at room temperature and RNA extraction can proceed exactly as described for a cell monolayer (step 2).

3.2.2.2. Cell Monolayer

1. The cell monolayer should be washed with ice cold PBS, followed by lysis in TRIzol reagent (1 ml per 10 cm^2 of culture dish). Lysed cells can be removed from the surface using a rubber cell scraper. The cell lysate is then passed several times through a P1000 pipette tip and transferred to a 1.5 ml microcentrifuge tube for vortexing. The homogenized sample is incubated for 5 min at room temperature to allow dissociation of nucleoprotein complexes. Any visible cell debris can then be removed by centrifugation.
2. Separation of aqueous phase: Add 0.2 ml of chloroform per 1 ml of TRIzol reagent, cap sample tubes securely and vortex vigorously for 15 s followed by 3 min incubation at room temperature. Samples are then centrifuged at 12,000×*g* for 15 min at 4°C. Following centrifugation, a lower red, phenol–chloroform phase, a thin white interface and a colourless upper aqueous phase can be seen. RNA is present in the aqueous phase. Transfer the aqueous phase carefully into a clean tube by pipetting, taking care not to aspirate any of the interface (*see* **Note 2**). The volume of aqueous phase transferred is usually 60% of the initial volume of TRIzol reagent used.
3. RNA precipitation: RNA is precipitated from the aqueous phase by addition of 0.5 ml isopropyl alcohol per 1 ml TRIzol reagent used initially. Samples are then incubated at room temperature for 10 min and centrifuged at 12,000×*g* for 10 min at 4°C (*see* **Note 3**).
4. RNA wash: Supernatant is completely removed from pellet. The RNA pellet is then washed once with 1 ml of 75% ethanol per 1 ml of TRIzol reagent used initially. Samples are mixed by gentle agitation and centrifuged at 7,500×*g* for 5 min at 4°C. This washing step is repeated once, followed by complete removal of ethanol (*see* **Note 4**).
5. Redissolving RNA: The RNA pellet is air-dried for 5–10 min, bearing in mind that a completely dry RNA pellet has a greatly decreased solubility. The RNA is then dissolved in the desired quantity of RNase-free water by gentle pipetting.

3.3. RNA Quantification and Quality Control

Several methods are available for RNA quantification and quality control. For quantification one of the most reliable and widely used methods is spectrophotometry using the Nanodrop system. Assessment of RNA quality is usually done by inspection of ribosomal RNA band integrity, either by visualization on an agarose–formaldehyde gel or using the virtual gel image supplied by the Agilent Bioanalyser, which also provides a numerical measure of RNA integrity.

3.3.1. Quantification of RNA by Spectrophotometry

RNA concentration can be determined by spectrophotometric measurement of absorbance at 260 nm, the convention being that a solution of 40 μg/ml RNA gives an optical density (OD) of 1. OD can be measured at 260 and 280 nm for calculation of sample purity. The *A*260/280 absorbance ratio gives a primary measure of nucleic acid purity and should be above 1.6 and ideally between 1.8 and 2.0. An absorbance ratio (*A*260/280) lower than 1.6 may indicate the presence of protein contamination (*see* **Note 5**).

3.3.2. Quantification of RNA by Nanodrop Spectrophotometry

The Nanodrop spectrophotometer, used according to manufacturer's instructions (Nanodrop.com), provides an immediate measurement of nucleic acid concentration from a volume of 1 μl, making dilution of the sample unnecessary. Otherwise, the use and interpretation of data are exactly as a conventional spectrophotometer (*see* **Note 6**).

3.3.3. Quality Control Using Agarose–Formaldehyde RNA Gel

The following protocol for RNA electrophoresis is adapted from (4).

1. Prepare a 5× formaldehyde gel running (FGR) buffer containing 0.1 M MOPS (pH 7.0), 40 mM sodium acetate and 5 mM EDTA (pH 8.0).
2. Prepare the agarose gel by mixing 1 part formaldehyde solution (3.7% stock) with 3.5 parts of agarose in water and 1.1 parts of 5× FGR buffer (*see* **Note 7**). The agarose should be dissolved in the water first and then cooled to 60°C. The gel should be cast in a chemical fume hood and allowed to set for at least 30 min.
3. RNA samples should be prepared by mixing in a sterile centrifuge tube: 4.5 μl RNA (up to 30 μg), 2 μl 5× FGR buffer, 3.5 μl formaldehyde (3.7% stock) and 10 μl formamide. Samples are then incubated at 65°C for 15 min, chilled on ice and centrifuged briefly.
4. About 2 μl of sterile, RNase-free gel loading buffer containing 50% glycerol, 1 mM EDTA (pH 8.0) and a trace of bromophenol blue is added to each sample.
5. The gel is pre-run for 5 min at 5 V/cm, the samples are then loaded onto the gel and the gel is run at 3–4 V/cm

until the bromophenol blue has migrated approximately 8 cm. Visualization of RNA samples is by UV transillumination, and EtBr staining can either be achieved by immersion of the gel in EtBr solution (0.5 μg/ml in 0.1 M ammonium acetate) for 30 min following the run, or by addition of 1 μl EtBr (1 mg/ml) to each sample prior to the run.

6. Generally, an RNA sample with two intact rRNA bands and a faint smear of mRNA between them is considered to be suitable for experimental purposes. In a degraded sample, the rRNA bands disappear and a large quantity of staining is observed at low molecular weight.

3.3.4. Quality Control Using Bioanalyser

Quality of RNA can also be tested on an Agilent Model 2,100 Bioanalyzer (Agilent Technologies). The bioanalyser report not only gives an electropherogram and a virtual gel image from which it is possible to estimate rRNA band integrity but also provides an RNA integrity number (RIN). Samples with a RIN higher than 7.0 are considered to be suitable for microarray analysis and are therefore also suitable for other mRNA quantification procedures (*see* **Note 8**).

3.4. cDNA Preparation

Three different types of primers can be used for preparation of cDNA. An oligo-dT primer can be used to transcribe all mRNAs simultaneously using their 3′-poly-A tails as template, whereas using a mixture of random primers produces non-full-length cDNAs from all mRNAs. Finally, a sequence-specific primer can be used if only one cDNA sequence is desired. The major benefit of random primers over oligo-dT is the production of cDNA fragments with an increased representation of the 5′-ends of mRNA sequences. Use of the oligo-dT primer may bias the 3′-end of the mRNA sequence; however, for general purposes the oligo-dT can still be used and can be substituted for random primers in the protocol given below.

Reverse transcription using random primers (5).

1. Add 1 μl of random primers (100 pmol/μl) to 11.1 μl of RNA and incubate at 60°C for 10 min. Include negative controls (no-RNA and no-reverse transcriptase)
2. Prepare a pre-mix, as in **Table 9.1** (*see* **Note 9**).
3. Remove tubes containing RNA from thermocycler, place on ice and add 6.9 μl of pre-mix to each tube.
4. Incubate for 2 min at 42°C.
5. Add 1 μl of Superscript^{TM}II RNase H$^-$ Reverse Transcriptase (RT) to every tube and incubate for 60 min at 42°C.
6. Incubate at 70°C for 15 min to inactivate the RT enzyme.
7. Store at –20°C until further use.

Table 9.1
Reagents pre-mixed for reverse transcription

Reagents: Invitrogen	Unitary quantities (μl)
First-strand RT buffer (5×)	4
DTT (0.1 M)	2
dNTPs (10 mM mixture of A,C,G and T)	0.4
RNAsin RNase inhibitor	0.5

3.5. Quantification Methods Based on Traditional RT-PCR

3.5.1. Primers

Careful design of the primers is a very important step to ensure accuracy of CFTR transcript quantification by RT-PCR. This can be done manually by examining the sequence to be amplified and applying the rules of primer design or by using software packages either freely available online [e.g. http://genome-www2.stanford.edu/cgi-bin/SGD/web-primer/ or http://www.changbioscience.com/primo/primo.html] or included with certain real-time thermocycler machines (e.g., PrimerExpress^{TM}, Applied Biosystems).

3.5.2. RT-PCR Quantification of CFTR Transcripts in Native Tissues from CF Patients with One F508del Allele

This RT-PCR protocol allows the relative quantification of CFTR transcripts from F508del carriers or CF patients possessing the F508del mutation in one allele. This strategy also allows us to distinguish between transcripts with or without skipping of exon 9 (6) and quantify the amount of transcripts with and without exon 9 skipped. PCR amplification in the region of exons 8–10 is performed using the following primers (*see* **Section 3.6.1** for comments on primer design):

- 6-Fam-B3F: 5′-AATGTAACAGCCTTCTGGGAG-3′ in exon 8 (positions 1,318–1,338 numbering as in Genebank Ac# M28668)
- C16D: 5′-GTTGGCATGCTTTGATGACGCTTC-3′ in exon 10 (positions 1,685–1,708)

Before starting, *see* **Note 10**.

1. Before starting the PCR reaction, prepare the "pre-mix" as indicated in **Table 9.2** and place on ice (*see* **Note 11**).
2. Pipette the pre-mix to each PCR tube and place on ice.
3. Still on ice, add 5 μl of each cDNA sample (final volume 50 μl), using one tube as control without cDNA (same volume of water instead: "no DNA control"), and 1 tube with a CFTR exon 9+/9– plasmid (6) to control for the PCR efficiency between templates with different sizes.

Table 9.2
Reagents pre-mixed for RT-PCR for CFTR

Unitary quantities (per tube)

PCR buffer I 10× (Applied Biosystems)	5.0 μl
dNTPs (10 mM mixture)	0.16 μl
6-Fam-labelled primer B3F (10 pmol/μl)	1.0 μl
Primer C16D (10 pmol/μl)	1.0 μl
H_2O (sterile, nuclease-free)	37.49 μl
Taq polymerase 5 U/μl (Applied Biosystems)	0.35 μl
Total volume per tube	45 μl

Table 9.3
Conditions for RT-PCR for CFTR

1×	94°C 5 min
n,(*n*+1),(*n*+2),(*n*+3)×	94°C 1 min
	60°C 1 min
	72°C 2 min
1×	72°C 30 min

4. PCR conditions should be as indicated in **Table 9.3**.
5. Programme the thermocycler and stabilize it to 94°C and then transfer the tubes from ice to the thermocycler block (*see* **Note 12**). Allow reaction to proceed.
6. Collect aliquots from each PCR tube at different cycle numbers namely at *n*, *n*+1, *n*+2, *n*+3 (to verify if the reaction is still in the exponential phase) to different tubes that must be then kept in another thermocycler (or water bath) at 72°C for 30 min, to allow completion of product extension.
7. Separate the products by capillary electrophoresis in a high-resolution automated DNA sequencer.
8. Analyse the results using the GeneScan® software (Applied Biosystems) to integrate peak areas corresponding to the amount of PCR products (*see* **Fig. 9.2**).
9. Estimate levels of full-length CFTR transcripts. The difference in amplification efficiencies between transcripts with and without exon 9 are corrected through the use of a control plasmid. The percentage of each mRNA species is estimated relative to the total CFTR transcripts present, by the integration of the corresponding PCR product peaks using GeneScan® software. The absolute amount of transcripts

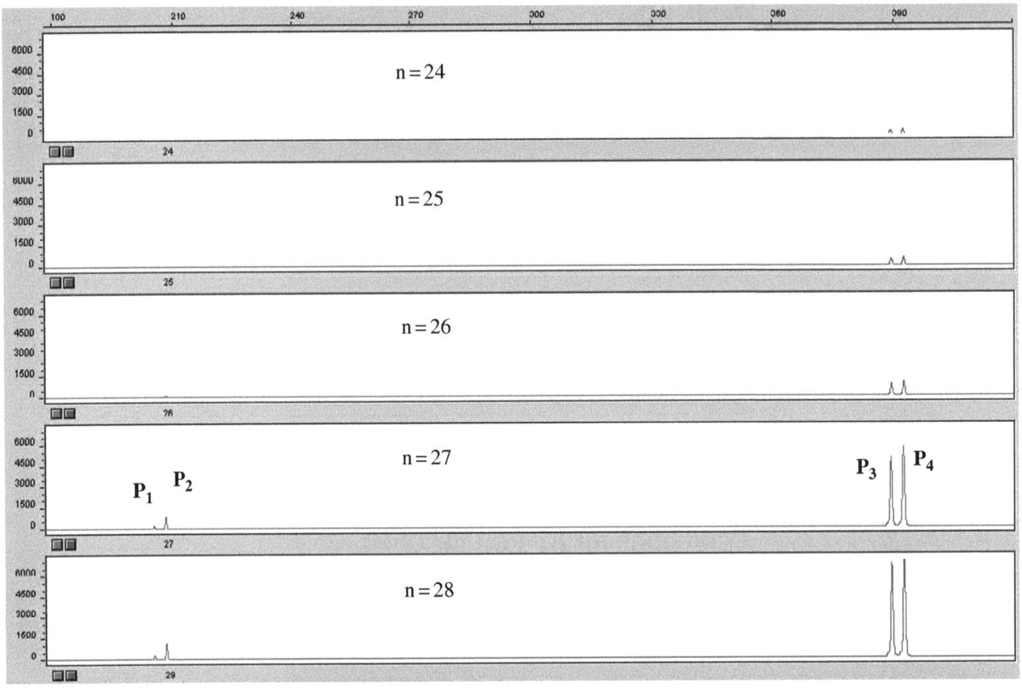

Fig. 9.2. Typical result after analysis by GeneScan after different number of PCR cycles (indicated in each electropherogram). Peaks P1 and P2 correspond to RT-PCR products of the CFTR transcripts without exon 9 from the F508del allele and from the non-F508del allele, respectively. P3 and P4 peaks correspond to RT-PCR products of the CFTR transcripts with exon 9 from the F508del allele and from the non-F508del allele, respectively.

from the non-F508del CFTR allele is then calculated, using raw data obtained from integration of peak areas from separate analysis of samples from each individual (CF carrier or patient) (6). Here, F508del transcripts are considered as internal standards, i.e., assumed as non-variant among individuals (*see* **Note 13**).

3.5.3. Relative Quantification of CFTR mRNA by RT-PCR Using β-Actin as an Internal Standard

This is a variation of the previous protocol, allowing relative quantification of CFTR transcripts by comparison with the abundance of β-actin, a housekeeping gene assumed to be expressed in roughly equal levels in different cell types and under different conditions (*see* **Note 14**). Unlike in the protocol above, the presence of the F508del allele is not required and therefore this is a more general method for detection of differences in CFTR mRNA abundance between different samples. The full protocol is available online (7).

1. A duplex RT-PCR is performed using FAM-labelled primers to amplify CFTR and β-actin cDNAs from the same RNA samples, originating products of similar (but unequal) size to minimize differences in amplification efficiency. β-Actin primers originating a product of 385 bp (ACT-F: 5′-GCA CTC TTC CAG CCT TCC-3′: Fam-labelled; ACT-R2:

Table 9.4
Reagents pre-mixed for duplex PCR (CFTR/actin)

Unitary quantities (per tube)

PCR buffer I 10× (Applied Biosystems)	5.0 μl
dNTPs (10 mM mixture)	0.16 μl
6-Fam-labelled CFTR primer B3F (10 pmol/μl)	1.0 μl
CFTR primer C16D (10 pmol/μl)	1.0 μl
6-Fam-labelled β-actin primer ACT-F (10 pmol/μl)	1.0 μl
β-Actin primer ACT-R (10 pmol/μl)	1.0 μl
H_2O (sterile, nuclease-free)	35.49 μl
Taq polymerase 5 U/μl (Applied Biosystems)	0.35 μl
Total volume per tube	45 μl

5′-AGA AAG GGT GTA ACG CAA CTA AG-3′) can be used in duplex with the CFTR primers shown in **Section 3.5.2**, which give a product of 391 bp. The PCR pre-mix is set up according to **Table 9.4** (*see* **Note 11**).

2. Repeat steps 2–5 of **Section 3.5.2**.
3. Aliquots of 6 μl are removed from the PCR reaction at the end of the annealing phase of increasing numbers of PCR cycles (*see* **Note 15**). The aliquots are immediately transferred into new microtubes and incubated at 72°C in a separate hot block or waterbath to allow complete product extension.
4. The products are run on an automatic sequencer, and PCR product abundance is estimated by integration of the corresponding peak areas using the GeneScan® software. Provided both products are still in the logarithmic phase of amplification, which can be confirmed by plotting peak areas against number of cycles for each product (*see* **Note 16**). CFTR mRNA abundance is then calculated as a percentage of β-actin expression (*see* **Note 17**).

3.5.4. Detection and Quantification of CFTR Splicing Variants

The splicing mechanism (intron removal from pre-mRNA) is a very complex process regulated by several elements. The well-known consensus sequences flanking the intron are the donor sequence (5′-GU), the acceptor (3′-AG) and the branch site. However, other non-canonical sequences (intronic and exonic enhancer and silencer sequences) can influence the splicing process, and these are difficult to detect by sequence analysis alone (8). It is therefore very important to analyse the effect at the mRNA level of each and every mutation, and not only mutations that abolish the well-recognized splicing sequences or create new putative splicing sequences. Even missense or silent mutations (9) can have an unexpected effect on mRNA abundance.

To analyse the effect of a mutation on the mRNA transcript, we can first inspect the mutated sequence using software that allows a splicing prediction (e.g. http://www.fruitfly.org/seq_tools/splice.html) or one that finds regulatory elements (e.g. http://rulai.cshl.edu/cgi-bin/tools/ESE3/esefinder.cgi). Then, for the detection of putative CFTR splice variants the CFTR transcripts can be analysed by RT-PCR using primers that amplify the mutation flanking sequence. If we have a prediction of total or partial exon skipping or creation of a cryptic exon we can use primers that flank the alternative spliced sequence in order to test the theoretical prediction. If no prediction is obtained we should use a forward primer that hybridizes at least one exon upstream of the exon where the mutation is localized, and a reverse primer that hybridizes at least one exon downstream of this exon (10, 11). The quantification of the alternative transcripts of CFTR can be obtained by fluorescent RT-PCR analysis. One of the primers used in the RT-PCR reaction is 6-Fam-fluorescent labelled, which allows the quantification of the RT-PCR products in an automated sequencer using the GeneScan™ software as described in **Section 3.5.2**. The relative abundance of any given transcript (aberrantly or correctly spliced) is determined as the signal peak area of the corresponding PCR product divided by the sum of the signal peak areas of both aberrantly and correctly spliced PCR products. The RT-PCR products taken for quantification are first ensured to be in the log phase of amplification. Values obtained must be validated by experimental replication (at least $n = 3$) followed by statistical analysis.

3.6. Quantitative Real-Time (qRT)-PCR

3.6.1. Primer and Amplicon Design

Primers used in qRT-PCR should amplify relatively short products (75–150 bp) and have a T_m of approximately 60°C. Care should be taken to exclude complementary sequences which might result in the formation of primer–dimers, and primers should ideally span exon boundaries to reduce the probability of amplification of residual genomic DNA. Suitability of primers for real-time quantitative PCR amplification should always be tested by amplifying a product from test cDNAs using the chosen primer pairs in a conventional PCR reaction, and confirming the absence of non-specific PCR products and primer–dimers for all targets by electrophoretic separation of the products in 2% ethidium bromide stained agarose gels.

CFTR was amplified using primer pair 6995996a2 (Fwd: 5′-ATG CCC TTC GGC GAT GTT TT-3′; Rev: 5′-TGA TTC TTC CCA GTA AGA GAG GC-3′: 105 bp), and GAPDH was amplified using primer pair 7669492a1 (Fwd: 5′-ATG GGG AAG GTG AAG GTC G-3′; Rev: 5′-GGG GTC ATT GAT GGC AAC AAT A-3′: 108 bp: *see* **Note 18**).

3.6.2. Reaction Set-Up

Quantitative real-time PCR is performed in a sealed 96-well plate (e.g., Hard Shell Thin Wall PCR plates sealed with Microseal B film), with experimental and control samples arranged as in **Fig. 9.3**, where it is shown that both CFTR and the reference gene GAPDH are amplified in triplicate from the same cDNA samples. In this example, expression in five independent experimental samples is compared with expression in five independent control samples. For statistical confidence, at least three technical replicates (rows A, B and C for CFTR and rows D, E and F for GAPDH, **Fig. 9.3**) and three biological replicates should be used (in this example five are used: columns 1–5 for experimental samples and 6–10 for controls).

The standards are a duplicate series of fivefold dilutions of a cDNA sample known to express both the CFTR and GAPDH in abundance (*see* **Note 19**). No-template controls have the water used in standard dilutions in the place of cDNA, but other controls can also be added, such as cDNA from which RT enzyme

	1	2	3	4	5	6	7	8	9	10	11	12
A	Ex1 CFTR	Ex2 CFTR	Ex3 CFTR	Ex4 CFTR	Ex5 CFTR	Ctr1 CFTR	Ctr2 CFTR	Ctr3 CFTR	Ctr4 CFTR	Ctr5 CFTR	-	-
B	Ex1 CFTR	Ex2 CFTR	Ex3 CFTR	Ex4 CFTR	Ex5 CFTR	Ctr1 CFTR	Ctr2 CFTR	Ctr3 CFTR	Ctr4 CFTR	Ctr5 CFTR	-	-
C	Ex1 CFTR	Ex2 CFTR	Ex3 CFTR	Ex4 CFTR	Ex5 CFTR	Ctr1 CFTR	Ctr2 CFTR	Ctr3 CFTR	Ctr4 CFTR	Ctr5 CFTR	-	-
D	Ex1 GAP	Ex2 GAP	Ex3 GAP	Ex4 GAP	Ex5 GAP	Ctr1 GAP	Ctr2 GAP	Ctr3 GAP	Ctr4 GAP	Ctr5 GAP	-	-
E	Ex1 GAP	Ex2 GAP	Ex3 GAP	Ex4 GAP	Ex5 GAP	Ctr1 GAP	Ctr2 GAP	Ctr3 GAP	Ctr4 GAP	Ctr5 GAP	-	-
F	Ex1 GAP	Ex2 GAP	Ex3 GAP	Ex4 GAP	Ex5 GAP	Ctr1 GAP	Ctr2 GAP	Ctr3 GAP	Ctr4 GAP	Ctr5 GAP	-	-
G	Std1 CFTR	Std2 CFTR	Std3 CFTR	Std4 CFTR	Std5 CFTR	Std1 GAP	Std2 GAP	Std 3 GAP	Std4 GAP	Std5 GAP	-	NTC CFTR
H	Std1 CFTR	Std2 CFTR	Std3 CFTR	Std4 CFTR	Std5 CFTR	Std1 GAP	Std2 GAP	Std 3 GAP	Std4 GAP	Std5 GAP	-	NTC GAP

Fig. 9.3. 96-Well plate layout for qRT-PCR reaction. Ex: experimental samples, Ctr: control samples, Std: standard samples, NTC: no template controls.

Table 9.5
Reagents pre-mixed for duplex RT-PCR (CFTR/actin)

Component	Volume per well
1. 2× SYBR Green master mix (Applied Biosystems)	10 μl
2. Mixture of forward and reverse primers at 1 μM concentration	5 μl
3. A 1:5 dilution of sample cDNA (or standard curve sample[a])	5 μl
Total volume per well	20 μl

[a] *See* **Note 21**

was omitted, to test for amplification of residual genomic DNA in the RNA sample.

Each well of the PCR plate contains the reagents listed in **Table 9.5**, added in the order shown (*see* **Note 20**).

3.6.3. PCR Reaction

Once the PCR reaction is set up, the 96-well plate is inserted into a real-time PCR machine. Examples include the ABI 7000 Sequence Detection System (Applied Biosystems) and the Bio-Rad Cx96. These instruments, and their associated software, allow the simultaneous measurement of the fluorescence of SYBR Green in all wells of a 96-well plate throughout the course of a PCR reaction. The cycling protocol is shown in **Table 9.6**.

Fluorescence is measured after each extension phase at 60°C for detection of SYBR Green dye whose fluorescence increases during its intercalation in double-stranded DNA.

A melting curve analysis with a temperature gradient from 60 to 95°C is programmed following the PCR amplification, to confirm that real-time PCR reactions have amplified without contamination or primer–dimer formation and to ensure reaction specificity and uniformity among all samples. Following amplification, melting curves for every well are first checked to ensure the presence of only one major peak of one size per primer pair, before proceeding with data analysis (*see* **Fig. 9.4**).

Table 9.6
Conditions for quantitative real-time RT-PCR

Step	Temperature (°C)	Time	Notes
1.	95	10 min	
2.	95	15 s	
3.	60	60 s	Return to step 2, 39 times

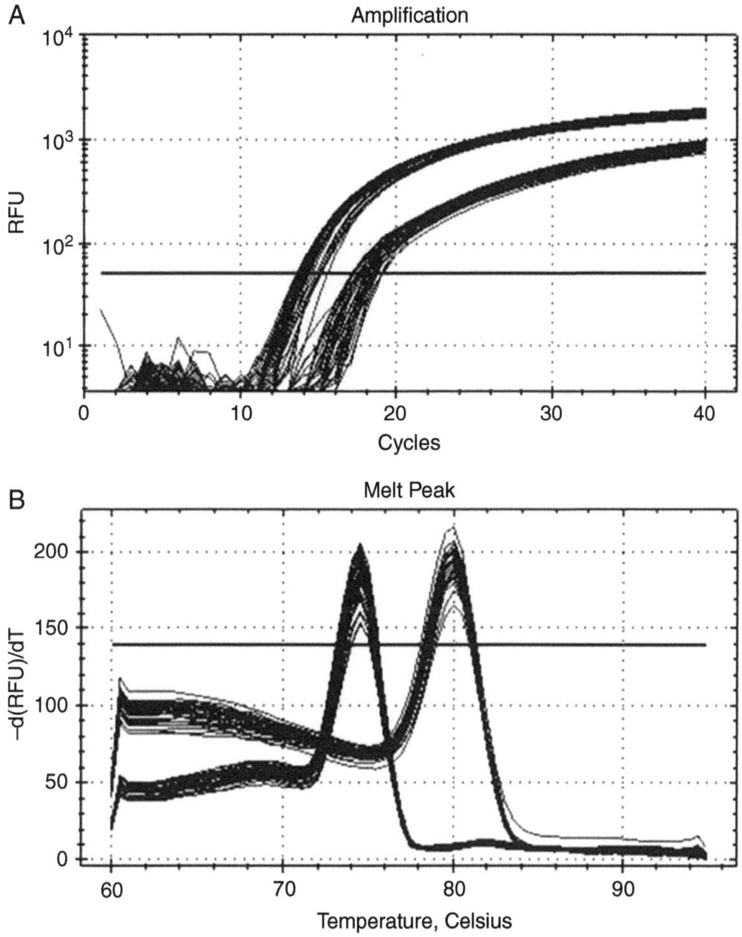

Fig. 9.4. Examples of qRT-PCR amplification and melt curves. (**a**) Amplification curves for GAPDH (left-hand cluster) and CFTR (right-hand cluster) from 3 replicates of 12 cDNA samples on one 96-well plate. Fluorescence is plotted on a log scale against cycle number. Each amplification curve crosses the horizontal cycle threshold line at a certain cycle threshold number (C_T) which is then used for quantification. (**b**) Melting peaks for GAPDH (*right*) and CFTR (*left*) PCR products produced in (**a**). The single peak for each product in all samples indicates lack of contamination and primer–dimers.

3.6.4. Data Analysis I: Standard Curve Comparison

The log of each known concentration in the dilution series is plotted against the C_T value for that concentration to produce standard curves for CFTR and GAPDH. Various parameters of the standard curves are checked to assess reaction efficiency: removal of poorly performing individual technical replicates may improve these values if necessary. The correlation coefficient (R^2) of each curve should be as close as possible to 1, although generally 0.99 is the maximum achievable value. The slope of the log-linear phase of the amplification can be used to calculate reaction efficiency ($E = 10^{(-1/\text{slope})} - 1$). A slope of –3.32 corresponds to 100% PCR efficiency. When it is confirmed that the efficiency of amplification of both genes is similarly high, relative quantification can then be performed. When using ABI or Bio-Rad real-time PCR analysis software packages, standard curves are automatically calculated, but C_T thresholds can be altered to optimize the fit between the two standard curves.

3.6.5. Data Analysis II: Relative Quantification of CFTR Expression

The signal curves of unknowns, measured in the same run (*see* **Fig. 9.4**), are used for quantification. In brief, the cycle number C_T, which indicates where the signal curve crosses an arbitrary threshold intersecting the signal curves in their exponential phases, is determined. The C_T values are proportional to the logarithms of the initial target concentrations. The $\Delta\Delta C_T$ method is a simple way of quantifying fold change in expression of the test gene CFTR in experimental vs. control samples using expression levels of a housekeeping gene (GAPDH) for normalization. The calculation is performed as follows, on means of C_T values for the three technical replicates of each condition:

1. ΔC_T is calculated for the experimental condition:

$$\Delta C_T^{EXP} = C_T\text{CFTR}^{EXP} - C_T\text{GAPDH}^{EXP}$$

2. ΔC_T is calculated for the control condition:

$$\Delta C_T^{CTRL} = C_T\text{CFTR}^{CTRL} - C_T\text{GAPDH}^{CTRL}$$

3. $\Delta\Delta C_T$ is calculated:

$$\Delta\Delta C_T = \Delta C_T^{EXP} - C_T^{CTRL}$$

4. Normalized fold change of CFTR expression for experimental vs. control condition is calculated:

   Normalized fold change of CFTR^{EXP} vs . $\text{CFTR}^{CTRL} = 2^{(-\Delta\Delta C_T)}$

A mean overall experimental vs control fold change for CFTR expression can then be calculated from the five biological replicates tested.

4. Notes

1. Cell lysates can be stored in RTL buffer at –80°C for several months. RNA samples dissolved in RNase-free H_2O can be stored for a few days at –20°C or up to a year at –80°C. For longer term storage (more than a year) RNA may be stored at –20°C as a precipitate in ethanol.

2. If visible interface transfer occurs an additional, identical chloroform purification may be needed for satisfactory purity of the final sample.
3. The RNA will form a fragile, translucent pellet at the side of the tube, and it is important to note tube orientation during centrifugation to facilitate pellet identification and avoid its aspiration during subsequent steps.
4. After the second ethanol wash the pellet is usually loose and great care is needed to avoid aspiration at this step. Therefore, removal of the final drop of ethanol should be with a fine (10 μl) micropipette tip.
5. A secondary measure of RNA sample purity is the *A*260/230 ratio which should also be around 2.0 and may indicate contamination with extraction buffer reagents (e.g., guanidinium ions or phenol) if it is low.
6. Care must be taken when using the Nanodrop to use an appropriate blank solution, i.e., the one used for dissolving your RNA sample. The measuring platform should be wiped between samples, and RNA must be chosen in the options menu.
7. For example, a 1% agarose gel with a final volume of 56 ml would contain 10 ml formaldehyde, 35 ml water with 0.56 g agarose dissolved in it, and 11 ml FGR buffer.
8. The RIN of a poor RNA sample may be raised by performing an RNA cleanup protocol, for example, using the Qiagen RNeasy Mini Kit.
9. Multiply the quantities shown in the table by the number of RNA samples +1.
10. Preparation of samples for PCR (Steps 1 and 2 in **Section 3.6.1**) should be performed in a separate room (low DNA) with complete absence of high concentration of DNA, plasmids and PCR products.
11. An $(n+1)\times$ volume of pre-mix should be prepared, where n is the total number of experimental plus control samples.
12. Before proceeding with PCR reaction check that thermocycler hot lid is on.
13. Almost all F508del chromosomes detected in CF patients and carriers all over the world are associated with the same extended haplotype and TG10T9 (12). Each RT-PCR analysis is repeated at least three times to ensure accurate quantification.
14. Other commonly used control genes such as GAPDH may also be used successfully.
15. The number of cycles can be determined empirically, but during a 30- to 35-cycle PCR reaction the amplification is

usually in the logarithmic phase between cycles 15 and 25. Therefore aliquots could be taken during cycles 16, 18, 20, 22 and 24.

16. For very low abundance mRNAs (e.g., CFTR in many cell types), the logarithmic phase of amplification may not correspond to that of β-actin. In this case, competitive (non-extendable) β-actin primers, which are identical in sequence to those shown above, but which are synthesized with 3′-dideoxynucleotides to prevent PCR product extension, can be added to the normal β-actin primers in an empirically determined proportion. This has the effect of delaying the β-actin amplification reaction and thereby synchronizing the logarithmic amplification phases to enable comparison (13).
17. Values obtained by the semi-quantitative PCR methods shown in **Sections 3.5.2** and **3.5.3** should be validated by experimental replication and may only be compared with others obtained by exactly the same method, particularly if competitive β-actin primers have been added.
18. The primers used in this example for amplification of CFTR and the control gene GAPDH were taken from the Harvard Primerbank database (http://pga.mgh.harvard.edu/primerbank/), an extensive online source of primer pairs already optimized for use in qRT-PCR.
19. A suitable sample for this purpose is the Calu-3 cell line.
20. For pipetting accuracy, an electronic pipette (Biopette E, Labnet International) is used to dispense identical 10 μl aliquots of 2× SYBR green master mix to all wells to be used, followed by 5 μl aliquots of the relevant primer mix. Finally, individual cDNA samples are added with a standard pipette using one tip per well, to avoid any cross-contamination.
21. The template DNA of both unknowns and Std1 are generally diluted 1:5 in sterile, nuclease-free water following reverse transcription. Stds 2–5 are then diluted 1:5 from Std1.

References

1. Riordan, J. R., Rommens, J. M., Kerem, B., Alon, N., Rozmahel, R., Grzelczak, Z., et al. (1989) Identification of the cystic fibrosis gene: cloning and characterization of complementary DNA. *Science* **245**, 1066–1073.
2. Bremer, S., Hoof, T., Wilke, M., Busche, R., Scholte, B., Riordan, J. R., et al. (1992) Quantitative expression patterns of multidrug-resistance P-glycoprotein (MDR1) and differentially spliced cystic-fibrosis transmembrane- conductance regulator mRNA transcripts in human epithelia. *Eur. J. Biochem.* **206**, 137–149.
3. Harris, C. M., Mendes, F., Dragomir, A., Doull, I. J. M., Carvalho-Oliveira, I.,

Bebok, Z., et al. (2004) Assessment of CFTR localisation in native airway epithelial cells obtained by nasal brushing. *J. Cyst. Fibros.* **3**(Suppl 2), 43–48.

4. Sambrook, J., Fritsch, E. F., and Maniatis, T. (1989) *Molecular Cloning: A Laboratory Manual*, 2nd edn. Cold Spring Harbor Laboratory Press, Cold Spring Harbor, NY.
5. Ramalho, A. S., Beck, S., Farinha, C. M., Clarke, L. A., Heda, G. D., Steiner, B., et al. (2004) Methods for RNA extraction, cDNA preparation and analysis of CFTR transcripts. *J. Cyst. Fibros.* **3**(Suppl 2), 11–15.
6. Ramalho, A. S., Beck, S., Meyer, M., Penque, D., Cutting, G. R., and Amaral, M. D. (2002) Five percent of normal cystic fibrosis transmembrane conductance regulator mRNA ameliorates the severity of pulmonary disease in cystic fibrosis. *Am. J. Respir. Cell Mol. Biol.* **27**, 619–627.
7. Clarke, L. A., and Amaral, M. D. (2004) Semi-Quantitative RT-PCR Analysis of CFTR mRNA Abundance. European working group on CFTR expression, virtual repository. http://central.igc.gulbenkian.pt/cftr/vr/a/clarke_semi_quantitative_rt_pcr_analysis_cftr_mrna.pdf
8. Chasin, L. A. (2007) Searching for splicing motifs. *Adv. Exp. Med. Biol.* **623**, 85–106.
9. Pagani, F., Buratti, E., Stuani, C., and Barelle, F. E. (2003) Missense, nonsense, and neutral mutations define juxtaposed regulatory elements of splicing in cystic fibrosis transmembrane regulator exon 9. *J. Biol. Chem.* **278**, 26580–26588.
10. Ramalho, A. S., Beck, S., Penque, D., Gonska, T., Seydewitz, H. H., Mall, M., et al. (2003) Transcript analysis of the cystic fibrosis splicing mutation 1525-1G>A shows use of multiple alternative splicing sites and suggests a putative role of exonic splicing enhancers. *J. Med. Genet.* **40**, e88.
11. Tzetis, M., Efthymiadou, A., Doudounakis, S., and Kanavakis, E. (2001) Qualitative and quantitative analysis of mRNA associated with four putative splicing mutations (621+3A→G, 2751+2T→A, 296+1G→C, 1717-9T→C-D565G) and one nonsense mutation (E822X) in the CFTR gene. *Hum. Genet.* **109**, 592–601.
12. Dork, T., Fislage, R., Neumann, T., Wulf, B., and Tümmler, B. (1994) Exon 9 of the CFTR gene: splice site haplotypes and cystic fibrosis mutations. *Hum. Genet.* **93**, 67–73.
13. Zink, D., Amaral, M. D., Englmann, A., Lang, S., Clarke, L. A., Rudolph, C., et al. (2004) Transcription-dependent spatial arrangements of CFTR and adjacent genes in human cell nuclei. *J. Cell. Biol.* **166**, 815–825.

Chapter 10

Nonsense-Mediated mRNA Decay and Cystic Fibrosis

Liat Linde and Batsheva Kerem

Abstract

Approximately one-third of the alleles causing genetic diseases carry premature termination codons (PTCs). Therapeutic approaches for mutations generating in-frame PTCs are aimed at promoting translational readthrough of the PTC, to enable the synthesis and expression of full-length functional proteins. Interestingly, readthrough studies in tissue culture cells, mouse models, and clinical trials revealed a wide variability in the response to the readthrough treatments. The molecular basis for this variability includes the identity of the PTC and its sequence context, the chemical composition of the readthrough drug, and, as we showed recently, the level of PTC-bearing transcripts. One post-transcriptional mechanism that specifically regulates the level of PTC-bearing transcripts is nonsense-mediated mRNA decay (NMD). We have previously shown a role for NMD in regulating the response of CF patients carrying CFTR PTCs to readthrough treatment. Here we describe all the protocols for analyzing CFTR nonsense transcript levels and for investigating the role of NMD in the response to readthrough treatment. This includes inhibition of the NMD mechanism, quantification of CFTR nonsense transcripts and physiologic NMD substrates, and analysis of the CFTR function.

Key words: Premature termination codons, nonsense-mediated mRNA decay, readthrough, gentamicin, PTC124.

1. Introduction

Approximately one-third of the alleles causing genetic diseases carry premature termination codons (PTCs). PTCs originate from mutations such as nonsense mutations, frame-shift deletions and insertions, or aberrant splicing, generating mRNA isoforms with truncated reading frames. PTCs can lead to the production of truncated nonfunctional proteins or proteins with deleterious function, due to dominant-negative or gain-of-function

M.D. Amaral, K. Kunzelmann (eds.), *Cystic Fibrosis*, Methods in Molecular Biology 741,
DOI 10.1007/978-1-61779-117-8_10, © Springer Science+Business Media, LLC 2011

effects (1). In the last years there has been an attempt to develop pharmacological approaches for mutations generating in-frame PTCs. These therapeutic approaches are aimed at promoting translational readthrough of the PTCs, to enable the synthesis and expression of full-length functional proteins at sufficient levels. In most of these studies the readthrough drugs were aminoglycosides, mainly gentamicin. The clinical benefit of gentamicin is limited since high concentrations and/or long-term treatments have severe side effects such as kidney damage and hearing loss. Therefore, high-throughput screen was performed to identify compounds that promote readthrough of PTCs. This analysis identified PTC124 (Ataluren), a small organic molecule that promotes selective and specific readthrough of disease-causing PTCs without adverse side effects (2). Interestingly, studies using aminoglycosides and PTC124 in tissue culture cells, mouse models, and even clinical trials revealed a wide variability in the response to these readthrough treatments. The molecular basis for this variability (reviewed in (3)) includes the identity of the PTC and its sequence context, the chemical composition of the readthrough drug, and, as we showed recently, the level of PTC-bearing transcripts (4).

The level of transcripts is regulated by several mechanisms including transcription, pre-mRNA processing, and mRNA degradation. One post-transcriptional mechanism that specifically regulates the level of PTC-bearing transcripts is nonsense-mediated mRNA decay (NMD). NMD detects and degrades PTC-bearing transcripts in order to prevent the synthesis of truncated proteins. We have previously shown a role for NMD in regulating the response to readthrough treatment, since the level of nonsense transcripts might be a limiting factor in readthrough of PTCs. In cases of efficient NMD, the level of nonsense transcripts is markedly reduced and it is expected that there are not enough cystic fibrosis transmembrane conductance regulator (CFTR) nonsense transcripts to produce sufficient CFTR proteins, even if readthrough drug is provided. By contrast, in cases of less-efficient NMD, the level of CFTR nonsense transcripts is higher, expected to enable response to readthrough treatment. Hence, analyzing the level of CFTR nonsense transcripts may indicate the CF patients with a potential to respond to readthrough treatment.

Here we describe all the protocols for investigating the role of NMD in the response of CF patients carrying nonsense mutations to readthrough treatment (e.g., PTC124 or gentamicin). This includes analysis of CFTR nonsense transcript levels, inhibition of NMD mechanism, quantification of physiologic NMD substrates, and analysis of CFTR chloride efflux.

2. Materials

2.1. Scraping of Nasal Cells for RNA Analysis of CFTR Transcript Levels

1. Rhino-probe nasal curettes should be used for curettage.
2. RNase-free Eppendorf tubes.

2.2. Cell Culture

1. All cell lines originated from human epithelium and are grown as detailed below:
   (a) HeLa cells, which were derived from cervical carcinoma, MCF7 cells, derived from breast adenocarcinoma, and IB3-1 cells, derived from a primary culture of bronchial epithelia isolated from a CF patient (5), are grown in 100 mm tissue dishes (Nunc) and maintained in Dulbecco's modified Eagle's medium (DMEM, Biological Industries) supplemented with 20 mM glutamine, 50 mg/l streptomycin, 50,000 units/l penicillin, and 10% fetal calf serum (Biological Industries).
   (b) Nasal epithelial cell lines were established by the group of Prof. J. Yankaskas from nasal polyps of CF patients (6–8): CFP22a by using the E6/E7 genes of the human papilloma virus 18 and hTERT; CFP15a by using E6/E7 genes alone; and CFP15b by LT-hTERT. These cells are grown in 100 mm tissue dishes (Falcon, Becton Dickinson) coated with collagen (*see* **Section 2.2, step 2**) and maintained in bronchial epithelial cell basal medium (BEBM, Lonza).
   (c) T84 cells, derived from lung metastases from colorectal carcinoma, are grown in 100 mm tissue dishes (Nunc) and maintained in DMEM-F12 (Biological Industries) supplemented with 20 mM glutamine, 50 mg/l streptomycin, 50,000 units/l penicillin, and 10% fetal calf serum (Biological Industries).
2. Collagen (rat tail, Roche) is dissolved in 5 ml filtrated 0.2% acetic acid (100 μl acetic acid glacial (Frutarom) in 50 ml double distilled water (DDW)) for a stock solution and stored at 4°C. A total of 1.17 ml collagen is diluted in 49 ml DDW. To coat 100 mm dish, 6 ml of the diluted collagen is used, and to coat 6-well, 1 ml is used. Following the addition of the diluted collagen, the dishes should be dried overnight in hood ventilation and then placed under UV light for about 20 min.
3. Trypsin–EDTA (Biological Industries).
4. Phosphate-buffered saline (PBS, Gibco).

2.3. CFTR Plasmid Construction

1. pCMVbeta vector (ATCC), in which sequences of the beta-gal are deleted.
2. CFTR primers are designed for three PCR reactions with flanking tail sequences in order to enable the ligation of these PCR fragments. In addition, these primers contain restriction sites to enable the insertion of the PCR fragments into the vector. Sequences for the primer pairs are as follows (5′–3′):

   oligo 1 CTCTTGGGAAGAACTGGATCAGG (these nucleotides are specific to the gene sequence at exon 20).

   oligo 2 CTAATCCCGATATCCAAAAGCCCAAGGCTCC CA (the first eight nucleotides are complementary to nucleotides 15–22 of oligo 3, the following six nucleotides are the restriction site of *Eco*RV enzyme, the next eight nucleotides are complementary to nucleotides 1–8 of oligo 3, and the rest of the nucleotides are specific to the gene sequence at intron 20).

   oligo 3 GGCTTTTGGATATCGGGATTAGAAAAATGTT CACAAGGGAC (the first eight nucleotides are complementary to nucleotides 15–22 of oligo 2, the following six nucleotides are the restriction site of *Eco*RV enzyme, the next eight nucleotides are complementary to nucleotides 1–8 of oligo 2, and the rest of the nucleotides are specific to the gene sequence at intron 20).

   oligo 4 GTGCCAGGTTCGAAGTACTCCATTTTGAAGT TGTGCACAG (the first eight nucleotides are complementary to nucleotides 14–21 of oligo 5, the following six nucleotides are the restriction site of *Bst*BI enzyme, the next seven nucleotides are complementary to nucleotides 1–7 of oligo 5, and the rest of the nucleotides are specific to the gene sequence at intron 21).

   oligo 5 GGAGTACTTCGAACCTGGCACGTAATAGACA CTCATTG (the first seven nucleotides are complementary to nucleotides 15–21 of oligo 5, the following six nucleotides are the restriction site of *Bst*BI enzyme, the next eight nucleotides are complementary to nucleotides 1–8 of oligo 4, and the rest of the nucleotides are specific to the gene sequence at intron 21).

oligo 6 GCACTGGGTTCATCAAGCAGCAAG (these nucleotides are specific to the gene sequence at exon 22).

3. The template for these PCR reactions is DNA from HT-29 cells, carrying normal CFTR alleles, or DNA from KM cells, homozygous for the W1282X mutation.
4. The CFTR plasmids are generated by cloning the fragment between *Bpu*10I and *Bst*XI (Fermentas) restriction sites in the vector.
5. PCR reactions are performed using the DNA polymerase Accuprime Pfx (Invitrogen) for the smaller PCR products and with Platinum PCR SuperMix High Fidelity (Invitrogen) for the bigger PCR products.

2.4. CFTR Plasmid Transfections into Non-CFTR Expressing Cells

1. Transfections of HeLa and MCF7 cells are performed by using calcium chloride precipitation method. CFTR WT or mutant constructs (*see* **Section 2.3**) are co-transfected with a plasmid encoding enhanced green fluorescence protein (pEGFP, Clontech) for normalization.
2. $CaCl_2$ (Merck) is dissolved at 2.5 M in DDW, filtrated, and stored in aliquots at –20°C.
3. For BBS preparation: 0.533 g BES (Sigma, cell culture tested) is dissolved in 30 ml DDW. A total of 2.8 ml of 5 M NaCl (Frutarom) and 500 μl of 0.15 M Na_2HPO_4 (Sigma, cell culture tested) are added. The pH should be adjusted exactly to 6.96. DDW is added to a final volume of 50 ml.

2.5. Gentamicin Treatment and NMD Inhibition in Nasal Epithelial Cell Lines Carrying CFTR Nonsense Alleles

1. Gentamicin sulfate salt (Sigma) is dissolved at 50 mg/ml in DDW, filtrated, and stored in aliquots at –20°C.
2. Cycloheximide (CHX) (Sigma) is dissolved at 10 mg/ml in DDW, filtrated, and stored in aliquots at –20°C.
3. siRNA transfection is performed using oligofectamine reagent (Invitrogen) and Opti-MEM+GlutaMAX (Gibco) with MEM non-essential amino acids (Gibco) (for 500 ml Opti-MEM+GlutaMAX 5 ml MEM non-essential amino acids is added).
4. The targeted nucleotides of siRNA oligos (Dharmacon) are as follows: UPF1: AAGATGCAGTTCCGCTCCATTTT; UPF2: AAGGCTTTTGTCCCAGCCATCTT; Luciferase: AACGUACGCGGAAUACUUCGATT. The non-specific control oligo contains 52% GC content, similar to the GC content in both UPF1- and UPF2-specific oligos.

2.6. RNA Analysis for Quantification of Transcript Levels in Primary and Transformed Nasal Epithelial Cells Obtained from CF Patients

1. RNeasy extraction kit (Qiagen) or Tri-Reagent-LS (MRC) is used for total RNA extraction.
2. SuperScript II Reverse transcriptase (RT, Invitrogen).
3. Real-time polymerase chain reaction (PCR) is performed using the LightCycler system (software version 3.5) with FastStart DNA Master SYBR Green I kit (Roche Diagnostics) for the samples of cell lines or the ABI PRISM 7900HT system with Power SYBR Green PCR Master Mix (Applied Biosystems) for the samples of patients.
4. *Primers (5′–3′) for the cDNA samples of the patients:*
   (a) "Non-F508del" transcripts: forward GGCACCATTAAAGAAAATATCATCTT, reverse TTGTCTTTCTC TGCAAACTTGG.
   (b) Keratin 18 (KRT18): forward TGATGACACCAATATCACACGA, reverse GGGGCCATCTACCTCCAC.
   (c) RNA polymerase II subunit A (RPII): forward GTC CAGTTCGGAGTCTGAG, reverse GCCAGTCCGCTCAACA.
5. *Primers (5′–3′) for the cDNA samples of HeLa and MCF7 transfected with CFTR constructs:*
   (a) pCFTR: forward (exon 20) ATGGTGTGTCTTGGGA, reverse (exon 22) ACAAGGACAAAGTCAAGC.
   (b) pEGFP (enhanced green fluorescence protein): forward GCAACTACAAGACCCGC, reverse GTCGGCCATGATATAGACG.
6. *Primers (5′–3′) for the cDNA samples of CFP15a, CFP15b, and CFP22a cell lines:*
   (a) CFTR: forward GAGGGTAAAATTAAGCACAGT, reverse TGCTCGTTGACCTCCA.
   (b) Ribosomal protein S9 (RPS9): forward AGACCCTTCGAGAAATCTCGTCTCG, reverse TGGGTCCTTCTCATCAAGCGTCAGC.
7. *Primers (5′–3′) for quantification of physiologic NMD substrates:*
   (a) Ribosomal protein L3 (RPL3): forward GGCATTGTG GGCTACGTG, reverse CTTCAGGAGCAGAGCAGA.
   (b) Splicing component 35 kDa (SC35) 1.6 kb: forward CGGTGTCCTCTTAAGAAAATGATGTA, reverse CT GCTACACAACTGCGCCTTTT.
   (c) SC35 1.7 kb: forward GGCGTGTATTGGAGCAGATGTA, reverse – the same as for SC35 1.6 kb.
   (d) Asparagine synthetase (ASNS): forward TCAGGTTGA TGATGCAATG, reverse CAGCTGACTTG TAGTG GGTC.

(e) Cysteinyl-tRNA synthetase (CARS): forward AAATTAAATGAGACCACGGA, reverse TGACATCACAG CCAAGTGTA.

(f) Glyceraldehyde 3-phosphate dehydrogenase (GAPDH) (for normalization): forward TGAGCTTGACAAAG TGGTCG, reverse GGCTCTCCAGAACATCATCC.

2.7. Western Blot Analysis of UPF1 and UPF2 Proteins in Nasal Epithelial Cell Lines Carrying CFTR Nonsense Alleles

1. Extraction buffer containing 250 mM NaCl (Frutarom), 50 mM Tris (Sigma) at pH 8.0, 20 mM ethylene glycol-bis(2-aminoethylether)-*N,N,N′,N′*-tetraacetic acid EGTA (Sigma), 50 mM NaF (Sigma), and 1% NP-40 (Sigma).
2. Protease inhibitor cocktail (Sigma).
3. Protein ladder PageRuler Plus (Fermentas).
4. Bradford reagent (Sigma).
5. 10% polyacrylamide gel, containing 10% acrylamide mix (1:37.5, Sigma), 4× 1.5 M Tris–Cl at pH 8.8, 0.1% sodium dodecyl sulfate (SDS, Sigma), 0.05% ammonium persulfate (APS, Sigma), and 1,000× *N,N,N,N′*-tetramethylethylenediamine (TEMED, J.T. Baker).
6. Stacking gel containing 4% acrylamide mix (1:37.5, Sigma), 125 mM Tris–Cl at pH 6.8, 0.1% SDS (Sigma), 0.1% APS (Sigma), and 750× TEMED (J.T. Baker).
7. Sample buffer: 2% SDS (Sigma), 80 mM Tris–Cl at pH 6.8, 10% glycerol (Sigma), bromophenol blue (Sigma-Aldrich).
8. 10× TBS containing 80 g NaCl, 2 g KCl, 30 g Tris in 900 ml DDW. The pH should be adjusted exactly to 7.4. Fill up with DDW to final volume of 1 l. For 1× TBS-Tween (TBS-T), 50 ml 10× TBS is added to 450 ml DDW. Subsequently, 500 μl Tween is added.
9. 10× running buffer: 144 g glycine and 30 g Tris base (Sigma) in 1 l DDW. 1× running buffer: 360 ml DDW, 40 ml 10× running buffer, 2 ml of 20% SDS (Sigma).
10. Transfer buffer: 10% methanol (J.T. Baker), 10% 10× running buffer, 0.1% SDS (Sigma).
11. Blocking: 1 h in 8% non-fat skimmed milk powder in 1× TBS-T, at room temperature with constant agitation.
12. Primary antibodies are against UPF1 (1:2,000 dilution, a kind gift from A. E. Kulozik), UPF2 (1:1,000 dilution, a kind gift from J. Lykke-Andersen), β-catenin (1:5,000 dilution, BD Biosciences), and tubulin (1:50,000 dilution, Sigma). All the primary antibodies are diluted in 4% non-fat skimmed milk powder in TBS-T.
13. Secondary antibodies conjugated to horseradish peroxidase are used. For UPF1 and UPF2, donkey anti-rabbit

(Sigma) and for β-catenin and tubulin, donkey anti-mouse (Jackson) are used. All the antibodies are diluted in 4% non-fat skimmed milk powder in TBS-T.

14. Enhanced chemiluminescence (ECL) reagents (Santa Cruz).
15. Mini Trans-Blot electrophoretic transfer cell (Bio-Rad).

2.8. CFTR Functional Analysis Measured by Chloride Efflux in Nasal Epithelial Cells

1. A chloride-sensitive fluorescent indicator, *N*-(6-methoxyquinolyl)acetoethyl ester (MQAE) (Molecular Probes), is dissolved at 1 M in methanol (Merck) for a stock solution and stored in dark at –20°C. Working solution of 10 mM is diluted in medium.
2. The Cl^- buffer containing 137 mM NaCl (Frutarom), 2.7 mM KCl (Frutarom), 0.7 mM $CaCl_2$(Merck), 1.1 mM $MgCl_2$ (Merck), 1.5 mM KH_2PO_4 (Merck), and 8.1 mM Na_2HPO_4 (Merck), at a total pH of 7.4.
3. The NO_3^- buffer containing 137 mM $NaNO_3$ (Sigma-Aldrich), 2.7 mM KNO_3 (Sigma), 0.7 mM $Ca(NO_3)_2$ (Merck), 1.1 mM $Mg(NO_3)_2$ (Sigma-Aldrich), 1.5 mM KH_2PO_4, and 8.1 mM Na_2HPO_4, at a total pH of 7.4.
4. cAMP agonist, forskolin (Sigma), is dissolved at 100 mM in dimethyl sulfoxide (DMSO) for a stock solution and stored in dark at –20°C. The stock solution is diluted to 5 mM in DMSO and stored in dark at room temperature. For working solution, the latter should be diluted to 5 μM in NO_3^- buffer.
5. Collagen I coated 96-well black plates with clear bottom (Sigma).
6. FLUOstar galaxy fluorescent reader (BMG LABTECH).

3. Methods

3.1. Scraping of Nasal Cells for RNA Analysis of CFTR Transcript Levels

1. The patients should blow their nose before starting the curettage.
2. The Rhino-probe nasal curette should be placed on the inferiomedial surface, from where the nasal cells are obtained.
3. The curette should gently be pulled forward and replaced two to three times to obtain cells.
4. Then the cells are released into an RNase-free Eppendorf tube.
5. For RNA extraction please *see* **Section 3.6**.

3.2. Cell Culture

1. All cell lines are passaged with trypsin–EDTA when approaching confluence, to provide new maintenance cultures on 100 mm tissue dishes and experimental cultures on 6-well plates.
2. Before splitting, cells are washed with PBS.
3. For CHX experiments in HeLa and MCF7 cells, transfected with CFTR constructs, 2×10^5 cells are seeded in 6-well plates.
4. For CHX experiments in CFP15a, CFP15b, CFP22a and IB3-1 cells, 5×10^5 cells are seeded in 6-well plates.
5. For UPF1 and UPF2 downregulation experiments in all cell lines tested 1.4×10^5 cells are seeded for RNA analysis in 6-well plates and for protein analysis in 100 mm plates, 24 h before oligotransfection; 1×10^4 cells are plated for functional analysis in 96-well plates, 24 h before oligotransfection.

3.3. CFTR Plasmid Construction

1. Three primer pairs are used. PCR1: oligo 1 (forward) and oligo 2 (reverse); PCR2: oligo 3 (forward) and oligo 4 (reverse); PCR3: oligo 5 (forward) and oligo 6 (reverse). For these reactions the template is DNA derived from either HT-29 or KM cells, for CFTR WT or mutant construct, respectively.
2. These PCR fragments are connected by performing two PCR reactions using the primer pairs oligo 1 and oligo 4; oligo 3 and oligo 6. The template for these PCR reactions is the PCR products from the former reactions PCR1+PCR2 and PCR2+PCR3, respectively.
3. These two PCR fragments are connected by performing another PCR reaction using the primer pair oligo 1 and oligo 6. The template for these PCR reactions is the PCR products from the former reactions: PCR(1+2)+PCR3 or alternatively PCR1+PCR(2+3). Using this strategy, connection of the three PCR fragments containing exons 20 and part of its downstream intronic sequence (264 bp), exon 21 and part of its flanking introns (240 bp at intron 20 and 289 bp at intron 21), and exon 22 and part of its upstream intronic sequence (260 bp) is performed (9).
4. Both CFTR plasmids, WT and mutant, are generated by cloning the fragment between *Bpu*10I and *Bst*XI (Fermentas) restriction sites in the vector.

3.4. CFTR Plasmid Transfections for Non-CFTR Expressing Cells

1. The DNA mix for the CFTR transfections contains 2 μg DNA per 6 well of WT or W1282X CFTR constructs together with 0.2 μg DNA of GFP. DDW is added to a total volume of 90 μl.

2. 8 μl of 2.5 M $CaCl_2$ and 100 μl of BBS are added to the DNA mix.
3. Vortex.
4. 10–15 min incubation at room temperature.
5. The mix is added to the cells with 2 ml fresh medium (has been replaced maximum 4 h before).
6. The cells are grown overnight at 3% CO_2 and 37°C.
7. On the next day, 24 h following the transfection, the cells are washed with PBS and are grown in fresh medium in regular conditions including 5% CO_2 and 37°C for an additional 48 h.
8. For RNA extraction please *see* **Section 3.6**.

3.5. Gentamicin Treatment and NMD Inhibition in Nasal Epithelial Cell Lines Carrying CFTR Nonsense Alleles

1. Cells are treated with 50–200 μg/ml gentamicin for 18–24 h.
2. Indirect NMD inhibition is performed using 200 μg/ml CHX for 5 h.
3. Direct NMD inhibition is achieved by silencing the expression of UPF1 or UPF2 using siRNA oligos. Either siRNA oligo for luciferase or non-specific oligo is used as control.
4. For CHX experiments in HeLa and MCF7 cells transfected with CFTR constructs: 48 h following the transfection (*see* **Section 3.4**) CHX is added to the cells.
5. For UPF1 downregulation experiments in HeLa and MCF7 cells transfected with CFTR constructs:
   (a) siRNA transfection is performed using 10 μl of siRNAs (20 μM stock) in 175 μl Opti-MEM (in one Eppendorf tube) and 3 μl oligofectamine reagent in 15 μl Opti-MEM (in another Eppendorf tube).
   (b) Following incubation for 5 min at room temperature the oligofectamine mix is added to the siRNA mix.
   (c) This mix is incubated for 15 min at room temperature.
   (d) Then, the mix is added to cells with 800 μl Opti-MEM.
   (e) The cells are grown overnight at 3% CO_2 and 37°C.
   (f) After 4 h, 1 ml DMEM supplemented with 20% FCS is added to the cells.
   (g) 24 h following the transfection with UPF1 siRNA, transfection of the CFTR constructs is performed (*see* **Section 3.4**).
   (h) On the next day the medium should be changed to fresh medium.

(i) On the next day (72 h after knockdown and 48 h after CFTR transfection) cells are harvested for RNA and protein analyses.

6. For UPF1 and UPF2 downregulation experiments in CFP15a, CFP15b, CFP22a and IB3-1 cells:
   (a) siRNA transfection is performed using 20 μl of siRNAs (20 μM stock) in 350 μl medium lacking serum and 8 μl oligofectamine reagent in 30 μl medium lacking serum (per 6 well).
   (b) Following incubation for 10 min at room temperature the oligofectamine preparation is added to the siRNA preparation.
   (c) This mix is incubated for 20 min at room temperature.
   (d) Then, the mix is added to cells with 1.6 ml medium with serum.
   (e) The cells are grown for 48 h at regular conditions including 5% CO_2 and 37°C.
   (f) Gentamicin is added to the cells for 18–24 h prior to the harvesting, for RNA or protein (western blot) analyses or for measurements of CFTR chloride efflux.
7. For RNA extraction please *see* **Section 3.6.**

3.6. RNA Analysis for Quantification of Transcript Levels in Primary and Transformed Nasal Epithelial Cells Obtained from CF Patients

1. For the patients' samples

   Scraped nasal epithelial cells are obtained from the patients and total RNA is extracted according to the manufacturer's protocol. RT reactions are performed to obtain cDNA. Real-time PCR is performed using the ABI PRISM 7900HT system with the Power SYBR Green PCR Master Mix. RNA-less and reverse-transcriptase-less reactions are used as controls. The level of CFTR transcripts carrying nonsense mutations is quantified using the "non-F508del" transcripts. The level of "non-F508del" transcripts is normalized to that of two genes: KRT18, a gene expressed specifically at ciliated and secretory epithelial cells, and RPII, a housekeeping gene. The level of CFTR nonsense transcripts is calculated relative to the level of CFTR mRNA of a healthy control individual who does not carry a known CFTR mutation (10). An example of the results produced, based on (10), is shown in **Fig. 10.1**.

2. For quantification of CFTR W1282X transcript levels in HeLa and MCF7 cells, transfected with the CFTR constructs

   RNA is extracted according to the manufacturer's protocol and RT reactions are performed to obtain cDNA. Real-time PCR is performed using the LightCycler with the

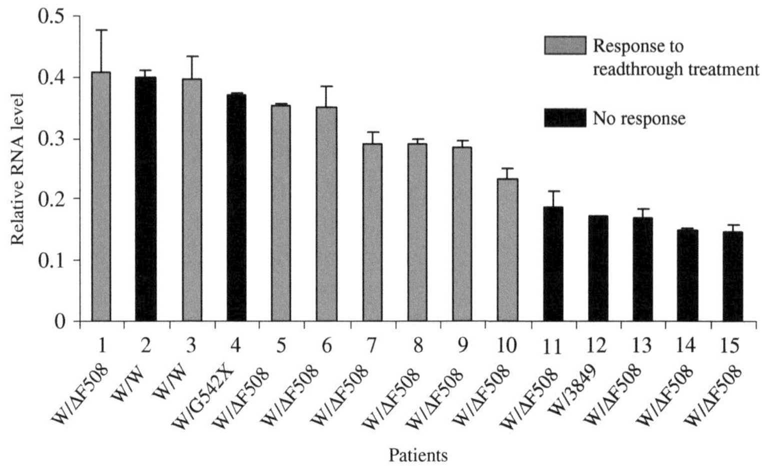

Fig. 10.1. Levels of *CFTR* nonsense transcripts in nasal epithelium obtained from CF patients. The levels of CFTR nonsense transcripts were normalized to the level of KRT18 and RPII and compared to the normalized level obtained from a control individual with normal *CFTR* alleles. The levels are shown as mean ± SEM. The genotype of each patient is indicated at the *bottom* of the figure. W – the W1282X mutation; 3849 – the 3849+10 kb C→T mutation.

FastStart DNA Master SYBR Green I kit. The level of RNA transcribed from the WT or W1282X CFTR constructs is normalized to the RNA level of GFP (which is used as a reference for transfection efficiency). Subsequently, the ratio between the normalized RNA level transcribed from the mutant and the WT constructs is calculated. An example of the results produced following CHX treatment is shown in **Fig. 10.2**.

3. For CFP15a, CFP15b, and CFP22a cell lines

   RNA is extracted according to the manufacturer's protocol and RT reactions are performed to obtain cDNA. Real-time PCR is performed using the LightCycler with the FastStart DNA Master SYBR Green I kit. The CFTR mRNA levels are normalized to those transcribed from a control gene RPS9. The level of the normalized CFTR transcripts is compared to the normalized level of untreated cells. An example of the results produced following NMD inhibition is shown in **Fig. 10.3**.

4. For quantification of physiologic NMD substrates, RPL3, SC35 1.6 kb, SC35 1.7 kb, ASNS, and CARS:

   RNA is extracted according to the manufacturer's protocol and RT reactions are performed to obtain cDNA. Real-time PCR is performed. The levels of each transcript are normalized to those transcribed from GAPDH. Then, the level of the normalized transcripts following NMD

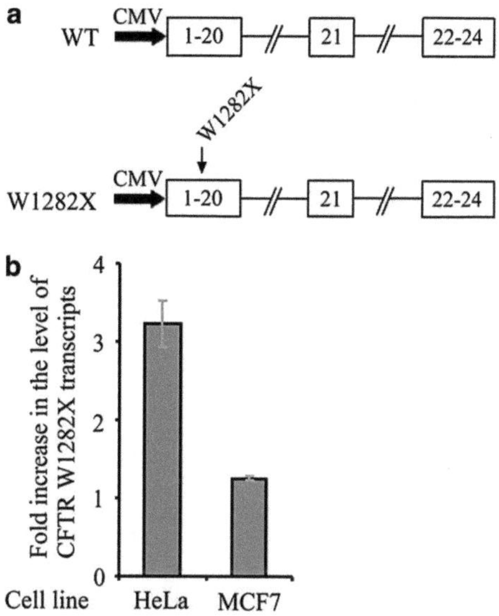

Fig. 10.2. Effect of CHX treatment on the level of CFTR mRNA transcribed from constructs carrying the W1282X PTC. (**a**) A scheme of the wild-type (WT) (*upper panel*) and W1282X (*lower panel*) constructs, which contain all CFTR exons (*marked in the boxes by numbers*) and part of the intronic sequences between exons 20 and 22. The CMV promoter is marked by *a thick horizontal arrow*. (**b**) Real-time PCR analysis of CFTR transcripts following CHX treatment. The level of mRNA transcribed from CFTR constructs carrying either the normal sequence or the W1282X PTC was normalized to the mRNA level of GFP. The ratio between these normalized levels following CHX treatment was calculated and compared with the ratio in untreated cells. The fold increase in the level of CFTR W1282X transcripts is shown as mean ± SEM (reproduced from (9)).

inhibition is compared to the normalized level of untreated cells. An example of the results produced following NMD inhibition is shown in **Fig. 10.4**.

3.7. Western Blot Analysis for UPF1 and UPF2 Proteins in Nasal Epithelial Cell Lines Carrying CFTR Nonsense Alleles

1. Extraction buffer and protease inhibitor in a ratio of 100:1 are added to the cells for protein extractions.
2. Incubation of 30 min on ice.
3. Centrifugation of 13,000 rpm for 15 min at 4°C.
4. Upper phase is transferred to a new tube.
5. Protein concentration should be measured in each sample using Bradford reagent (2 μl sample with 600 μl Bradford reagent).
6. 10% polyacrylamide gel is prepared. The gel is poured, while leaving space for a stacking gel, and is overlaid with DDW. The gel should polymerize in about 20 min.
7. DDW is then poured and the stacking gel is prepared without the TEMED. Then, the TEMED is added and

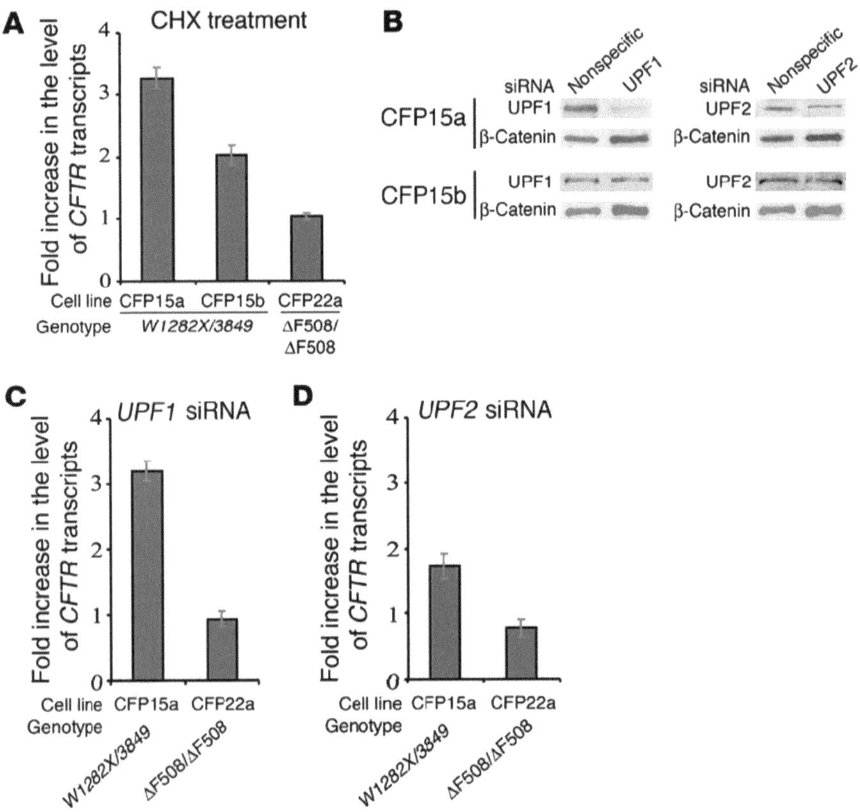

Fig. 10.3. Effect of NMD inhibition on the level of endogenous CFTR transcripts. (**a**) Effect of indirect NMD inhibition by CHX on the level of CFTR transcripts. The level was measured by real-time PCR and normalized to that of RPS9, and the ratio between these normalized levels following treatment was calculated and compared to the ratio in untreated cells. (**b**) Western blot analysis in CFP15a (*upper panel*) and CFP15b (*lower panel*) cells following sequence-specific downregulation of UPF1 and UPF2. (**c** and **d**) Effect of direct NMD inhibition by siRNA directed against UPF1 (**c**) and UPF2 (**d**) on the level of CFTR transcript. The level was measured and normalized as described in (**a**). The increase in the level of CFTR transcripts is shown as mean ± SEM (reproduced from (4)).

the stacking gel is immediately poured. The comb should be inserted. The stacking gel should polymerize within 20 min.

8. 6× sample buffer is added to each sample and then the samples are boiled at 100°C for 5 min.
9. Once the stacking gel has set, it should be laid inside the gel unit and 1× running buffer should be filled. The comb needs to be carefully removed and the wells should be washed with running buffer using needle.
10. Proteins and molecular weight markers are loaded.
11. The gel unit is connected to a power supply and run at 180 V for about 45 min.
12. The stacking gel is removed and one corner cut from the separating gel to allow its orientation to be tracked.

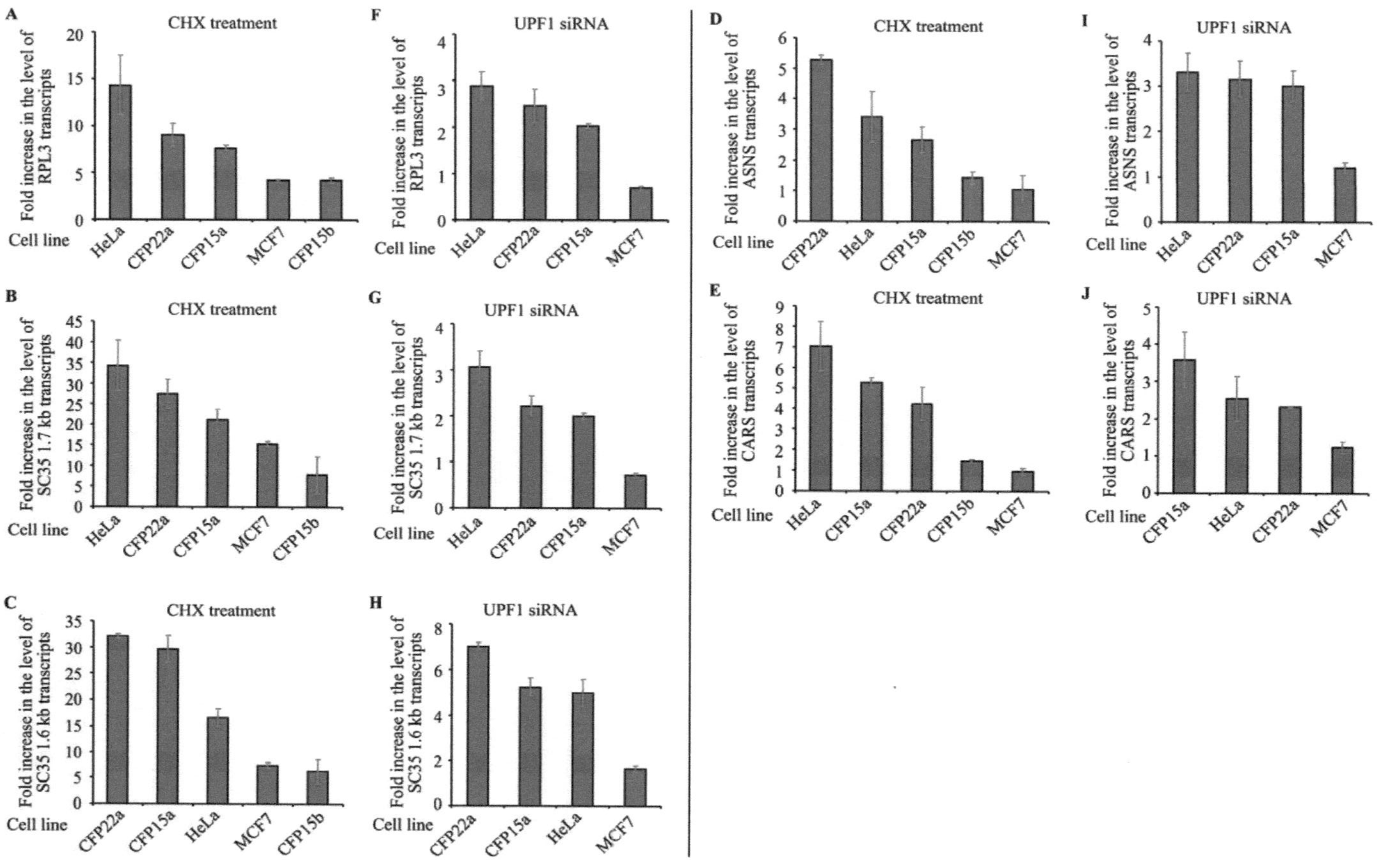

Fig. 10.4. Effect of NMD inhibition on the transcript level of physiologic NMD substrates in epithelial cell lines. The level of each analyzed transcript was measured by real-time PCR and normalized to that of GAPDH, and the ratio between these normalized levels following treatment was calculated and compared to the ratio in untreated cells. (**a–e**) Effect of indirect NMD inhibition by CHX on the level of RPL3 (**a**), SC35 1.7 kb (**b**), SC35 1.6 kb (**c**), ASNS (**d**), and CARS (**e**) transcripts. (**f–j**) Effect of direct NMD inhibition by UPF1 downregulation on the level of RPL3 (**f**), SC35 1.7 kb (**g**), SC35 1.6 kb (**h**), ASNS (i), and CARS (**j**) transcripts. The increase in the level of CFTR transcripts is shown as mean ± SEM (reproduced from (4, 9)).

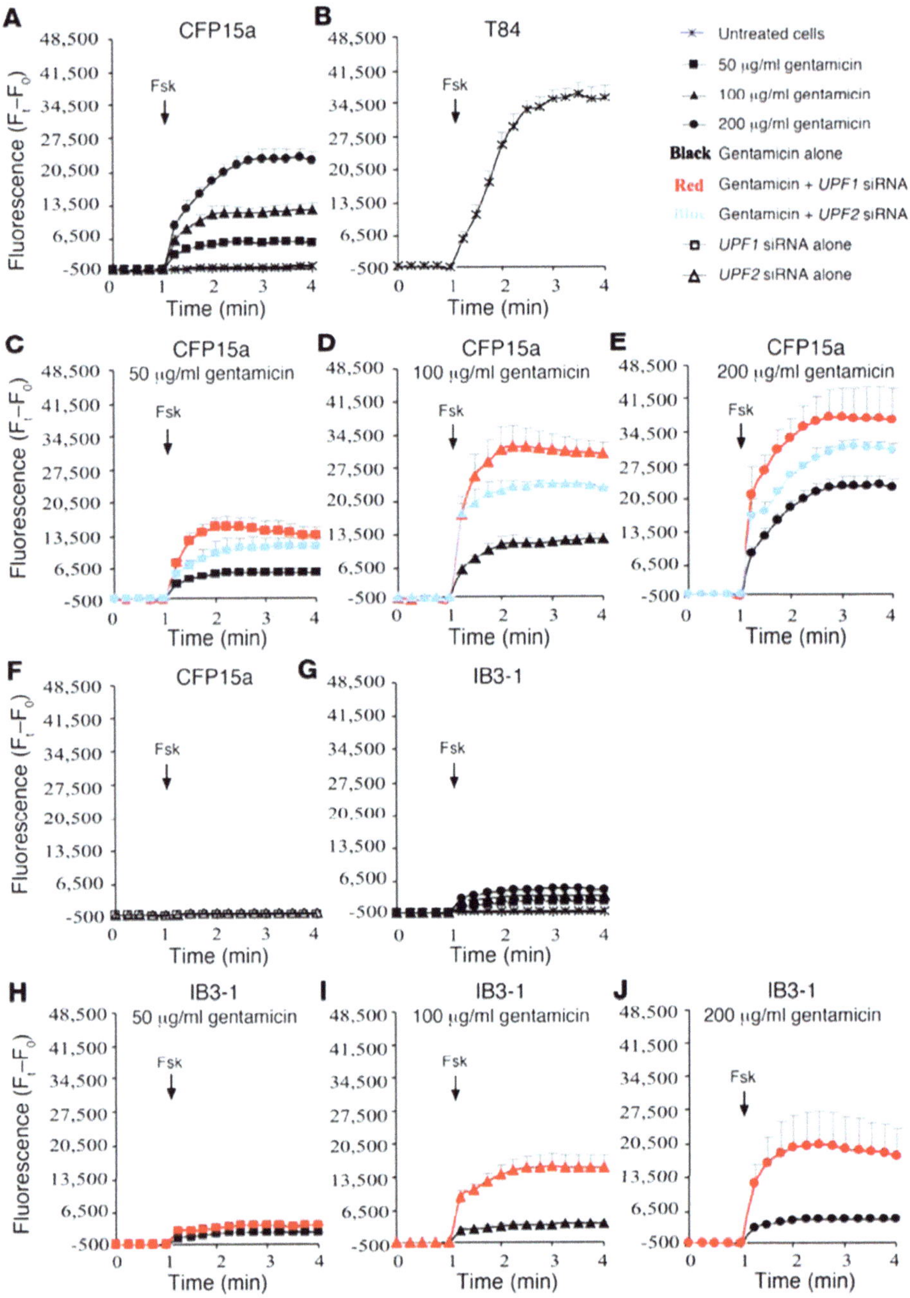

Fig. 10.5. Effect of NMD downregulation on the CFTR chloride efflux following gentamicin treatment. (**a**) CFP15a cells treated with 50–200 μg/ml gentamicin. (**b**) Chloride efflux in T84 cells. (**c–e**) CFP15a cells treated with siRNA directed against UPF1 and UPF2 following gentamicin treatment with 50 μg/ml (**c**), 100 μg/ml (**d**), and 200 μg/ml (**e**). (**f**) CFP15a cells treated with siRNA directed against UPF1 or UPF2 alone. (**g**) IB3-1 cells treated with 50–200 μg/ml gentamicin. (**h–j**) IB3-1 cells treated with siRNA directed against UPF1 following gentamicin treatment with 50 μg/ml (**h**), 100 μg/ml (**i**), and 200 μg/ml (**j**). Fsk, forskolin. The *arrow* indicates the time of forskolin administered. The increase in chloride efflux is shown as mean ± SEM. F_t, fluorescence intensity at the reading time; F_0, fluorescence intensity at the beginning of the experiment (reproduced from (4)).

13. A sponge with transfer buffer is placed. Two wet Whatman papers (with transfer buffer) are laid on it, then the gel is set, and on it the nitrocellulose membrane. Another two Whatman papers soaked with transfer buffer and a wet sponge are placed.
14. The gel unit is connected to a power supply at 280 mamp for about 1.5 h to enable proteins to be transferred to the membrane. Transfer buffer is poured to the gel unit.
15. Once the transfer is complete, the membrane is incubated in blocking buffer for 1 h.
16. The membrane is incubated with the primary antibody for 1 h at room temperature (with anti-β-catenin and anti-tubulin) or overnight at 4°C (with anti-UPF1 and anti-UPF2), with constant agitation.
17. The membrane is washed with TBS-T three times at room temperature for 10 min, each wash with constant agitation.
18. Then the membrane is incubated for 1 h with the secondary antibody at room temperature with constant agitation.
19. Three washes with TBS-T at room temperature for 10 min are performed, each wash with constant agitation.
20. An ECL reaction is performed and the membrane is exposed to X-ray film. An example of the results produced following NMD inhibition is shown in **Fig. 10.3**.

3.8. CFTR Functional Analysis Measured by Chloride Efflux in Nasal Epithelial Cells

1. Cells are loaded overnight with 10 mM MQAE in medium.
2. Cells are washed twice with PBS and loaded with100 μl Cl^- buffer for 15 min at 5% CO_2 and 37°C.
3. Fluorescent measurements are performed.
4. The extracellular chloride is exchanged with nitrate, which passes through the CFTR but unlike Cl^- does not quench the fluorescence of the indicator. Two washes followed by fluorescent measurements for the rate of chloride efflux are performed.
5. Exchange to nitrate with 5 μM forskolin to activate the CFTR chloride channel is performed, and immediately after, fluorescent measurements are taken place.
6. For evaluation of CFTR activation the difference between fluorescent intensity at the reading time (F_t) and that at the beginning of the experiment (F_0) is calculated. An example of the results produced following NMD inhibition is shown in **Fig. 10.5**.

4. Notes

1. RNA extraction from nasal epithelial cells scraped from CF patients should be performed using a highly sensitive kit, which enables extraction from only dozens of cells as the input material. We tried many kits and found that the Qiagen kit was the best for this purpose. More recently, several kits designed especially to extract RNA from small amounts of cells became available (such as Quick-RNA MicroPrep of Zymo Research), hence one could also try these kits.
2. BBS which is used for the plasmid transfection should be split into aliquots after preparation and not be re-freezed. We found that thaw–freeze cycles of BBS dramatically reduced the transfection efficiency.

References

1. Frischmeyer, P. A., and Dietz, H. C. (1999) Nonsense-mediated mRNA decay in health and disease. *Hum. Mol. Genet.* **8**, 1893–1900.
2. Hirawat, S., Welch, E. M., Elfring, G. L., Northcutt, V. J., Paushkin, S., Hwang, S. et al. (2007) Safety, tolerability, and pharmacokinetics of PTC124, a nonaminoglycoside nonsense mutation suppressor, following single- and multiple-dose administration to healthy male and female adult volunteers. *J. Clin. Pharmacol.* **47**, 430–444.
3. Linde, L., and Kerem, B. (2008) Introducing sense into nonsense in treatments of human genetic diseases. *Trends Genet.* **24**, 552–563.
4. Linde, L., Boelz, S., Nissim-Rafinia, M., Oren, Y. S., Wilschanski, M., Yaacov, Y. et al. (2007) Nonsense-mediated mRNA decay affects nonsense transcript levels and governs response of cystic fibrosis patients to gentamicin. *J. Clin. Invest.* **117**, 683–692.
5. Zeitlin, P. L., Lu, L., Rhim, J., Cutting, G., Stetten, G., Kieffer, K. A. et al. (1991) A cystic fibrosis bronchial epithelial cell line: Immortalization by adeno-12-SV40 infection. *Am. J. Respir. Cell Mol. Biol.* **4**, 313–319.
6. Yankaskas, J. R., Haizlip, J. E., Conrad, M., Koval, D., Lazarowski, E., Paradiso, A. M. et al. (1993) Papilloma virus immortalized tracheal epithelial cells retain a well-differentiated phenotype. *Am. J. Physiol.* **264**, C1219–1230.
7. Lundberg, A. S., Randell, S. H., Stewart, S. A., Elenbaas, B., Hartwell, K. A., Brooks, M. W. et al. (2002) Immortalization and transformation of primary human airway epithelial cells by gene transfer. *Oncogene* **21**, 4577–4586.
8. Nissim-Rafinia, M., Aviram, M., Randell, S. H., Shushi, L., Ozeri, E., Chiba-Falek, O. et al. (2004) Restoration of the cystic fibrosis transmembrane conductance regulator function by splicing modulation. *EMBO Rep.* **5**, 1071–1077.
9. Linde, L., Boelz, S., Neu-Yilik, G., Kulozik, A. E., and Kerem, B. (2007) The efficiency of nonsense-mediated mRNA decay is an inherent character and varies among different cells. *Eur. J. Hum. Genet.* **15**, 1156–1162.
10. Kerem, E., Hirawat, S., Armoni, S., Yaakov, Y., Shoseyov, D., Cohen, M. et al. (2008) Effectiveness of PTC124 treatment of cystic fibrosis caused by nonsense mutations: A prospective phase II trial. *Lancet* **372**, 719–727.

Chapter 11

Approaches to Study CFTR Pre-mRNA Splicing Defects

Elisa Goina, Eugenio Fernandez-Alanis, and Franco Pagani

Abstract

In cystic fibrosis, genomic variants can result in defective processing of the CFTR precursor mRNA. Due to the complexity of the splicing process, the evaluation of their pathological effect is an important aspect both in the diagnostic field and in the study of basic regulatory mechanism. Efficient and correct splicing of CFTR relies on a complex process that includes recognition within the nascent transcripts of a series of different splicing regulatory elements that frequently overlap with the coding sequences. Identification of these elements is essential to determine the pathological impact of splicing-affecting genomic variants. In this chapter, to evaluate the effect of CFTR DNA variations on the pre-mRNA splicing process, different tools based on hybrid minigenes will be described.

Key words: Pre-mRNA splicing, hybrid minigenes, siRNA, splicing regulatory elements, splicing factors.

1. Introduction

1.1. Regulatory Elements in Pre-mRNA Splicing and Mutations That Can Affect Them

Correct pre-mRNA processing, with splicing of intron sequences and joining of coding exonic sequences, requires the classical consensus splice sites: the 5′-splice site (5′ss, AG|GURAGU), the branch point sequence (CURAY), the polypyrimidine (Py) tract (a run of polypyrimidines located between the 3′-splice site and the branch point), and the 3′-splice site (3′ss, YAG). These consensus splice sites are overrepresented in pre-mRNAs and thus not sufficient to define the correct intron–exon boundaries. To direct the splicing machinery on the correct splice sites additional splicing regulatory sequences called exonic splicing enhancers (ESE) and silencers (ESS) and intronic splicing enhancers (ISE) and silencers (ISS) are required. In general, enhancers are binding sites for serine/arginine-rich (SR) proteins,

M.D. Amaral, K. Kunzelmann (eds.), *Cystic Fibrosis*, Methods in Molecular Biology 741,
DOI 10.1007/978-1-61779-117-8_11, © Springer Science+Business Media, LLC 2011

whereas silencers interact mainly with members of the heterogeneous nuclear ribonucleoprotein (hnRNP) family (1). These *cis*-acting regulatory elements can also have an overlapping function as reported for the cystic fibrosis transmembrane conductance regulator gene (CFTR) exons 9 and 12 (2, 3). In this case, it may be more appropriate to talk about composite exonic regulatory elements of splicing (CERES).

These regulatory sequences are characterized by highly degenerate sequence motifs making their identification by sequence inspection alone difficult. Considering the complexity of the pre-mRNA process and the large amount of splicing regulatory sequences involved, it is not surprising that mutations may cause aberrant splicing (4, 5). In fact the pathological effect of a mutation on pre-mRNA processing may not be immediately evident. Mutations that affect the canonical splice sites at the nearly invariant AG and GT dinucleotides disrupt splicing in the majority of cases but mutations at nearby intronic sequences (genomic variants near the 3′ss or the 5′ss) or at exonic or intronic regulatory elements are more difficult to evaluate. Interestingly, several sequence variations listed in the CFTR Mutation Database (http://www.genet.sickkids.on.ca/cftr/app) are located near the 3′ss or 5′ss and their possible effect on splicing is not clearly established. The same problem may occur for synonymous or missense changes. If mutation affects an exonic splicing regulatory element (independent of the effect on the amino acidic sequence) it may cause aberrant splicing (5, 6).

The analysis of RNA samples from affected patients is the ideal way to assess whether a suspected genomic variation impairs splicing. In CF, patients' nasal brushing can be useful for screening but it is not always available. Moreover, some CF mutations may restrict the analysis of aberrant splicing expression to a specific tissue. Consequently, the use of a minigene system and the development of functional splicing assays become essential when it comes to discriminate between benign polymorphisms and disease-causing mutations. A transient transfection of a minigene is also useful in order to identify the mechanism behind aberrant RNA processing and explore novel therapeutic strategies.

1.2. Identification of Splicing Defects Using the Hybrid Minigene Assay

A minigene is a "simplified" version of a gene and usually contains the genomic region from the gene of interest that includes the exon along with its flanking intronic sequences. For practical cloning reasons relatively short intronic sequences (~100–200 bp) are preferred but sometimes longer sequences are required (*see* **Note 1**). The genomic segment cloned in the minigene derives by direct PCR amplification of the target DNA. The oligonucleotides used contain restriction enzyme sites at their ends that match restriction sites in the recipient plasmid (7). When it comes to determining whether a genomic variant plays a role in altering splicing processing, both wild-type (WT) and mutant minigenes must be built and later on their splicing patterns compared. Mutant minigenes must include the suspected genomic variant and WT minigene should replicate as far as possible the splicing pattern found in vivo. For a reliable analysis it is imperative to sequence final minigenes in order to ensure that they differ only in the genomic variation of interest. The splicing pattern of a genomic segment under study is obtained after expression of minigene pre-mRNAs by transient transfection into appropriate cell lines and subsequent RT-PCR (**Fig. 11.1b, c**). A widely used hybrid minigene is the pTB, whose basic scaffold has been successfully adapted to study different systems (**Fig. 11.1a**) (2, 3). pTB minigene transcription is under the control of minimal α-globin promoter and a simian virus 40 enhancer (SV40). The reporter minigene is composed of α-globin and fibronectin exons, while at the 3′-end it contains a functionally competent polyadenylation site, derived from the α-globin gene. A unique *Nde*I site allows cloning of genomic variant-containing exons/introns whose effect on splicing processing is unknown (**Fig. 11.1a**). The hybrid minigene assay has been extensively used for the study of several naturally occurring mutations in CFTR exon 12. Skipping of this exon renders the CFTR protein non-functional (3, 8).

As an example of a typical analysis with minigenes, here we focus on disease-causing mutations in CFTR exon 12. The CF Mutation Database reports more than 40 mutations in CFTR exon 12 and interestingly 6 of them are concentrated in a short stretch of five nucleotides between positions 1,835 and 1,839, relative to the cDNA sequence. These natural substitutions are predicted to change two amino acids creating four missense and two nonsense mutations (**Fig. 11.2b**). To study their potential effect on splicing, the six natural mutations were introduced in the CFTR exon 12 hybrid minigene and analysed in splicing functional assays (**Fig. 11.2a, c**). Details of the transfection and splicing assays are provided in **Section 3**. In comparison with the WT construct, which produced as reported in vivo (3) about 80% of CFTR exon 12 inclusion, transfection experiments showed that some mutants induced a change in the splicing pattern. Three mutants showed an increase in splicing inclusion (T1837C, T1837G, and A1838C), two a significant exon skipping (T1835A and G1836T), whereas one did not change the splicing pattern (T1839A; **Fig. 11.2c, d**).

1.3. Evaluating the Regulatory Role of a Splicing Factor Using siRNA-Mediated Silencing

Once a genomic variant has been found to affect pre-mRNA splicing it is important to investigate the mechanism of the aberrant splicing and clarify the splicing factors involved. In general, splicing mutations can abolish or promote binding to mRNA of regulatory *trans*-acting splicing factors with positive or negative

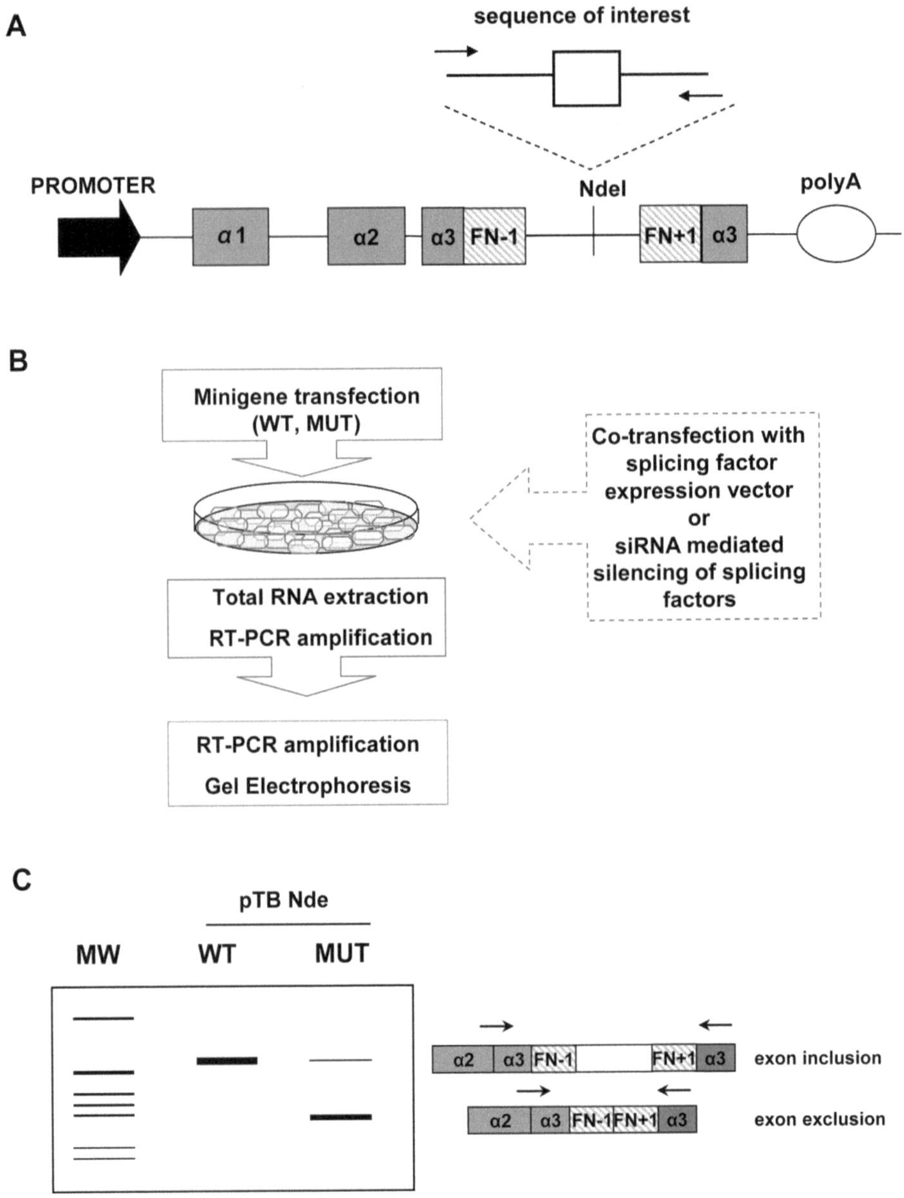

Fig. 11.1 **Functional splicing assay using hybrid minigene.** (**a**) The typical pTB hybrid minigene contains a promoter region (*black arrow, left end*), exonic (*boxes*) and intronic (*lines*) segments, and a functional polyadenylation site (polyA; *circle, right end*). The promoter region includes the α-globin promoter and the SV40 enhancer sequence and is followed by three α-globin exons (*grey boxes*), two fibronectin exons (*shaded boxes*), and the α-globin polyA site. The gene segment of interest (wild type, WT, and/or containing a particular mutation, MUT) is generated by PCR amplification directly from genomic DNA using oligonucleotides with restriction enzyme site (*Nde*I) overhangs and subsequently cloned in the recipient plasmid. (**b**) Functional splicing assay steps. Minigenes are transiently transfected in eucaryotic cell lines, followed by total RNA extraction, RT-PCR with specific primers, and gel electrophoresis analysis. To study the effect of a particular *trans*-acting factor an expression vector can be co-transfected or siRNA-mediated silencing can also be performed. (**c**) Splicing pattern analysis. In the picture a schematic representation of the functional splicing analysis of transcripts derived from the WT and MUT minigenes is shown. In this hypothetical example, the WT sequence shows complete exon inclusion and the MUT sequence prevalent exon skipping. The *small black superimposed arrows* represent the position of the primers used for the RT-PCR analysis after transient transfection and the identity of the amplified band is indicated.

A

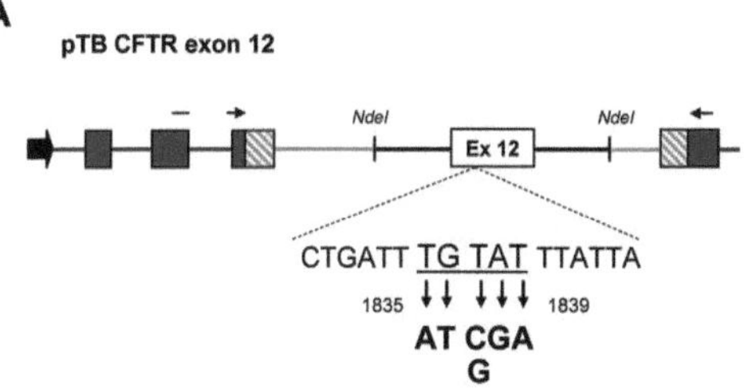

C

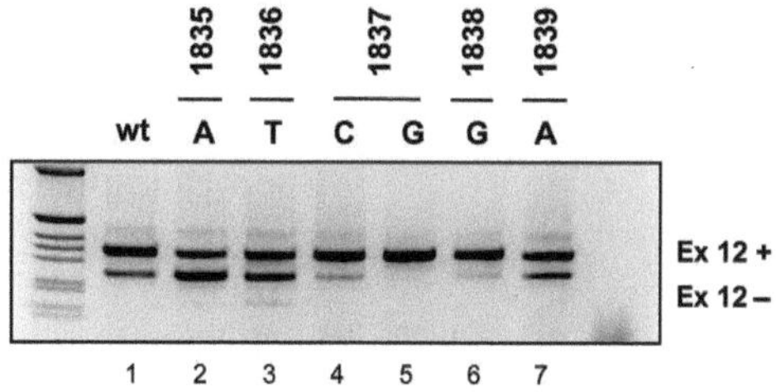

B

Aminoacid Change	Nucleotide change
L568X	T to A at 1835
L568F	G to T at 1836
Y569H	T to C at 1837
Y569D	T to G at 1837
Y569C	A to C at 1838
Y569X	T to A at 1839

D

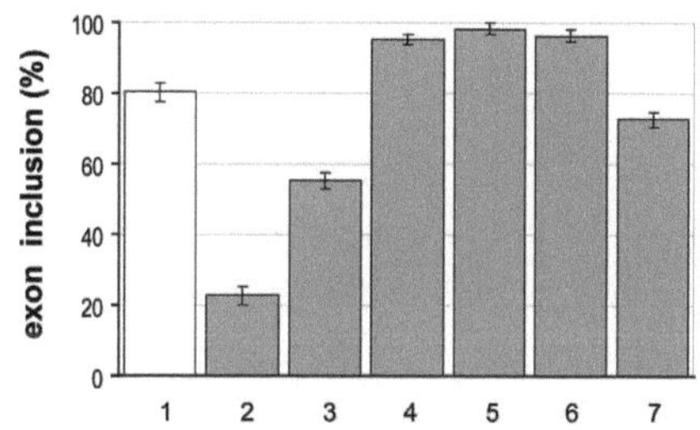

Fig. 11.2. **Identification of splicing-affecting mutations in CFTR exon 12 using the hybrid minigene system.** (**a**) Schematic representation of pTB CFTR exon 12 minigene. *Dark grey*, *shaded*, and *white boxes*, respectively, represent α-globin, fibronectin EDB exons, and human CFTR exon 12, with introns shown as *lines*. Exon 12 and parts of its flanking introns were cloned in the pTB plasmid. The *small black superimposed arrows* represent the position of the primers used for the RT-PCR analysis after transient transfection. The central part of CFTR exon 12 sequence is *highlighted* and the *black arrows*, from position 1,835 to 1,839, indicate the natural point mutations. (**b**) The table shows the CFTR exon 12 variants analysed: the *first column* shows the amino acid changes prediction and the *second column* the relative cDNA position. The natural mutations indicated are listed in CF database (http://www.genet.sickkids.on.ca/cftr/app). (**c**) Splicing pattern analysis. The agarose gel shows the RT-PCR products of WT and mutant minigenes after transient transfection into HeLa cell line. The position of the two splicing forms corresponding to exon 12 inclusion (ex12+) and exclusion (ex12–) are indicated on the right. (**d**) Percentage of CFTR exon 12 inclusion. The histogram shows the average value for the percentage of exon 12 skipping ± standard deviation, based on three independent experiments.

effect on splicing. Dozens of protein factors can bind exonic or intronic regulatory elements or serve as scaffold or mediate for protein–protein interactions. So how to begin looking for a responsible *trans*-splicing factor? An initial approach would imply the use of bioinformatic tools, such as enhancers/silencers prediction software (*see* **Note 2**). To prove in vivo the involvement of a splicing factor two complementary minigene-derived procedures are useful: overexpression and depletion of the candidate factor(s) in cell cultures. Overexpression is accomplished through co-transfection of the minigene along with an expression vector containing the full-length cDNA sequence of candidate factor(s), which is normally tagged with an epitope in order to be distinguished from the endogenous protein. Details of this strategy are not described here but can be found elsewhere (2, 3, 7). On the other hand, small interfering RNA (siRNA) silencing is the ideal tool for depletion of candidate factor(s) for its specificity and efficacy (9). Knockdown of target protein levels is verified using Western blot and/or immunostaining analysis. Northern blot analysis or quantitative RT-PCR can also be carried out to check mRNA levels when no antibody is available.

Research on alternative splicing of CFTR exon 9 constitutes a good example of mapping of an intronic regulatory element and identification of *trans*-acting splicing factors. Exon 9 definition is regulated at the 3′ss by a polymorphic TG_m repeat (9–13 UG) immediately followed by T_n tract (a polypyrimidine tract of 5, 7, or 9 Us) (10).

The $(TG)_{11-13}T_{3-5}$ polymorphism is associated with non-classical or mild CF and increasing the number of UG repeats increases the amount of aberrant exon 9 skipping (11, 12). The UG repeats were shown in vitro to bind a novel splicing factor TDP43 (13, 14). To test the effect of TDP43 on CFTR exon 9 splicing, depletion of this protein was carried out through RNA interference (15, 16). Western blotting analysis indicated that more than 90% of TDP43 was successfully silenced (**Fig. 11.3b**). As shown in **Fig. 11.3c**, lane 2, a high proportion of exon skipping is detected after transfection of HeLa cells with a pTB CFTR

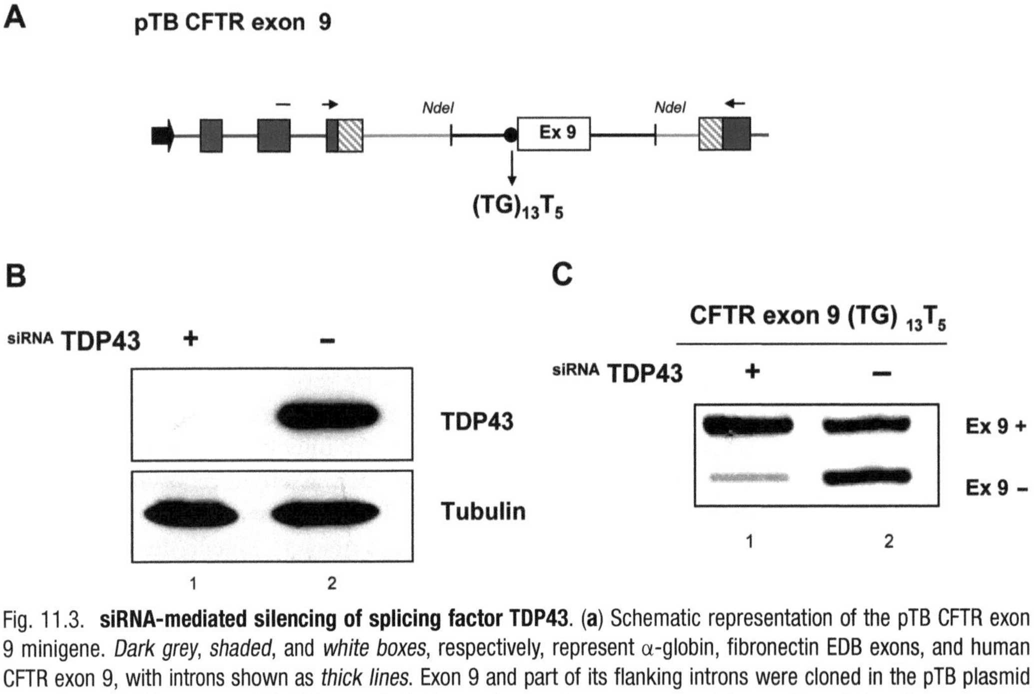

Fig. 11.3. **siRNA-mediated silencing of splicing factor TDP43.** (**a**) Schematic representation of the pTB CFTR exon 9 minigene. *Dark grey*, *shaded*, and *white boxes*, respectively, represent α-globin, fibronectin EDB exons, and human CFTR exon 9, with introns shown as *thick lines*. Exon 9 and part of its flanking introns were cloned in the pTB plasmid using the restriction enzyme *NdeI*. The *small black superimposed arrows* represent the position of the primers used for the RT-PCR analysis after transient transfection. The *black dot* indicates the $TG_{13}T_5$ polymorphism near the 3′-splice site. (**b**) The *panel* shows the Western blot analysis of protein extracts from HeLa cells treated with either TDP43 siRNA (+) or a control siRNALuc (–). The normalization of the protein loaded was checked using an antibody against tubulin, as reported in the lower panel. (**c**) The gel picture shows the RT-PCR products after transfection of the pTB CFTR exon 9 $TG_{13}T_5$ minigene into TDP43 siRNA-treated (+) and siRNALuc-treated (–) HeLa cells. On the *right* the mRNA processing outcomes, Ex 9+ and Ex 9–, are shown. An increase of exon 9 inclusion was observed in the siRNA-treated cells (*lane 1*), indicating that TDP43 is involved in exon 9 recognition.

exon 9 minigene containing the $(TG)_{13}T_5$ polymorphism (14, 17, 18). Silencing of TDP43 by siRNA resulted in a significant increase of exon 9 inclusion (**Fig. 11.3c**, lane 1) (15), indicating its direct involvement in aberrant exon skipping (16).

2. Materials

2.1. Cell Culture

1. Hep3B cells, human hepatocellular carcinoma (ATCC Number: HB-8064).
2. HeLa cells, human cervical cancer cells (ATCC Number: CCL-2).
3. Standard 100 mm tissue culture dishes.
4. Dulbecco's modified Eagle's medium (DMEM) 1X liquid (Gibco BRL, Gaithersburg, MD) with GlutaMAX^{TM} I, 4,500 mg/L D-glucose (high glucose), and sodium pyruvate. For cell culture, supplement it with 10% foetal bovine serum (Gibco) and 1X antibiotic/antimycotic. Store at 4°C.
5. Antibiotic antimycotic solution 100X stabilized (Sigma-Aldrich, St. Louis, MO), store aliquoted at –20°C. Dilute with DMEM medium to obtain 1X final concentration before use.
6. Phosphate-buffered saline (PBS) 10X solution: dissolve 2 g KCl, 80 g NaCl, 17.8 g Na_2HPO_4, and 2.4 g KH_2PO_4 in distilled H_2O up to 1 L. Autoclave and prepare 1X working solution.
7. Trypsin solution 10X: 0.2% ethylenediamine tetraacetic acid (EDTA) and 0.5% trypsin in PBS 1X, store aliquoted at –20°C. Prepare 2X working solution with PBS 1X.

2.2. Transfection of Recombinant DNA

1. Plasmid DNA: process MIDI prep using JetStar purification kit (Genomed, Löhne, Germany) and dilute to a final concentration of 100 ng/μL.
2. Effectene transfection reagent kit (Qiagen Inc., Valencia, CA, USA): Buffer EC, enhancer, and Effectene transfection reagent.
3. 35 mm tissue culture dishes or 6-well plates, as applicable.

2.3. RNA Isolation

1. PBS 1X.
2. TRI reagent for RNA isolation of high quality (Ambion, Foster City, CA, USA).
3. Chloroform.
4. Isopropanol.

5. Glycogen 20 mg/mL (Roche Diagnostics, Indianapolis, IN, USA).
6. 70% ethanol.
7. Nuclease-free H_2O.
8. RNase-free recombinant DNase I and 10X DNase incubation buffer (Roche).
9. RNeasy Mini Kit (Qiagen): buffer RLT, buffer RPE, and 100% ethanol (not supplied).
10. 10% hydrogen peroxide (H_2O_2) solution (diluted with distilled H_2O).
11. Morpholino-propanesulfonic acid (MOPS) 10X buffer: 0.2 M MOPS pH 7.0, 0.01 M EDTA pH 8.0, and 0.05 M sodium acetate, pH 8.0.
12. Denaturing agarose gel: agarose powder, 10X MOPS, and 37% formaldehyde.
13. Denaturing running buffer: 10X MOPS and 37% formaldehyde.
14. Loading dye 6X: 25 mg bromophenol blue (0.25%), 25 mg xylene cyanol (0.25%), 4 g sucrose (40%), adjust volume to 10 mL with distilled H_2O. Store at –20°C.
15. RNA sample buffer: 10X MOPS, 37% formaldehyde, deionized formamide, ethidium bromide 10 mg/mL, and loading dye 6X. Store at –20°C.

2.4. RT-PCR Analysis

1. Random primers: pd(N)6 Random Hexamer (GE Healthcare), dissolve at 100 ng/μL in distilled H_2O and store aliquoted at –20°C.
2. dNTP set: dATP, dCTP, dGTP, dTTP, 100 mM each (EuroClone SpA, Siziano, Italy). Take 25 μL apiece, mix, and dilute with distilled H_2O to a final concentration of 10 mM. Store aliquoted at –20°C.
3. M-MLV Reverse Transcriptase set (Invitrogen, San Diego, CA): 5X First strand buffer, 0.1 M DTT, and M-MLV RT enzyme 200 U/μL.
4. RNase inhibitor, 40 U/μL (Ambion).
5. Taq DNA Polymerase set (Roche): 10X PCR reaction buffer (with 15 mM $MgCl_2$) and Taq DNA polymerase, 5 U/μL.
6. DNA primers (Sigma-Aldrich): α2,3 (forward primer: 5′-CAACTTCAAGCTCCTAAGCCACTGC-3′) and Bra2 (reverse primer: 5′-TAGGATCCGGTCACCAGGAAGTTG GTTAAATCA-3′). Dissolve in autoclaved H_2O (or 1X TE) to 100 μM as stock solution and to 10 μM as working solution. Store at –20°C.

2.5. Small Interfering RNA (siRNA) Analysis

1. Opti-MEM I Reduced Serum media (Gibco).
2. Oligofectamine Transfection Reagent (Invitrogen).
3. Duplex RNA oligonucleotides (Dharmacon Inc., Lafayette, CO, USA): siRNA against TDP43 (AAG-CAAAGCCAAGAUGAGCCU) and siRNA against firefly luciferase gene (siCONTROL Non-Targeting siRNA #2) as non-specific control. Resuspend the RNA oligos in 1X siRNA Universal Buffer to 75 μM as stocking solution and to 40 μM as working solution. Store at –80°C.
4. 60 mm tissue culture dishes.

2.6. Protein Analysis

1. Protein lysis buffer 2X: 30 mM HEPES, pH 7.6, 0.5 M NaCl, 1% NP-40, and 20% glycerol. Before use dilute to 1X with distilled H_2O and add complete protease inhibitor cocktail (Roche) to a final concentration of 2X.
2. Running gel: 1.5 M Tris–HCl, pH 8.8, 30% Protogel acrylamide mix (National Diagnostics Inc., Atlanta, GA, USA), 10% SDS, 10% APS (Amersham Biosciences, Fairfield, CT, USA), and TEMED (Fluka, Sigma-Aldrich).
3. Stacking gel: 0.5 M Tris–HCl, pH 6.8, 30% Protogel acrylamide mix (National Diagnostics Inc.), 10% SDS, 10% APS (Amersham Biosciences), and TEMED (Fluka, Sigma-Aldrich).
4. Running buffer 5X: dissolve 30 g Tris base, 144.0 g glycine, and 5 g SDS in 1 L with distilled H_2O. Store at room temperature and dilute to 1X before use.
5. Transfer buffer 10X: dissolve 30 g Tris base, 144.0 g glycine with distilled H_2O. Dilute to 1X and add 20% methanol before use. Store at 4°C.
6. Hybond-P PVDF membrane (Amersham Biosciences).
7. Phosphate-buffered saline (PBS-T): 0.1% Tween in PBS 1X.
8. Blocking buffer: 5% (w/v) non-fat dry milk in PBS-T.
9. Primary antibody dilution: 1:1,000 polyclonal rabbit anti-TDP43, 1:2,000 monoclonal mouse anti-tubulin.
10. Secondary antibody: 1:2,000 polyclonal goat anti-rabbit immunoglobulin HRP, 1:2,000 polyclonal goat anti-mouse immunoglobulin HRP (DakoCytomation, Glostrup, Denmark).
11. Enhanced chemiluminescent (ECL) Western blotting substrate (Pierce, Thermo Fisher Scientific LSR, Rockford, IL, USA): Peroxide solution and luminol enhancer solution.

3. Methods

3.1. Transfection of Recombinant DNA

The following transfection protocol is a modified version of the Effectene transfection reagent handbook. Usually, transfection protocol takes about 3 days.

Day 1: Collect Hep3B or HeLa cells grown confluent in a 100 mm dish and seed 3 × 10^5 cells in 2 mL of supplemented DMEM medium on 35 mm dishes (or wells, when working with plates). Incubate them for 24 h at 37°C, 5% CO_2. Cells must have reached a 50–70% of confluence in order to proceed with transfection.

Day 2: Use 1.5 mL microfuge tubes to dilute 500 ng of plasmidic DNA with 100 μL of DNA condensation buffer (Buffer EC), pre-warmed at 37°C almost 30 min before use (Note: plasmidic DNA quality strongly influences transfection efficiency.).

In co-transfection experiments, transfect 0.5 μg of the plasmidic DNA together with an increasing amount (0.1–0.25–0.50 μg) of the protein expression plasmid (Note: it is also important to include controls in which the same amounts of control empty vector are co-transfected.).

Add 4 μL of enhancer to DNA–Buffer EC mixture for each transfection sample, vortex for 10 s, and incubate at room temperature for 5 min to allow DNA condensate (Note: the ratio DNA/enhancer should not be altered since it is proportional to the tissue culture dish area.).

Add 5 μL of Effectene to the mixture, vortex for 10 s, and incubate for 10 min at room temperature to allow transfection complex formation (Note: the ratio DNA complex/Effectene must be optimized for each cell line and plasmidic DNA. Different ratios can be used: 1:10; 1:25; 1:50. For Hep 3B and HeLa a 1:10 ratio is recommended.).

Remove the medium and wash the cells twice with 1 mL PBS 1X. Then add 1.5 mL of supplemented DMEM on each dish/well.

Add 500 μL of supplemented DMEM to transfection mixture, transfer the whole volume to each 35 mm dish/well, and incubate them at 37°C for up to 24 h.

Day 3: Wash the cells twice with PBS 1X and proceed with total RNA extraction protocol.

3.2. Total RNA Extraction and RT-PCR

Total RNA extraction and RT-PCR are performed with standard procedures. Although DNase treatment may be needed for removal of contaminant DNA, this procedure is normally not required (Note: digestion with DNase–RNase free can be required for minigenes that have short intronic sequences or when there is the interest in evaluating precursor mRNA levels. In these cases, the eventual presence of contaminant plasmid DNA which can compete with the spliced products should be removed with the DNase treatment.).

The analysis of the amplified products after RT-PCR is performed by gel electrophoresis on a 1.5 or 2% agarose gel. The identity of the resulting splicing pattern has to be verified by direct sequence analysis. ImageJ 1.38 software (http://rsb.info.nih.gov/ij/) can be used to quantify the ratio between exon inclusion and skipping. Alternatively, the RT-PCR can be performed with FAM-labelled oligonucleotides and analysed with denaturant capillary electrophoresis.

3.3. siRNA Transfection

Both Dharmacon, Inc. (Lafayette, CO, USA) and Sigma-Aldrich are trustworthy suppliers of siRNA oligos. The whole procedure usually takes 3 days.

Day 1: Collect HeLa or Hep3B cells grown confluent and seed 2.5×10^5 HeLa cells in 4 mL of DMEM (not supplemented) on 60 mm dishes. Incubate for 24 h at 37°C, 5% CO_2. Cells must have a 30–50% of confluence on the day of transfection.

Day 2: Dilute 6 μL of oligofectamine with 24 μL of Opti-MEM I medium in 1.5 mL microfuge tubes, mix gently, and incubate for 5–10 min at room temperature (reaction 1) (Note: prepare a master mix for all the samples.). Meanwhile and in another tube dilute 10 μL of 40 μM siRNA duplex oligo in 360 μL of Opti-MEM I medium (reaction 2) (Note: the amount of siRNA transfected has to be set up for each kind of siRNA and cell type. A 20–75 μM is the range normally tested.).

Add reaction 1 (30 μL) with reaction 2 (370 μL), mix gently, and incubate at room temperature for 20 min, allowing the siRNA oligo–oligofectamine complex to form.

In the meantime, remove DMEM from cells, wash twice with 2 mL PBS 1X, and then add 1.6 mL of Opti-MEM I to each 60 mm dish. Finally, load the siRNA oligo–oligofectamine mixture (400 μL) onto each dish and let incubate for 12–24 h, at 37°C, 5% CO_2. To improve the silencing efficiency a second round of siRNA transfection can be performed (*see* **Note 3**).

Day 3: Wash cells twice with PBS 1X, collect them, and separate them into two aliquots: one half for RNA extraction and the other half for protein extraction.

Perform standard RNA extraction and RT-PCR procedures and whole protein analysis as described earlier.

3.4. Protein Analysis

Prepare whole protein extracts by sonicating half of the cell pellet with 100 μL of lysis buffer (15 mM HEPES, pH 7.5, 250 mM NaCl, 0.5% NP-40, 10% glycerol, and 1 mM PMSF) three times for 10 s (Note: put the sample in ice after each round of sonication.). Splicing factors' endogenous expression and knockout are analysed by immunoblot analysis using the specific antibodies. Tubulin can be used as protein loading control.

4. Notes

1. Minigenes:
   Minigenes may not reproduce the endogenous splicing pattern. For instance, an exon that is normally included in vivo may show partial or total skipping in the minigene context. Several approaches can be useful:
   (a) To create a more physiological context inserting additional intronic or exonic sequences: In some cases, the inclusion of intronic elements initially excluded from the cloned fragments is required for proper exon definition and/or the presence of the flanking exons. In addition, sometimes pseudo-splice sites are brought together during minigene construction leading to their activation and inclusion of a cryptic exon in the final transcript. The elimination of cryptic splice sites can be achieved by changing the cloning strategy: clone a shorter or longer intronic region or simply remove the pseudo-splice sites by PCR site-directed mutagenesis.
   (b) To change promoter sequences: Since splicing processing can be affected by the composition of the promoter it can be useful to change its sequence and re-evaluate the splicing pattern.
   (c) Transfect minigenes into a different cell line: Expression levels of many splicing factors vary among different tissues and splicing often shows tissue-specific patterns. Consequently it could be useful to utilize different cell lines so as to set up the adequate one where the endogenous splicing pattern is faithfully reproduced.
2. Computer-assisted analysis of splicing factor-binding sequences:
   Several web-based, enhancer/silencer bioinformatic tools have been developed to predict the presence of regulatory splicing elements in the pre-mRNA sequence. For example, the ESEfinder web programme (http://rulai.cshl.edu/tools/ESE/) (19) predicts the location of SR protein-specific putative ESEs. RESCUE-ESE, another prediction programme (relative enhancer and silencer classification by unanimous enrichment), identifies putative ESE motifs by selecting hexamers that are enriched in exons against introns and in weak exons against strong ones (20, 21). Similarly, the PESX approach (putative exonic splicing enhancers/silencers) allows the identification of putative exonic splicing regulatory elements (22, 23).

   Although these tools are very popular in defining potential disease-causing mutations, the following aspects must be taken into account: (a) most of them offer predictive scores restricted to few splicing factors (only the SR protein family comprises more than 10 members); (b) changes in RNA secondary structure might affect the binding of splicing factors; and (c) the influence of the sequence context is usually not considered.

3. Overexpression and siRNA:
   (a) No effect on the splicing pattern after overexpression: This might be due to the fact that the splicing factor does not regulate the exon under study. However, it is important to consider that high levels of splicing factors are endogenously expressed in some cell lines. Therefore, overexpressing them could have no effect on splicing. In this case, silencing of the splicing factor is a better experimental approach.
   (b) No effect on splicing pattern after siRNA-mediated depletion: When planning siRNA experiment it is important to use a cell line that produces sufficient levels of the target splicing factor(s). In general, splicing factors are variably expressed in different cell lines and in a few cases they can be present at very low levels. In addition, it should be considered that one sequence motif can be recognized by different splicing factors. As a result, the depletion of only one splicing factor may not be sufficient to produce an effect on the splicing pattern (24). A typical case is represented by hnRNP-A1 and hnRNP-A2, two homologous inhibitory splicing factors. In some cases they have to be depleted together in order to affect splicing pattern (25).
   (c) No depletion of the siRNA target protein: If endogenous levels of the target protein are high or its turnover rate is low, longer incubation times and sometimes two sequential siRNA treatments are recommended to achieve a significant depletion. Additionally, in the absence of previous data it is better to test at least two or three siRNA sequences targeting different regions of the mRNA to choose the most effective.
   (d) To choose a good control for siRNA-mediated splicing regulation like an endogenous gene already known to be affected by the splicing factor: The splicing response of the endogenous gene to both depletion and overexpression experiments is generally considered as a strong evidence for regulation by the candidate protein. Alternatively, a minigene already known to respond to the splicing factor overexpression or silencing can be used as a control.

(e) It is important to remark that responsiveness to over-expression and siRNA treatments does not necessarily imply direct binding of the splicing factor to a regulatory motif in the pre-mRNA. To establish direct interaction in vitro RNA-binding assays and UV crosslinking experiments should be eventually performed (14, 17, 25).

References

1. Cartegni, L., Chew, S. L., and Krainer, A. R. (2002) Listening to silence and understanding nonsense: Exonic mutations that affect splicing. *Nat. Rev. Genet.* **3**, 285–298.
2. Pagani, F., Buratti, E., Stuani, C., and Baralle, F. E. (2003) Missense, nonsense and neutral mutations define juxtaposed regulatory elements of splicing in CFTR Exon 9. *J. Biol. Chem.* **278**, 26580–26588.
3. Pagani, F., Stuani, C., Tzetis, M., Kanavakis, E., Efthymiadou, A., Doudounakis, S. et al. (2003) New type of disease causing mutations: The example of the composite exonic regulatory elements of splicing in CFTR exon 12. *Hum. Mol. Genet.* **12**, 1111–1120.
4. Faustino, N. A., and Cooper, T. A. (2003) Pre-mRNA splicing and human disease. *Genes Dev.* **17**, 419–437.
5. Pagani, F., and Baralle, F. E. (2004) Genomic variants in exons and introns: Identifying the splicing spoilers. *Nat. Rev. Genet.* **5**, 389–396.
6. Buratti, E., Baralle, M., and Baralle, F. E. (2006) Defective splicing, disease and therapy: Searching for master checkpoints in exon definition. *Nucleic Acids Res.* **34**, 3494–3510.
7. Cooper, T. A. (2005) Use of minigene systems to dissect alternative splicing elements. *Methods* **37**, 331–340.
8. Pagani, F., Raponi, M., and Baralle, F. E. (2005) Synonymous mutations in CFTR exon 12 affect splicing and are not neutral in evolution. *Proc. Natl. Acad. Sci. USA* **102**, 6368–6372.
9. Park, J. W., and Graveley, B. R. (2005) Use of RNA interference to dissect the roles of trans-acting factors in alternative pre-mRNA splicing. *Methods* **37**, 341–344.
10. Hefferon, T. W., Broackes-Carter, F. C., Harris, A., and Cutting, G. R. (2002) Atypical 5′ splice sites cause CFTR exon 9 to be vulnerable to skipping. *Am. J. Hum. Genet.* **71**, 294–303.
11. Cuppens, H., Lin, W., Jaspers, M., Costes, B., Teng, H., Vankeerberghen, A. J. et al. (1998) Polyvariant mutant cystic fibrosis transmembrane conductance regulator genes. The polymorphic (Tg)m locus explains the partial penetrance of the T5 polymorphism as a disease mutation. *J. Clin. Invest.* **101**, 487–496.
12. Chu, C. S., Trapnell, B. C., Curristin, S., Cutting, G. R., and Crystal, R. G. (1993) Genetic basis of variable exon 9 skipping in cystic fibrosis transmembrane conductance regulator mRNA. *Nat. Genet.* **3**, 151–156.
13. Buratti, E., and Baralle, F. E. (2001) Characterization and functional implications of the RNA binding properties of nuclear factor TDP-43, a novel splicing regulator of CFTR exon 9. *J. Biol. Chem.* **276**, 36337–36343.
14. Buratti, E., Dörk, T., Zuccato, E., Pagani, F., Romano, M., and Baralle, F. E. (2001) Nuclear factor TDP-43 and SR proteins promote in vitro and in vivo CFTR exon 9 skipping. *EMBO J.* **20**, 1774–1784.
15. Ayala, Y. M., Pagani, F., and Baralle, F. E. (2006) TDP43 depletion rescues aberrant CFTR exon 9 skipping. *FEBS Lett.* **580**, 1339–1344.
16. D'Ambrogio, A., Buratti, E., Stuani, C., Guarnaccia, C., Romano, M., Ayala, Y. M. et al. (2009) Functional mapping of the interaction between TDP-43 and hnRNP A2 in vivo. *Nucleic Acids Res.* **37**, 4116–4126.
17. Pagani, F., Buratti, E., Stuani, C., Romano, M., Zuccato, E., Niksic, M. et al. (2000) Splicing factors induce cystic fibrosis transmembrane regulator exon 9 skipping through a nonevolutionary conserved intronic element. *J. Biol. Chem.* **275**, 21041–21047.
18. Niksic, M., Romano, M., Buratti, E., Pagani, F., and Baralle, F. E. (1999) Functional analysis of cis-acting elements regulating the alternative splicing of human CFTR exon 9. *Hum. Mol. Genet.* **8**, 2339–2349.
19. Cartegni, L., Wang, J., Zhu, Z., Zhang, M. Q., and Krainer, A. R. (2003) ESEfinder: A web resource to identify exonic splicing enhancers. *Nucleic Acids Res.* **31**, 3568–3571.
20. Fairbrother, W. G., Yeh, R. F., Sharp, P. A., and Burge, C. B. (2002) Predictive

identification of exonic splicing enhancers in human genes. *Science* **297**, 1007–1013.

21. Fairbrother, W. G., Holste, D., Burge, C. B., and Sharp, P. A. (2004) Single nucleotide polymorphism-based validation of exonic splicing enhancers. *PLoS Biol.* **2**, E268.
22. Zhang, X. H., and Chasin, L. A. (2004) Computational definition of sequence motifs governing constitutive exon splicing. *Genes Dev.* **18**, 1241–1250.
23. Zhang, X. H., Kangsamaksin, T., Chao, M. S., Banerjee, J. K., and Chasin, L. A. (2005) Exon inclusion is dependent on predictable exonic splicing enhancers. *Mol. Cell. Biol.* **25**, 7323–7332.
24. Venables, J. P., Koh, C. S., Froehlich, U., Lapointe, E., Couture, S., Inkel, L. et al. (2008) Multiple and specific mRNA processing targets for the major human hnRNP proteins. *Mol. Cell. Biol.* **28**, 6033–6043.
25. Goina, E., Skoko, N., and Pagani, F. (2008) Binding of DAZAP1 and hnRNPA1/A2 to an exonic splicing silencer in a natural BRCA1 exon 18 mutant. *Mol. Cell. Biol.* **28**, 3850–3860.

Chapter 12

Impact of MicroRNA in Normal and Pathological Respiratory Epithelia

Lisa Giovannini-Chami, Nathalie Grandvaux, Laure-Emmanuelle Zaragosi, Karine Robbe-Sermesant, Brice Marcet, Bruno Cardinaud, Christelle Coraux, Yves Berthiaume, Rainer Waldmann, Bernard Mari, and Pascal Barbry

Abstract

Extensive sequencing efforts, combined with ad hoc bioinformatics developments, have now led to the identification of 1222 distinct miRNAs in human (derived from 1368 distinct genomic loci) and of many miRNAs in other multicellular organisms. The present chapter is aimed at describing a general experimental strategy to identify specific miRNA expression profiles and to highlight the functional networks operating between them and their mRNA targets, including several miRNAs deregulated in cystic fibrosis and during differentiation of airway epithelial cells.

Key words: Lung, microRNA, cystic fibrosis, cancer.

1. Introduction

In 1993, a new type of small regulatory RNA was described in the nematode *Caenorhabditis elegans*: the heterochronic gene lin-4, encoding a small RNA with partial antisense complementarity to lin-14 (1, 2), corresponds to the first ever reported miRNA. Extensive sequencing efforts (3, 4), combined with ad hoc bioinformatics developments (5), have now led to the identification of 1222 distinct miRNAs in human and of many miRNAs in other multicellular organisms (accessible through miRBase, version 16, the main miRNA online registry) (6). It is currently postulated that the total number of human miRNAs should not exceed 2000.

M.D. Amaral, K. Kunzelmann (eds.), *Cystic Fibrosis*, Methods in Molecular Biology 741,
DOI 10.1007/978-1-61779-117-8_12, © Springer Science+Business Media, LLC 2011

Mature miRNAs, approximately 22 nucleotides long (7, 8), are usually derived from a primary transcript called pri-miRNA, usually transcribed by a type II RNA polymerase (transcription by type III RNA polymerase has also been suggested for some miRNAs (9, 10); but see also (11–14)). Pri-miRNAs are cleaved into the nucleus by Microprocessor, a hetero-dimer composed of Drosha, an RNase III endonuclease, and DGCR8 (DiGeorge syndrome critical region gene 8)/Pasha. This first cleavage liberates the pre-miRNA (formed by a hairpin of about 70 nucleotides that includes an overhang of 2–3 nucleotides at the 3′ end). Pre-miRNAs are then exported to the cytoplasm via exportin-5 in a Ran GTP-dependent manner. In the cytoplasm, cleavage of each pre-miRNA near the hairpin by Dicer, a second RNase III endonuclease, generates two short RNA sequences: one sequence corresponds to the mature miRNA, while the second is usually degraded (15–17). The final effector able to interact with the target mRNAs is the RNA-induced silencing complex (RISC). The efficient transfer of nascent miRNAs from Dicer to this complex necessitates that Dicer assembles with the RNA-binding protein TRBP and members of the Argonaute family to form a RISC-loading complex, before loading of the miRNA on Argonautes (18). Each resulting RISC complex can directly interact with its target mRNA(s) (19). The cytoplasmic steps of miRNA biosynthesis largely overlap with those of siRNA biosynthesis. More specifically, human AGO1 and AGO2, but not AGO3 and AGO4, possess strand-dissociating activity of miRNA duplexes. They function as RNA chaperones, capable of performing multiple rounds of strand dissociation, while only AGO2 has target RNA cleavage activity (also called slicer activity) (20).

Animal miRNAs and siRNAs differ by their mode of interaction with their targets: while siRNAs fully match their target mRNA sequences, perfect complementarity is not required between a miRNA and its target(s). Target recognition follows a complex set of rules that is usually dominated by the existence of a perfect match between six and eight nucleotides located in the 5′ region of the miRNA (called the seed) and the target mRNA (21–23). Recent experimental evidences demonstrate convincingly that interactions take place within the 3′-non-coding region in 40% of the cases (especially at proximity of the stop codon and near the poly A tail, 23a) within the CDS in 25% of the cases, and within the 5′-non-coding region in 1% of the cases, the rest of the hybridizations being located within non-coding RNAs and intronic, intergenic, or other sequences (24).

Based on relative complexities of seeds and targets, each miRNA can potentially interact with hundreds of mRNAs. Estimation is that up to 30% of human genes could potentially be regulated by miRNAs (25). This view, implying that miRNAs can "tune" the expression of most of their putative targets, needs probably to be reappraised, since miRNAs and their predicted targets are not necessarily co-expressed into the same cell, nor within the same subcellular compartment. The ability of the miRNA to interact with many targets, together with the possibility for several miRNAs to share a same target, represents a powerful mechanism to increase tremendously the complexity of biological networks. Challenges in miRNA research are currently to improve the prediction of miRNA targets and to integrate their complex modes of regulation into already existing biological networks.

miRNA regulates protein synthesis at a post-transcriptional level, by affecting mRNA translation or stability. More specifically, miRNA base pairing to a target mRNA can induce post-transcriptional gene repression by deadenylation (26–28), inhibition of translation (29, 30), or mRNA cleavage (31). In some cases, miRNA can also relocalize target mRNA to cytoplasm *foci* called P-bodies for storage or degradation (32). A careful comparison between gene expression and proteomic measurements after overexpression of a specific miRNA has shown that most of the proteins which were deregulated at a protein level were also affected at an mRNA level (33). This observation implies that analysis at a transcript level can often be sufficient to identify relevant miRNA::mRNA complexes.

1.1. miRNAs in Normal and Pathological Respiratory Tissues

Lung development and ageing. Tissue-specific inactivation of Dicer in lung epithelium led to the conclusion that Dicer is essential for proper lung morphogenesis (34). During lung development, a maternally imprinted miRNA cluster located at human chromosome 14q32.21 (mouse chromosome 12F2) is upregulated in neonatal mouse as well as in fetal human lung. This locus includes the miR-154 and miR-335 families and is situated within the imprinted Gtl2-Dio3 domain. Several miRNAs are upregulated in adult compared to neonatal/fetal lung, including miR-29a and miR-29b. Williams et al. observed no significant changes in the expression of 256 miRNAs, over lung ageing up to 18 months of age in female BALB/c mice (35). A parallel by Navarro et al. between embryonic lung and lung tumors reported a downregulation of members of the let-7 family and an overexpression of members of the miR-17-92 cluster and of miR-221 (36). More recently, Marcet et al. (36a) have established miRNA expression profiles specific of in vitro regeneration of airway epithelial cells. The most dramatic variations occurred at the onset of ciliogenesis, with the increased expression of 12 microRNAs (miR-449a, miR-449b, miR-449b*, miR-449c, miR-34a, miR-34b-3p, miR-34b-5p, miR-34c-5p, miR-92b, miR-191, miR-1975, miR-125a), and the decreased expression of 11 microRNAs (miR-17, miR-193b, miR-31, miR-31*, miR-130a, miR-205, miR-21, miR-24-1, miR-24-2, miR-210, miR-29a).

Asthma. In an attempt to identify the role of miRNA during the development of asthma, Williams et al. found no significant differences between normal and mild asthmatic patients, and no effect after 1 month treatment with the corticosteroid budesonide after examining airway biopsies obtained from normal and mild asthmatic patients by quantitative RT-PCR (37). On the other hand, lipopolysaccharides (LPS) alone induced a fast increase in the expression of 46 miRNAs which peaked at 3 h (including miR-21, miR-25, miR-27b, miR-100, miR-140, miR-142-3p, miR-181c, miR-187, miR-194, miR-214, miR-223, and miR-224), while dexamethasone had no effect on miRNA expression.

Lung inflammation. miRNAs, such as miR-10a, miR-106a-363, miR-130a, miR-133, miR-142, miR-146, miR-150, miR-155, miR-181a, miR-17-92, miR-221, miR-222, miR-223, miR-424, or miR-451, can affect the immune responses to infection and the development of diseases of immunological origin. Impact of these miRNAs in the context of the immune system has been well-described elsewhere (38, 39), but recent reports more directly have involved some of these "immunological" miRNAs into respiratory tissues (36, 40–44).

MiR-155 is contained within the only phylogenetically conserved region of BIC RNA (45, 46). It has been linked to cancer (47–50), viral infection (51), and immunity (52–55). MiR-155 has been shown to be induced by pro-inflammatory stimuli such as LPS, Toll-like receptors (TLRs), IL-1, and TNF-α in macrophages and dendritic cells (56–58), in particular through NF-κB and AP-1 transcription factors (56, 59, 60). It has also been detected in fibroblasts from different origins (61) including lung (62) in which miR-155 was also found to be upregulated by IL-1β and TNF-α (63) as well as overexpressed in a mouse model of bleomycin-induced lung fibrosis (63). Multiple targets for miR-155 have been identified in several cell types and linked with the regulation of B- and T-cell differentiation (53, 54, 64–66), TLR signaling in inflammatory cells (58), or cellular adhesion in epithelial malignancies (67). Interestingly, BIC-deficient mice displayed significant remodeling of lung airways with age, associated with increased bronchiolar subepithelial collagen deposition and increased cell mass of sub-bronchiolar myofibroblasts. Recently, Pottier et al. (63) have found that miR-155 targets keratinocyte growth factor (KGF, FGF-7), a paracrine-acting, epithelial mitogen and a central mediator of epithelial–mesenchymal interaction. Overall miR-155 would be involved in the attenuation of the inflammatory signaling pathway (58) and epithelial regeneration (63), making it a potential key player during lung injuries. Bhattacharyya et al. (67a) have shown that miR-155 was also more than 5-fold elevated in CF IB3-1 lung epithelial cells in culture, compared to control IB3-1/S9 cells. They also detected it in CF lung epithelial cells, and in circulating CF neutrophils. They propose that elevated miR-155 could contribute to pro-inflammatory expression of IL-8 in CF lung epithelial cells by lowering SHIP1 expression and activating the PI3K/Akt signaling pathway.

Viral infection. Respiratory viruses, such as influenza virus, respiratory syncytial virus (RSV), severe acute respiratory syndrome coronavirus (SARS-CoV), rhinovirus, parainfluenza virus, and adenovirus, induce acute infections of the respiratory tract that lead to clinical pictures going from rhinitis, otitis, bronchiolitis or pneumonia. Respiratory epithelial cells represent the primary targets that initially detect the viruses. Their resistance to infection depends on their capacity to detect and restrict virus replication. From that perspective, degradation of the viral genome appears as an ad hoc mechanism for efficient antiviral defense. The contribution of small non-coding RNA to this mechanism has been well-established in plants and invertebrates (68), but rarely in mammals, where the innate antiviral response is rather mediated by a robust type I interferon (IFN-α, β, and λ)-mediated response (69, 70). In that case, virus recognition occurs through the detection of pathogen-associated molecular patterns (PAMPs, usually viral nucleic acids) by pathogen-recognition receptors (PRRs) (71). Interactions within the cytoplasm or at the host cell surface lead to robust cytokine and chemokine responses, via several distinct pathways of activation (72, 73). Interestingly, Otsuka et al. have reported that a mouse mutant with hypomorphic Dicer1 expression (Dicer1(d/d)) was more prone to infection by vesicular stomatitis virus (VSV) (74). These authors detected that host miR-24 and miR-93 were increasing VSV replication in Dicer1-deficient cells after interfering with viral transcripts, without altering VSV genome-derived siRNA pathways and interferon-mediated antiviral responses. miR-122, on the contrary, was required for hepatitis C proliferation in liver (75).

At the moment, there is no report associating any cellular miRNA response to infections by rhinovirus, parainfluenza virus, RSV, or adenovirus in human. On the other hand, Wang et al. have investigated the impact of an infection by the low pathogenic H5N3 influenza virus in chicken. They found a large number of differentially expressed miRNAs between infected and non-infected tissues (73 in lungs and 36 in tracheae) (76). Alteration of the expression of several miRNAs in bronchioalveolar stem cells (BASCs) at the onset of infection by SARS-CoV, which causes acute infectious disease associated with pulmonary fibrosis and lung failure, has been described by Mallick et al., who suggest that BASCs correspond to the primary site of infection (77). Such variations may participate in the suppression of SARS-CoV replication, thus favoring successful transmission of the virus.

Responses to environmental and external stresses. Expression of several miRNAs appears sensitive to environmental and external stresses. Rat and mouse lungs exposed to environmental cigarette smoke show a downregulation by a factor at least equal to 2 for 30% of the miRNAs tested (78, 79). Schembri et al. have found 28 miRNAs downregulated in human bronchial epithelium from current smokers in comparison to never smokers (80). Four miRNAs were found at the same time in human and in rodent: miR-125b, miR-146, miR-223, and miR-99a. miRNA response to stress has been well-documented in the context of the hypertrophy of adult cardiomyocytes where altered expression of miR-23a, miR-23b, miR-24, miR-195, and miR-214 has been observed. Transgene expression of miR-195 indeed triggers heart failure in mice (81).

miRNAs and lung cancer. A strong link has been established between miRNAs and cancers since the initial report by Calin et al. of frequent deletions of mir-15 and mir-16 in chronic lymphocytic leukemia (82). A large number of studies have demonstrated since then that deregulation of miRNAs is often associated with cancer development and progression (83, 84). Indeed, some miRNAs can be defined as bona fide tumor suppressors or oncogenes. miRNA expression appears in various tumors as a more robust method for classifying cancer subtypes than mRNA expression profiles (85). Numerous publications have documented aberrant expression of miRNAs in cancers (83, 86–89). Specific reviews about miRNAs and lung cancer can be found elsewhere (90–92). Of note, Puisségur et al. (92a) have highlighted the importance of miR-210 and of its transcriptional regulation by the transcription factor hypoxia-inducible factor-1 at late stages of non-small cell lung cancer, and its association with an aberrant mitochondrial phenotype.

Cystic fibrosis. Finally, a paper from Oglesby et al. has just reported variations of miR-126 expression during cystic fibrosis in airway epithelial cells (93) and showed that miR-126 was regulating TOM1, a protein that may have an important role in regulating innate immune responses. Increased expression of miR-155 in CF epithelial cells has been also reported (67a and see above).

The present chapter is aimed at describing a general experimental strategy to identify specific miRNA expression profiles and to highlight the functional networks operating between them and their mRNA targets. This approach is based on several methodological developments previously published by our group (63, 94, 95).

2. Materials

2.1. Identification of miRNome

2.1.1. Total RNA Extraction and Quality Controls

- Trizol® reagent (Invitrogen, the Netherlands),
- Chloroform,
- Ethanol 100%,
- Qiagen RNeasy kit column (Qiagen, France),
- NanoDrop spectrophotometer (Labtech, Palaiseau, France),
- Bioanalyzer System (RNA nano-chip, Agilent Technologies, France).

2.1.2. miRNA High-Throughput Sequencing (HTS)

- SOLiD™ sequencing system (Applied Biosystems, France),
- SOLiD™ Small RNA Expression Kit (Applied Biosystems, France),
- Statistical analysis is based on statistical libraries freely accessible on Bioconductor (http://www.bioconductor.org/).

2.1.3. MicroRNA Microarrays

- Human miRNA Microarray v2 (Agilent Technologies, France),
- miRNA complete labeling and hybridization kit (Agilent Technologies, France),
- Agilent DNA microarray scanner, using Feature Extraction and Analysis software (Agilent Technologies, France).

2.1.4. Quantitative RT-PCR of Mature miRNA

- TaqMan MicroRNA Assay (Applied Biosystems, Foster City, CA),
- GeneAmp Fast PCR Master Mix (Applied Biosystems, Foster City, CA),
- Lightcycler 480 (Roche) real-time PCR machine.

2.1.5. In Situ Hybridization of miRNAs

- 4% paraformaldehyde (Electron Microscopy Sciences) solution in sterile PBS,
- acetylation solution (2.33 ml triethanolamine, 500 μl acetic anhydride, volume up to 200 ml in sterile water),
- miRNA digoxigenin-labeled LNA probe (Locked nucleic acid) or scramble miR digoxigenin-labeled LNA probe (Exiqon, Woburn, MA),
- hybridization mixture consisting to 50% deionized formamide, 0.3 M NaCl, 20 mM Tris–HCl pH 8.0, 5 mM

EDTA, 10 mM $NaPO_4$ pH 8.0, 10% dextran sulfate, 1× Denhardt's solution, and 0.5 mg/ml yeast RNA,

- washing solution: formamide 50%, 0.1% Tween-20, 1× SSC, for 15 min at RT in 0.2× SSC,
- horseradish peroxidase conjugated with sheep anti-digoxigenin antibodies (1:100, Roche, Mannheim, Germany),
- Tyramide Signal Amplification Plus DNP AP System (Perkin Elmer, Shelton, CT),
- BCIP/NBT substrate (DakoCytomation, Glostrup, Denmark),
- Nuclear Fast Red (Sigma-Aldrich),
- Eukitt mounting medium (Electron Microscopy Sciences).

2.2. Combined In Silico and Experimental Approaches to Identify miRNA Targets

2.2.1. Transcriptome Analysis Combined with Ectopic Expression of miRNAs in Cells

2.2.1.1. Ectopic Expression of miRNA

- Lipofectamine RNAi MAX Reagent (Invitrogen) in OPTI-MEM (Invitrogen, Gibco product)

2.2.1.2. Analysis of RNA Expression Using DNA Microarray

- DNA GeneChip® Human Gene 1.0 ST Array (Affymetrix),
- Whole Transcript (WT) Sense Target Labeling and Control Reagents (Affymetrix),
- GeneChip Fluidics Station 450,
- GeneChip Scanner 3000 7G (Affymetrix),
- Expression Console software (Affymetrix).

2.2.1.3. Bioinformatics Analysis of miRNA Targets

- Bioconductor statistical suite developed by the R consortium (http://www.bioconductor.org),
- Mediante (http://www.microarray.fr:8080/merge/index),
- Ingenuity Pathway Analysis (IPA) software (Ingenuity Systems, Mountain View, CA),
- MicroCible and MicroTopTable (http://www.microarray.fr:8080/merge/index),
- Sylamer.

2.3. Validation of miRNA Targets

2.3.1. Reporter Plasmid Assay

2.3.1.1. Molecular Constructs

- psiCHECK™-2 (Promega),
- QuickChange Kit (Stratagene),
- 10× Oligo Annealing Buffer (Invitrogen).

2.3.1.2. Transfection and Luciferase Assays

Pre-miRNA overexpression in cultured cells:
- Pre-miRNA and control miRNA (miR-Neg #1) (Ambion),
- Lipofectamine™ RNAi MAX™ (Invitrogen).

Pre-miRNA and psiCHECK™-2 plasmid construct co-transfection:
- Lipofectamine 2000™ (Invitrogen),
- Dual-Glo™ Luciferase Assay (Promega),
- Luminometer (Luminoskan Ascent, Thermolab system).

3. Methods

3.1. Identification of miRNome

Abundance of miRNA ranges from a few copies to 50,000 copies per cell. Distinct technologies can detect the abundance of specific miRNAs. Mature miRNAs and their precursors can be analyzed by Northern blot, quantitative real-time PCR (96), microarrays (94, 97–103), flow cytometric assays (85), padlock probes and rolling circle amplification (104), or deep-sequencing technologies (5, 105).

3.1.1. Total RNA Extraction and Quality Controls

Cells are lyzed by the addition of Trizol® reagent (Invitrogen, the Netherlands) directly on the cells. Total RNAs containing small RNA fraction are then purified on a Qiagen RNeasy kit column (Qiagen, France) according to the manufacturer's instructions (*see* **Note 1**). Total RNAs are first evaluated using NanoDrop spectrophotometer (Labtech, Palaiseau, France). Ratios 260/280 and 260/230 are checked to be near a value of 2. Integrity of the RNA is controlled on a Bioanalyzer System (RNA nano-chip, Agilent Technologies, France).

3.1.2. miRNA High-Throughput Sequencing (HTS)

Ad hoc high-throughput sequencing approaches are now commercially available. We use the SOLiD™ Small RNA Expression Kit (Applied Biosystems, France) that provides a simple and robust means to convert small RNAs into a library of double-stranded DNA molecules. Sequencing is performed according to the manufacturer's instructions. Briefly, total RNAs containing the small RNA fraction are hybridized (65°C for 10 min, then at 16°C for 5 min) and ligated (at 16°C for 2–16 h in a thermal cycler) to Adaptor Mix A to produce template for sequencing the 5′ ends of small RNAs, or to Adaptor Mix B to sequence the 3′ ends. The samples are then reverse transcribed (at 42°C for 30 min) to synthesize cDNA. Small RNA Library Amplification is realized by PCR and size selection of amplified small RNA Library by polyacrylamide gel extraction is carried out as indicated by the manufacturer's instructions (https://www3.appliedbiosystems.com/cms/groups/mcb_marketing/documents/generaldocuments/cms_054973.pdf). The 105–150 bp material is excised from the gel, eluted, and then re-suspended in nuclease-free water. Multiplexing can be done by using modified adaptors, thus allowing the sequencing of up to 20 different libraries in parallel. In that case, the DNA concentrations of all libraries are normalized by qPCR before operating the final preparation of the analytes.

Statistical analysis is based on statistical libraries freely accessible on Bioconductor (http://www.bioconductor.org/). For each sequenced miRNA, the number of sequences for 5p- and 3p-arm of each miRNA is counted, and the total number of sequences is normalized to 10^6 for each library. Data are normalized following the limma protocol (106). For further analysis, we usually retain those miRNAs whose percent of expression was >1% of the total miRNA expression in at least one condition, with a $|\log_2 \text{ratio}| > 0.5$ and an adjusted P-value < 0.05.

3.1.3. MicroRNA Microarrays

Direct and sensitive miRNA profiling from the same total RNA samples can also be performed using miRNA microarrays (Human miRNA Microarray v2, containing 866 human and 89 human viral distinct miRNA sequences, derived from the Sanger miRBase v.12.0, Agilent Technologies, France). Total RNAs are labeled and hybridized using miRNA complete labeling and hybridization kit (Agilent Technologies, France) following the manufacturer's instructions. Slides are then analyzed on Agilent DNA microarray scanner, using Feature Extraction and Analysis software (Agilent Technologies, France).

3.1.4. Quantitative RT-PCR of Mature miRNA

MiRNA expression level can also be assessed by the TaqMan MicroRNA Assay (Applied Biosystems, Foster City, CA) according to the supplier's protocol. Real-time PCR is performed using GeneAmp Fast PCR Master Mix (Applied Biosystems, Foster City, CA) on a Lightcycler 480 (Roche) real-time PCR machine. All reactions are performed in duplicate. Expression levels of mature microRNAs were evaluated using comparative

CT method (2-deltaCT), using transcript levels of RNU44 as endogenous control.

3.1.5. In Situ Hybridization of miRNAs

The exact cellular localization of miRNAs can be determined by in situ hybridization (ISH) (90, 107, 108). Some specific adaptations are, however, necessary, due to the short size of the miRNAs (109). A first method uses LNA oligonucleotide probes (110–114). A second method developed by Thompson et al. used RNA probes to detect mature miRNAs in tissue sections (107, 115). Both approaches may detect primarily mature miRNAs (116).

Ten-micrometer frozen sections of tissues are stored at –80°C until use for in situ hybridization of miRNA. Slides are air-dried for 30 min, and then sections are fixed in 4% paraformaldehyde (Electron Microscopy Sciences) solution in sterile PBS at 4°C for 10 min. After washes in PBS at room temperature (RT), sections are incubated in acetylation solution (2.33 ml triethanolamine, 500 μl acetic anhydride, volume up to 200 ml in sterile water) for 10 min at RT and then washed in PBS. Slides are then exposed overnight at T_m –20°C to either 0.3 ng/μl miRNA digoxigenin-labeled LNA probe (Locked nucleic acid) or 0.3 ng/μl scramble miR digoxigenin-labeled LNA probe (Exiqon, Woburn, MA) in hybridization mixture consisting of 50% deionized formamide, 0.3 M NaCl, 20 mM Tris–HCl pH 8.0, 5 mM EDTA, 10 mM $NaPO_4$ pH 8.0, 10% dextran sulfate, 1× Denhardt's solution, and 0.5 mg/ml yeast RNA. Slides are then sequentially washed for 30 min at T_m –20°C in solution composed of formamide 50%, 0.1% Tween-20, 1× SSC for 15 min at RT in 0.2× SSC and finally for 15 min at RT in PBS. After incubation with horseradish peroxidase conjugated with sheep anti-digoxigenin antibodies (1:100, Roche, Mannheim, Germany) for 1 h at RT, detection of probes is realized using Tyramide Signal Amplification Plus DNP AP System (Perkin Elmer, Shelton, CT) and BCIP/NBT substrate (DakoCytomation, Glostrup, Denmark). Sections are finally counterstained using Nuclear Fast Red (Sigma Aldrich), dehydrated through graded ethanol concentrations, and mounted using Eukitt mounting medium (Electron Microscopy Sciences).

3.2. Combined In Silico and Experimental Approaches to Identify miRNA Targets

Identification of genes targeted by miRNAs in a specific cellular model requires a combination of in silico and experimental approaches. Many computational algorithms have been developed to predict potential genes targeted by miRNAs (21, 22, 117–121). They are generally based on the fact that the "seed" region forms perfect base pairing with the target sites and that this seed pairing is conserved across species (122). It is important to notice that analyses performed with different algorithms usually overlap poorly. This implies that a careful experimental validation of the predicted targets is mandatory.

3.2.1. Transcriptome Analysis Combined with Ectopic Expression of miRNAs in Cells

The easiest approach combines ectopic expression of synthetic miRNA with mRNA expression studies. Enrichments at an RNA level of predicted targets in the set of genes that are downregulated after overexpression of a specific miRNA or in the set of genes that are upregulated after silencing of a specific miRNA have been clearly demonstrated (53, 54, 63, 123), suggesting that many miRNAs can indeed trigger some degradation of their mRNA targets. Transfection of small RNA duplexes at a high copy number does not perturb globally the regulation by endogenous miRNAs (124 , 125). A combination of measurements of the expression profiles at miRNA and mRNA levels is powerful to identify functional miRNA::mRNA relationships and to provide an experimental counterpart to pure computational approaches (126).

3.2.1.1. Ectopic Expression of miRNA

Cells are grown until 30% confluency is reached and then transfected with miRNAs of interest (10 nM) using Lipofectamine RNAi MAX Reagent (Invitrogen) in OPTIMEM (Invitrogen, Gibco product) following the manufacturer's instructions. Transfected cells are lyzed in Trizol® 48 h later for total RNA extraction.

3.2.1.2. Analysis of RNA Expression Using DNA Microarray

Total RNAs are purified, quantified, and quality controlled as above. RNAs are then analyzed on a DNA GeneChip® Human Gene 1.0 ST Array (Affymetrix®). Each of the 28,869 genes is represented on the array by approximately 26 probes spread across the full length of the gene (http://www.affymetrix.com). Total RNAs are labeled and hybridized using the Whole Transcript (WT) Sense Target Labeling and Control Reagents, fluidics and scanning instrumentation, and basic analysis software, as indicated by the manufacturer's instructions. Slides are quantified using Expression Console software (Affymetrix). Data analyses are performed using the statistical suite Bioconductor developed by the R consortium (http://www.bioconductor.org) and then data are visualized within Mediante, an information system developed for storing our microarray data (127). For Affymetrix microarrays, the data are processed using the RMA (Robust Multi-Chip Average) algorithm, which performs a background correction, a normalization step, and a probe-level summary. This method has been shown to have higher precision, particularly for low expression values, and higher specificity and sensitivity than many of the other commonly used methods (128). Data sets are further normalized following a linear model and an empirical Bayes method using R software. The Ingenuity Pathway Analysis (IPA) software (Ingenuity Systems, Mountain View, CA) is utilized to identify networks of interacting genes and other functional groups.

3.2.1.3. Bioinformatics Analysis of miRNA Targets

Two in-house bioinformatics tools have been developed to predict miRNA targets (http://www.microarray.fr:8080/merge/index; follow the link to microRNA and bioinformatics tools): (i) MicroCible is a miRNA target predictor that scans transcript sequences for the presence of complementary sequence to the "miRNA seed." This search can be performed for different "seed" match type (129), a minimal free energy binding cut-off, and the location of the potential targeting site (i.e., 3′UTR or the entire transcript); (ii) MicroTopTable is dedicated to the search of putative enrichments in predicted miRNA binding sites among a set of modulated genes, based on several prediction software. MicroTopTable ranks the transcripts into three categories ("upregulated," "downregulated," and "non-modulated"), according to thresholds for expression level and for differential expression. MicroTopTable then calculates the number of predicted targets for each miRNA, according to the prediction software selected, in each of the three categories. Enrichment in miRNA targets in each category is then tested using a hypergeometric law. More systematic analyses can be performed with Sylamer, which measures hypergeometric *P*-values for all short sequences of fixed length across a ranked gene list (130).

3.2.2. Other Approaches

Biochemical approaches combining RNA-induced silencing complex (RISC) purification, either combined with cloning (131), microarray analysis (Rip-Chip) (132–136), or high-throughput sequencing approaches (137), have also been proposed. Interestingly, Chi et al. have decoded microRNA::mRNA interaction maps by a technique called "Argonaute HITS-CLIP." These authors used high-throughput sequencing of RNAs isolated by immunoprecipitation of covalent crosslink between the Argonaute protein and RNA complexes (i.e., miRNA::mRNA). This produced two simultaneous data sets – Ago–miRNA and Ago–mRNA binding sites – that were electronically combined to identify interaction sites between miRNA and target mRNA. "Argonaute HITS-CLIP" provides a general platform for exploring the specificity and range of miRNA action in vivo and identifies precise sequences interacting into pertinent miRNA::mRNA interactions. A systematic use of such a technology may help unravel the precise interactions existing in vivo between miRNAs and mRNAs. Azuma-Mukai et al. have used a simpler approach that identifies miRNAs associated with hAgo2 and hAgo3 (138). Proteomic approaches, based on differential labeling of the biological samples, have shown that a single miRNA can repress the production of hundreds of proteins. Surprisingly, this repression appears usually relatively mild (see above) (33, 139). Interestingly, changes in translation efficiencies of targeted mRNAs were highly correlated with changes in the abundance of those RNAs, suggesting a functional link between microRNA-mediated repression of translation and mRNA decay (134).

3.3. Validation of miRNA Targets

When a specific miRNA::mRNA interaction is detected, validations can include direct functional assay, Western blot analysis, and/or reporter plasmid assay. In the latter case, the 3′UTR of the predicted target mRNA is inserted into an expression plasmid to control the level of production of a reporter gene. Experiments are performed in the presence or absence of the miRNA of interest to measure the impact of the miRNA on reporter expression (63, 119, 140).

3.3.1. Reporter Plasmid Assay

3.3.1.1. Molecular Constructs

Molecular constructs are derived from psiCHECK™-2 (Promega) by cloning behind the renilla luciferase ORF sequences from target 3′UTR mRNA in the *Xho*I and *Not*I restriction sites. Mutations are introduced by site-directed mutagenesis of target 3′UTR miRNA putative binding sites using the QuickChange Kit (Stratagene). Complementary oligonucleotides (50 μM final concentrations) are mixed with 10× Oligo Annealing Buffer (Invitrogen), heated to 95°C for 4 min, and allowed to cool at room temperature for 10 min. Diluted (10 nM) dsDNA are subsequently cloned in *Xho*I/*Not*I restriction sites in psiCHECK™-2 (Promega).

3.3.1.2. Transfection and Luciferase Assays

Pre-miRNA overexpression in cultured cells: Pre-miRNA and control miRNA (miR-Neg #1) are purchased from Ambion. Cells are transfected at 50% confluency in 6-well plates using Lipofectamine™ RNAi MAX™ (Invitrogen) with pre-miRNA at a final concentration of 10 nM.

Pre-miRNA and psiCHECK™-2 plasmid construct co-transfection: Cells are cultured in regular medium until confluency. Then cells are plated into 48-well plates at a density of 26.5 × 10^3 cells/well and co-transfected using 1 μl of lipofectamine 2000™ (Invitrogen) with 0.4 μg of psiCHECK™-2 plasmid construct and pre-miRNA or control miRNA at a final concentration of 10 nM. The medium is replaced 8 h after transfection with fresh medium supplemented with penicillin and streptomycin. Forty-eight hours after transfection, firefly and renilla luciferase activities are assayed using the Dual-Glo™ Luciferase Assay (Promega) and measured with a luminometer (Luminoskan Ascent, Thermolab system).

4. Conclusion

Protein-coding genes probably correspond to the tip of an iceberg corresponding to all RNAs generated by a living cell.

With 15,908, 20,158, 22,974, 23,438, and 24,408 protein-coding genes reported by Ensembl (http://www.ensembl.org) in chicken, *Caenorhabditis elegans*, mouse, human, and *Arabidopsis thaliana*, respectively, while genome sizes vary from 0.1×10^9 nucleotides to 3.4×10^9 nucleotides, it is clear that a large fraction of the genome indeed exerts its biological functions independently of its translation into protein(s) (141, 142). Though the focus of this review was limited to microRNAs (miRNA), which constitute a tiny subclass of regulatory non-coding RNAs, many more works will be necessary to unravel the many roles played by non-coding RNAs in biological processes. It remains that miRNAs deserve a special interest due to their already established association with many biological processes and to the already ongoing efforts to transfer them into new useful prognosis markers, therapeutic targets, or targeted drugs.

5. Note

1. Total RNAs containing small RNA fraction can be isolated using either miRNeasy Minikit or RNeasy Minikit. Columns (RNeasy Mini Spin Columns) are identical. The point is to add 1.5 volume 100% ethanol to provide appropriate binding conditions for all RNA molecules from 18 nucleotides (nt) upward.

Acknowledgments

This work is supported by CNRS, "Vaincre la Mucoviscidose," CHU of Nice, ANR-09-GENO-039, European Community (MICROENVIMET, FP7-HEALTH-F2-2008-201279), the Canceropole PACA, and the Association de Recherche contre le Cancer.

References

1. Lee, R. C., Feinbaum, R. L., and Ambros, V. (1993) The C. elegans heterochronic gene lin-4 encodes small RNAs with antisense complementarity to lin-14. *Cell* **75**, 843–854.
2. Wightman, B., Ha, I., and Ruvkun, G. (1993) Posttranscriptional regulation of the heterochronic gene lin-14 by lin-4 mediates temporal pattern formation in C. elegans. *Cell* **75**, 855–862.
3. Bentwich, I., Avniel, A., Karov, Y., Aharonov, R., Gilad, S., Barad, O., et al. (2005) Identification of hundreds of conserved and nonconserved human microRNAs. *Nat. Genet.* **37**, 766–770.
4. Landgraf, P., Rusu, M., Sheridan, R., Sewer, A., Iovino, N., Aravin, A., et al. (2007) A mammalian microRNA expression atlas based on small RNA library sequencing. *Cell* **129**, 1401–1414.

5. Friedlander, M. R., Chen, W., Adamidi, C., Maaskola, J., Einspanier, R., Knespel, S., et al. (2008) Discovering microRNAs from deep sequencing data using mirdeep. *Nat. Biotechnol.* **26**, 407–415.
6. Griffiths-Jones, S., Grocock, R. J., van Dongen, S., Bateman, A., and Enright, A. J. (2006) Mirbase: MicroRNA sequences, targets and gene nomenclature. *Nucleic Acids Res.* **34**, D140–144.
7. Lee, R., Feinbaum, R., and Ambros, V. (2004) A short history of a short RNA. *Cell* **116**, S89–92, 81 p following S96.
8. Bartel, D. P. (2004) MicroRNAs: Genomics, biogenesis, mechanism, and function. *Cell* **116**, 281–297.
9. Borchert, G. M., Lanier, W., and Davidson, B. L. (2006) RNA polymerase iii transcribes human microRNAs. *Nat. Struct. Mol. Biol.* **13**, 1097–1101.
10. Gu, T. J., Yi, X., Zhao, X. W., Zhao, Y., and Yin, J. Q. (2009) Alu-directed transcriptional regulation of some novel miRNAs. *BMC Genomics* **10**, 563.
11. Bortolin-Cavaille, M. L., Dance, M., Weber, M., and Cavaille, J. (2009) C19mc microRNAs are processed from introns of large pol-ii, non-protein-coding transcripts. *Nucleic Acids Res.* **37**, 3464–3473.
12. Berezikov, E., Chung, W. J., Willis, J., Cuppen, E., and Lai, E. C. (2007) Mammalian mirtron genes. *Mol. Cell* **28**, 328–336.
13. Ruby, J. G., Jan, C. H., and Bartel, D. P. (2007) Intronic microRNA precursors that bypass drosha processing. *Nature* **448**, 83–86.
14. Babiarz, J. E., Ruby, J. G., Wang, Y., Bartel, D. P., and Blelloch, R. (2008) Mouse es cells express endogenous shRNAs, siRNAs, and other microprocessor-independent, dicer-dependent small RNAs. *Genes Dev.* **22**, 2773–2785.
15. Lee, Y., Jeon, K., Lee, J. T., Kim, S., and Kim, V. N. (2002) MicroRNA maturation: Stepwise processing and subcellular localization. *EMBO J.* **21**, 4663–4670.
16. Gregory, R. I., Yan, K. P., Amuthan, G., Chendrimada, T., Doratotaj, B., Cooch, N., et al. (2004) The microprocessor complex mediates the genesis of microRNAs. *Nature* **432**, 235–240.
17. Denli, A. M., Tops, B. B., Plasterk, R. H., Ketting, R. F., and Hannon, G. J. (2004) Processing of primary microRNAs by the microprocessor complex. *Nature* **432**, 231–235.
18. Wang, H. W., Noland, C., Siridechadilok, B., Taylor, D. W., Ma, E., Felderer, K., et al. (2009) Structural insights into RNA processing by the human RISC-loading complex. *Nat. Struct. Mol. Biol.* **16**, 1148–1153.
19. Peters, L., and Meister, G. (2007) Argonaute proteins: Mediators of RNA silencing. *Mol. Cell* **26**, 611–623.
20. Wang, B., Li, S., Qi, H. H., Chowdhury, D., Shi, Y., and Novina, C. D. (2009) Distinct passenger strand and mRNA cleavage activities of human argonaute proteins. *Nat. Struct. Mol. Biol.* **16**, 1259–1266.
21. Lewis, B. P., Burge, C. B., and Bartel, D. P. (2005) Conserved seed pairing, often flanked by adenosines, indicates that thousands of human genes are microRNA targets. *Cell* **120**, 15–20.
22. Brennecke, J., Stark, A., Russell, R. B., and Cohen, S. M. (2005) Principles of microRNA-target recognition. *PLoS Biol.* **3**, e85.
23. Doench, J. G., and Sharp, P. A. (2004) Specificity of microRNA target selection in translational repression. *Genes Dev.* **18**, 504–511.
23a. Le Brigand, K., Robbe-Sermesant, K., Mari, B., and Barbry, P. (2010) MiRonTop: mining microRNAs targets across large scale gene expression studies. *Bioinformatics* **26**, 3131–3132.
24. Chi, S. W., Zang, J. B., Mele, A., and Darnell, R. B. (2009) Argonaute hits-clip decodes microRNA-mRNA interaction maps. *Nature* **460**, 479–486.
25. Xie, X., Lu, J., Kulbokas, E. J., Golub, T. R., Mootha, V., Lindblad-Toh, K., et al. (2005) Systematic discovery of regulatory motifs in human promoters and 3′ UTRs by comparison of several mammals. *Nature* **434**, 338–345.
26. Wu, L., Fan, J., and Belasco, J. G. (2006) MicroRNAs direct rapid deadenylation of mRNA. *Proc. Natl. Acad. Sci. USA* **103**, 4034–4039.
27. Eulalio, A., Huntzinger, E., and Izaurralde, E. (2008) Gw182 interaction with argonaute is essential for miRNA-mediated translational repression and mRNA decay. *Nat. Struct. Mol. Biol.* **15**, 346–353.
28. Chen, C. Y., Zheng, D., Xia, Z., and Shyu, A. B. (2009) Ago-tnrc6 triggers microRNA-mediated decay by promoting two deadenylation steps. *Nat. Struct. Mol. Biol.* **16**, 1160–1166.
29. Pillai, R. S., Artus, C. G., and Filipowicz, W. (2004) Tethering of human ago proteins to mRNA mimics the miRNA-mediated repression of protein synthesis. *RNA* **10**, 1518–1525.
30. Kozak, M. (2008) Faulty old ideas about translational regulation paved the way for

current confusion about how microRNAs function. *Gene* **423**, 108–115.
31. Wang, Y., Juranek, S., Li, H., Sheng, G., Wardle, G. S., Tuschl, T., et al. (2009) Nucleation, propagation and cleavage of target RNAs in ago silencing complexes. *Nature* **461**, 754–761.
32. Filipowicz, W., Bhattacharyya, S. N., and Sonenberg, N. (2008) Mechanisms of post-transcriptional regulation by microRNAs: Are the answers in sight? *Nat. Rev. Genet.* **9**, 102–114.
33. Selbach, M., Schwanhausser, B., Thierfelder, N., Fang, Z., Khanin, R., and Rajewsky, N. (2008) Widespread changes in protein synthesis induced by microRNAs. *Nature* **455**, 58–63.
34. Harris, K. S., Zhang, Z., McManus, M. T., Harfe, B. D., and Sun, X. (2006) Dicer function is essential for lung epithelium morphogenesis. *Proc. Natl. Acad. Sci. USA* **103**, 2208–2213.
35. Williams, A. E., Perry, M. M., Moschos, S. A., and Lindsay, M. A. (2007) MicroRNA expression in the aging mouse lung. *BMC Genomics* **8**, 172.
36. Navarro, A., Marrades, R. M., Vinolas, N., Quera, A., Agusti, C., Huerta, A., et al. (2009) MicroRNAs expressed during lung cancer development are expressed in human pseudoglandular lung embryogenesis. *Oncology* **76**, 162–169.
36a. Marcet, B., Chevalier, B., Luxardi, G., Coraux, C., Zaragosi, L. E., Cibois, M., Robbe-Sermesant, K., Jolly, T., Cardinaud, B., Moreilhon, C., Giovannini-Chami, L., Nawrocki-Raby, B., Birembaut, P., Waldmann, R., Kodjabachian, L., and Barbry, P. (2011) Control of vertebrate multiciliogenesis by miR-449 through direct repression of the Delta/Notch pathway. *Nat. Cell Biol.* In Press.
37. Williams, A. E., Larner-Svensson, H., Perry, M. M., Campbell, G. A., Herrick, S. E., Adcock, I. M., et al. (2009) MicroRNA expression profiling in mild asthmatic human airways and effect of corticosteroid therapy. *PLoS One* **4**, e5889.
38. Baltimore, D., Boldin, M. P., O'Connell, R. M., Rao, D. S., and Taganov, K. D. (2008) MicroRNAs: New regulators of immune cell development and function. *Nat. Immunol.* **9**, 839–845.
39. Sheedy, F. J., and O'Neill, L. A. (2008) Adding fuel to fire: MicroRNAs as a new class of mediators of inflammation. *Ann. Rheum. Dis.* **67**(Suppl 3), iii50–55.
40. Busacca, S., Germano, S., De Cecco, L., Rinaldi, M., Comoglio, F., Favero, F., et al. (2010) MicroRNA signature of malignant mesothelioma with potential diagnostic and prognostic implications. *Am. J. Respir. Cell. Mol. Biol.* **42**, 312–319.
41. Qian, S., Ding, J. Y., Xie, R., An, J. H., Ao, X. J., Zhao, Z. G., et al. (2008) MicroRNA expression profile of bronchioalveolar stem cells from mouse lung. *Biochem. Biophys. Res. Commun.* **377**, 668–673.
42. Melkamu, T., Zhang, X., Tan, J., Zeng, Y., and Kassie, F. (2010) Alteration of microRNA expression in vinyl-carbamate-induced mouse lung tumors and modulation by the chemopreventive agent indole-3-carbinol. *Carcinogenesis* **31**, 252–258.
43. Chen, J. F., Mandel, E. M., Thomson, J. M., Wu, Q., Callis, T. E., Hammond, S. M., et al. (2006) The role of microRNA-1 and microRNA-133 in skeletal muscle proliferation and differentiation. *Nat. Genet.* **38**, 228–233.
44. Chiba, Y., Tanabe, M., Goto, K., Sakai, H., and Misawa, M. (2009) Down-regulation of mir-133a contributes to up-regulation of rhoA in bronchial smooth muscle cells. *Am. J. Respir. Crit. Care Med.* **180**, 713–719.
45. Tam, W., Ben-Yehuda, D., and Hayward, W. S. (1997) Bic, a novel gene activated by proviral insertions in avian leukosis virus-induced lymphomas, is likely to function through its noncoding RNA. *Mol. Cell. Biol.* **17**, 1490–1502.
46. Tam, W. (2001) Identification and characterization of human bic, a gene on chromosome 21 that encodes a noncoding RNA. *Gene* **274**, 157–167.
47. Iorio, M. V., Ferracin, M., Liu, C. G., Veronese, A., Spizzo, R., Sabbioni, S., et al. (2005) MicroRNA gene expression deregulation in human breast cancer. *Cancer Res.* **65**, 7065–7070.
48. Eis, P. S., Tam, W., Sun, L., Chadburn, A., Li, Z., Gomez, M. F., et al. (2005) Accumulation of mir-155 and bic RNA in human b cell lymphomas. *Proc. Natl. Acad. Sci. USA* **102**, 3627–3632.
49. Kluiver, J., Poppema, S., de Jong, D., Blokzijl, T., Harms, G., Jacobs, S., et al. (2005) Bic and mir-155 are highly expressed in Hodgkin, primary mediastinal and diffuse large b cell lymphomas. *J. Pathol.* **207**, 243–249.
50. Jung, I., and Aguiar, R. C. (2009) MicroRNA-155 expression and outcome in diffuse large b-cell lymphoma. *Br. J. Haematol.* **144**, 138–140.
51. Yin, Q., McBride, J., Fewell, C., Lacey, M., Wang, X., Lin, Z., et al. (2008) MicroRNA-155 is an Epstein-Barr virus-induced gene

that modulates Epstein-Barr virus-regulated gene expression pathways. *J. Virol.* **82**, 5295–5306.

52. Thai, T. H., Calado, D. P., Casola, S., Ansel, K. M., Xiao, C., Xue, Y., et al. (2007) Regulation of the germinal center response by microRNA-155. *Science* **316**, 604–608.
53. Vigorito, E., Perks, K. L., Abreu-Goodger, C., Bunting, S., Xiang, Z., Kohlhaas, S. et al. (2007) MicroRNA-155 regulates the generation of immunoglobulin class-switched plasma cells. *Immunity* **27**, 847–859.
54. Rodriguez, A., Vigorito, E., Clare, S., Warren, M. V., Couttet, P., Soond, D. R., et al. (2007) Requirement of bic/microRNA-155 for normal immune function. *Science* **316**, 608–611.
55. Kohlhaas, S., Garden, O. A., Scudamore, C., Turner, M., Okkenhaug, K., and Vigorito, E. (2009) Cutting edge: The foxp3 target mir-155 contributes to the development of regulatory t cells. *J. Immunol.* **182**, 2578–2582.
56. O'Connell, R. M., Taganov, K. D., Boldin, M. P., Cheng, G., and Baltimore, D. (2007) MicroRNA-155 is induced during the macrophage inflammatory response. *Proc. Natl. Acad. Sci. USA* **104**, 1604–1609.
57. Tili, E., Michaille, J. J., Cimino, A., Costinean, S., Dumitru, C. D., Adair, B., et al. (2007) Modulation of mir-155 and mir-125b levels following lipopolysaccharide/tnf-alpha stimulation and their possible roles in regulating the response to endotoxin shock. *J. Immunol.* **179**, 5082–5089.
58. Ceppi, M., Pereira, P. M., Dunand-Sauthier, I., Barras, E., Reith, W., Santos, M. A., et al. (2009) MicroRNA-155 modulates the interleukin-1 signaling pathway in activated human monocyte-derived dendritic cells. *Proc. Natl. Acad. Sci. USA* **106**, 2735–2740.
59. Kluiver, J., van den Berg, A., de Jong, D., Blokzijl, T., Harms, G., Bouwman, E., et al. (2007) Regulation of pri-microRNA bic transcription and processing in Burkitt lymphoma. *Oncogene* **26**, 3769–3776.
60. Yin, Q., Wang, X., McBride, J., Fewell, C., and Flemington, E. (2008) B-cell receptor activation induces bic/mir-155 expression through a conserved ap-1 element. *J. Biol. Chem.* **283**, 2654–2662.
61. Stanczyk, J., Pedrioli, D. M., Brentano, F., Sanchez-Pernaute, O., Kolling, C., Gay, R. E., et al. (2008) Altered expression of microRNA in synovial fibroblasts and synovial tissue in rheumatoid arthritis. *Arthritis Rheum.* **58**, 1001–1009.
62. Martin, M. M., Lee, E. J., Buckenberger, J. A., Schmittgen, T. D., and Elton, T. S. (2006) MicroRNA-155 regulates human angiotensin ii type 1 receptor expression in fibroblasts. *J. Biol. Chem.* **281**, 18277–18284.
63. Pottier, N., Maurin, T., Chevalier, B., Puissegur, M. P., Lebrigand, K., Robbe-Sermesant, K., et al. (2009) Identification of keratinocyte growth factor as a target of microRNA-155 in lung fibroblasts: Implication in epithelial-mesenchymal interactions. *PLoS One* **4**, e6718.
64. Rai, D., Karanti, S., Jung, I., Dahia, P. L., and Aguiar, R. C. (2008) Coordinated expression of microRNA-155 and predicted target genes in diffuse large b-cell lymphoma. *Cancer Genet. Cytogenet.* **181**, 8–15.
65. Dorsett, Y., McBride, K. M., Jankovic, M., Gazumyan, A., Thai, T. H., Robbiani, D. F., et al. (2008) MicroRNA-155 suppresses activation-induced cytidine deaminase-mediated myc-igh translocation. *Immunity* **28**, 630–638.
66. Teng, G., Hakimpour, P., Landgraf, P., Rice, A., Tuschl, T., Casellas, R., et al. (2008) MicroRNA-155 is a negative regulator of activation-induced cytidine deaminase. *Immunity* **28**, 621–629.
67. Kong, W., Yang, H., He, L., Zhao, J. J., Coppola, D., Dalton, W. S., et al. (2008) MicroRNA-155 is regulated by the transforming growth factor beta/smad pathway and contributes to epithelial cell plasticity by targeting rhoA. *Mol. Cell. Biol.* **28**, 6773–6784.

67a. Bhattacharyya, S., Balakathiresan, N. S., Dalgard, C., Gutti, U., Armistead, D., Jozwik, C., Srivastava, M., Pollard, H. B., and Biswas, R. (2011) Elevated miR-155 promotes inflammation in cystic fibrosis by driving hyper-expression of interleukin-8. *J. Biol. Chem.* In Press.

68. Gitlin, L., and Andino, R. (2003) Nucleic acid-based immune system: The antiviral potential of mammalian RNA silencing. *J. Virol.* 77, 7159–7165.
69. Samuel, C. E. (2001) Antiviral actions of interferons. *Clin. Microbiol. Rev.* **14**, 778–809.
70. Grandvaux, N., TenOever, B. R., Servant, M. J., and Hiscott, J. (2002) The interferon antiviral response: From viral invasion to evasion. *Curr. Opin. Infect. Dis.* **15**, 259–267.
71. Barral, P. M., Sarkar, D., Su, Z. Z., Barber, G. N., DeSalle, R., Racaniello, V. R., et al. (2009) Functions of the cytoplasmic RNA sensors rig-i and mda-5: Key regulators of innate immunity. *Pharmacol. Ther.* **124**, 219–234.

72. Kawai, T., and Akira, S. (2008) Toll-like receptor and rig-i-like receptor signaling. *Ann. N Y Acad. Sci.* **1143**, 1–20.
73. Kumar, H., Kawai, T., and Akira, S. (2009) Toll-like receptors and innate immunity. *Biochem. Biophys. Res. Commun.* **388**, 621–625.
74. Otsuka, M., Jing, Q., Georgel, P., New, L., Chen, J., Mols, J., et al. (2007) Hypersusceptibility to vesicular stomatitis virus infection in dicer1-deficient mice is due to impaired mir24 and mir93 expression. *Immunity* **27**, 123–134.
75. Jopling, C. L., Yi, M., Lancaster, A. M., Lemon, S. M., and Sarnow, P. (2005) Modulation of hepatitis c virus RNA abundance by a liver-specific microRNA. *Science* **309**, 1577–1581.
76. Wang, Y., Brahmakshatriya, V., Zhu, H., Lupiani, B., Reddy, S. M., Yoon, B. J., et al. (2009) Identification of differentially expressed miRNAs in chicken lung and trachea with avian influenza virus infection by a deep sequencing approach. *BMC Genomics* **10**, 512.
77. Mallick, B., Ghosh, Z., and Chakrabarti, J. (2009) MicroRNome analysis unravels the molecular basis of sars infection in bronchoalveolar stem cells. *PLoS One* **4**, e7837.
78. Izzotti, A., Calin, G. A., Arrigo, P., Steele, V. E., Croce, C. M., and De Flora, S. (2009) Downregulation of microRNA expression in the lungs of rats exposed to cigarette smoke. *FASEB J.* **23**, 806–812.
79. Izzotti, A., Calin, G. A., Steele, V. E., Croce, C. M., and De Flora, S. (2009) Relationships of microRNA expression in mouse lung with age and exposure to cigarette smoke and light. *FASEB J.* **23**, 3243–3250.
80. Schembri, F., Sridhar, S., Perdomo, C., Gustafson, A. M., Zhang, X., Ergun, A., et al. (2009) MicroRNAs as modulators of smoking-induced gene expression changes in human airway epithelium. *Proc. Natl. Acad. Sci. USA* **106**, 2319–2324.
81. van Rooij, E., Sutherland, L. B., Liu, N., Williams, A. H., McAnally, J., Gerard, R. D., et al. (2006) A signature pattern of stress-responsive microRNAs that can evoke cardiac hypertrophy and heart failure. *Proc. Natl. Acad. Sci. USA* **103**, 18255–18260.
82. Calin, G. A., Dumitru, C. D., Shimizu, M., Bichi, R., Zupo, S., Noch, E., et al. (2002) Frequent deletions and down-regulation of micro- RNA genes mir15 and mir16 at 13q14 in chronic lymphocytic leukemia. *Proc. Natl. Acad. Sci. USA* **99**, 15524–15529.
83. Esquela-Kerscher, A., and Slack, F. J. (2006) Oncomirs – microRNAs with a role in cancer. *Nat. Rev. Cancer* **6**, 259–269.
84. Croce, C. M. (2009) Causes and consequences of microRNA dysregulation in cancer. *Nat. Rev. Genet.* **10**, 704–714.
85. Lu, J., Getz, G., Miska, E. A., Alvarez-Saavedra, E., Lamb, J., Peck, D., et al. (2005) MicroRNA expression profiles classify human cancers. *Nature* **435**, 834–838.
86. Volinia, S., Calin, G. A., Liu, C. G., Ambs, S., Cimmino, A., Petrocca, F., et al. (2006) A microRNA expression signature of human solid tumors defines cancer gene targets. *Proc. Natl. Acad. Sci. USA* **103**, 2257–2261.
87. Jemal, A., Siegel, R., Ward, E., Hao, Y., Xu, J., Murray, T., et al. (2008) Cancer statistics 2008. *CA Cancer J. Clin.* **58**, 71–96.
88. D'Amico, T. A. (2008) Molecular biologic staging of lung cancer. *Ann. Thorac. Surg.* **85**, S737–742.
89. Harpole, D. H, Jr. (2007) Prognostic modeling in early stage lung cancer: An evolving process from histopathology to genomics. *Thorac. Surg. Clin.* **17**, 167–173.
90. Ortholan, C., Puissegur, M. P., Ilie, M., Barbry, P., Mari, B., and Hofman, P. (2009) MicroRNAs and lung cancer: New oncogenes and tumor suppressors, new prognostic factors and potential therapeutic targets. *Curr. Med. Chem.* **16**, 1047–1061.
91. Wang, Q. Z., Xu, W., Habib, N., and Xu, R. (2009) Potential uses of microRNA in lung cancer diagnosis, prognosis, and therapy. *Curr. Cancer Drug Targets* **9**, 572–594.
92. Wu, X., Piper-Hunter, M. G., Crawford, M., Nuovo, G. J., Marsh, C. B., Otterson, G. A., et al. (2009) MicroRNAs in the pathogenesis of lung cancer. *J. Thorac. Oncol.* **4**, 1028–1034.
92a. Puisségur, M. P., Mazure, N. M., Bertero, T., Pradelli, L., Grosso, S., Robbe-Sermesant, K., Maurin, T., Lebrigand, K., Cardinaud, B., Hofman, V., Fourre, S., Magnone, V., Ricci, J. E., Pouysségur, J., Gounon, P., Hofman, P., Barbry, P., and Mari, B. (2010) miR-210 is overexpressed in late stages of lung cancer and mediates mitochondrial alterations associated with modulation of HIF-1 activity. *Cell Death Differ.* **18**, 465–478.
93. Oglesby, I. K., Bray, I. M., Chotirmall, S. H., Stallings, R. L., O'Neill, S. J., McElvaney, N. G., et al. (2010) Mir-126 is downregulated in cystic fibrosis airway epithelial cells and regulates tom1 expression. *J. Immunol.* **184**, 1702–1709.
94. Triboulet, R., Mari, B., Lin, Y. L., Chable-Bessia, C., Bennasser, Y., Lebrigand, K., et al. (2007) Suppression of microRNA-silencing

pathway by hiv-1 during virus replication. *Science* **315**, 1579–1582.
95. Saumet, A., Vetter, G., Bouttier, M., Portales-Casamar, E., Wasserman, W. W., Maurin, T., et al. (2009) Transcriptional repression of microRNA genes by pml-rara increases expression of key cancer proteins in acute promyelocytic leukemia. *Blood* **113**, 412–421.
96. Shi, R., and Chiang, V. L. (2005) Facile means for quantifying microRNA expression by real-time PCR. *Biotechniques* **39**, 519–525.
97. Liu, C. G., Calin, G. A., Meloon, B., Gamliel, N., Sevignani, C., Ferracin, M., et al. (2004) An oligonucleotide microchip for genome-wide microRNA profiling in human and mouse tissues. *Proc. Natl. Acad. Sci. USA* **101**, 9740–9744.
98. Liu, C. G., Calin, G. A., Volinia, S., and Croce, C. M. (2008) MicroRNA expression profiling using microarrays. *Nat. Protoc.* **3**, 563–578.
99. Shingara, J., Keiger, K., Shelton, J., Laosinchai-Wolf, W., Powers, P., Conrad, R., et al. (2005) An optimized isolation and labeling platform for accurate microRNA expression profiling. *RNA* **11**, 1461–1470.
100. Sun, Y., Koo, S., White, N., Peralta, E., Esau, C., Dean, N. M., and Perera, R. J. (2004) Development of a micro-array to detect human and mouse microRNAs and characterization of expression in human organs. *Nucleic Acids Res.* **32**, e188.
101. Wang, H., Ach, R. A., and Curry, B. (2007) Direct and sensitive miRNA profiling from low-input total RNA. *RNA* **13**, 151–159.
102. Castoldi, M., Schmidt, S., Benes, V., Noerholm, M., Kulozik, A. E., Hentze, M. W., et al. (2006) A sensitive array for microRNA expression profiling (michip) based on locked nucleic acids (lna). *RNA* **12**, 913–920.
103. Nelson, P. T., Baldwin, D. A., Scearce, L. M., Oberholtzer, J. C., Tobias, J. W., and Mourelatos, Z. (2004) Microarray-based, high-throughput gene expression profiling of microRNAs. *Nat. Methods* **1**, 155–161.
104. Jonstrup, S. P., Koch, J., and Kjems, J. (2006) A microRNA detection system based on padlock probes and rolling circle amplification. *RNA* **12**, 1747–1752.
105. Ansorge, W. J. (2009) Next-generation DNA sequencing techniques. *Nat. Biotechnol.* **25**, 195–203.
106. Gentleman, R. C., Carey, V. J., Bates, D. M., Bolstad, B., Dettling, M., Dudoit, S., et al. (2004) Bioconductor: Open software development for computational biology and bioinformatics. *Genome Biol.* **5**, R80.
107. Thompson, R. C., Deo, M., and Turner, D. L. (2007) Analysis of microRNA expression by in situ hybridization with RNA oligonucleotide probes. *Methods* **43**, 153–161.
108. Lassalle, S., Bonnetaud, C., Hofman, V., Puisségur, M. P., Brest, P., Loubatier, C., et al. (2009) MicroRNA signature of thyroid tumors of uncertain malignancy (ttump). *Submitted.*
109. Pena, J. T., Sohn-Lee, C., Rouhanifard, S. H., Ludwig, J., Hafner, M., Mihailovic, A., et al. (2009) MiRNA in situ hybridization in formaldehyde and edc-fixed tissues. *Nat. Methods* **6**, 139–141.
110. Wienholds, E., Kloosterman, W. P., Miska, E., Alvarez-Saavedra, E., Berezikov, E., de Bruijn, E., et al. (2005) MicroRNA expression in zebrafish embryonic development. *Science* **309**, 310–311.
111. Kloosterman, W. P., Wienholds, E., de Bruijn, E., Kauppinen, S., and Plasterk, R. H. (2006) In situ detection of miRNAs in animal embryos using lna-modified oligonucleotide probes. *Nat. Methods* **3**, 27–29.
112. Darnell, D. K., Kaur, S., Stanislaw, S., Konieczka, J. H., Yatskievych, T. A., and Antin, P. B. (2006) MicroRNA expression during chick embryo development. *Dev. Dyn.* **235**, 3156–3165.
113. Nelson, P. T., Baldwin, D. A., Kloosterman, W. P., Kauppinen, S., Plasterk, R. H., and Mourelatos, Z. (2006) Rake and lna-ish reveal microRNA expression and localization in archival human brain. *RNA* **12**, 187–191.
114. Wulczyn, F. G., Smirnova, L., Rybak, A., Brandt, C., Kwidzinski, E., Ninnemann, O., et al. (2007) Post-transcriptional regulation of the let-7 microRNA during neural cell specification. *FASEB J.* **21**, 415–426.
115. Deo, M., Yu, J. Y., Chung, K. H., Tippens, M., and Turner, D. L. (2006) Detection of mammalian microRNA expression by in situ hybridization with RNA oligonucleotides. *Dev. Dyn.* **235**, 2538–2548.
116. Obernosterer, G., Leuschner, P. J., Alenius, M., and Martinez, J. (2006) Post-transcriptional regulation of microRNA expression. *RNA* **12**, 1161–1167.
117. Kiriakidou, M., Nelson, P. T., Kouranov, A., Fitziev, P., Bouyioukos, C., Mourelatos, Z., et al. (2004) A combined computational-experimental approach predicts human microRNA targets. *Genes Dev.* **18**, 1165–1178.
118. Krek, A., Grun, D., Poy, M. N., Wolf, R., Rosenberg, L., Epstein, E. J., et al. (2005) Combinatorial microRNA target predictions. *Nat. Genet.* **37**, 495–500.

119. Lewis, B. P., Shih, I. H., Jones-Rhoades, M. W., Bartel, D. P., and Burge, C. B. (2003) Prediction of mammalian microRNA targets. *Cell* **115**, 787–798.
120. Miranda, K. C., Huynh, T., Tay, Y., Ang, Y. S., Tam, W. L., Thomson, A. M., et al. (2006) A pattern-based method for the identification of microRNA binding sites and their corresponding heteroduplexes. *Cell* **126**, 1203–1217.
121. Rajewsky, N., and Socci, N. D. (2004) Computational identification of microRNA targets. *Dev. Biol.* **267**, 529–535.
122. Rajewsky, N. (2006) MicroRNA target predictions in animals. *Nat. Genet* **38(Suppl)**, S8–13.
123. Lim, L. P., Lau, N. C., Garrett-Engele, P., Grimson, A., Schelter, J. M., Castle, J., et al. (2005) Microarray analysis shows that some microRNAs downregulate large numbers of target mRNAs. *Nature* **433**, 769–773.
124. Khan, A. A., Betel, D., Miller, M. L., Sander, C., Leslie, C. S., and Marks, D. S. (2009) Transfection of small RNAs globally perturbs gene regulation by endogenous microRNAs. *Nat. Biotechnol.* **27**, 549–555.
125. Wang, W. X., Wilfred, B. R., Hu, Y., Stromberg, A. J., and Nelson, P. T. (2010) Anti-argonaute rip-chip shows that miRNA transfections alter global patterns of mRNA recruitment to microribonucleoprotein complexes. *RNA* **16**, 394–404.
126. Huang, J., Liang, Z., Yang, B., Tian, H., Ma, J., and Zhang, H. (2007) Derepression of microRNA-mediated protein translation inhibition by apolipoprotein b mRNA-editing enzyme catalytic polypeptide-like 3 g (apobec3g) and its family members. *J. Biol. Chem.* **282**, 33632–33640.
127. Le Brigand, K., and Barbry, P. (2007) Mediante A web-based microarray data manager. *Bioinformatics* **23**, 1304–1306.
128. Irizarry, R. A., Hobbs, B., Collin, F., Beazer-Barclay, Y. D., Antonellis, K. J., Scherf, U., and Speed, T. P. (2003) Exploration, normalization, and summaries of high density oligonucleotide array probe level data. *Biostatistics* **4**, 249–264.
129. Bartel, D. P. (2009) MicroRNAs: Target recognition and regulatory functions. *Cell* **136**, 215–233.
130. van Dongen, S., Abreu-Goodger, C., and Enright, A. J. (2008) Detecting microRNA binding and siRNA off-target effects from expression data. *Nat. Methods* **5**, 1023–1025.
131. Beitzinger, M., Peters, L., Zhu, J. Y., Kremmer, E., and Meister, G. (2007) Identification of human microRNA targets from isolated argonaute protein complexes. *RNA Biol.* **4**, 76–84.
132. Karginov, F. V., Conaco, C., Xuan, Z., Schmidt, B. H., Parker, J. S., Mandel, G., et al. (2007) A biochemical approach to identifying microRNA targets. *Proc. Natl. Acad. Sci. USA* **104**, 19291–19296.
133. Keene, J. D., Komisarow, J. M., and Friedersdorf, M. B. (2006) Rip-chip: The isolation and identification of mRNAs, microRNAs and protein components of ribonucleoprotein complexes from cell extracts. *Nat. Protoc.* **1**, 302–307.
134. Hendrickson, D. G., Hogan, D. J., Herschlag, D., Ferrell, J. E., and Brown, P. O. (2008) Systematic identification of mRNAs recruited to argonaute 2 by specific microRNAs and corresponding changes in transcript abundance. *PLoS One* **3**, e2126.
135. Easow, G., Teleman, A. A., and Cohen, S. M. (2007) Isolation of microRNA targets by mirnp immunopurification. *RNA* **13**, 1198–1204.
136. Landthaler, M., Gaidatzis, D., Rothballer, A., Chen, P. Y., Soll, S. J., Dinic, L., et al. (2008) Molecular characterization of human argonaute-containing ribonucleoprotein complexes and their bound target mRNAs. *RNA* **14**, 2580–2596.
137. Chi, S. W., Zang, J. B., Mele, A., and Darnell, R. B. (2009) Argonaute hits-clip decodes microRNA-mRNA interaction maps. *Nature* **460**, 479–486.
138. Azuma-Mukai, A., Oguri, H., Mituyama, T., Qian, Z. R., Asai, K., Siomi, H., et al. (2008) Characterization of endogenous human argonautes and their miRNA partners in RNA silencing. *Proc. Natl. Acad. Sci. USA* **105**, 7964–7969.
139. Baek, D., Villen, J., Shin, C., Camargo, F. D., Gygi, S. P., and Bartel, D. P. (2008) The impact of microRNAs on protein output. *Nature* **455**, 64–71.
140. Cimmino, A., Calin, G. A., Fabbri, M., Iorio, M. V., Ferracin, M., Shimizu, M., et al. (2005) Mir-15 and mir-16 induce apoptosis by targeting bcl2. *Proc. Natl. Acad. Sci. USA* **102**, 13944–13949.
141. Mattick, J. S., and Makunin, I. V. (2005) Small regulatory RNAs in mammals. *Hum. Mol. Genet.* **14(S 1)**, R121–132.
142. Kapranov, P. (2009) From transcription start site to cell biology. *Genome Biol.* **10**, 217.

Chapter 13

Genomic Approaches to Studying *CFTR* Transcriptional Regulation

Christopher J. Ott and Ann Harris

Abstract

The *CFTR* gene was identified over 20 years ago, and yet how the gene is transcriptionally regulated is not fully understood. Completion of the human genome sequence has encouraged a new generation of genomic techniques that can be used to identify and characterize the regulatory elements of the genome, which are often hidden in non-coding regions. In this chapter we describe two techniques that we have used to identify regulatory regions of the *CFTR* locus: DNase-chip, which utilizes DNase I-digested chromatin hybridized to tiled microarrays in order to locate regions of the *CFTR* locus that are "open" and thus likely regions of transcription factor binding; and quantitative chromosome conformation capture (q3C), which uses quantitative PCR analysis of digested and ligated, crosslinked chromosomes to measure physical interactions between distal genomic regions. When used together, these methods provide a powerful avenue to discover transcriptional regulatory elements within large genomic regions.

Key words: *CFTR*, DNase-chip, chromosome conformation capture, enhancers, regulatory elements.

1. Introduction

The expression of genes depends on the activity of regulatory elements that recruit the necessary nuclear factors and co-factors required for transcriptional activation and repression. These regulatory elements are especially important for activating genes that display specific spatial and temporal expression patterns. While these elements are often found within or adjacent to promoter regions of genes, they can also reside at large genomic distances away from promoters, within intergenic and intronic regions of the genome. The cystic fibrosis transmembrane conductance

M.D. Amaral, K. Kunzelmann (eds.), *Cystic Fibrosis*, Methods in Molecular Biology 741,
DOI 10.1007/978-1-61779-117-8_13,

regulator (*CFTR*) gene is expressed primarily in specialized epithelial cells of the airway, sweat glands, pancreas, intestine, and genital duct (1–5). The *CFTR* core promoter only weakly activates transcription and does not seem to possess the elements necessary for the cell- and tissue-specific expression profile of the gene (6–8). Thus, it is a goal of our laboratory to locate and characterize regions of the *CFTR* locus outside the promoter that contribute to its transcriptional regulation. Strategies to define these elements have traditionally utilized chromatin digestion by nucleases in order to reveal nucleosome-depleted or "open" regions that mark putative sites for *trans* factor association (for example, *see* (9–12)). These nuclease hypersensitivity assays were performed by incubating cellular chromatin with DNase I, followed by digestion with a specific restriction enzyme and Southern blotting with probes for individual restriction fragments. While this method can identify DNase I hypersensitive sites (DHS) within targeted regions, it is not completely accurate. Moreover, identifying DHS comprehensively across a large region of the genome is very labor and time intensive and requires a large number of cells. Herein we describe DNase-chip (**Fig. 13.1**) (13), a method for mapping DHS across the entire *CFTR* locus and beyond using tiled microarrays. This method was developed by Gregory Crawford and colleagues (13) and

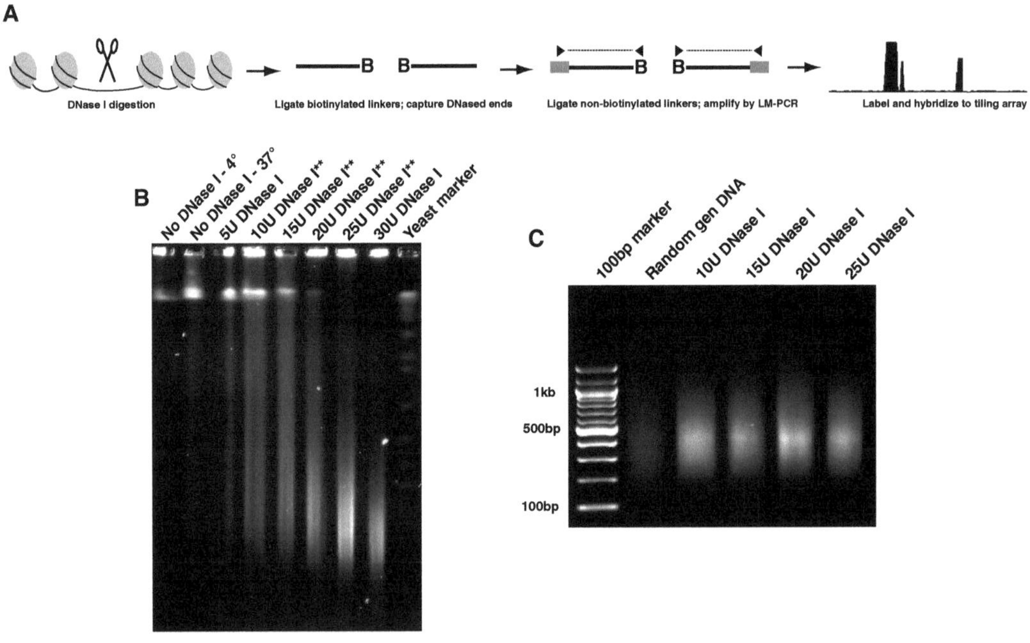

Fig. 13.1. (**a**) An overview of the DNase-chip procedure. (**b**) A sample pulsed field gel of DNase I-digested chromatin samples obtained from Caco2 cells exposed to increasing amounts of DNase I. The 10, 15, 20 and 25 U (marked with **) samples are adequately digested for use in DNase-chip. (**c**) Final purified LM-PCR product obtained from each digested sample and the randomly sheared genomic DNA control.

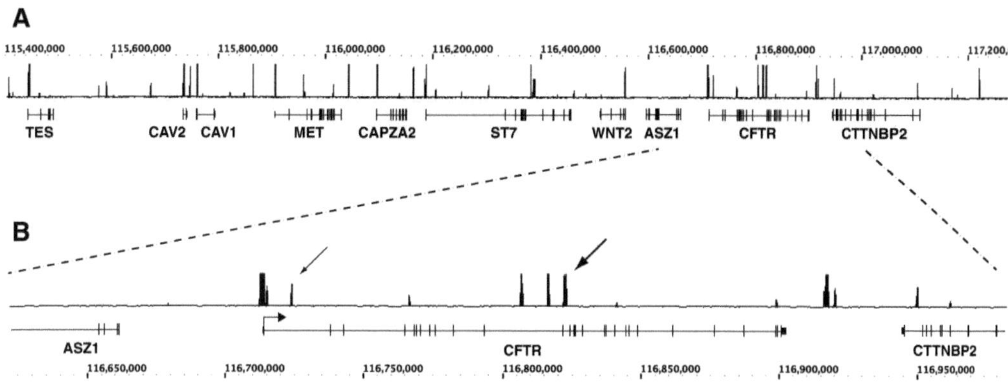

Fig. 13.2. DNase-chip results for Caco2 cells. (**a**) This track shows about 2 Mb of human chromosome 7 corresponding to ENCODE region 1 (see genome.ucsc.edu/ENCODE/pilot.html for details on the ENCODE pilot project). Coordinates correspond to human genome build 17 (May 2004). This DNase-chip track above the line is the average of three separate Caco2 experiments processed with the ACME algorithm. (**b**) A closer look at about 400 kb of the extended *CFTR* locus. Notice prominent DHS located within introns 1 and 11 of *CFTR* (*arrows*), which correspond to major enhancers of *CFTR* expression (14, 21).

we applied it to the study of *CFTR*-expressing primary cells and human cell lines (**Fig. 13.2**) (14). Furthermore, we describe quantitative chromosome conformation capture (referred to as q3C), a method developed by Job Dekker and colleagues (15) which allows the identification of physically interacting elements of chromosomes, for example, promoters and their cognate distal enhancers. The digestion of crosslinked chromatin with a specific restriction enzyme, ligation of the digested ends, and measurement of ligation frequencies of specific regions with quantitative PCR (**Fig. 13.3**) generate data on the interaction frequency of these regions. The use of DNase-chip coupled with q3C allowed us to discover a strong enhancer of *CFTR* gene expression that lies 100 kb distal to the promoter (14). Together with other weaker intronic enhancers that we identified previously, this element may prove useful when incorporated into gene therapy vectors or in future studies aimed at elucidating the cellular pathways that influence *CFTR* expression.

2. Materials

2.1. Cell Culture (See Note 1)

1. Human colon carcinoma cells Caco2 (ATCC #HTB-37)
2. DMEM media (Hyclone #SH0021.FS) (add 10% fetal calf serum)
3. Trypsin/EDTA (Cellgro #25-053-CI)

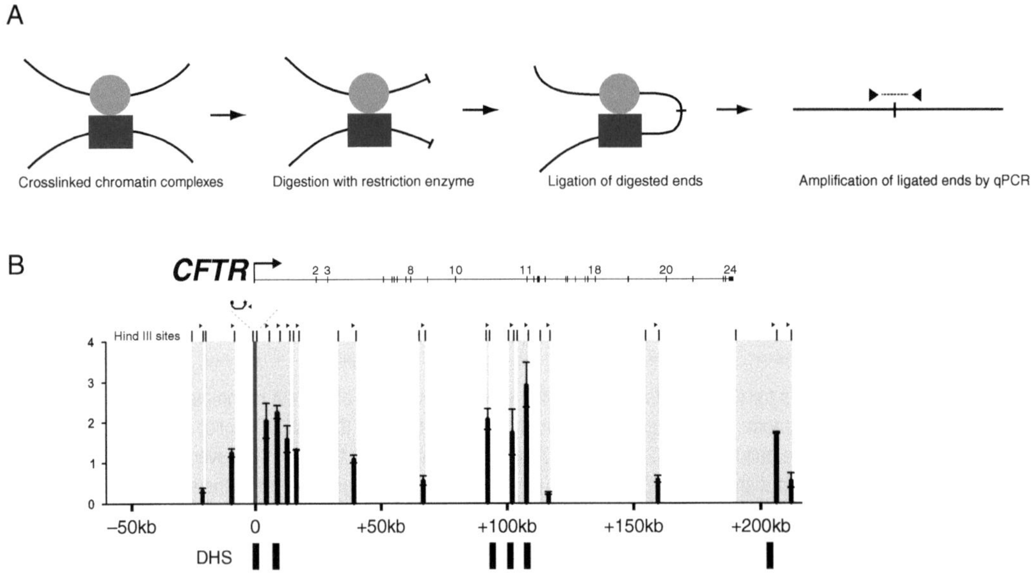

Fig. 13.3. (**a**) An overview of the q3C procedure. (**b**) q3C results for Caco2 cells using *Hin*dIII restriction enzyme (from (14), data generated by Dr. N. Blackledge). Each assayed *Hin*dIII fragment is represented by a *light gray* bar, with the restriction sites and associated primer displayed above. The *dark gray* bar represents the promoter-associated *Hin*dIII fragment, or "bait" region, with the associated reverse primer and probe adjacent to the 5′ *Hin*dIII site indicated above; this region spans the identified *CFTR* transcriptional start sites. The *x*-axis represents the position relative to the translational start site; the *y*-axis represents the interaction frequency relative to the interaction frequency between two *Hin*dIII fragments within the ubiquitously expressed *ERCC3* gene. Below the graph the locations of the major DHS are indicated (*see* **Fig. 13.2**). Data are from a single representative q3C experiment; error bars are ±SEM of at least two qPCR reactions for each fragment.

2.2. Oligonucleotides

1. 5′Biotin-GCG GTG ACC CGG GAG ATC TGA ATT C-3′
2. 5′Phos-GAA TTC AGA TC-3′AmM
3. oJW102C: 5′-GCG GTG ACC CGG GAG ATC TGA ATT C-3′
4. oJW103B: 5′-GAA TTC AGA TC-3′
   Set A: $^1/_2$
   Set B: $^3/_4$
5. For details on q3C oligos, please *see* **Note 2**.

2.3. Buffers and Solutions

1. 1× phosphate-buffered saline
2. Resuspension buffer (RSB) (10 mM Tris–Cl pH 7.4, 10 mM NaCl, 3 mM $MgCl_2$)
3. 100 mM EDTA pH 8.0
4. 50 mM EDTA pH 8.0
5. LIDS buffer (1% (w/v) LIDS [lauryl sulfate, lithium salt: Sigma #L4632], 10 mM Tris–Cl pH 7.4, 100 mM EDTA pH 8.0)
6. New England Biolabs Buffer #2 (NEB #B7002S)

7. DNA polymerase buffer (50 mM NaCl, 10 mM Tris–Cl pH 7.4, 10 mM $MgCl_2$, 1 mM dithiothreitol (DTT, Fisher #BP172-5)) (store at 4°C)
8. 1× Tris/EDTA (TE) buffer
9. 5× ligase buffer (Invitrogen #46300018)
10. Binding buffer (1 M NaCl diluted with 1× TE)
11. New England Biolabs ThermoPol buffer (NEB #B9004S)
12. 0.5× Tris/boric acid/EDTA (TBE) buffer
13. 3 M NaOAc pH 5.6
14. Lysis buffer for gDNA prep (100 mM NaCl, 10 mM Tris–HCl pH 8, 25 mM EDTA pH 8, 0.5%SDS, 0.1 mg/ml proteinase K (must be added fresh))
15. q3C lysis buffer (10 mM Tris–HCl pH 8, 10 mM NaCl, 0.2% NP-40)
16. q3C ligation buffer – 10× (660 mM Tris–HCl pH 7.5, 50 mM $MgCl_2$, 50 mM DTT, 10 mMATP)
17. 1 M glycine
18. 20% SDS
19. 37% formaldehyde (Sigma #F8775)
20. 20% Triton X-100 (Sigma #T8787)
21. 1× q3C PK buffer (5 mM EDTA pH 8, 10 mM Tris–HCl pH 8, 0.5% SDS)

2.4. Reagents

1. NP-40 (Igepal CA-630) (Sigma #I8896)
2. DNase I (NEB #MO303S)
3. InCert agarose (Lonza #50121)
4. SeaKem agarose (Lonza #50071)
5. Yeast chromosome PFG marker (NEB #NO345S)
6. dNTP mix (NEB #NO447S)
7. T4 DNA polymerase (NEB #MO203L)
8. BSA (NEB #B9001S)
9. UltraPure Buffer-Saturated Phenol (Invitrogen #15513-039)
10. UltraPure phenol:chloroform:isoamyl alcohol (25:24:1 v/v) (Invitrogen #15593-031)
11. Chloroform (MPBiomedicals #194002)
12. Glycogen (Roche #901393)
13. 100% ethanol
14. 70% ethanol
15. T4 DNA ligase (NEB #MO202S)
16. Dynabeads M-280 (Invitrogen #112.06D)

17. Taq DNA polymerase (NEB #MO267S)
18. Electrophoresis-grade agarose (Invitrogen #15510-027)
19. Ethidium bromide
20. Protease inhibitors (Roche #11-697-498-001)
21. q3C restriction enzyme of choice and appropriate buffer (*see* **Note 2**)
22. T4 DNA ligase (Roche #10799009001)
23. Proteinase K (20 μg/μl Roche #03-115-887-001)
24. RNase (DNase-free) (Roche #11-119-915-001)
25. *Power* SYBR Green qPCR 2× Master Mix (Applied Biosystems #4367659)
26. Taqman qPCR 2× Master Mix (Applied Biosystems #4352042)
27. *CFTR* BAC (BAC1,2,3 (16))
28. *ERCC3* BAC (RP11-313N8)

2.5. Equipment

1. Tissue culture incubators (37°C, 5% CO_2)
2. Pulsed field gel apparatus (we use the Bio-Rad CHEF-DR III system)
3. Agarose plug molds (Bio-Rad #1703-706)
4. Screened caps (Bio-Rad #170-3711)
5. Sonicator (we use a Cole-Parmer Ultrasonic Processor with a stepped microtip, #630-0422)
6. Magnetic tube rack (DYNAL MPC-S)
7. Phase lock tubes, high density (Qiagen #129056)
8. Fluorescent probe purification kit (Array IT #FPP)
9. NimbleGen arrays (we use NimbleGen hg17 ENCODE arrays)
10. Temperature-controlled shaker (Labnet Vortemp 56)
11. Real-time PCR thermocycler (Applied Biosystems Fast 7500)

3. Methods

3.1. DNase-Chip Methods

3.1.1. Cell Culture

Caco2 cells are grown and cultured as per instructions provided by ATCC and harvested when cells are post-confluent, when *CFTR* is maximally expressed (17).

3.1.2. DNase I Digestion of Chromatin

1. Harvest 5 × 10^7 cells (this corresponds to approximately 8–10 confluent 10 cm tissue culture plates) by trypsinization (*see* **Note 3**).
2. Spin cells in a 15 ml conical tube, 800 rpm for 5 min at 4°C.
3. Wash cells 2× with ice-cold 1× PBS, spin and pellet as above.
4. Resuspend the washed pellet in 500 μl RSB. In a separate 15 ml conical tube, add 14 μl NP-40 to 14 ml RSB (0.1% solution). Mix well until NP-40 is completely dissolved. Add NP-40 solution to resuspended cells. Gently invert ~10× until cells look white and fluffy (*see* **Note 4**).
5. Spin cells, 500 rpm for 10 min at 4°C. During spin, add various amounts of DNase I to eight 1.5 ml tubes and keep on ice. Keep two tubes for control reactions without DNase I. With NEB DNase I, we set up reactions with 5, 10, 15, 20, 25, and 30 U DNase I (*see* **Note 5**). Equate volumes in each tube with addition of RSB.
6. Carefully discard supernatant with pipette or vacuum. The nuclear pellet should be white and fluffy. Resuspend nuclei in 1 ml RSB and mix gently with a cutoff pipette tip.
7. Aliquot 120 μl of resuspended nuclei into each tube using a cutoff pipette tip and mix well by gently pipetting up and down.
8. Incubate tubes at 37°C for 10 min (keep the 4°C control tube on ice).
9. During incubation, prepare InCert agarose. Add 50 mg of agarose powder to 5 ml of 50 mM EDTA (for 1% agarose gel) using a small glass beaker or flask. Dissolve in microwave using short heating times (5–10 s is usually enough to dissolve powder and heat solution). Put agarose at 55°C to equilibrate.
10. After DNase I incubation, stop the reaction by adding 330 μl of 100 mM EDTA and invert tubes a few times to mix. Tubes can be kept at room temperature until ready to be embedded into agarose plugs (while agarose temperature is equilibrating).
11. Equilibrate DNase I-digested DNA at 55°C for 1 min.
12. Add 450 μl agarose to each tube and invert three to four times to mix.
13. Add 80 μl of the mixture to plug mold using a cutoff tip. Make 10 molds for each DNase I concentration sample. Let the agarose set at 4°C for 5 min.

14. Release plugs into 50 ml LIDS buffer (in 50 ml conical tubes; use a separate tube for each DNase I concentration) and incubate tubes on their sides for 2 h at room temperature while rocking very gently.
15. Wash out LIDS using screened plug caps, add 50 ml fresh LIDS, and incubate overnight at 37°C (not rocking, but keep tubes lying on their sides).

3.1.3. Pulsed Field Gel Analysis of Digested Chromatin

1. Wash out LIDS a second time using screened plug caps. Add 35 ml of 50 mM EDTA pH 8.0 and gently rock tubes on their sides for 1 h. Repeat EDTA wash 4× for a total of five 1-h washes. After the final wash the plugs can be stored indefinitely in 50 mM EDTA at 4°C.
2. Set up pulsed field gel with 1% SeaKem agarose in 0.5× TBE. Add 0.5× TBE to gel system and chill buffer to 14°C. After agarose has solidified, add a slice of plug from each DNase I concentration (about 1/3 of the plug) to the gel wells with a small clean spatula or scalpel blade. Load a slice of the yeast chromosomal DNA as a marker.
3. Set the gel running conditions to 20/60 s switch times, 6 V/cm, 18 h run time, pump speed 60-70, temperature 14°C. Run the gel overnight.
4. Stain gel in ethidium bromide H_2O. Determine adequately digested samples to use for arrays (**Fig. 13.1b**).

3.1.4. In-Gel Blunting of DNase I-Digested DNA and Ligation of Biotinylated Linkers

1. Remove two to five plugs from EDTA and place in a 50 ml conical tube. Use only plugs from adequately digested samples for the arrays. A total of 5 μg of total DNA will need to be extracted from plugs of each digested sample – this is usually obtained from two plugs although for some cell types/preparations more plugs will need to be processed.
2. Wash the plugs 3× with 50 ml of fresh T4 polymerase buffer (1 h each, gently rocking with tubes on their sides).
3. Carefully remove all liquid from tubes after final wash (use vacuum line and pipettes to remove residual buffer after using screened plug caps).
4. Make up blunting mix:

10× polymerase buffer (NEB #2)	12 μl/plug
dNTP mix (10 mM)	5 μl/plug
T4 DNA polymerase	6 μl/plug
BSA (100×)	2 μl/plug
H_2O	100 μl/plug

Add 125 μl blunting mix/plug to each tube; make sure plugs are completely submerged by gently shaking.

Incubate at room temperature for 3–4 h (gently mix the tubes every hour).

5. As a control sample for the arrays, we use purified genomic DNA from the same cell type being analyzed. Genomic DNA is prepared by harvesting a single confluent plate of cells, pelleting and washing in 1× PBS as above, and resuspending in 500 μl Lysis buffer. Cells are lysed overnight at 37°C with gentle shaking. The lysed cells are then phenol extracted: phenol, phenol:chloroform, then chloroform, and precipitated with ethanol. Genomic DNA can be resuspended in 1× TE. To set up control reaction, use 25 μg genomic DNA and add the following:

12 μl	NEB Buffer #2
5 μl	dNTP mix (10 mM)
1 μl	T4 DNA polymerase
2 μl	BSA (100×)

   up to 120 μlH_2O

   This blunting reaction needs to be incubated for 1 h at room temperature; thus, begin this reaction 2–3 h after the start of the DNase I-digested DNA blunting reaction.
6. Remove plugs from blunting solution and add to 1.5 ml tubes. Add 1× TE to bring total volume to 600 μl.
7. Heat tubes at 65°C for 10 min. Flick the tubes every few minutes to assist disruption of the gel pieces. The plugs should be completely melted.
8. Phenol extract by adding 600 μl phenol, shaking vigorously and centrifuging tubes at top speed for 1 min. Repeat phenol extraction, then extract with phenol:chloroform:isoamyl alcohol (25:24:1 v/v) and once with chloroform. Bring the volume of the genomic DNA control sample to 600 μl with 1× TE and extract as above.
9. Ethanol precipitate DNA with addition of one-tenth the volume of 3 M NaOAc, two volumes of 100% EtOH and 1 μl glycogen. Precipitate DNA at −20°C for at least 30 min.
10. Spin tubes at 16,000×*g* at 4°C for 15 min. After spin, wash DNA pellet with 70% EtOH and spin again for 10 min.
11. Carefully aspirate off all residual liquid, let pellet dry for no longer than 5 min. Resuspend pellet in 40 μl 1× TE, flick tube gently to resuspend (do not pipette up and down, this will shear the DNA). Let DNA hydrate for 30–60 min at 4°C. After hydration, use a spectrophotometer to obtain concentration of DNA in each sample.

12. Linker oligo pairs must be annealed (Set A: 1/2, Set B: 3/4, *see* **Section 2.2**). To anneal linkers:

50 μl	1 M Tris–HCl pH 7.6
375 μl	40 μM oligo #1 or #3
375 μl	40 μM oligo #2 or #4
200 μl	H_2O

Put mix in boiling water, shut off heat, and let tubes sit in water until it reaches room temperature. Then put oligo mixes at 4°C overnight. Aliquot and store at –20°C. Always thaw slowly on ice.

13. Set up biotinylated linker ligations:

DNA	5 μg
5× ligase buffer (use cut tip)	10 μl
Annealed linkers (1/2)	6.7 μl (Oligo set A, must be thawed on ice)
T4 ligase	0.5 μl
H_2O	up to 50 μl

14. Incubate overnight at 14°C.

3.1.5. Shearing DNA, Blunt-Ending Sheared Ends, Ligation of Non-biotinylated Linkers

1. Add ligation mixtures to 1.5 ml 1× TE in 15 ml conical tubes. Place the tubes on ice.
2. Keeping tubes in an ice bath, sonicate each 8× for 25 s. We use a Cole-Parmer sonicator with a stepped microtip at 25% amplitude. Keep tip almost at the bottom of the tube and cool tip on ice after each round of sonication.
3. Bind DNA/linker mixtures to streptavidin beads:
   Use 100 μl per sample

   First, wash beads with 1 ml binding buffer 3× using magnetic tube holder

   Add 300 μl 5 M NaCl to each sonicated DNA sample

   Add 100 μl washed beads to each sample

   Rock gently with tubes lying on their sides for 15 min at room temperature

   Use magnetic holder to capture beads

   Wash beads 3× with 1 ml binding buffer

   After the last wash step, aspirate residual liquid from tube
4. Resuspend beads in blunt-ending mix:

H_2O	97.3 μl
NEB Buffer #2	11 μl
dNTP mix (10 mM)	1 μl
T4 DNA polymerase	0.2 μl
BSA (100×)	0.5 μl

Incubate for 1 h at 16°C (resuspend beads with a cut tip once during incubation).

5. Wash beads 3× with 1 ml binding buffer; after last wash aspirate off residual buffer.
6. Resuspend beads in non-biotinylated linker ligation mix:

H_2O	32.8 μl
5× ligase buffer (use cut tip)	10 μl
Annealed linkers (3/4)	6.7 μl (Oligo set B; must be thawed on ice)
T4 ligase	0.5 μl

7. Incubate overnight at 14°C (resuspend beads once during incubation using a cut tip).

3.1.6. Amplification of DNase I-Digested Ends

1. Wash beads 3× with 1 ml binding buffer; aspirate off residual buffer after final wash. Resuspend the beads in 50 μl 1× TE.
2. Set up LM-PCR reaction (we generally set up eight reactions per sample):

H_2O	32.5 μl
10× ThermoPol Buffer	4 μl
dNTP mix (10 mM)	1.25 μl
Oligo #3 (40 μM)	1.25 μl
Beads	1 μl

Place tubes in PCR machine and start program – put on hold when block reaches 50°C and add Taq mixture:

Taq DNA polymerase	0.5 μl
H_2O	8.5 μl
10× ThermoPol Buffer	1 μl

LM-PCR cycling conditions:

55°C – 4 min (add Taq mixture at 50°C for hot start)

72°C – 3 min

95°C – 2 min

95°C – 30 s
60°C – 30 s } >> 25 cycles
72°C – 1 min

72°C – 5 min

4°C – hold

3. Run 5–10 μl of each sample on a 2% agarose gel. There should be a smear visible at ~300–700 bp (**Fig. 13.1c**).

4. Clean up LM-PCR product: combine like PCR samples into 400 μl 1× TE. Extract with phenol:chloroform:isoamyl alcohol using 2.0 ml Phase lock high-density tubes.
5. EtOH precipitate DNA with one-tenth the volume of 3 M NaOAc, two volumes of 100% EtOH, and 1 μl glycogen. Precipitate at –20°C for at least 30 min.
6. Spin samples at 16,000×*g* for 15 min at 4°C. Wash pellet with 70% EtOH and repeat spin. Aspirate off EtOH and resuspend pellet in 50 μl 1× TE.
7. Clean up samples on Array IT columns:
   a. Add 150 μl blue FPP binding buffer to each sample
   b. Split samples into two binding columns, 100 μl into each
   c. Spin columns for 30 s at 2.0 rpms
   d. Wash 3× with 140 μl FPP wash buffer (after each wash, spin for 30 s at 2.0 rpms)
   e. After final wash, empty collection tube and spin again for 1 min at 2.0 rpms
   f. Aspirate any residual liquid from inside of column (be careful not to touch the membrane)
   g. Place columns into collection tubes, elute DNA with 50 μl molecular-grade H_2O; let thecolumns sit at room temperature for 5 min
   h. Spin columns for 1 min at 2.0 rpms
   i. Consolidate like samples and spec each to determine concentration

3.1.7. Processing Samples, Analyzing Data

1. Raw material can be shipped directly to NimbleGen whose technical staff will label and hybridize the material to the appropriate arrays. The array data will then be sent directly to the investigator.
2. Raw data can be analyzed by a variety of peak-calling algorithms. We use the ACME program (18) which runs on the R statistical analysis platform and is freely available through the Bioconductor consortium (www.bioconductor.org).

3.2. Chromosome Conformation Capture (q3C) Methods

3.2.1. Restriction Enzyme Selection and q3C Primer Design

1. Ideal restriction enzymes for use in q3C will cut regularly along the locus of interest so that specific putative regulatory elements can be analyzed separately. For our analysis of *CFTR* we have used either *Eco*RI or *Hin*dIII, which are both enzymes with a 6 bp recognition sequence (6-cutters) that digests regularly along the locus.

2. For q3C PCR analysis, several oligonucleotides need to be designed: a Taqman probe and reverse primer in the "bait" region, forward primers adjacent to the 3′ end of each restriction fragment to be assayed for interaction frequency with the "bait," and cognate reverse primers for each forward primer that allows for amplification across the restriction sites to assay for digestion efficiencies. A more detailed discussion of enzyme choice and primer design and optimization can be found in a comprehensive review of qPCR 3C by Hagège et al. (15).
3. The amplification efficiency of each forward primer with the "bait" reverse primer/probe set must be assayed to ensure that differences are minimal and will not bias the q3C results. To do this we use a bacterial artificial chromosome (BAC) that contains the entire human *CFTR* locus. The BAC is digested with the chosen 3C restriction enzyme and religated. The DNA is then purified and serial dilutions of the religated BAC are analyzed by qPCR with each primer set to determine the amplification efficiency. We also use primer sets for the ubiquitously expressed excision repair cross-complementing rodent repair deficiency, complementation group 3 (*ERCC3*) gene locus as a normalizing control in our q3C experiments (19) and thus use an *ERCC3*-containing BAC to determine the amplification efficiency of these primer sets. A detailed explanation of this procedure can be found in Hagège et al. (15).

3.2.2. Cell Harvest and Chromatin Digestion

1. Caco2 cells should be cultured and harvested as in **Section 3.1**. For a single q3C experiment, use 1×10^7 cells. Resuspend cells in 12 ml of media.
2. Add 649 μl of 37% formaldehyde (final concentration 2%) and rotate cells at room temperature for 10 min to crosslink the chromatin and protein complexes.
3. Quench the crosslinking by adding 1.5 ml of 1 M glycine. Then spin down the cells at 1,300 rpm for 8 min at 4°C.
4. Wash the cell pellet with 10 ml cold 1× PBS and spin down again at 1,300 rpm for 8 min at 4°C.
5. Discard PBS wash and resuspend the pellet in 5 ml of cold q3C lysis buffer; incubate cells for 10 min on ice.
6. Spin cells at 1,800 rpm for 5 min at 4°C. Discard lysis buffer supernatant, then resuspend the cell pellet in 500 μl 1.2× restriction enzyme buffer (60 μl 10× buffer + 440 μl H_2O) and transfer to a 1.5 ml tube that locks securely.
7. Add 7.5 μl 20% SDS; shake the tube horizontally in Vortemp for 1 h at 37°C.
8. Add 50 μl 20% Triton X-100; shake horizontally for 1 h at 37%. (After each incubation step, the extract may appear

clumpy due to nuclei aggregation. Gently resuspend with a cut pipette tip to homogenize the sample.)

9. Take a 5 μl aliquot and label as UNDIGESTED – store this at –20°C.
10. Add 400 U of appropriate restriction enzyme and shake horizontally overnight at 37°C.

3.2.3. Ligation of Digested Chromatin

1. Take 5 μl from the sample and label as DIGESTED.
2. Add 40 μl 20% SDS to the remaining sample; shake the tube horizontally for 20 min at 65°C to inactivate the restriction enzyme.
3. Transfer the sample to a 50 ml tube; add 6.125 ml 1.15× q3C ligation buffer.
4. Add 375 μl 20% Triton X-100; incubate for 1 h at 37°C with gentle shaking.
5. Cool down on ice for 2 min, then add 100 U T4 DNA ligase; incubate for 4 h at 14°C and then 30 min at room temperature.
6. Add 300 μg proteinase K and incubate overnight at 65°C to reverse the crosslinks.
7. To the 5 μl UNDIGESTED and DIGESTED samples add 500 μl of 1× q3C PK buffer and 20 μg proteinase K and incubate at 65°C overnight.

3.2.4. q3C Library Purification, Quantification, and qPCR Analysis of Interaction Frequency

1. To q3C sample add 30 μl of 10 mg/ml RNase and incubate for 1 h at 37°C.
2. Add 7 ml phenol:chloroform:isoamyl alcohol (25:24:1 v/v) and mix well. Spin sample at 2,200×*g* for 15 min at room temperature.
3. Transfer supernatant to a new 50 ml tube and add 7 ml H_2O, 1 ml of 3 M NaOAc, and 35 ml 100% EtOH; mix and place at –80°C for 1 h.
4. Spin sample at 4,200×*g* for 1 h at 4°C, then remove supernatant and add 10 ml cold 70% EtOH. Spin sample again at 4,200×*g* for 15 min at 4°C. Briefly dry DNA pellet at room temperature. Resuspend pellet in 150 μl H_2O – this is the purified q3C library.
5. To the UNDIGESTED and DIGESTED samples add 1 μl RNase and incubate at 37°C for 2 h. Extract DNA with phenol:chloroform:isoamyl alcohol (25:24:1 v/v), ethanol precipitate, and resuspend DNA in 100 μl H_2O. These samples will be used to determine the digestion efficiency at each restriction site.
6. The precise concentration of the 3C library must be determined by qPCR. To do this, the 3C sample must

be compared to a reference sample of genomic DNA of a known concentration. Use a 1:50 dilution of the 3C library and a serial dilution of the reference genomic DNA (10–0.1 ng/μl) to generate a standard curve. For the qPCR reactions, use an "internal" primer set that amplifies an undigested region of the *CFTR* locus. After determining the concentration of the 3C library, adjust the concentration to 100 ng/μl.

7. Determine the interaction frequency for each chosen primer set by Taqman qPCR. We set up our reactions as follows: 10 μl 2× Taqman master mix, 2.5 μl Taqman probe (1 μM), 1 μl forward primer (5 μM), 1 μl reverse "bait" primer (5 μM), 2 μl q3C template (200 ng), 3.5 μl H_2O. PCR cycling reactions we use are 95°C, 20 s (1 cycle); 95°C, 3 s (40 cycles); 60°C, 30 s (1 cycle). In order to control for variation between experiments and cell types, we normalize our data to the interaction frequencies measured at the ubiquitously expressed *ERCC3* locus (19). To display the data, we use a bar chart with the *x*-axis aligned to the *CFTR* locus coordinates and corresponding *Hin*dIII sites (**Fig. 13.3**). Take care to clearly mark the analyzed restriction fragments and the fragment used as "bait."

3.2.5. Determining Digestion Efficiency

1. Perform qPCR using SYBR Green dye on the UNDIGESTED (UND) and DIGESTED (DIG) samples using primers that amplify across the restriction sites of interest (this will give the Ct_R DIG and Ct_R UND values). Use 2 μl of the UNDIGESTED and DIGESTED samples per reaction.
2. Also use the same "internal" primer set used above to amplify a region that does not contain a restriction site (this will give Ct_C DIG and Ct_C UND values. For each restriction site of interest, calculate the digestion efficiency as

$$\% \text{ digestion} = 100 - \left(\frac{100}{2^{((Ct_R - Ct_C)\text{DIG} - (Ct_R - Ct_C)\text{UND})}}\right)$$

Ideally, the digestion efficiency at each measured restriction site will be >80%.

4. Notes

1. The procedure here describes analysis of the *CFTR*-expressing Caco2 human colon carcinoma cell line; however, these techniques can be applied to most cultured primary human cells and cell lines, either adherent or

suspension cultures, provided an adequate number of cells can be harvested (cells from other species may require a custom-built tiled microarray for DNase-chip).

2. The design of oligonucleotide primer sets for q3C requires extensive preparation before experimentation. Their design is first dependent upon the choice of restriction enzyme to be used for the q3C assays, and the number of oligos to be generated depends upon the number of restriction fragments of the locus to be assayed. A list of primers we have used in experiments using *Hin*dIII and *Eco*RI digestions can be found in Blackledge et al. (20, 14). Specific guidelines concerning the design of q3C oligos can be found in Hagège et al. (15).
3. The total cell number required for the procedure can vary by cell type and can be determined empirically. We have successfully titrated cell number down to ~1×10^7 total cells harvested by adjusting the number of cell equivalents for each DNase I concentration and adjusting other aspects of the protocol such as the range of DNase I concentrations used and the number of agarose plugs made for each concentration.
4. Some cell types may become overly damaged with 0.1% NP-40. The nuclei of damaged cells do not completely resuspend in RSB. If this occurs, try reducing the concentration of NP-40 used to lyse cells. Cell lysis efficiency can be monitored by staining with Trypan blue and viewing on a hemocytometer.
5. The amount of DNase I needed to adequately digest chromatin samples can also vary depending on cell type, cell number, and the activity of the DNase I used in the experiment. Thus it is important to use a range of DNase I to digest the samples and then to assay them for adequate digestion by pulsed field gel electrophoresis. We generally select a range of digested samples to proceed with in the protocol (*see* **Fig. 13.1b**), which are pooled together just prior to the array hybridization step.

Acknowledgments

We would like to thank Dr. Neil Blackledge (Department of Biochemistry, Oxford University) for generating data shown in **Fig. 13.3b** and Dr. Greg Crawford (Institute for Genome Sciences & Policy, Duke University) for assistance with the DNase-chip technique.

References

1. Harris, A., Chalkley, G., Goodman, S., and Coleman, L. (1991) Expression of the cystic fibrosis gene in human development. *Development* **113**, 305–310.
2. Crawford, I., Maloney, P. C., Zeitlin, P. L., Guggino, W. B., Hyde, S. C., Turley, H., et al. (1991) Immunocytochemical localization of the cystic fibrosis gene product CFTR. *Proc. Natl. Acad. Sci. USA* **88**, 9262–9266.
3. Engelhardt, J. F., Zepeda, M., Cohn, J. A., Yankaskas, J. R., and Wilson, J. M. (1994) Expression of the cystic fibrosis gene in adult human lung. *J. Clin. Invest.* **93**, 737–749.
4. Kreda, S. M., Mall, M., Mengos, A., Rochelle, L., Yankaskas, J., Riordan, J. R., et al. (2005) Characterization of wild-type and deltaF508 cystic fibrosis transmembrane regulator in human respiratory epithelia. *Mol. Biol. Cell* **16**, 2154–2167.
5. Strong, T. V., Boehm, K., and Collins, F. S. (1994) Localization of cystic fibrosis transmembrane conductance regulator mRNA in the human gastrointestinal tract by in situ hybridization. *J. Clin. Invest.* **93**, 347–354.
6. Chou, J. L., Rozmahel, R., and Tsui, L. C. (1991) Characterization of the promoter region of the cystic fibrosis transmembrane conductance regulator gene. *J. Biol. Chem.* **266**, 24471–24476.
7. Koh, J., Sferra, T. J., and Collins, F. S. (1993) Characterization of the cystic fibrosis transmembrane conductance regulator promoter region. Chromatin context and tissue-specificity. *J. Biol. Chem.* **268**, 15912–15921.
8. Yoshimura, K., Nakamura, H., Trapnell, B. C., Dalemans, W., Pavirani, A., Lecocq, J. P., et al. (1991) The cystic fibrosis gene has a "housekeeping"-type promoter and is expressed at low levels in cells of epithelial origin. *J. Biol. Chem.* **266**, 9140–9144.
9. Nuthall, H. N., Moulin, D. S., Huxley, C., and Harris, A. (1999) Analysis of DNase-I-hypersensitive sites at the 3′ end of the cystic fibrosis transmembrane conductance regulator gene (CFTR). *Biochem. J.* **341**, 601–611.
10. Phylactides, M., Rowntree, R., Nuthall, H., Ussery, D., Wheeler, A., and Harris, A. (2002) Evaluation of potential regulatory elements identified as DNase I hypersensitive sites in the CFTR gene. *Eur. J. Biochem.* **269**, 553–559.
11. Smith, A. N., Barth, M. L., McDowell, T. L., Moulin, D. S., Nuthall, H. N., Hollingsworth, M. A., et al. (1996) A regulatory element in intron 1 of the cystic fibrosis transmembrane conductance regulator gene. *J. Biol. Chem.* **271**, 9947–9954.
12. Smith, D. J., Nuthall, H. N., Majetti, M. E., and Harris, A. (2000) Multiple potential intragenic regulatory elements in the CFTR gene. *Genomics* **64**, 90–96.
13. Crawford, G. E., Davis, S., Scacheri, P. C., Renaud, G., Halawi, M. J., Erdos, M. R., et al. (2006) DNase-chip: A high-resolution method to identify DNase I hypersensitive sites using tiled microarrays. *Nat. Methods* **3**, 503–509.
14. Ott, C. J., Blackledge, N. P., Kerschner, J. L., Leir, S. H., Crawford, G. E., Cotton, C. U., et al. (2009) Intronic enhancers coordinate epithelial-specific looping of the active CFTR locus. *Proc. Natl. Acad. Sci. USA* **106**, 19934–19939.
15. Hagège, H., Klous, P., Braem, C., Splinter, E., Dekker, J., Cathala, G., et al. (2007) Quantitative analysis of chromosome conformation capture assays (3C-qPCR). *Nat. Protoc.* **2**, 1722–1733.
16. Kotzamanis, G., Abdulrazzak, H., Gifford-Garner, J., Haussecker, P. L., Cheung, W., Grillot-Courvalin, C., et al. (2008) CFTR expression from a BAC carrying the complete human gene and associated regulatory elements. *J. Cell. Mol. Med.* **13**, 2938–2948.
17. Mouchel, N., Henstra, S. A., McCarthy, V. A., Williams, S. H., Phylactides, M., and Harris, A. (2004) HNF1alpha is involved in tissue-specific regulation of CFTR gene expression. *Biochem. J.* **378**, 909–918.
18. Scacheri, P. C., Crawford, G. E., and Davis, S. (2006) Statistics for ChIP-chip and DNase hypersensitivity experiments on NimbleGen arrays. *Methods Enzymol.* **411**, 270–282.
19. Vernimmen, D., De Gobbi, M., Sloane-Stanley, J. A., Wood, W. G., and Higgs, D. R. (2007) Long-range chromosomal interactions regulate the timing of the transition between poised and active gene expression. *EMBO J.* **26**, 2041–2051.
20. Blackledge, N. P., Ott, C. J., Gillen, A. E., and Harris, A. (2009) An insulator element 3′ to the CFTR gene binds CTCF and reveals an active chromatin hub in primary cells. *Nucleic Acids Res.* **37**, 1086–1094.
21. Ott, C. J., Suszko, M., Blackledge, N. P., Wright, J. E., Crawford, G. E., and Harris, A. (2009) A complex intronic enhancer regulates expression of the CFTR gene by direct interaction with the promoter. *J. Cell. Mol. Med.* **13**, 680–692.

Section III

CFTR Protein Biogenesis, Folding, Degradation, and Traffic

Chapter 14

Introduction to Section III: Biochemical Methods to Study CFTR Protein

Margarida D. Amaral and Gergely L. Lukacs

Abstract

This section of *Cystic Fibrosis: Diagnosis and Protocols* is focussed on methods aimed at detecting expression, localization, endocytic sorting and metabolism (biogenesis and turnover), as well as interacting partners of the cystic fibrosis transmembrane conductance regulator (CFTR), the protein product of the gene mutated in cystic fibrosis (CF). An overview of the protocols to be found in subsequent chapters of this book section is provided here, as well as the rationale for utilizing these protocols (also as a workflow) explaining which scientific question(s) each of them helps to address. Protocols included in other sections of this book are also cross-referenced.

Key words: Cystic fibrosis, CFTR, biochemical methods.

The gene which is mutated in cystic fibrosis (CF) encodes the CF transmembrane conductance regulator (CFTR) protein, a 1480-amino acid, glycosylated membrane protein, functioning as a cAMP-dependent and phosphorylation-regulated Cl^- channel. CFTR (or ABCC7) belongs to the family of ATP-binding cassette (ABC) transporters, being thus formed by two membrane-spanning domains (MSD1 and MSD2), two nucleotide-binding domains (NBD1 and NBD2), and a regulatory domain (RD). CFTR is mainly expressed in secretory epithelia and besides its Cl^- channel activity has been proposed many other roles in the cell, most notably as a regulator of other channels and transporters.

The F508del-CFTR protein, which results from the mutant gene found in 70% of CF chromosomes and ~90% of CF patients, is aberrantly folded, thus failing to acquire a native conformation. Therefore, its traffic to the plasma membrane is mostly blocked at the level of the endoplasmic reticulum (ER) by still not fully

M.D. Amaral, K. Kunzelmann (eds.), *Cystic Fibrosis*, Methods in Molecular Biology 741,
DOI 10.1007/978-1-61779-117-8_14,

identified components of the ER quality control (ERQC) which target it for proteolysis via the ubiquitin (Ub)–proteasome pathway (UPP). Since this mutant is partially functional as a cAMP-dependent Cl^- channel, intense research efforts focus on designing strategies to restore the biosynthetic processing and permit the mutant accumulation at the plasma membrane.

The wild-type (wt) and various mutant CFTR proteins have been extensively studied using biochemical and biophysical approaches in order to characterize their intrinsic properties and cellular metabolism in addition to map the composite of their interacting proteins. Through these studies which have been developed for the last 20 years, many key questions in the field have been addressed, but new challenges also emerged.

Whereas the biophysical and structural approaches to investigate CFTR are dealt with elsewhere in this book (*see* **Section IV**), the biochemical protocols have been included within the current section. As some of the questions which biochemical methods address can also be tackled by other methods, namely cell biology methods, the reader is also referred to additional sections of the book.

Proteomic approaches have been developed to gain insights into differential protein expression pattern in CF vs non-CF cells/tissues and determine the protein interactome of CFTR/F508del-CFTR that may be involved in the regulation of this channel trafficking, degradation, and function. These methods are presented elsewhere in this book (*see* **Section II, Chapters 13** and **14, Volume II**).

Chapters within this section include both basic and cutting-edge biochemical techniques currently used in CFTR research. Additional assays can be found at the previous edition of this book (1) and at a special supplement of the *Journal of Cystic Fibrosis*, entirely dedicated to CF-related methodologies (2). References are included to those consensus protocols that are accessible at the *European Working Group on CFTR Expression* Web site (3), a previous initiative to provide a methodological "consensus" compendium for basic research in the CF field.

A critical evaluation of anti-CFTR antibodies, required for most of the techniques below, has been presented in several reports (4–7).

The aim here is to provide a series of methodologies that will be useful both to the novice and experienced researchers alike by reducing effort and research time of all with an interest in this field.

A workflow of protocols to be found in this section chapters is provided in **Fig. 14.1** as a roadmap to the rationale for utilizing these approaches in concert with pertinent questions that they help to address.

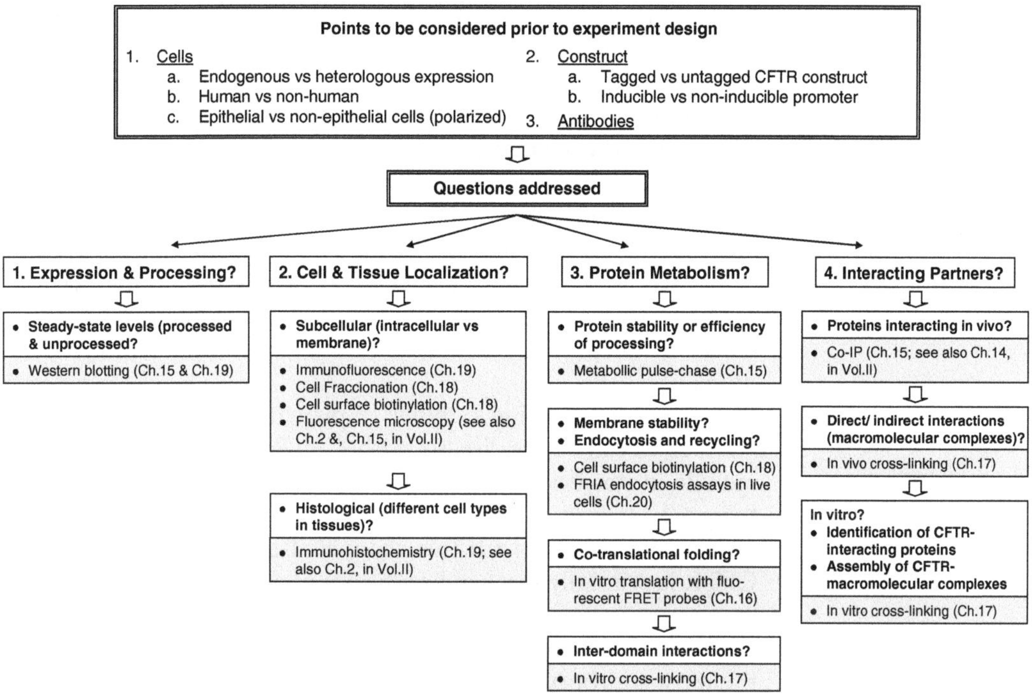

Fig. 14.1. Workflow of protocols included in the subsequent chapters within this section serving as a roadmap to use these methodological approaches to address scientific questions.

Since misfolding and premature degradation are the major problems associated with F508del-CFTR, the mutant which occurs in most CF patients, several groups have identified and functionally characterized the components of the UPP as well as chaperones which act either at the ER membrane or in the cytoplasm to select misfolded CFTR conformers for degradation. **Chapter 15** describes methods to study the impact of UPP modulation on the early biogenesis (folding and degradation) of wild-type (wt)- and F508del-CFTR at the ER. Methods to detect complexes formed between CFTR folding intermediates and ER quality control factors are also discussed. The biochemical assays described in **Chapter 15** include metabolic pulse chase; Western blot (WB); co-immunoprecipitation (co-IP) of CFTR with chaperones and ERQC factors (both endogenous and exogenous, epitope-tagged factors).

Cell-free expression systems constitute powerful tools to uncover and manipulate the molecular machinery involved in CFTR biosynthesis and degradation. In **Chapter 16**, on "*Novel Mammalian Based Systems for In Vitro CFTR Expression*" by Skach and colleagues, novel protocols resulting from technical advances in systems for in vitro translation are described. These cell-free translation systems, obtained from cultured cell lysates, represent better alternatives to classical rabbit reticulocyte lysate (RRL) methods, often with even greater synthetic capacity, providing a well-defined environment for production of correctly folded proteins or their domains. Through novel design and exploitation, they also allow “ribosome display” approaches permitting the characterization of domain folding during the polypeptide chain biogenesis and detection of protein–protein interactions. The biochemical assays described in **Chapter 16** include the preparation of classical and improved lysates for in vitro translation, measurement of relative translation efficiency, as well as the discussion of their strengths and limitations for synthesis of full-length CFTR and its transmembrane and cytosolic domains.

Given the growing number of protein partners described to interact directly or indirectly with CFTR, it is most relevant to include in this book methodological approaches aimed at identifying CFTR-interacting proteins (CIPs) and characterizing their physical interaction with this channel. Because in native tissues, CFTR is primarily localized at the apical surface of epithelial cells lining the airway, gut, exocrine glands, etc., methods to elucidate such interactions in physiologically relevant systems in vivo are the most appropriate to be reported. **Chapter 17** describes cross-linking methods for CFTR-containing macromolecular complexes aimed at identifying their components as well as their assembly and regulation at the plasma membrane (**Chapter 15** deals with methods to characterize early secretory pathway protein complexes). Since the large cytoplasmic domains are predominantly involved in regulatory interactions of the CFTR channel gating, most heterologous protein associations take place primarily at the amino (N)- and carboxyl (C)-termini of the channel either directly or mediated through various PDZ domain-containing proteins. The C-terminal PDZ domain-binding motif of CFTR is responsible for at least four distinct protein interactions. In **Chapter 17**, methods to characterize physical interactions between proteins binding to both the N- and C-termini of CFTR are introduced. The assays described in **Chapter 17** thus include a combination of in vivo and in vitro methods to characterize both intra-CFTR and intermolecular CFTR–CIP interactions, namely in vivo chemical cross-linking of CFTR and its interacting partners; expression and purification of recombinant tagged fusion proteins in bacteria; CFTR:NHERF stoichiometry in apical plasma membrane; and in vitro CFTR-containing macromolecular complex assembly (CFTR–NHERF2–LPA2 complex).

The amount of CFTR that is present at the cell surface at any time point results from the balance between the portion which is being endocytosed vs that resulting from both de novo biogenesis along the secretory pathway and effective recycling from early endosomes. **Chapter 18** examines current methods employed to measure the cell surface expression of CFTR, as well as assays to monitor CFTR movement through the endocytic pathway.

As CFTR endocytosis and recycling are tightly regulated processes with multiple intervenients (Ras GTPases, SNAREs, PDZ domain-containing proteins, myosin motors, lipids, etc.) the methods described in **Chapter 18** are thus most appropriate to elucidate the functional role of a given putative regulator of these processes. Biochemical methods included in **Chapter 18** for the detection and quantification of apical membrane abundance of CFTR and follow-up of its intracellular trafficking through the endocytic pathway include a cell surface biotinylation-based endocytosis, a recycling assay and an OptiPrep gradient fractionation method to separate subcellular compartments.

To address the similar questions, but complementary to methods described in this section, additional microscopy-based assays using extracellular epitope tagging for screening purposes are described elsewhere in the book (*see* **Chapter 15, Volume II**).

An emergent role for CFTR in the kidney has become recently clear through demonstration of its presence in endosomes of the cells lining the terminal part of the proximal tubule, in addition to its plasma membrane location. Given the specificity of this organ which has not been extensively studied in the context of CF, a complete chapter of the current book section is dedicated to methodologies aimed at characterizing CFTR and its endocytosis in native tissues, being kidney its major focus. Thus, **Chapter 19** includes antigen retrieval and immunoperoxidase labeling procedures with paraffin-embedded serial sections of mouse kidney; and analytical subcellular fractionation of mouse kidney and immunoblotting for CFTR.

To address CFTR localization questions in other cells and tissues, additional microscopy methods are described elsewhere in the book (*see* **Chapter 2, Volume II**).

A growing body of evidence indicates that constitutive internalization and recycling of CFTR at the plasma membrane are conformation sensitive, implying that additional checkpoints for the quality control of the secretory pathway exist beyond those at the ER. **Chapter 20** describes a sophisticated fluorescence imaging technique which, when coupled to genetic manipulation, enables to identify molecular determinants of CFTR post-endocytic fate: either recycling back to the plasma membrane or ubiquitination-dependent targeting for lysosomal degradation. This method takes advantage of the different pH values found in distinct endocytic compartments, which alter emission of pH-sensitive fluorophore probes coupled to the wild-type or mutant CFTR.

References

1. Skach, W. R. (2002) *Cystic Fibrosis Methods and Protocols.* Methods in Molecular Medicine. Humana Press, Totowa, NJ, pp. 1–631.
2. Amaral, M. D. (2004) *Special Supplement.* Journal of Cystic Fibrosis. Elsevier, Kindlington, UK, pp. 1–250
3. European Working Group on CFTR Expression (2003) website http://central.igc.gulbenkian.pt/cftr/vr/index.html.
4. Doucet, L., Mendes, F., Montier, T., Delepine, P., Penque, D., Ferec, C., and Amaral, M. D. (2003) Applicability of different antibodies for the immunohistochemical localization of CFTR in respiratory and intestinal tissues of human and murine origin. *J. Histochem. Cytochem.* **51**, 1191–1199.
5. Mendes, F., Farinha, C. M., Roxo, R. M., Fanen, P., Edelman, A., Dormer, R., McPherson, M., Davidson, H., Puchelle, E., de Jonge, H. R., Heda, G. D., Gentzsch, M., Lukacs, G. L., Penque, D., and Amaral, M. D. (2004) Antibodies for CFTR studies. *J. Cyst. Fibros.* **3**(S2), 73–77.
6. Carvalho-Oliveira, I., Efthymiadou, A., Malho, R., Nogueira, P., Tzetis, M., Kanavakis, E., Amaral, M. D., and Penque, D. (2004) CFTR localization in native airway cells and cell lines expressing wild-type or F508del-CFTR by a panel of different antibodies. *J. Histochem. Cytochem.* **52**, 193–203.
7. Farinha, C. M., Mendes, F., Roxo-Rosa, M., Penque, D., and Amaral, M. D. (2004) A comparison of 14 antibodies for the biochemical detection of the cystic fibrosis transmembrane conductance regulator protein. *Mol. Cell Probes* **18**, 235–242.

Chapter 15

Analysis of CFTR Folding and Degradation in Transiently Transfected Cells

Diane E. Grove, Meredith F.N. Rosser, Richard L. Watkins, and Douglas M. Cyr

Abstract

Misfolding and premature degradation of F508del-CFTR is the major cause of cystic fibrosis. Components of the ubiquitin-proteasome system function on the surface of the endoplasmic reticulum to select misfolded proteins for degradation. The folding status of F508del-CFTR is monitored by at least two ER quality control checkpoints. The ER-associated Derlin-1/RMA1 E3 complex appears to recognize folding defects in CFTR that involve misassembly of NBD1 into a complex with the R-domain. In contrast, the cytosolic Hsp70/CHIP E3 complex appears to sense folding defects that occur after synthesis of NBD2. Herein we describe methods that allow for the study of how modulation of these ER quality control factors by siRNA impacts CFTR folding and degradation. The experimental system described employs transiently transfected HEK293 cells and is utilized to monitor the biogenesis of CFTR by both Western blot and pulse chase studies. Methods to detect complexes formed between CFTR folding intermediates and ER quality control factors will also be described.

Key words: F508del, pulse chase, Western blot, folding, degradation.

1. Introduction

Proper folding and interdomain contact formation between membrane and cytosolic sub-domains of CFTR is critical for channel activity (1–3). CFTR synthesis takes around 10 min and affords chaperones and ER quality control factors sufficient time in which to monitor the progression of CFTR folding intermediates (4). However, CFTR folding is a relatively inefficient process with approximately 70–85% of wild-type and 99% of the F508del mutant being partitioned from a folding to the ubiquitin-proteasome degradation pathway (5).

M.D. Amaral, K. Kunzelmann (eds.), *Cystic Fibrosis*, Methods in Molecular Biology 741,
DOI 10.1007/978-1-61779-117-8_15,

The attempt to fold CFTR into a native conformation that is no longer recognized by the ER quality control machinery involves the cooperation of both ER-localized and cytosolic chaperones. The Hdj-2/Hsp70 chaperone pair mediates early or co-translational folding of CFTR sub-domains (4). Calnexin's contribution to CFTR folding involves facilitating proper interactions between the membrane and cytosolic domains of CFTR (6). Terminal steps of CFTR folding appear to be mediated by Hsp90 and its co-factors (7, 8).

Selection of nascent forms of CFTR and F508del-CFTR for proteasomal degradation is also facilitated by molecular chaperones. Misfolded forms of CFTR are recognized by at least two ER quality control complexes. The cytosolic E3 ubiquitin ligase CHIP interacts with Hsp70 to form a quality control machine that utilizes the polypeptide binding activity of Hsp70 to target misfolded CFTR for proteasomal degradation (9). In addition, the ER-associated E3 RMA1/RNF5 acts in association with Derlin-1 and the E2 Ubc6e to ubiquitinate CFTR (10). Other co-factors, including Gp78, BAP31, and p97, are then responsible for delivering the ubiquitinated CFTR to the proteasome (11–13). How selection of CFTR for degradation by the RMA1 E3 machinery and the CHIP E3 complex is synergized is not entirely clear. However, the RMA1 E3 complex may act co-translationally to recognize folding defects in CFTR that involve misassembly of NBD1 into a complex with the R-domain (6, 10). In contrast, the CHIP E3 may act post-translationally to recognize misfolded regions of CFTR that include NBD2 (10).

Herein we describe methods that allow for modulation of the ubiquitin ligase complexes which select F508del-CFTR for degradation that can be used in efforts to permit cell surface expression of F508del-CFTR. The experimental system described employs transiently transfected HEK293 cells to study the biogenesis of CFTR and its folding mutants. We describe how to deplete levels of ER quality control factors by siRNA. Next, biochemical methods to analyze CFTR steady-state levels by Western blot and folding/degradation kinetics by pulse chase studies are detailed. Finally, methods to detect complexes formed between CFTR folding intermediates and ER quality control factors will also be described.

2. Materials

2.1. General Reagents

1. Phenylmethylsulfonyl fluoride (PMSF): 100 mM stock of PMSF in 100% molecular-grade ethanol. Store at –20°C.
2. Protease inhibitor cocktail (PI): Complete™ Protease inhibitor cocktail (Roche, 11697498001).

3. Phosphate-buffered saline (PBS), pH 7.4: 135 mM NaCl, 2.7 mM KCl, 10 mM Na_2HPO_4, 1.8 mM KH_2PO_4. Store at 4°C. Supplement PBS with 1% Triton X-100 (PBS-Tr (1%)), 1 mM PMSF, and PI just prior to use in cell lysis.
4. 10% bovine serum albumin (BSA) in PBS.
5. Antibodies: CFTR clone MM13-4 (Millipore, 05-581) and RMA1 (Santa Cruz Biotechnology, sc81716).
6. Protein G-agarose (PG beads) (Roche, 11243233001): resuspend PG beads in PBS supplemented with 1% Triton and 1% BSA. Incubate PG beads on a rotator for 24 h at 4°C to block non-specific binding sites on the beads. Pellet the beads with a microcentrifuge and resuspend them as a 50% v/v slurry in PBS supplemented with 1% Triton. Store at 4°C.

2.2. Reagents and Buffers

2.2.1. SDS-PAGE

1. Sodium dodecyl sulfate-polyacrylamide gel electrophoresis (SDS-PAGE) 2× sample buffer (2× SB): 125 mM Tris–HCl, pH 6.8, 4% SDS, 20% glycerol, 0.05% of Coomassie blue, and distilled water. This solution can be stored at room temperature. Prior to use add 80 μl of β-mercaptoethanol and 10 μl PI to 1 ml of 2× SB.
2. SDS-PAGE electrode buffer, pH 8.3: 10 mM Tris–HCl, 75 mM glycine, and 0.1% SDS.
3. Acrylamide-*bis*-acrylamide solution: 30% acrylamide, 0.8% *N,N*-methylene *bis*-acrylamide. Store in an aluminum foil-covered glass bottle at 4°C.
4. 4× SDS-PAGE resolving gel buffer, pH 8.8: 1.5 M Tris–HCl, 8 mM EDTA, and 0.4% SDS. Adjust to pH 8.8 and store at room temperature.
5. 4× SDS-PAGE stacking gel buffer, pH 6.8: 0.5 M Tris–HCl, 8 mM EDTA, and 0.4% SDS. Adjust to pH 6.8 and store at room temperature.
6. 10% ammonium persulfate (APS).
7. *N,N,N′,N′*-Tetramethylethylenediamine (TEMED) (Fisher Scientific, BP150).
8. Different percentage SDS-PAGE gels are used to resolve proteins of varying size. SDS-PAGE gels are made by combining the above SDS-PAGE buffers and reagents as follows: 2.35 ml acrylamide, 5.15 ml distilled water, and 2.5 ml 4× resolving gel buffer for a 7% gel; 3.2 ml acrylamide, 4.3 ml distilled water, and 2.5 ml 4× resolving gel buffer for a 10% gel; and 4.2 ml acrylamide, 3.23 ml distilled water, and 2.5 ml 4× resolving gel buffer for a

12.5% gel. To polymerize these gel mixtures add 100 μl of 10% APS and 7.5 μl of TEMED. The combined solution is mixed and then poured between the glass plates of a mini-gel apparatus (Bio-Rad). A layer of water-saturated *N*-butanol is added to the top surface of the gel to obtain a flat smooth surface and to prevent the resolving gel from drying out. Polymerization should be complete by 30 min. When the resolving gel is polymerized, pour off the butanol layer, rinse top of gel with distilled water, and then add the stacking gel mixture. The stacking gel is composed of the following: 0.6 ml of acrylamide, 2.35 ml of distilled water, 1 ml of 4× stacking gel buffer, 75 μl of 10% APS, and 5 μl of TEMED. The stacking gel mixture should be mixed well and then added to the top of the resolving gel. Immediately insert well combs and stacking gel polymerization should occur within 15 min.

9. SDS-PAGE gel stain: 25% methanol, 10% glacial acetic acid, 2.5 g/l of Coomassie blue. In order to minimize the formation of precipitates use distilled water to prepare this stain.
10. SDS-PAGE gel destain: 10% methanol, 10% acetic acid, and distilled water.
11. Fluorography reagent: 0.5 M sodium salicylate, pH 7.4.

2.2.2. Western Blot

1. Western blot transfer buffer: 20 mM Tris-base, 150 mM glycine–HCl, 20% methanol, and 0.02% SDS.
2. Ponceau S protein stain: Dissolve 1 g of Ponceau S in 2 ml of glacial acetic acid and 198 ml of water.
3. PBSTrX-100: PBS supplemented with 0.1% Triton X-100.
4. Western blot blocking solution: PBSTrX-100 and 10% non-fat dry milk.
5. Antibody solutions: antibody diluted into PBSTrX-100 supplemented with 3% BSA and 0.2% sodium azide.
6. 0.45-μm nitrocellulose membrane (GE Water and Process Technologies, WP4HY00010).
7. 3M Whatman filter paper.

2.3. Cell Culture

1. HEK293 cells are grown in Dulbecco's modified Eagle's medium (Sigma, D6429) supplemented with 10% fetal bovine serum (FBS; Mediatech, 35010CV) and antibiotics (100 U/ml penicillin and 100 μg/ml streptomycin; Mediatech, 30002CI) (DMEM) at 37°C in an atmosphere of 5% CO_2 to approximately 100% confluency in T-75 flasks (Corning, 430641). Each flask contains approximately 8.4×10^6 cells.

2. Citric saline: 135 mM KCl, 15 mM Na-citrate, pH 7.4.
3. Minimum essential medium without L-methionine (MEM) (Gibco, 21013) supplemented with 5 ml glutamine (Cellgro, 25-0005-Cl) and 5 ml pyruvate (Mediatech; 25000CI): pre-warm media to 37°C prior to use. Cells are incubated in this media to deplete intracellular methionine prior to incubation with Trans ^{35}S-Label.
4. Trans ^{35}S-Label (1200 Ci/mmol; MP Biomedicals, 51006). Trans ^{35}S-Label is a mixture of ^{35}S-methionine and ^{35}S-cysteine utilized for radiolabeling of cellular proteins. Supplement MEM with 100 μCi Trans ^{35}S-Label per 35 mm well.
5. 0.05% trypsin-EDTA (Gibco, 25300).
6. Transfection reagents: Effectene (Qiagen, 301427); Lipofectamine 2000 (Invitrogen, 11668-019).
7. High-quality plasmid DNA (*see* **Note 1**).

3. Methods

3.1. Expression of CFTR in HEK293 Cells

3.1.1. Growth of HEK293 Cells for Transfection

1. Grow HEK293 cells to approximately 100% confluency in T-75 flasks.
2. Aspirate growth media and gently rinse cells with 6 ml of PBS. Remove PBS from cells.
3. Add 1.5 ml of trypsin-EDTA and incubate cells for approximately 1 min at 37°C to detach cells from the bottom of the flask.
4. After the cells have detached, dilute the trypsin-EDTA with 32 ml of DMEM. Pipet several times to break up large clumps of cells.
5. Pipet 2 ml of cell suspension into each 35-mm well. A confluent T-75 flask will provide enough cells for 16 wells. Allow 12–14 h for these cells to adhere to the bottom of the 35-mm wells.
6. The cells will be at approximately 40–50% confluency and are now ready to transfect.

3.1.2. Transfection of HEK293 Cells for Overexpression Analysis

1. The mammalian expression plasmid pcDNA3.1(+)-CFTR or F508del-CFTR is introduced into HEK293 cells with the Effectene transfection reagent. For each 35-mm well of cells add 1 μg of pcDNA3.1(+)-CFTR to 100 μl of EC buffer

and mix well. Next, add 4 μl of Enhancer reagent/μg of DNA, mix the cocktail well, and incubate the mixture at room temperature for 5 min. Add 5 μl of Effectene/μg of DNA, vortex for 10 s, and incubate for 20 min. Dilute the transfection mixture with 800 μl of DMEM.

2. Aspirate the DMEM from the HEK293 cells and gently add the transfection mixture down the side of the 35-mm well of cells. Incubate the cells with the transfection mixture for 4–5 h at 37°C and 5% CO_2. Replace the transfection mixture with DMEM and incubate for 18–24 h (*see* **Note 2**).

3.1.3. Isolation of Transfected HEK293 Cells

1. To harvest HEK293 cells remove the DMEM and add 1 ml citric saline.
2. Detach the cells by repeatedly pipetting the citric saline over the cells. Once the cells have become detached remove them from the 35-mm well and place in a microcentrifuge tube.
3. Rinse the 35-mm well with 0.5 ml of citric saline and add the solution to the microcentrifuge tube.
4. Pellet the cells by centrifugation at 3,000×*g* for 2 min. Aspirate supernatant. Cell pellets can either be placed on ice prior to lysis or frozen in liquid nitrogen for storage and later lysis.

3.2. Impact of ER Quality Control Factors on CFTR Biogenesis

The fate of CFTR and F508del-CFTR is dependent on ER quality control factors. Modulation of the levels of known quality control factors allows us to assess how each protein impacts the folding of CFTR. Here we describe the general procedure for depleting endogenous quality control proteins, using the RMA1 E3 ligase as an example.

1. Prepare HEK293 cells for transfection as described in **Section 3.1.1**.
2. Introduce siRNA oligonucleotides (oligos) into HEK293 cells using Lipofectamine 2000 as the transfection reagent. In tube A, oligos directed against RMA1 (sequence 1, GCGCGACCUUCGAAUGUAA; sequence 2, CGGCAAGAGUGUCCAGUAU) or a non-specific control (Dharmacon) are mixed with 250 μl/reaction of Opti-MEM (Invitrogen). In tube B, 10 μl/reaction of Lipofectamine 2000 and 240 μl/reaction of Opti-MEM are combined.

   The siRNA oligos and Lipofectamine 2000 reagent can be added to the tubes outside of a tissue culture hood but Opti-MEM addition and subsequent transfection steps should be carried out within the hood. Incubate tubes A and B for 7 min. Combine 250 μl/reaction of tube B with 250 μl/reaction of tube A and incubate for 25 min. During this incubation remove media from cells in 35-mm wells and replace with 2 ml DMEM supplemented with 10% FBS but lacking antibiotics (no penicillin or streptomycin). Add

500 μl of the combined tube A and B mixture to each well. We have found that using a final total concentration of 100 nM with the RMA1 siRNA oligos is sufficient to obtain greater than 90% knockdown of endogenous RMA1 levels.

3. Incubate the cells with the transfection mixture for 4–5 h at 37°C and 5% CO_2. Replace the transfection mixture with DMEM supplemented with FBS and antibiotics.
4. Twenty-four hours post-transfection, remove the media and wash the cells with 1 ml PBS.
5. Aspirate off the PBS, add 200 μl trypsin-EDTA, and incubate cells at 37°C for approximately 1 min to detach cells from the bottom of the wells.
6. Add 800 μl DMEM to the cells and pipet several times to break up clumps of cells.
7. Take 350–400 μl of resuspended cells and add to a new 35-mm well. Add 1.5 ml of DMEM to the new wells. Thus, one well of siRNA cells can be divided into two new wells. Allow the cells to attach to the bottom of the wells overnight.
8. Transfect siRNA cells with pcDNA3.1(+)-CFTR or pcDNA3.1(+)-F508del-CFTR and harvest these cells as described in **Sections 3.1.2** and **3.1.3**.
9. For CFTR steady-state analysis, harvest the siRNA cells 24 h post-transfection and add 250 μl 2× SDS SB. To lyse the cells sonicate the samples (intensity 5) for 10 s × 2. To prevent overheating of the samples it is important to keep them on ice during sonication. Normalize samples to contain the same total amount of protein (*see* **Note 3**). Analyze the levels of CFTR and the efficiency of RMA1 knockdown via Western blot as described in **Section 3.3.1**.
10. For CFTR pulse chase studies follow the procedure outlined in **Section 3.3.2**.

3.3. Analysis of CFTR and F508del-CFTR Folding and Degradation in HEK293 Cells

3.3.1. Analysis of CFTR Levels by Western Blot

Steady-state levels of transiently transfected CFTR and F508del-CFTR in HEK293 cells can be determined by Western blots (**Fig. 15.1**).

1. Transfect HEK293 cells with pcDNA3.1(+)-CFTR or pcDNA3.1(+)-F508del-CFTR and harvest these cells as described in **Sections 3.1.1 – 3.1.3**.

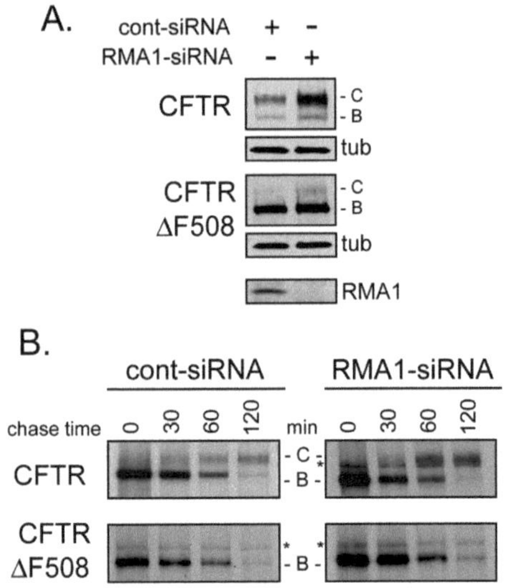

Fig. 15.1. Impact of RMA1 siRNA on CFTR folding in HEK293 cells. RMA1 siRNA and transient transfection of CFTR or F508del-CFTR are described in **Section 3.2**. Steady-state levels (**a**) and stability (**b**) of CFTR and F508del-CFTR in the presence or absence of the E3 ligase RMA1 are indicated by Western blot (**Section 3.3.1**) and pulse chase assays (**Section 3.3.2**), respectively. Bands B and C represent the ER-localized immaturely glycosylated form and the maturely glycosylated plasma membrane form of CFTR, respectively. The band marked with a $*$ denotes a background band.

2. Add 200 μl 2× SB to each cell pellet, sonicate as described in **Section 3.2**, and normalize samples to contain the same total amount of protein (*see* **Note 3**).
3. Heat samples at 37°C for 10 min. Load an equal volume from each sample to a 10% SDS-PAGE gel and electrophorese samples by applying a constant voltage of 120 V to gels for approximately 90 min.
4. To prepare for the wet transfer of proteins in the SDS-PAGE gel to a nitrocellulose membrane using a Bio-Rad mini-gel transfer apparatus
   a. Cut 3 M Whatman filter paper to the same size as the apparatus sponges and soak the paper in Western blot transfer buffer.
   b. Soak the transfer apparatus sponges in Western blot transfer buffer.
   c. Cut a nitrocellulose membrane to the size of the mini-gel and soak this membrane in Western blot transfer buffer.
5. On completion of the electrophoresis, assemble the gel into the transfer apparatus with a nitrocellulose membrane.
6. Transfer the protein in the gel to the nitrocellulose by applying a constant voltage of 110 V for 70 min. The transfer can be run either at room temperature or at 4°C.

7. After completion of the transfer, remove the nitrocellulose membrane from the transfer apparatus. Stain the proteins on the membrane with Ponceau S for 2–3 min and then destain with distilled water. This staining step allows for comparison of protein loads in each lane.
8. Block sites on the nitrocellulose membrane that bind antibodies non-specifically via incubation of the membrane on a shaker with Western blot blocking solution. This blocking step can be carried out at room temperature for minimally 1 h and can be extended overnight with incubation at 4°C.
9. Rinse membrane with PBSTrX-100 a few times to remove excess block solution.
10. Incubate the membrane with the monoclonal primary antibody α-CFTR MM13-4 at a 1:1000 dilution in PBSTrX-100 supplemented with 3% BSA and 0.2% sodium azide. To determine the efficiency of RMA1 knockdown use the α-RMA1 monoclonal antibody at a 1:1000 dilution. α-tub (1:2000 dilution) can be used to indicate loading consistency. The nitrocellulose membrane(s) and primary antibody solution(s) should be incubated on a shaker for minimally 1 h at room temperature or overnight at 4°C.
11. Wash the membrane with PBSTrX-100 3 × 5 min on a shaker.
12. Incubate the membrane with goat anti-mouse sera conjugated to horseradish peroxidase (Bio-Rad) that is diluted 1:3000 with PBSTrX-100 and 1% non-fat dry milk on a shaker for 60 min at room temperature.
13. Wash the nitrocellulose membrane 3 × 5 min with PBSTrX-100 on a shaker.
14. Incubate the membrane with enhanced chemiluminescent reagent (GE Healthcare). Wrap the membrane in saran wrap, expose membrane to X-ray film, and develop the film. Exposure times may vary to observe a signal in the linear range; thus we typically take a few exposures usually between 30 s and 2 min.

3.3.2. Pulse Chase Analysis

Pulse chase experiments are used to analyze the folding efficiency of CFTR folding and the rate of F508del-CFTR degradation (**Fig. 15.1b**).

1. Transfect HEK293 cells with pcDNA3.1(+)-CFTR or pcDNA3.1(+)-F508del-CFTR as described in **Sections 3.1.1** and **3.1.2**.
2. Approximately 18–24 h post-transfection remove the media, wash the cells with 0.5 ml of pre-warmed MEM minus methionine, and then methionine-starve the cells

with 1 ml MEM for 20 min at 37°C in a 5% CO_2 atmosphere.

3. Replace the MEM minus methionine with 750 μl MEM minus methionine supplemented with 100 μCi Trans ^{35}S-Label. Incubate the cells for 20 min at 37°C and 5% CO_2.
4. Remove the labeling media and start the chase by adding 1 ml of DMEM supplemented with 5 mM methionine. Incubate the ^{35}S-labeled cells for 0–3 h at 37°C and 5% CO_2.
5. At each chase time point, remove chase media from the cells and add 1 ml ice-cold citric saline. Collect the detached cells and place into pre-chilled 1.5 ml microcentrifuge tubes. Pellet the cells and aspirate off the supernatant. Freeze the cell pellets with liquid nitrogen and store in freezer until all time points have been collected.
6. When all time points have been harvested, cells can be lysed in 400 μl of cold PBS-Tr (1%) supplemented with PI and 1 mM PMSF. Cells are resuspended in the PBS-Tr (1%) buffer by mixing with a pipet. Incubate samples for 1 h at 4°C on a rotator.
7. Obtain the soluble cell lysate by centrifuging the samples at 36,000×*g* for 10 min at 4°C. Transfer the supernatant to a new precooled microcentrifuge tube.
8. Normalize each sample to contain the same total amount of protein (*see* **Note 3**).
9. Add 3 μl of CFTR MM13-4 antibody and 0.2% BSA to the normalized samples and incubate for 30 min on a rotator at 4°C.
10. Add 30 μl of a 50% Protein G-agarose slurry to each sample and incubate for 30 min on a rotator at 4°C.
11. Pellet the Protein G beads by centrifugation at 1,500×*g* for 2 min at 4°C.
12. Aspirate off the supernatant being careful not to disturb the beads. Resuspend the pelleted beads with 500 μl cold PBS-Tr (1%) and transfer to a new 1.5 ml microcentrifuge tube. Changing the tubes helps to get rid of any radiolabeled proteins that may be stuck to the sides of the microcentrifuge tube.
13. Pellet the Protein G beads again, remove the supernatant, then resuspend and wash the pelleted beads two times with 500 μl cold PBS-Tr (1%) supplemented with 0.2% SDS. After the last wash, aspirate off the buffer and remove all remaining buffer from around the Protein G beads using a Hamilton syringe.

14. To each pellet add 15 μl 2× SB and heat samples at 55°C for 10 min.
15. Pellet the Protein G beads by centrifugation at 1,500×*g* for 1 min at room temperature. Load all the supernatant using a Hamilton syringe onto a 7% SDS-PAGE gel.
16. Electrophorese the samples by applying a constant voltage of 120 V for 70 min.
17. After electrophoresis, fix and stain the protein in the gel by incubation in SDS-PAGE gel stain for 5 min.
18. Remove the stain, rinse the gel with distilled water, and then soak the gel with SDS-PAGE gel destain until protein bands on the gel are clearly visible.
19. Rinse the gel with distilled water and then soak the gel in 0.5 M sodium salicylate for at least 20 min (*see* **Note 4**).
20. Rinse the gel with distilled water and place it on a wet piece of Whatman paper to be dried on a slab type gel dryer for 1 h at 80°C.
21. Expose the dried SDS-PAGE gel to X-ray film for 1–3 days at –80°C. Develop the film with a processor.

3.4. Co-immunoprecipitation of CFTR with ER Quality Control Factors

Complexes formed between CFTR folding intermediates and ER quality control factors can be detected by co-immunoprecipitation studies (**Fig. 15.2**).

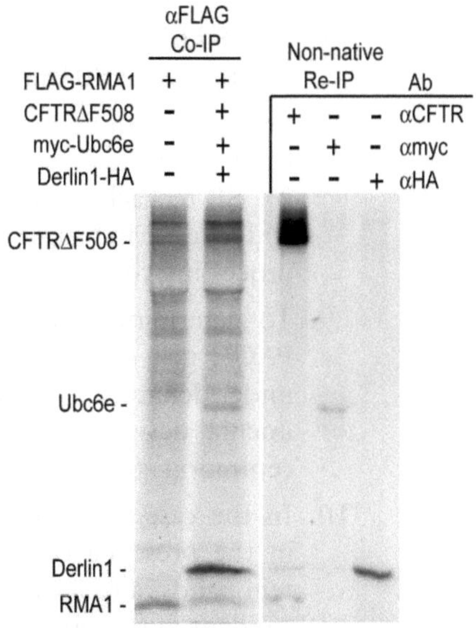

Fig. 15.2. Co-immunoprecipitation of components of the RMA1 E3 complex with F508del-CFTR. Using the method described in **Section 3.4**, the complex of interest was isolated by co-immunoprecipitation through FLAG-RMA1. The other potential components of this complex were then identified by a re-immunoprecipitation step.

1. Follow **Section 3.1.2** for the transient transfection of HEK293 cells with CFTR and epitope-tagged ER quality control factors. For co-immunoprecipitation reactions we usually transfect 1 μg of CFTR and 0.2 μg of the other factors into the HEK293 cells. If necessary, use the empty vector pcDNA3.1(+) to ensure equal microgram quantities of DNA are used in all transfection reactions.
2. Metabolically label transfected cells with ^{35}S as described in **Section 3.3.2**.
3. After the ^{35}S-labeling step, harvest the cells as indicated in **Section 3.1.3**. All subsequent steps are carried out at 4°C.
4. Lyse the samples with 250 μl of cold PBS-Tr (1%) supplemented with PI, 1 mM PMSF, and 0.2% BSA. Incubate samples for 1 h on a rotator.
5. Soluble cell lysate is obtained by centrifuging samples at 36,000×*g* for 10 min. Transfer supernatant to a new microcentrifuge tube.
6. Add antibody to the soluble cell lysate and incubate for 30 min on a rotator. For this experimental setup, we typically use 2 μl of antibody against the protein we want to immunoprecipitate. For example, to assess which factors are interacting with RMA1 we would use 2 μl of anti-RMA1. To monitor the background binding of overexpressed proteins a good control to include is co-immunoprecipitation samples that do not have antibody added to them.
7. Add 30 μl of 50% Protein G-agarose slurry to each sample and rotate for 30 min.
8. Pellet the Protein G beads by centrifugation, wash the isolated complex 3 × 500 μl with PBS-Tr (1%), add 15 μl 2× SB to each sample, heat samples at 55°C for 10 min, and load all the supernatant onto a SDS-PAGE gel. Finish processing the gel as detailed in **Section 3.3.2**.
9. To determine where a given protein runs on the SDS-PAGE gel, a direct immunoprecipitation of the protein under denaturing conditions can be included in the experimental design. For this control, add SDS (0.2% final concentration) to the buffer in the wash steps.
10. In the case that the co-immunoprecipitation step results in the presence of a large number of radiolabeled protein bands, a re-immunoprecipitation reaction can be used to identify the other potential components of the isolated complex. Add 2× SB to the complex isolated by co-immunoprecipitation and heat the samples at 55°C to disrupt the interacting proteins. Dilute the samples with PBS-Tr (1%) supplemented with PI, 1 mM PMSF, 0.2%

SDS, and 0.5% BSA. Antibodies against the proteins of interest are next added to the samples and the remainder of this immunoprecipitation reaction is processed as described in **Section 3.3.2**.

4. Notes

1. Transfection efficiency is dependent on the quality of the DNA expression constructs. We suggest using Qiagen reagents to obtain high-quality plasmid DNA. Expression can vary between different preparations of the same plasmid; therefore, we also recommend preparing a large quantity of the expression plasmid of interest and to use the same material for each experiment.
2. Continually overgrowing HEK293 cells (exceeding 100% confluence) can result in reduced transfection efficiencies. In addition, surpassing 30 passes of HEK293 cells can result in variable transfection efficiency.
3. To determine the protein concentration of our samples we use the colorimetric detergent compatible (DC) protein assay (Bio-Rad). To minimize the amount of sample that is used for protein determination we follow the modified assay for a 96-well plate as supplied by Bio-Rad. A standard protein curve is generated using dilutions of BSA ranging from 0.5 to 2.5 mg/ml that are prepared in the same buffer as the sample. As a side note, if the samples that need to be normalized are to be lysed in 2× SB, leave the β-mercaptoethanol out of the SB as the DC protein assay is incompatible with this chemical. The β-mercaptoethanol can be added after the samples are normalized.
4. After the SDS-PAGE gel has been destained, rinsing the gel with distilled water is a necessary step. Failure to sufficiently remove the acetic acid (a component of the destain solution) may cause a precipitate to form on the gel when it is soaked in sodium salicylate. This precipitate is caused by the low pH of the gel and can be re-dissolved by adding 1 M Tris–HCl, pH 8.0. After the precipitate is dissolved, add fresh sodium salicylate to the gel.

References

1. Cui, L., Aleksandrov, L., Chang, X. B., Hou, Y. X., He, L., Hegedus, T., et al. (2007) Domain interdependence in the biosynthetic assembly of CFTR. *J. Mol. Biol.* **365**, 981–994.
2. Du, K., Sharma, M., and Lukacs, G. L. (2005) The DeltaF508 cystic fibrosis mutation impairs domain-domain interactions and arrests post-translational folding of CFTR. *Nat. Struct. Mol. Biol.* **12**, 17–25.

3. Serohijos, A. W., Hegedus, T., Aleksandrov, A. A., He, L., Cui, L., Dokholyan, N. V., et al. (2008) Phenylalanine-508 mediates a cytoplasmic-membrane domain contact in the CFTR 3D structure crucial to assembly and channel function. *Proc. Natl. Acad. Sci. USA* **105**, 3256–3261.
4. Meacham, G. C., Lu, Z., King, S., Sorscher, E., Tousson, A., and Cyr, D. M. (1999) The Hdj-2/Hsc70 chaperone pair facilitates early steps in CFTR biogenesis. *EMBO J.* **18**, 1492–1505.
5. Ward, C. L., and Kopito, R. R. (1994) Intracellular turnover of cystic fibrosis transmembrane conductance regulator. Inefficient processing and rapid degradation of wild-type and mutant proteins. *J. Biol. Chem.* **269**, 25710–25718.
6. Rosser, M. F., Grove, D. E., Chen, L., and Cyr, D. M. (2008) Assembly and misassembly of CFTR: Folding defects caused by deletion of F508 occur before and after the calnexin-dependent association of MSD1 and MSD2. *Mol. Biol. Cell* **19**, 4570–4579.
7. Loo, M. A., Jensen, T. J., Cui, L., Hou, Y., Chang, X. B., and Riordan, J. R. (1998) Perturbation of Hsp90 interaction with nascent CFTR prevents its maturation and accelerates its degradation by the proteasome. *EMBO J.* **17**, 6879–6887.
8. Wang, X., Venable, J., LaPointe, P., Hutt, D. M., Koulov, A. V., Coppinger, J., et al. (2006) Hsp90 cochaperone Aha1 downregulation rescues misfolding of CFTR in cystic fibrosis. *Cell* **127**, 803–815.
9. Meacham, G. C., Patterson, C., Zhang, W., Younger, J. M., and Cyr, D. M. (2001) The Hsc70 co-chaperone CHIP targets immature CFTR for proteasomal degradation. *Nat. Cell. Biol.* **3**, 100–105.
10. Younger, J. M., Chen, L., Ren, H. Y., Rosser, M. F., Turnbull, E. L., Fan, C. Y., et al. (2006) Sequential quality-control checkpoints triage misfolded cystic fibrosis transmembrane conductance regulator. *Cell* **126**, 571–582.
11. Dalal, S., Rosser, M. F., Cyr, D. M., and Hanson, P. I. (2004) Distinct roles for the AAA ATPases NSF and p97 in the secretory pathway. *Mol. Biol. Cell* **15**, 637–648.
12. Morito, D., Hirao, K., Oda, Y., Hosokawa, N., Tokunaga, F., Cyr, D. M., et al. (2008) Gp78 cooperates with RMA1 in endoplasmic reticulum-associated degradation of CFTR{Delta}F508. *Mol. Biol. Cell* **19**, 1328–1336.
13. Wang, B., Heath-Engel, H., Zhang, D., Nguyen, N., Thomas, D. Y., Hanrahan, J. W., et al. (2008) BAP31 interacts with Sec61 translocons and promotes retrotranslocation of CFTRDeltaF508 via the derlin-1 complex. *Cell* **133**, 1080–1092.

Chapter 16

In Vitro Methods for CFTR Biogenesis

Yoshihiro Matsumura, LeeAnn Rooney, and William R. Skach

Abstract

Cell-free expression systems provide unique tools for understanding CFTR biogenesis because they reconstitute the cellular folding environment and are readily amenable to biochemical and pharmacological manipulation. The most common system for this purpose is rabbit reticulocyte lysate (RRL), supplemented with either canine pancreatic microsomes or semi-permeabilized cells, which has yielded important insights into the folding of CFTR and its individual domains. A common problem in such studies, however, is that biogenesis of large proteins such as CFTR is often inefficient due to low translation processivity, ribosome stalling, and/or premature termination. The first part of this chapter therefore describes parameters that affect in vitro translation of CFTR in RRL. We have found that CFTR expression is uniquely dependent upon 5′- and 3′-untranslated regions (UTRs) of the mRNA. Full-length CFTR expression can be markedly increased using mRNA lacking a 5′-cap analog (G(5′)ppp(5′)G), whereas the reverse usually holds for smaller proteins and individual CFTR domains. In the context of the full-length mRNA, translation was further stimulated by the presence of a long 3′-UTR. The second part of this chapter describes CFTR translation in lysates derived from cultured mammalian cells including human bronchial epithelial cells. Unfortunately, mammalian cell-derived lysates showed limited ability to sustain full-length CFTR synthesis. However, they provide a unique opportunity to examine specific CFTR domains (i.e., nucleotide-binding domain 1 and transmembrane domain 1) under conditions that more closely resemble the native folding environment.

Key words: Bronchial epithelial cells, canine pancreatic microsomes, cystic fibrosis transmembrane conductance regulator (CFTR), endoplasmic reticulum (ER), in vitro translation, membrane protein, molecular chaperone, protein folding, rabbit reticulocyte lysate (RRL).

1. Introduction

1.1. Principles and Limitations of Cell-Free Translation Systems

In order to function properly, proteins must be synthesized, folded, and assembled in the crowded cellular environment. This process begins as the nascent polypeptide emerges from ribosomal exit tunnel and encounters a variety of molecular chaperones

M.D. Amaral, K. Kunzelmann (eds.), *Cystic Fibrosis*, Methods in Molecular Biology 741,
DOI 10.1007/978-1-61779-117-8_16, © Springer Science+Business Media, LLC 2011

and co-chaperones that facilitate folding by inhibiting aggregation and formation of misfolded off-pathway intermediates. Membrane proteins require additional machinery for endoplasmic reticulum (ER) targeting, translocation, and integration into the lipid bilayer (1). Therefore, two key considerations are necessary for accurate in vitro reconstitution of protein biogenesis: (i) robust translational activity of ribosomes and (ii) the chaperone environment in which protein folding and assembly occur.

We have previously reported details for in vitro CFTR translation in rabbit reticulocyte lysate (RRL) and use of this system to study aspects of ER-associated degradation (2, 3). In the course of these studies we noted that the efficiency and processivity of CFTR translation was uniquely affected by 5′- and 3′-untranslated regions (UTRs) of mRNA. Notably, translation of full-length CFTR in RRL was paradoxically improved several fold using mRNA lacking the G(5′)ppp(5′)G cap analog, whereas high concentrations of capped mRNA were strongly inhibitory. In addition removal of the 3′-UTR, which usually enhances translation of other substrates, completely abolished CFTR synthesis. Thus translation properties of CFTR mRNA in vitro are markedly different than other proteins expressed to date, and translation reactions should be optimized accordingly.

Stress-induced phosphorylation of the translation initiation factor eIF2α is one of the major obstacles in preparing highly active cell-free translation extracts. eIF2α is a G protein required to bring the 40 S ribosomal subunit to the 5′-cap (7-methyl-diguanosine triphosphate) on the mRNA (4). eIF2α is phosphorylated under numerous stress conditions and once phosphorylated, it inhibits the guanine nucleotide exchange factor eIF2β. In RRL, the major eIF2α kinase (HRI) is inhibited by hemin, which maintains translation during the final stages of globin synthesis (5–7). Addition of exogenous hemin inhibits HRI and has enabled RRL to be widely used for the in vitro translation and folding of many protein substrates (8, 9). For reasons that remain unclear, however, biogenesis of large proteins such as CFTR (>100 kDa) often results in partial length N-terminal fragments due to ribosome stalling and/or premature release (2, 3, 10). Other mammalian systems (e.g., HeLa S3 cell lysates) have also been used for in vitro translation (11), although translation efficiency is generally low due to eIF2α phosphorylation during lysate preparation and incubation. To overcome this limitation, Zeenko et al. recently developed a novel in vitro translation system using mouse embryonic fibroblasts homozygous for the S51A mutation in eIF2α (MEF-AA) (12). Lysates prepared from MEF-AA cells were highly efficient in producing small cytosolic and secretory proteins such as luciferase and β-lactamase. However, the utility of such systems for synthesizing larger proteins such as CFTR has not been tested.

Eukaryotic cytosol contains diverse molecular chaperones and co-chaperones that cotranslationally bind client substrates and collectively facilitate folding and/or prevent aggregation of newly synthesized proteins (13). Many chaperones are also linked via co-chaperones to the ubiquitin proteasome pathway by their ability to bind to recruit E3 ligases. Thus, composition of the cellular chaperone pool establishes a global folding environment that monitors and maintains homeostasis of newly synthesized proteins (14, 15). This cellular proteostasis environment is dependent upon cellar differentiation, stress, age, etc., such that the fate of client proteins can be cell type specific. The environment is particularly important for proteins with marginal thermodynamic stability and/or folding kinetics such as CFTR which is easily recognized by ER quality control machinery. Because of the clinical importance of CFTR function in the lungs, an important challenge is to develop systems in which to study CFTR biogenesis in a cellular environment that resembles its native environment.

Here we provide updated protocols for CFTR expression in RRL and preparation of cell lysates. Strategies and limitations for optimizing CFTR biosynthesis in RRL and novel mammalian cell-free expression systems are discussed.

2. Materials

2.1. Preparation of RRL

2.1.1. Reticulocyte Induction

1. New Zealand white rabbits (~6 months old, ≥3 kg).
2. 3 cc syringes (no. of rabbits × 3).
3. 26-Gauge needles.
4. Clinical centrifuge with rotor suitable for hematocrit determination (e.g., IEC rotor no. 927).
5. Hematocrit reader, hematocrit tubes, clay plugs.
6. Acetyl phenyl hydrazine (APH) solution: add 2.5 g of APH to 20 ml of ethanol and then add 50 ml of water. Adjust pH to 7.0 with approx. 1 ml of 1 M KOH and bring to 100 ml with water. Filter the solution (0.22 μm), aliquot, and store at –20°C.

2.1.2. Processing of Reticulocyte Lysate

1. Rabbit restrainer.
2. Pentobarbital/nembutal, 50 mg/ml (4–5 ml per rabbit).
3. Heparin 1,000 U/ml (2 ml per rabbit).

4. IV tubing (e.g., extension set no. ET-20L (472010) from B/Braun – 21-in. long tubing), IV butterfly 23-gauge needle.
5. Reticulocyte wash buffer: 5 mM glucose, 0.14 M NaCl, 0.05 M KCl, 5 mM $MgCl_2$ (approx 500 ml per rabbit).
6. S7 nuclease (*Staphylococcus aureus*), 15 U/μl: dissolve in 10 mM Tris–HCl, pH 8.0. Store in aliquots at –80°C (Roche Diagnostics Corporation, Indianapolis, IN).
7. 0.1 M $CaCl_2$.
8. 0.1 M EGTA-KOH, pH 7.5.
9. 1 mM hemin stock solution. Combine reagents in the following order: 6.44 mg of hemin (bovine crystalline type I, Sigma, St. Louis, MO), 0.25 ml of 1 M KOH, 0.5 ml of 0.2 M Tris–HCl, pH 7.0–8.0, 8.9 ml of ethylene glycol, 0.19 ml of 1 N HCl, 0.05 ml ddH_2O. Filter (0.22 μm) and store at –20°C.

2.2. Preparation of Canine Pancreatic Microsomal Membranes

1. Freshly excised pancreas.
2. 50 ml Potter-Elvehjem tissue homogenizer with Teflon pestles (one loose fitting and one snug).
3. 25 ml Potter-Elvehjem tissue homogenizer (Teflon pestle).
4. Hand-held coarse food grinder.
5. 10× stock buffer (100 ml): 0.5 M KOAc, 60 mM $Mg(OAc)_2$, 10 mM EDTA, 0.5 M triethanolamine acetate, pH 7.5.
6. Buffer A: 1:10 dilution of 10× stock buffer containing 0.25 M sucrose, 1 mM dithiothreitol (DTT), 0.5 mM phenylmethylsulfonyl fluoride (PMSF). Add DTT and PMSF immediately before use.
7. Buffer B: 1:10 dilution of 10× stock buffer containing 1.3 M sucrose.
8. Buffer C (100 ml): 0.25 M sucrose, 1 mM DTT, 50 mM triethanolamine acetate, pH 7.5. Add DTT immediately before use.
9. 1% sodium dodecyl sulfate (SDS), 0.1 M Tris–HCl, pH 8.0.
10. Ti 50.2 rotor and polycarbonate tubes (Beckman Coulter, Brea, CA).

2.3. Preparation of Capped and Non-capped RNA

2.3.1. Preparation of Capped RNA

1. 5× cap transcription buffer: 30 mM $MgCl_2$, 10 mM spermidine, 200 mM Tris–HCl, pH 7.5.

2. 10× NTPs for cap: 5 mM ATP, 5 mM CTP, 5 mM UTP, 1 mM GTP, 20 mM Tris–HCl, pH 8.0 (nucleotides from Roche Molecular Biochemicals, Indianapolis, IN). Store at –20 to –80°C.
3. 5 mM of G(5′)ppp(5′)G RNA cap structure analog (New England Biolabs, Ipswich, MA). Store at –20 to –80°C.
4. 0.1 M DTT (Roche Molecular Biochemicals).
5. 10 U/μl of RNase inhibitor (Fermentas, Glen Burnie, MD).
6. 10 U/ml of SP6 RNA polymerase (Epicenter, Madison, WI) or 0.1 mg/ml recombinant His-tagged SP6 RNA polymerase.
7. 7.5 M LiCl, 50 mM EDTA.

2.3.2. Preparation of Non-capped RNA

1. 5× non-cap transcription buffer: 400 mM *N*-(2-hydroxyethylpiperazine-*N*′-2-ethanesulfonic acid) (HEPES)-NaOH, pH 7.5, 80 mM $MgCl_2$, 10 mM spermidine.
2. 5× NTPs for non-cap: 15 mM ATP, 15 mM CTP, 15 mM UTP, 15 mM GTP, 20 mM HEPES-NaOH, pH 7.5 (final).
3. 0.1 M DTT.
4. 10 U/μl of RNase inhibitor.
5. 10 U/ml of SP6 RNA polymerase or 0.1 mg/ml His-tagged SP6 RNA polymerase.
6. 7.5 M LiCl, 50 mM EDTA.

2.4. In Vitro Translation in RRL

2.4.1. Linked In Vitro Transcription–Translation in RRL

1. 20× linked translation buffer: 2 M KOAc, 16 mM $Mg(OAc)_2$, 40 mM Tris-acetate, pH 7.5.
2. 5× Emix: 5 mM ATP, 5 mM GTP, 60 mM creatine phosphate, 1 mM mixture of 19 amino acids except methionine, and 5 μCi/μl Trans ^{35}S-label (ICN, Costa Mesa, CA). Aliquots are typically made in 100 to 200 μl volumes, adjusted to pH 7.5 with Tris base, and stored at –80°C.
3. RRL (hemin- and nuclease-treated; *see* **Section 3.1**, step 6).
4. 10 mg/ml of bovine liver tRNA (type XI, Sigma).
5. 10 U/μl of RNase inhibitor.
6. 4 mg/ml of creatine kinase (Sigma): dissolve in 50% glycerol, 10 mM Tris-acetate, pH 7.5.
7. Microsomal membranes (nuclease-treated; *see* **Section 3.2**, step 6).
8. Non-capped or capped RNA (*see* **Sections 3.3.1**, step 4, and **3.3.2**, step 4).

2.4.2. Unlinked In Vitro Translation in RRL

1. 20× unlinked translation buffer for RRL: 2 M KOAc, 40 mM $Mg(OAc)_2$, 200 mM Tris-acetate, pH 7.5, 3 mM spermidine, 40 mM DTT.
2. 5× Emix: 5 mM ATP, 5 mM GTP, 60 mM creatine phosphate, 1 mM mixture of 19 amino acids except methionine, and 5 μCi/μl Trans ^{35}S-label.
3. RRL (hemin- and nuclease-treated; *see* **Section 3.1**, step 6).
4. 10 mg/ml of bovine liver tRNA.
5. 10 U/μl of RNase inhibitor.
6. 4 mg/ml of creatine kinase.
7. Microsomal membranes (nuclease-treated; *see* **Section 3.2**, step 6).
8. Non-capped or capped RNA (*see* **Sections 3.3.1**, step 4, and **3.3.2**, step 4).

2.5. Preparation of MEF-AA and CFBE Lysates

1. Dulbecco's modified eagle's medium (DMEM) with high glucose supplemented with 10% fetal bovine serum, 2 mM L-glutamine, and 100 U/ml penicillin/streptomycin (reagents from Invitrogen, Carlsbad, CA).
2. Minimal essential medium (MEM) with Earl's salts supplemented with 10% fetal bovine serum, 2 mM L-glutamine, and 100 U/ml penicillin/streptomycin (reagents from Invitrogen).
3. 0.25% trypsin-EDTA (Invitrogen).
4. 150 mm tissue culture plates (Corning, Corning, NY).
5. Dulbecco's phosphate-buffered saline (D-PBS) without calcium and magnesium (Thermo Scientific, Waltham, MA), 11 mM D-glucose.
6. Lysis buffer A: 20 mM HEPES-KOH, pH 7.4, 10 mM KOAc, 0.5 mM $Mg(OAc)_2$, 1 mM DTT, 1 mM PMSF, 1× protease inhibitor cocktail set III EDTA free (EMD Chemicals Inc., Gibbstown, NJ, cat. no. 539134). Add DTT, PMSF, and protease inhibitor immediately before use.
7. Cell scraper.
8. 26-Gauge needle with 1 ml syringe.
9. 1 ml Dounce tissue homogenizer (Wheaton Science Products, Millville, NJ).

2.6. In Vitro Translation in MEF-AA and CFBE Lysates

1. 20× unlinked translation buffer for MEF-AA and CFBE: 2 M KOAc, 35 mM $Mg(OAc)_2$, 200 mM Tris acetate, pH 7.5, 3 mM spermidine, 40 mM DTT.
2. 5× Emix: 5 mM ATP, 5 mM GTP, 60 mM creatine phosphate, 1 mM mixture of 19 amino acids except methionine, and 5 μCi/μl Trans ^{35}S-label.

3. MEF-AA and CFBE lysates (nuclease-treated; *see* **Sections 3.5.1**, step 11, and **3.5.2**, step 8).
4. 10 mg/ml of bovine liver tRNA.
5. 10 U/μl of RNase inhibitor.
6. 4 mg/ml of creatine kinase.
7. Microsomal membranes (nuclease-treated; *see* **Section 3.2**, step 6).

3. Methods

3.1. Preparation of RRL

The following procedure, used routinely in our laboratory, is based on a protocol previously described by Jackson et al. (16) and takes roughly 1 week from start to finish. Note that reagents used for all steps of transcription and translation reactions should be prepared following strict RNase-free protocols. Typically 5–10 rabbits are processed in parallel. While commercial preparations of RRL are available (Promega, Madison, WI), preparing RRL de novo allows the composition and quality of reaction conditions to be controlled and optimized. Because preparations vary significantly in terms of activity, lysate from each animal is processed, stored, and assayed independently. The reason for this variability remains unknown, but likely reflects biological differences between animals (*see* **Note 1**). If large numbers of experiments are to be performed it is also more economical to prepare this reagent since one rabbit yields between 20 and 40 ml of RRL.

1. All handling and care of animals should be approved by the institutional animal review board.
2. Inject rabbits subcutaneously on three consecutive days (d 1, 2, and 3) with 2 ml of APH solution.
3. On d 4–7 monitor animals for health, activity, and food intake. Hematocrits are monitored by ear vein puncture, collection of capillary tubes, and centrifugation at 8,000×*g* for 5 min. The hematocrit normally does not fall below 20%.
4. On d 8, place rabbits in a restrainer, cannulate an ear vein, and inject 2 ml of heparin (1,000 U/ml) followed by a lethal dose of pentobarbital (200–250 mg) 1 min later. When the rabbit has lost eyelid reflex and respiration has ceased, remove the animal from the restrainer, transect left ribs with a scalpel, open chest cavity, and puncture left ventricle directly with a 16-gauge needle attached to IV extension tubing. Collect blood in a 250 ml centrifuge bottle on ice. Any remaining blood is collected using a syringe inserted into the right ventricle. Perform all subsequent steps on ice.

5. Centrifuge blood at 2,500×*g* at 4°C for 10 min. Discard supernatant and wash cells three times with 150 ml of ice-cold reticulocyte wash buffer followed by centrifugation at 2,500×*g* for 10 min. After the third wash resuspend cells in a small volume of wash buffer, transfer to a 50 ml conical tube, and centrifuge at 3,000×*g* for 10 min. Remove supernatant, and carefully aspirate top layer of white blood cells. Add one volume of ice-cold ddH_2O and shake very vigorously for 30 s to lyse cells. Repeat shaking every 5 min three times. Centrifuge the lysate at 15,000×*g* for 10 min and carefully decant supernatant. Lysate can be frozen in liquid nitrogen at this stage and stored at –80°C for several years with minimal loss of activity. Set aside several small samples (0.5 ml) to test relative translation activity.
6. Prior to use, hemin is added to a final concentration of 40 μM. Endogenous mRNA is digested by thawing a 1 ml RRL aliquot in a 25°C water bath and adding 10 μl of 0.1 M $CaCl_2$ and 10 μl of S7 nuclease. The sample is incubated for 8–10 min at 25°C, and 20 μl of 0.1 M EGTA is added. Samples are aliquoted, frozen in liquid nitrogen, and stored at –80°C for 2–3 months.

3.2. Preparation of ER Microsomal Membranes

Canine pancreas microsomes are prepared based on the procedure described by Walter and Blobel (17). All procedures are carried out on ice in a 4°C cold room.

1. Quickly remove pancreas in its entirety from euthanized animal and immediately place into 100 ml of ice-cold buffer A (*see* **Note 2**). Trim away fat, connective tissue, and blood vessels and record weight. Grind pancreas by hand using a coarse food grinder until a pulpy consistency is achieved. Collect fragments together with 4 volumes (4 ml/g of original tissue) of ice-cold buffer A.
2. Homogenize this mixture in a 50 ml Potter-Elvehjem tissue homogenizer attached to a high-speed motor with three to four passes of a loose-fitting Teflon pestle and return homogenate to ice. Homogenize solution a second time with one to three passes of a tight-fitting Teflon pestle. Sample must be kept ice cold during the entire procedure.
3. Divide homogenate into 50 ml aliquots and centrifuge at 600×*g* for 10 min. Collect supernatant and centrifuge at 10,000×*g* for 10 min. Decant the resulting supernatant into a 150 ml beaker, taking care to avoid the loose pellet.
4. Carefully layer approx. 15–20 ml of this supernatant fraction over a 5–7 ml cushion of buffer B and centrifuge at 150,000×*g* for 3 h using Ti 50.2 rotor. Aspirate supernatant and gently resuspend pellets (by hand in a 25 ml

homogenizer) in buffer C (1/2 ml per gram of starting material). When the solution is uniform, aliquot and freeze 1 ml aliquots in liquid nitrogen. Microsomes are stable for several years when stored at –80°C.

5. Determine OD_{280} by dissolving 10 μl of membrane suspension in 990 μl of 1% SDS, 0.1 M Tris–HCl, pH 8.0. This provides a useful reference based on crude protein content. OD_{280} concentration of the final membrane preparations should be approx. 50–100.
6. Prior to use, digest endogenous mRNA with S7 nuclease as described for RRL (*see* **Section 3.1**, step 6). Typically, 1 ml of microsomes is treated, frozen in liquid nitrogen as 50–100 μl aliquots, and stored at –80°C for up to 3 months.
7. Test microsome translocation and glycosylation efficiencies (*see* **Note 3**).

3.3. Preparation of Capped and Non-capped RNA

Endogenous eukaryotic mRNAs are characterized by a 7-methyl-guanosine triphosphate (m^7G) cap at the 5′-UTR. For in vitro transcription, the cap analog G(5′)ppp(5′)G is typically used as a more economical alternative. In cells, the cap regulates nuclear export, stabilizes the mRNA, and enhances recruitment of eukaryotic initiation factors eIF4F and eIF3 and the 43S pre-initiation complex. Capped RNA also improves in vitro translation in RRL (18). The 3′-UTR of most mRNAs is also modified, in this case by addition of a poly-adenosine monophosphate (poly(A)) tail that recruits poly(A)-binding protein, which interacts with the eIF4G–eIF4E complex. While the 5′-cap and 3′-poly(A) tail stimulate translation synergistically in vivo, this effect is not typically observed in nuclease-treated RRL where efficient translation is observed for most mRNAs that lack a 3′-UTR. cDNA templates for RRL translation therefore commonly include non-linearized plasmid, linearized plasmid, or PCR products that can be truncated very close to the stop codon. Surprisingly, we found that the presence of a 5′-cap actually reduced full-length CFTR expression at high mRNA levels when compared to similar concentrations of uncapped mRNA. In contrast, the reverse was true for individual CFTR domains. Moreover, a long 3′-UTR (>0.2 kb) was absolutely required for full-length CFTR translation.

Capped mRNA transcripts can be used fresh or stored at –80°C followed by linked transcription–translation. Purification of RNA is not necessary in linked transcription–translation. Both capped and non-capped RNAs can be purified and stored at –80°C when multiple experiments on the same protein are to be performed or when defined concentrations of RNA are to be used. Although non-capped RNA is often less efficient than capped RNA for translation, it is more economical due to the high cost of the cap analog. Moreover, most substrates can be successfully synthesized in vitro using higher concentration of non-capped RNA (12).

The following conditions are used for SP6 RNA polymerase, which in our hands usually gives better results for translation than T7 RNA polymerase (*see* **Note 4**). Our standard plasmid vector (pSP64T) contains a 66 base 5′-UTR that includes 52 bases of 5′-UTR from the *Xenopus laevis* globin gene (GCTTGTTCTTTTTGCAGAAGCTCAGAATAAACGCTCAA CTTTGGCAGATACC**ATG**G) (19) immediately upstream of the ATG initiation codon (bold). Where possible, DNA constructs are ligated into this vector to place their start codon close to the end of the *X. laevis* 5′-UTR. This is best accomplished using an *Nco*I restriction site (underlined), which also creates an optimal Kozak consensus translation start site.

3.3.1. Capped RNA Preparation

1. mRNAs with 3′-UTRs of defined length are generated by digesting plasmids with restriction enzymes that cleave downstream of the stop codon. Alternatively, supercoiled DNA or amplified PCR products can be used as transcription templates after standard phenol/chloroform extraction and ethanol precipitation.
2. Typically a 20 μl cap transcription reaction is prepared on ice by mixing 4 μl of 5× cap transcription buffer, 2 μl of 10× NTPs for cap, 2 μl of 0.1 M DTT, 2 μl of G(5′)ppp(5′)G, 0.8 μl of RNase inhibitor, 0.8 μl of SP6 polymerase, 4 μg of plasmid DNA or 200 ng of PCR products, and ddH_2O bringing the total volume to 20 μl. ddH_2O is substituted for DNA in mock transcription reactions. Incubate for 1 h at 40°C and transfer to ice. Transcription reaction can be added directly to in vitro translation in RRL (*see* **Section 3.4.1**) or stored at –80°C.
3. Capped RNA is typically purified from an identical transcription reaction scaled up to 200 μl. Precipitate mRNA by addition of 120 μl of 7.5 M LiCl, 50 mM EDTA. Incubate for 1 h at –20°C and centrifuge at 16,000×*g* at 4°C for 20 min. Rinse RNA pellet three times with 1 ml of 70% ethanol followed by centrifugation at 16,000×*g* at 4°C for 1 min. Rinse RNA pellet with 1 ml of 95% ethanol followed by centrifugation at 16,000×*g* at 4°C for 1 min. Discard supernatant and dissolve pellet into ddH_2O.
4. Determine RNA concentration by measuring OD_{260} (1.0 OD_{260} = 40 ng/μl) and adjust RNA concentration to 500 ng/μl. Freeze in liquid nitrogen and store at –80°C.

3.3.2. Non-capped RNA Preparation

1. DNA templates are prepared as for capped RNA (*see* **Section 3.3.1**, step 1).

2. Assemble a 100 μl non-cap transcription reaction, by combining the following reagents on ice: 20 μl of 5× non-cap transcription buffer, 20 μl of 5× NTPs for non-cap, 40 μl of 0.1 M DTT, 2 μl of RNase inhibitor, 5 μl of SP6 polymerase, 5 μg of plasmid DNA or 1 μg of PCR products, and ddH_2O bringing up to 100 μl. Incubate for 2 h at 40°C and transfer to ice.
3. Precipitate non-capped RNA by adding 60 μl of 7.5 M LiCl and 50 mM EDTA as described for capped RNA (*see* **Section 3.3.1**, step 3). Rinse and dissolve RNA pellet into ddH_2O.
4. Determine RNA concentration by measuring OD_{260} and adjust RNA concentration to 500 ng/μl. Freeze in liquid nitrogen and store at –80°C.

3.4. Translation in RRL

Translation initiation and chain elongation are two key factors that limit in vitro CFTR translation. As these parameters are classically affected by potassium and magnesium, optimal concentrations are determined empirically, although 100 mM potassium acetate and 2.0 mM magnesium acetate usually work best for this protocol (16, 20). As noted above, CFTR translation is unusual in that initiation is paradoxically inhibited by a 5′-G(5′)ppp(5′)G cap at high mRNA concentration (>20 ng/μl), whereas translation elongation requires a long 3′-UTR. The protocols below therefore describe experimental conditions used to optimize CFTR expression using non-capped mRNA and compare effects of varying the length of the 3′-UTR.

3.4.1. Linked In Vitro Transcription–Translation in RRL

1. For linked in vitro transcription–translation, purification of RNA is not necessary because the transcription reaction is added directly to the translation reaction. The composition of translation buffers therefore takes into account the ionic contributions of the transcript. Assemble a translation master mix by combining 1/20 vol of 20× linked translation buffer, 1/5 vol of 5× Emix, 40% RRL (nucleased and hemin-treated), 1/100 vol RNase inhibitor, 1/100 vol creatine kinase, 1/100 vol bovine liver tRNA, and ddH_2O bringing to 70% of final reaction volume. Add 70% master mix to 20% cap transcription reaction. The amount of microsomes is determined empirically based on translocation and glycosylation activity (*see* **Section 3.2**, step 7). Normally, they are added to achieve ≥90% translocation of a control secretory protein to ensure that adequate Sec61 translocons are available for engaged ribosomes. Full-length CFTR translations are performed at 24°C for 2 h, while smaller proteins (30–70 kDa) are incubated for 1 h.
2. Analyze 1 μl aliquots of translation by SDS-PAGE followed by phosphorimaging or autoradiography.

3.4.2. Unlinked In Vitro Translation in RRL

Unlinked translation reactions are performed using purified mRNAs, and the 20× buffer is adjusted accordingly. In this instance, the amount of mRNA can be titrated to optimize protein expression.

1. Combine 1/20 vol of 20× unlinked translation buffer for RRL, 1/5 vol of 5× Emix, 40% v/v RRL (nucleased and hemin-treated), 1/100 vol RNase inhibitor, 1/100 vol creatine kinase, 1/100 vol bovine liver tRNA, and ddH_2O bringing to 70% of final reaction volume. Add 70% master mix to non-capped or capped RNA and the remaining volume with microsomes plus ddH_2O. The quantity of microsomes is determined empirically based on translocation and glycosylation activity. Incubate at 24°C for 1–2 h.
2. Analyze 1 μl aliquots of translation by SDS-PAGE followed by phosphorimaging or autoradiography.

3.4.3. Effect of the 3′-UTR on CFTR Translation

Because translation is usually not dependent on a 3′-poly(A) tail in RRL, linearized plasmids or PCR products are frequently used as templates for in vitro transcription and often translate more efficiently than mRNAs generated from non-linearized plasmids (21–23). For CFTR, however, mRNA transcribed from a supercoiled plasmid is best translated into full-length CFTR, whereas mRNA transcribed from plasmid linearized approx. 0.2 kb downstream from the stop codon in the CFTR 3′-UTR generated only partial length intermediates (**Fig. 16.1a**). Similar results were observed when only 51 bases of the CFTR 3′-UTR were present (not shown). In contrast, inclusion of additional 3′-UTR

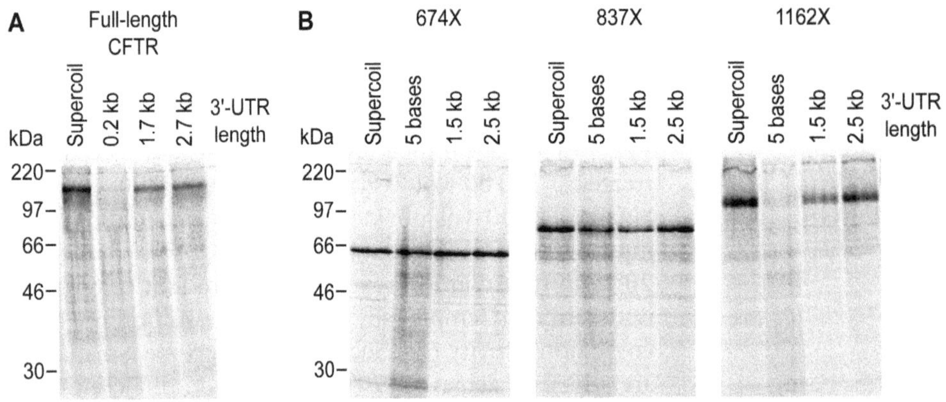

Fig. 16.1. Effect of 3′-UTR length on CFTR and CFTR domain expression in RRL. (**a**) Supercoiled or linearized plasmid encoding full-length CFTR was transcribed in vitro in the presence of G(5′)ppp(5′)G cap. *PstI*, *PvuI*, and *NheI* digestions produce 3′-UTR of approximately 0.2, 1.7, and 2.7 kb, respectively. Transcripts translated in linked RRL reactions supplemented with canine pancreatic microsomes. (**b**) Supercoiled or linearized plasmids encoding TMD1-NBD1 (674X), TMD1-NBD1-R (837X), or TMD1-NBD1-R-TMD2 (1162X) were transcribed and translated as in (**a**). In these constructs, *PstI* linearizes the plasmid 5 bases beyond the stop codon, whereas *PvuI* and *NheI* digestions produce approx. 1.5 and 2.5 kb 3′-UTR, respectively. Equal amounts of translation products were separated by SDS-PAGE on a 12–17% gel and analyzed by phosphorimaging.

(approx. 1.7 and 2.7 kb) transcribed from the plasmid vector restored translation of full-length CFTR. In each case CFTR mRNA was stable throughout the translation reaction (data not shown). To identify where CFTR translation was stalled, a stop codon was added after the first nucleotide-binding domain (NBD1, 674X), the regulatory (R) domain (837X), or transmembrane domain (TMD2, 1162X) after removing downstream CFTR sequence. Each construct was transcribed from either supercoiled (lane 1) or plasmids containing 5 bases, approx 1.5 or 2.5 kb of 3′-UTR (**Fig. 16.1b**). Constructs containing 673 aa and 836 aa were expressed from all templates regardless of the 3′-UTR length, whereas TMD1-NBD1-R-TMD2 required additional 3′-UTR sequences. Importantly, proteins generated are identical in size, and degradation does not occur at these temperatures or in the presence of hemin. Thus differences reflect translation efficiency rather than post-translational effects. For these reasons, CFTR transcripts are transcribed from non-linearized plasmids.

3.4.4. Effect of the 5′-Cap on CFTR Translation

The presence of a 5′-cap structure usually enhances protein expression in RRL by facilitating recruitment of translation initiation factors. For CFTR, however, capped mRNA produces maximal translation of full-length protein at a concentration of 5–20 ng/μl. Higher mRNA concentrations decrease the yield of full-length product (**Fig. 16.2a**). This effect was not observed for non-capped RNA, which produces full-length CFTR in a dose-dependent manner. Notably, the maximum yield obtained for non-capped mRNA was 2.5 times greater than capped RNA. We believe that more efficient translation initiation by capped RNA results in increased ribosome stalling. Note, however, that this property is specific for longer CFTR proteins, and that translation of isolated domains (NBD1 (**Fig. 16.2b**) and others, not shown) improved at every concentration of capped mRNA up to 100 ng/μl.

3.5. Preparation of MEF-AA and CFBE Lysates

3.5.1. Preparation of MEF-AA Lysate

Mouse embryo fibroblast cells homozygous for S51A eIF2α (MEF-AA) were kindly provided by Dr. Randal J. Kaufman (24). These cells are resistant to stress-induced eIF2α phosphorylation and therefore retain translation initiation activity during lysate preparation and in vitro incubation. Preparation of MEF-AA cell lysate is based on the procedure described by Zeenko et al. with minor modification (12). All procedures are carried out on ice.

1. Culture MEF-AA cells in DMEM, 10% FBS, 2 mM L-glutamine, and 100 U/ml penicillin/streptomycin in twenty 150 mm tissue culture plates at 37°C, 5% CO_2.

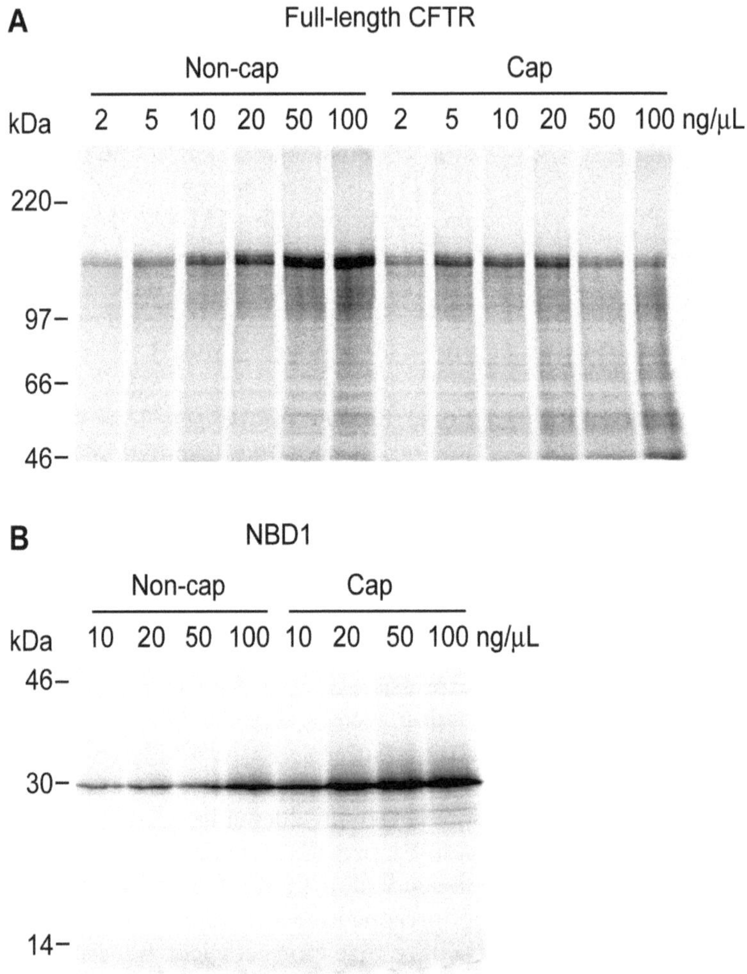

Fig. 16.2. Effect of 5′-cap on expression of NBD1 and full-length CFTR in RRL. (**a**) Full-length CFTR mRNA was transcribed from supercoiled plasmid in the presence or absence of cap analog. mRNA was purified and added at the indicated concentration to a RRL translation reaction supplemented with canine pancreatic microsomes. Products were analyzed by SDS-PAGE and phosphorimaging. (**b**) Non-capped and capped mRNAs encoding NBD1 (residues 389–673 aa) were transcribed from plasmid linearized 1 base beyond the stop codon. mRNA was purified and translated in RRL as in (**a**), and translation products were analyzed as in **Fig. 16.1**.

Grow to 100% confluency. Note that these cells exhibit little contact inhibition and will continue to grow and divide beyond 100% confluency (*see* **Note 5**).

2. Remove culture medium, wash cells with ice-cold D-PBS, 11 mM D-glucose, and harvest by scraping in 20 ml of D-PBS, 11 mM D-glucose per plate. Do not trypsinize.
3. Combine cells and spin at 1,000 rpm for 5 min at 4°C.
4. Wash cell pellet twice with 50 ml of D-PBS, 11 mM D-glucose.

5. Remove supernatant and estimate the cell pellet volume. Typical cell pellet volume should be 2–3 ml. Gently resuspend in equal volume of lysis buffer A.
6. Incubate on ice for 5 min. Cells should swell in this hypotonic solution.
7. Transfer cells to an ice-cold Dounce homogenizer and break the cells with 30–50 strokes, keeping on ice the entire time.
8. Pass broken cells through a 26-gauge needle attached to a 1 ml syringe three to five times.
9. Spin cell extract at 1,000×*g* for 5 min at 4°C and collect the supernatant (*see* **Note 6**).
10. Spin the supernatant at 10,000×*g* for 5 min at 4°C and collect the supernatant lysate.
11. Digest endogenous mRNA with S7 nuclease as described for RRL (*see* **Section 3.1**, step 6). Typically, 5 μl of 0.1 M $CaCl_2$ and 5 μl of S7 nuclease are added to 500 μl of MEF-AA lysate (*see* **Note 7**). The sample is incubated for 8–10 min at 25°C, and 10 μl of 0.1 M EGTA is added. Freeze aliquots in liquid nitrogen and store at −80°C.

3.5.2. Preparation of CFBE Lysate

The CFBE41o⁻ (CFBE) cell line was kindly provided by Dr. Dieter C. Gruenert (25). These cells are derived from human bronchial epithelial cells immortalized by SV40 large T antigen and thus provide a folding environment that mimics airway epithelium. Because they are sensitive to stress-induced phosphorylation of eIF2α, the following protocol is used to maintain translation initiation activity.

1. Culture CFBE cells in MEM, 10% FBS, 2 mM L-glutamine, and 100 U/ml penicillin/streptomycin onto ten 150 mm tissue culture plates at 37°C, 5% CO_2 (*see* **Note 8**). Grow to 90% confluency (*see* **Note 5**).
2. Place plates on ice, remove the culture medium, and rinse the cells twice with ice-cold D-PBS, 11 mM D-glucose.
3. Rapidly add approx. 10 ml of lysis buffer A to the plate and drain the buffer. Cells will remain attached and should swell but not lyse. Add lysis buffer A again and remove as much buffer as possible without drying the cells. Diluted lysates are less active in translation.
4. Pour approx. 10 ml of liquid nitrogen directly onto a plate, allow it to boil off and the frozen cells to thaw slightly. It is best to do this sequentially, one plate at a time.
5. Scrape and collect the cells directly into an ice-cold tube. This should yield an approximate volume of 300 μl per

150 mm plate. Pass through a 26-gauge needle attached to a 1 ml syringe 20 times on ice.

6. Spin extract at 1,000×*g* for 5 min at 4°C and collect the supernatant (*see* **Note 6**).
7. Spin the supernatant at 10,000×*g* for 5 min at 4°C and collect the supernatant lysate.
8. Digest endogenous mRNA with S7 nuclease similarly as above (*see* **Section 3.5.1**, step 11) except for adding 1.25 μl of S7 nuclease to 500 μl of CFBE lysate (*see* **Note** 7). Freeze in liquid nitrogen as 100 μl aliquots and store at –80°C.

3.6. In Vitro Translation in MEF-AA and CFBE Lysates

As described for RRL, magnesium and potassium concentrations in translation reaction must be determined empirically for optimal translation. Typical concentrations are 80–120 mM and 0.5–3 mM, respectively.

3.6.1. In Vitro Translation in MEF-AA and CFBE Lysate

1. Assemble a translation master mix by combining 1/20 vol of 20× unlinked translation buffer for MEF-AA and CFBE, 1/5 vol of 5× Emix, 40% MEF-AA or CFBE lysates (nucleased), 1/100 vol RNase inhibitor, 1/100 vol creatine kinase, 1/100 vol bovine liver tRNA, and ddH_2O bringing to 70% of final reaction volume. Add 70% master mix and non-capped or capped RNA at 50 ng/μl final concentration. ER microsomes if needed are determined empirically based on translocation and glycosylation activity (*see* **Note 9**). Incubate at 24°C for 1–2 h.
2. Analyze 1–4 μl aliquots of translation by SDS-PAGE followed by phosphorimaging or autoradiography.

3.6.2. CFTR Expression

1. In contrast to RRL, MEF-AA and CFBE lysates programmed with full-length, capped CFTR mRNA initiated translation but generate only partial length translation intermediates due to stalling and/or early termination (**Fig. 16.3a**). We believe that this is due to either depletion of cellular factor(s) or accumulation of inhibitory by-products during the translation reaction (26). mRNA titration between 2 and 100 ng/μl in MEF-AA and CFBE lysates increased partial length products but did not change the amount of full-length protein synthesis (data not shown). On the other hand, the NBD1 domain of CFTR was expressed in both MEF-AA and CFBE lysates (**Fig. 16.3b**). As in RRL, capped RNA was more efficient than non-capped RNA for NBD1 domain expression. We also noted that NBD1 was expressed more efficiently when canine pancreatic microsomes are added to MEF-AA and CFBE lysates. Preliminary results indicate that microsomes contain adsorbed factors that facilitate NBD1 translation

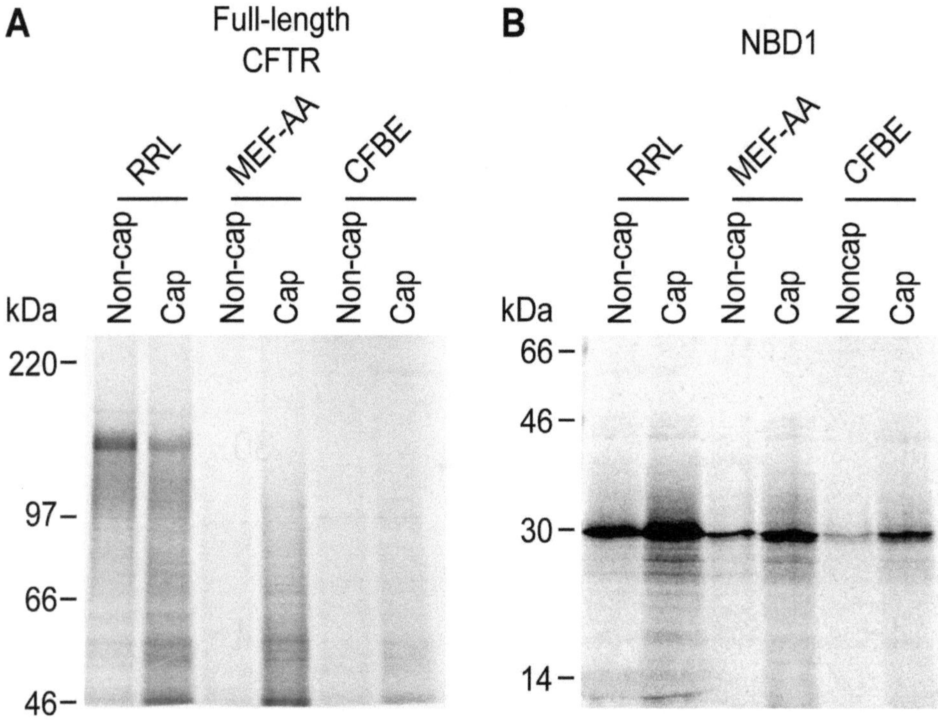

Fig. 16.3. Translation of NBD1 and full-length CFTR in mammalian cell lysates. (**a**) Non-capped and capped mRNA (50 ng/μl) encoding full-length CFTR was transcribed from supercoiled plasmid and translated in RRL, MEF-AA, or CFBE lysates as indicated. (**b**) Non-capped and capped mRNA (50 ng/μl) encoding NBD1 was transcribed from linearized plasmid 1 base beyond the stop codon and translated in RRL, MEF-AA, or CFBE lysates as indicated. All reactions were supplemented with canine pancreatic microsomes. Translation reactions (1 μl of RRL, 1 μl of MEF-AA, and 4 μl of CFBE) were analyzed by SDS-PAGE and imaged on a PhosphorImager.

although the identity of such factors remains unknown. MEF-AA and CFBE lysates are also suited for translating CFTR transmembrane domains (e.g., TMD1), although partial length translation intermediates were also generated, particularly in MEF-AA lysates (**Fig. 16.4a, b**). To date, the largest CFTR fragment we have expressed in CFBE lysate is TMD1-NBD1-R (837X); however, the efficiency is quite low (data not shown).

4. Notes

1. Repeated freeze–thaw cycles will decrease lysate activity, although three to four cycles are generally well tolerated as long as samples are thawed quickly and refrozen in liquid nitrogen. The quality of RRL also varies between rabbits

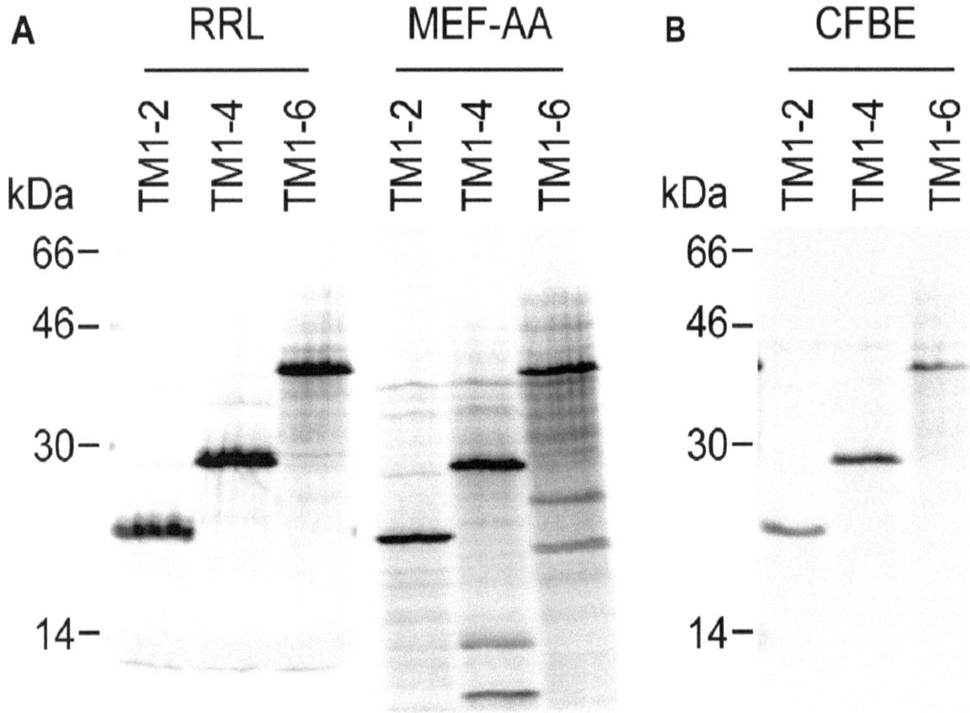

Fig. 16.4. Translation of CFTR TMD1 in mammalian cell lysates. (**a**) Capped mRNA (50 ng/μl) encoding CFTR transmembrane segments (TM) 1–2 (residues 1–187 aa), TM1–4 (residues 1–273 aa), or TM1–6 (residues 1–393 aa) was transcribed from PCR products and translated in RRL or MEF-AA lysate supplemented with canine pancreatic microsomes. (**b**) Capped mRNA (50 ng/μl) encoding TM1–2, TM1–4, or TM1–6 was translated in CFBE lysate supplemented with canine pancreatic microsomes. Translation reactions (1 μl of RRL, 4 μl of MEF-AA, and 4 μl of CFBE) were analyzed by SDS-PAGE and phosphorimaging. Exposure of CFBE lysate to the phosphorscreen (**b**) was approximately three times longer than in (**a**).

due to differences in age, maturity, and fraction of the reticulocytes harvested. Therefore, we process lysate from each rabbit separately. Lower yields can result from failure to completely exsanguinate the animal or inefficient lysis. The latter problem is usually due to inadequate shaking of the lysate and is accompanied by a large pellet in the second 15,000×*g* spin in the RRL protocol.

2. Traditionally canine pancreatic microsomes have been the major source of ER used to study in vitro translation of secreted and transmembrane proteins. However, preparations can also be made from pig or sheep pancreas by following essentially the same procedure (27). Proteolysis or autolysis of the pancreas can be a significant problem so the pancreas should be removed as quickly as possible following euthanasia.

3. Canine pancreas membrane preparations vary widely in translocation efficiency, and it may take several attempts to

achieve a satisfactory preparation. A suitable preparation, however, generates 10–30 ml of microsomes and is sufficient for many thousands of translation reactions. Optimal preparations yield ≥90% translocation and approx. 80% core glycosylation efficiency at a final OD_{280} concentration of 3–10 in the translation reaction.

4. If large numbers of transcription reactions are to be performed, it is more economical to use purified His-tagged SP6 RNA polymerase expressed in *Escherichia coli* BL21(DE3) than commercial SP6 RNA polymerase. Details for expression and purification of His-tagged proteins have been described previously (3).
5. We did not observe marked differences in translation efficiencies from lysates prepared from cells of different levels of confluency. However, we recommend using cells of similar confluency (80–100%) in order to maintain lysate consistency.
6. Low-speed supernatant at this step contains endogenous microsomal membranes and can also be used for in vitro translation after nuclease treatment. Microsomal membranes in MEF-AA low-speed lysate efficiently facilitate signal peptide processing and translocation of nascent polypeptides (12). However, the CFBE low-speed lysate does not support ER processing as efficiently as canine pancreatic microsomal membranes. This is likely due to different amounts of ER membranes present in the final lysate.
7. Optimal condition for S7 nuclease treatment will depend on lysate concentration. Excess nuclease will digest not only endogenous mRNAs but also tRNA and ribosomal RNA and thereby decrease translation activity. Nuclease conditions described here were determined by monitoring background translation of endogenous mRNAs present in lysates, while maintaining translation activity of exogenous (added) mRNA.
8. Collagen and fibronectin coating of culture plates or use of permeable support systems will help cell polarization and tight junction formation and provide a more physiological differentiated state of airway epithelium. However, we have opted to use uncoated culture plates which reduces cost. It is not yet known whether these plate treatments affect translation efficiency and folding environment.
9. The $10,000 \times g$ spin removes some but not all of the endogenous ER membranes from lysates and decreases ER targeting and processing of secretory and membrane proteins. ER microsomes are therefore added to translation reaction as a source of ER membranes when needed.

Acknowledgments

We thank Dr. Vladimir V. Zeenko for advice in developing mammalian cell lysates and Zhongying Yang for construction and preparation of plasmids. This work was supported by National Institutes of Health grant DK51818 and the Cystic Fibrosis Foundation Therapeutics (W.R.S.) and the Manpei Suzuki Diabetes Foundation (Y.M.).

References

1. Skach, W. R. (2009) Cellular mechanisms of membrane protein folding. *Nat. Struct. Mol. Biol.* **16**, 606–612.
2. Oberdorf, J., and Skach, W. R. (2002) In vitro reconstitution of CFTR biogenesis and degradation. *Methods Mol. Med.* **70**, 295–310.
3. Carlson, E., Bays, N., David, L., and Skach, W. R. (2005) Reticulocyte lysate as a model system to study endoplasmic reticulum membrane protein degradation. *Methods Mol. Biol.* **301**, 185–205.
4. Kaufman, R. J. (2004) Regulation of mRNA translation by protein folding in the endoplasmic reticulum. *Trends Biochem. Sci.* **29**, 152–158.
5. Adamson, S. D., Herbert, E., and Godchaux, W. (1968) Factors affecting the rate of protein synthesis in lysate systems from reticulocytes. *Arch. Biochem. Biophys.* **125**, 671–683.
6. Zucker, W. V., and Schulman, H. M. (1968) Stimulation of globin-chain initiation by hemin in the reticulocyte cell-free system. *Proc. Natl. Acad. Sci. USA* **59**, 582–589.
7. Farrell, P. J., Balkow, K., Hunt, T., Jackson, R. J., and Trachsel, H. (1977) Phosphorylation of initiation factor elF-2 and the control of reticulocyte protein synthesis. *Cell* **11**, 187–200.
8. Frydman, J., Nimmesgern, E., Ohtsuka, K., and Hartl, F. U. (1994) Folding of nascent polypeptide chains in a high molecular mass assembly with molecular chaperones. *Nature* **370**, 111–117.
9. Dalman, F. C., Bresnick, E. H., Patel, P. D., Perdew, G. H., Watson, S. J., Jr., and Pratt, W. B. (1989) Direct evidence that the glucocorticoid receptor binds to hsp90 at or near the termination of receptor translation in vitro. *J. Biol. Chem.* **264**, 19815–19821.
10. Xiong, X., Chong, E., and Skach, W. R. (1999) Evidence that endoplasmic reticulum (ER)-associated degradation of cystic fibrosis transmembrane conductance regulator is linked to retrograde translocation from the ER membrane. *J. Biol. Chem.* **274**, 2616–2624.
11. Carroll, R., and Lucas-Lenard, J. (1993) Preparation of a cell-free translation system with minimal loss of initiation factor eIF-2/eIF-2B activity. *Anal. Biochem.* **212**, 17–23.
12. Zeenko, V. V., Wang, C., Majumder, M., Komar, A. A., Snider, M. D., Merrick, W. C., et al. (2008) An efficient in vitro translation system from mammalian cells lacking the translational inhibition caused by eIF2 phosphorylation. *RNA* **14**, 593–602.
13. Hartl, F. U., and Hayer-Hartl, M. (2009) Converging concepts of protein folding in vitro and in vivo. *Nat. Struct. Mol. Biol.* **16**, 574–581.
14. Balch, W. E., Morimoto, R. I., Dillin, A., and Kelly, J. W. (2008) Adapting proteostasis for disease intervention. *Science* **319**, 916–919.
15. Hutt, D. M., Powers, E. T., and Balch, W. E. (2009) The proteostasis boundary in misfolding diseases of membrane traffic. *FEBS Lett.* **583**, 2639–2646.
16. Jackson, R. J., and Hunt, T. (1983) Preparation and use of nuclease-treated rabbit reticulocyte lysates for the translation of eukaryotic messenger RNA. *Methods Enzymol.* **96**, 50–74.
17. Walter, P., and Blobel, G. (1983) Preparation of microsomal membranes for cotranslational protein translocation. *Methods Enzymol.* **96**, 84–93.
18. Michel, Y. M., Poncet, D., Piron, M., Kean, K. M., and Borman, A. M. (2000) Cap-poly(A) synergy in mammalian cell-free extracts. Investigation of the requirements for poly(A)-mediated stimulation of translation initiation. *J. Biol. Chem.* **275**, 32268–32276.
19. Melton, D. A., Krieg, P. A., Rebagliati, M. R., Maniatis, T., Zinn, K., and Green, M. R. (1984) Efficient in vitro synthesis of bio-

logically active RNA and RNA hybridization probes from plasmids containing a bacteriophage SP6 promoter. *Nucleic Acids Res.* **12**, 7035–7056.
20. Jagus, R. (1987) Translation in cell-free systems. *Methods Enzymol.* **152**, 267–276.
21. Xiong, X., Bragin, A., Widdicombe, J. H., Cohn, J., and Skach, W. R. (1997) Structural cues involved in endoplasmic reticulum degradation of G85E and G91R mutant cystic fibrosis transmembrane conductance regulator. *J. Clin. Invest.* **100**, 1079–1088.
22. Lu, Y., Xiong, X., Helm, A., Kimani, K., Bragin, A., and Skach, W. R. (1998) Co- and posttranslational translocation mechanisms direct cystic fibrosis transmembrane conductance regulator N terminus transmembrane assembly. *J. Biol. Chem.* **273**, 568–576.
23. Carveth, K., Buck, T., Anthony, V., and Skach, W. R. (2002) Cooperativity and flexibility of cystic fibrosis transmembrane conductance regulator transmembrane segments participate in membrane localization of a charged residue. *J. Biol. Chem.* **277**, 39507–39514.
24. Scheuner, D., Song, B., McEwen, E., Liu, C., Laybutt, R., Gillespie, P., et al. (2001) Translational control is required for the unfolded protein response and in vivo glucose homeostasis. *Mol. Cell* 7, 1165–1176.
25. Gruenert, D. C., Willems, M., Cassiman, J. J., and Frizzell, R. A. (2004) Established cell lines used in cystic fibrosis research. *J. Cyst. Fibros.* **3**, 191–196.
26. Jackson, R. J., Campbell, E. A., Herbert, P., and Hunt, T. (1983) The preparation and properties of gel-filtered rabbit-reticulocyte lysate protein-synthesis systems. *Eur. J. Biochem.* **131**, 289–301.
27. Kaderbhai, M. A., Harding, V. J., Karim, A., Austen, B. M., and Kaderbhai, N. N. (1995) Sheep pancreatic microsomes as an alternative to the dog source for studying protein translocation. *Biochem. J.* **306**, 57–61.

Chapter 17

Analysis of CFTR Interactome in the Macromolecular Complexes

Chunying Li and Anjaparavanda P. Naren

Abstract

Cystic fibrosis transmembrane conductance regulator (CFTR) is a chloride channel localized primarily at the apical surface of epithelial cells lining the airway, gut, exocrine glands, etc., where it is responsible for transepithelial salt and water transport. A growing number of proteins have been reported to interact directly or indirectly with CFTR chloride channel, suggesting that CFTR might regulate the activities of other ion channels, receptors, and transporters, in addition to its role as a chloride conductor. Most interactions occur primarily between the opposing terminal tails (N or C) of CFTR and its binding partners, either directly or mediated through various PDZ domain-containing proteins. This chapter describes methods we developed to cross-link CFTR into a macromolecular complex to identify and analyze the assembly and regulation of CFTR-containing complexes in the plasma membrane.

Key words: CFTR, cross-linking, macromolecular complex, PDZ protein, interacting partner.

1. Introduction

Cystic fibrosis transmembrane conductance regulator (CFTR) is a plasma membrane cAMP-regulated Cl^- channel that is responsible for transepithelial salt and fluid transport (1–3). It is localized primarily to the luminal, or apical, membranes of epithelial cells in functionally diverse tissues including the airway, intestine, pancreas, kidney, vas deferens, and sweat duct (1–3). CFTR has been implicated in two major diseases: cystic fibrosis (CF) and secretory diarrhea (4, 5). In CF, the synthesis or the functional activity of the CFTR Cl^- channel is reduced. This autosomal recessive disorder affects approximately 1 in 2,500 Caucasians in the

M.D. Amaral, K. Kunzelmann (eds.), *Cystic Fibrosis*, Methods in Molecular Biology 741,
DOI 10.1007/978-1-61779-117-8_17,

United States (4, 5). Excessive CFTR activity has also been implicated in cases of toxin-induced secretory diarrhea (e.g., by cholera toxin and heat-stable *Escherichia coli* enterotoxin) that stimulates cAMP or cGMP production in the gut (5, 6). CFTR belongs to the superfamily of ATP-binding cassette transporters, which bind ATP and use the energy to drive the transport of a wide variety of substrates across cellular membrane (7). It is composed of two repeated motifs, each of which consists of a hydrophobic membrane-spanning domain containing six helices and a cytosolic hydrophilic region for binding with ATP (8). These two motifs are linked by a cytoplasmic regulatory domain that contains many charged residues and multiple consensus phosphorylation sites (substrates for various protein kinases, such as PKA, PKC, and PKG). Both the amino- and carboxyl-terminal tails of this membrane protein are cytoplasmically oriented and mediate the interaction between CFTR and a growing number of binding proteins (5, 9).

1.1. CFTR Forms Macromolecular Signaling Complexes with a Wide Variety of Proteins

A growing body of evidence suggest the existence of various physical and functional interactions between CFTR and many other proteins, including transporters, ion channels, receptors, kinases, phosphatases, signaling molecules, and cytoskeletal elements, and these interactions between CFTR and its binding proteins have been shown to play an important role in regulating CFTR-mediated transepithelial ion transport in vitro and most probably in vivo (10–24). Among these reported interactions, many are mediated through a physical interaction between these binding proteins with both the amino-/carboxyl-terminal tails of the CFTR chloride channel (21–24). The amino-terminal tail interacts directly with syntaxin-1A and is responsible in part for inhibiting CFTR Cl^- current activity (19, 20). In this chapter, we focus on only the methods and approaches that aid in the study of the interactions between CFTR carboxyl-terminal tail, which possesses a protein-binding motif, and a group of scaffolding proteins, which contain a specific binding module referred to as PDZ domains.

PDZ domains are composed of 80–90 amino acid residues that form peptide-binding clefts and mediate interactions, usually with the carboxyl termini of target proteins, which terminate in consensus PDZ-binding sequences (also referred to as PDZ motif) (5, 25–27). So far, six different PDZ scaffolding proteins have been reported to bind to the carboxyl-terminal tail of the CFTR channel with various affinities: NHERF1, NHERF2, PDZK1, PDZK2, CAL (CFTR-associated ligand), and Shank2 (28–34). Among these PDZ proteins, four (NHERF1, NHERF2, PDZK1, and PDZK2) possess multiple PDZ domains, whereas CAL and Shank2 have only one PDZ domain (27). NHERF1, NHERF2, PDZK1, PDZK2, and Shank2 have been reported to be localized to the apical membranes of epithelial cells where CFTR also resides, while CAL is localized primarily to Golgi. These CFTR-interacting scaffold proteins demonstrate different tissue distributions, thereby suggesting that different PDZ proteins might interact with CFTR in different tissues (27). The PDZ motif within CFTR that is recognized by PDZ proteins is the last four amino acids at the C terminus (i.e., 1477-DTRL-1480 in human CFTR) (28–34). Interestingly, CFTR can bind to more than one PDZ domain of both NHERFs and PDZK1, albeit with varying affinities (30). This multivalency with respect to CFTR binding has been shown to be functionally significant, suggesting that PDZ proteins may facilitate the formation of CFTR macromolecular signaling complexes (21–24). Protein–protein interactions that influence the expression or the functional activity of the CFTR channel at the plasma membrane have significant physiological importance, as this channel not only transports Cl^- and HCO_3^- but also regulates the activities of many other transporters and channels (27). The physiological significance of these interactions is that they not only provide a means to link CFTR activity to various epithelial functions and processes but also coordinate the CFTR chloride channel function with the overall physiologic demands of epithelial cells (5, 27).

1.2. Biochemical Assays Used to Analyze CFTR Interactome for Novel CFTR-Interacting Partners

Multiple biochemical assays have been developed to study CFTR-involving protein interactions, such as co-immunoprecipitation, pull-down assay, pair-wise binding assay, colorimetric pair-wise binding assay, and macromolecular complex assembly assay (19–24, 35, 36). Here we focus on the detailed procedures of analyzing and identifying the interacting partners in cross-linked CFTR-containing complex (36), which is used extensively by the Naren laboratory to study protein–protein or domain–domain interactions involving CFTR.

2. Materials

2.1. General Reagents

1. pGEX4T-1 vector (Amersham Pharmacia Biotech, Piscataway, NJ).
2. pMAL-C2 vector (New England BioLabs, Ipswich, MA).
3. pET30 vector (Novagen, Gibbstown, NJ).
4. pcDNA3 (Invitrogen, Carlsbad, CA).
5. Glutathione Sepharose beads (Amersham).
6. Amylose resin (New England BioLabs, Ipswich, MA).

7. Talon beads (Clontech, Mountain View, CA).
8. Restriction enzymes (Promega, Madison, WI).
9. PCR reagents (Stratagene, La Jolla, CA).
10. Oligonucleotide primers (Genemed Synthesis, San Antonio, TX).
11. ECL reagents (GE Health Care, Piscataway, NJ)

All other reagents were purchased from Sigma (St. Louis, MO) unless otherwise stated.

2.2. Media and Buffers

1. Luria-Bertani containing ampicillin (LB-Amp) or kanamycin (LB-Kan) medium (pH 7.0): 10 g bactotryptone, 5 g Bacto yeast extract, and 10 g NaCl per liter. Autoclave, cool, and add filter-sterilized ampicillin (50 μg/ml) or kanamycin (30 μg/ml).
2. Sucrose buffer: 50 mM Tris–HCl (pH 8.0), 1 mM EDTA, 1 mM PMSF, and 10% sucrose.
3. Elution buffer for GST fusion proteins: 25 mM Tris–HCl (pH 8.0), 140 mM NaCl, and 20 mM reduced glutathione.
4. Elution buffer for His fusion proteins: 20 mM Tris–HCl (pH 8.0), 500 mM NaCl, and 200 mM imidazole.
5. Elution buffer for MBP fusion proteins: 20 mM Tris–HCl (pH 8.0), 200 mM NaCl, 1 mM EDTA, 1 mM DTT, and 10 mM maltose.
6. Phosphate-buffered saline (PBS) (pH 7.4): 140 mM Na_2HPO_4, 1.5 mM KH_2PO_4, 2.7 mM KCl, and 140 mM NaCl.
7. PBS-C/M: PBS (pH 7.4), supplemented with 1 mM $MgCl_2$ and 0.1 mM $CaCl_2$.
8. Lysis buffer: PBS (pH 7.4)–0.2% Triton X-100 containing protease inhibitors (1 mM PMSF, 1 μg/μl leupeptin, 1 μg/μl aprotinin, and 1 μg/μl pepstatin).
9. RIPA buffer: 150 mM NaCl, 50 mM Tris–base (pH 8.0), 1% NP-40, 0.5% Na deoxycholate, and 0.1% SDS.
10. Sample buffer (5×): 0.6 M Tris–HCl (pH 6.8), 50% glycerol, 2% sodium dodecyl sulfate (SDS), and 0.1% bromophenol blue; add 5% β-mercaptoethanol (βME) before use.
11. Buffer A: 20 mM HEPES, pH 7.4, 1 mM EDTA, 250 mM sucrose, 1 mM DTT, and protease inhibitors.
12. Buffer B: 20 mM HEPES, pH 7.4, 1 mM EDTA, and protease inhibitors.

2.3. Cell Culture

1. All cell culture media and reagents are from Invitrogen (Carlsbad, CA) unless otherwise specified.

2. All cell lines except BHK cells are from American Type Culture Collection (Manassas, VA). BHK-parental, BHK-CFTR, and BHK-CFTR$_{his10}$ are from Dr. John Hanrahan (McGill University, Canada).
3. HEK293 (human embryonic kidney 293) cells, COS-7 cells (African green monkey kidney cells), and HT29-CL19A cells (human colonic epithelial origin) are grown in Dulbecco's modified Eagle's medium (DMEM) supplemented with 10% fetal bovine serum (FBS).
4. Calu-3 cells (serous gland epithelial cells) are grown in Eagle's minimal essential medium (MEM) supplemented with 15% FBS, 1 mM sodium pyruvate, and 1 mM nonessential amino acids.
5. T84 cells (human colonic epithelial origin), BHK (baby hamster kidney) cells stably expressing CFTR (BHK-CFTR), and C-terminal polyhistidine-tagged CFTR (BHK-CFTR$_{his10}$) are grown in DMEM and Ham's F-12 supplemented with 15 mM HEPES and 10% FBS.

Table 17.1
Various cross-linkers used to cross-link CFTR with its interacting partners

Cross-linkers	Acronym	MW	Spacer arm (Å)	Membrane permeable	Cleavable (by)	Soluble (in)
1, 5-Difluoro 2, 4-dinitrobenzene	DFDNB	204.1	3.0	Yes	No	DMSO
Disuccinimidyl tartrate	DST	344.24	6.4	Yes	Yes (periodate)	DMSO
Dimethyl pimelimidate·2 HCl	DMP	259.18	9.2	No	No	H_2O
Dimethyl-3,3′-dithiobispropionimidate·2 HCl	DTBP	309.28	11.9	No	Yes (thiols)	H_2O
Dithiobis (succinimidyl propionate)	DSP	404.42	12.0	Yes	Yes (thiols)	DMSO
3,3′-Dithiobis (sulfosuccinimidyl propionate)	DTSSP	608.51	12.0	No	Yes (thiols)	H_2O
Ethylene glycol bis (succinimidyl succinate)	EGS	456.37	16.1	Yes	Yes (hydroxylamine)	DMSO
Bis-[b-(4-azidosalicylamido) ethyl] disulfide	BASED	474.52	21.3	Yes	Yes (thiols)	DMSO
Disuccinimidyl suberate	DSS	368.35	11.4	Yes	No	DMSO

2.4. Antibodies, Constructs, and Uncommon Reagents

1. CFTR monoclonal antibodies R1104 mab recognizing the regulatory domain of CFTR (epitope at a.a. 722–734), GA1 mab (a.a. 1440–1460), and NBD1-R (a.a. 521–828) polyclonal antibody are custom-made (35, 36). Anti-CFTR IgG MM13-4 (a.a. 25–36) is from Millipore (Temecula, CA).
2. Anti-NHERF1 IgG is from BD-Transduction Laboratories (Lexington, KY).
3. Affinity-purified anti-syntaxin-1A IgG (14D8) is custom-made (19, 20).
4. Affinity-purified rabbit anti-G_{β} IgG is from Santa Cruz Biotechnology (Santa Cruz, CA).
5. Anti-NHERF2 antibody is from Dr. Emanuel Strehler (Mayo Clinic, Rochester, MN).
6. Sulfo-NHS-LC-biotin and various cross-linkers are from Pierce Biotechnology (Rockford, IL).
7. Cross-linkers used in the present chapter are listed in **Table 17.1**.

3. Methods

3.1. Expression and Purification of Recombinant Tagged Fusion Proteins in Bacteria

1. Amplify defined regions of CFTR-C tail (a.a. 1454–1480 or a.a. 1400–1480) and NHERFs (full-length or PDZ1 or PDZ2 domains) by PCR (containing appropriate restriction enzyme sites). Clone the PCR products into pGEX4T-1 vector (Pharmacia) for GST–NHERFs (or their PDZ1 or PDZ2 domains), pMAL-C2 vector (New England BioLabs) for MBP–CFTR-C tail or MBP–LPA2-C tail, and pET30 (Novagen) for His-S-CFTR-C tail.
2. Transform in a protease-deficient *E. coli* strain (BL21-DE3) as protein integrity is often an issue.
3. Grow the culture overnight (37°C) in LB with appropriate antibiotics (Amp or Kan). Dilute the overnight culture 1:10 and grow for further 2 h at 37°C. Induce with 0.5–1 mM IPTG for the next 4 h at 30°C. Pellet the cells by centrifugation at 8,000×*g* for 10 min at 4°C.
4. Lyse the cells in sucrose buffer (20 ml for cell pellet originating from 1 l of culture) containing lysozyme (1 mg/ml), 0.2% Triton X-100, and protease inhibitors (*see* **Section 2.2**). Mix on a rotary shaker for 30 min at 4°C.
5. Spin at 20,000×*g* for 30 min at 4°C. Collect the clear supernatant.
6. Into the clear supernatant, add 1 ml of the following resin/agarose beads (50% slurry in sucrose buffer):

- Glutathione Sepharose beads for GST fusion proteins.
- Talon beads for His-S fusion proteins.
- Amylose resin for MBP fusion proteins.

7. Mix for 4 h at 4°C on a rotary shaker.
8. Wash the beads by resuspending in PBS (15 ml), mix for 2 min, spin (800×*g* for 2 min), and decant. Repeat this step for six times.
9. Elute the protein from the beads by using respective elution buffer (2 ml elution buffer per 1 ml of beads; *see* **Sections 2.2, steps 3, 4,** and **5**; also *see* **Note 1**).
10. Dialyze the eluted proteins against 2 L of PBS. Change PBS every 4 h for four times. Concentrate the protein using a Centricon filter (10,000 MW cut-off; Millipore) and store as small aliquots at –80°C.
11. Determine the protein concentration by the Bradford method. Assess protein quality by SDS-PAGE using BSA as standard. If the integrity of the protein is not satisfactory, secondary purification procedures such as gel filtration or ion exchange may be used (e.g., we have used a G-75 Sepharose column to further purify GST fusion protein).

3.2. Preparation of Cross-linker Working Solutions

1. Always use freshly made cross-linkers to cross-link CFTR and its interacting partners.
2. Prepare the cross-linkers (*see* **Table 17.1**) on the day of the experiment.
3. Stocks are freshly prepared in DMSO for membrane-permeable cross-linkers (i.e., DSP and DFDNB) and in PBS-C/M (*see* **Section 2.2, step** 7) for membrane-impermeable cross-linkers (i.e., DMP and DTBP), respectively.
4. For example, to make 1 mM DSP solution, weigh 4.0 mg DSP into a 15-ml tube and add 200 μl of DMSO (dissolve completely). To this add 9.8 ml of warm PBS-C/M. Incubate at 37°C in dark until use.

3.3. Chemical Cross-linking of CFTR and Its Interacting Partners

1. Culture cells in 60- or 100-mm Petri dishes until the cells become confluent.
2. Wash cells for ~2 min with PBS-C/M (pH 7.4) at 22°C (alternatively, one could use membrane/vesicular preparation lacking Tris or amino group containing buffers). Repeat two more times.
3. Make cross-linker solution in PBS-C/M and incubate the solution at 37°C (prepare fresh each time, just before the incubation).

4. Incubate cells with cross-linker solution for varying times at 37°C (we typically incubate cells with cross-linkers for 10 min).
5. Treat control cells with prewarmed PBS-C/M (containing no cross-linkers).
6. Rinse cells with 10 ml of chilled TBS (Tris–base saline) for 1 min (this step is optional as RIPA has Tris, which acts as a quencher for cross-linking reaction – *see* **Note 2**).
7. Remove the buffer completely from the plate and add 1–2 ml of RIPA buffer (*see* **Section 2.2**, **step 9**) to each plate.
8. Scrape cells off the plate and transfer into a microcentrifuge tube (1.5 ml) and mix (10 min at 4°C).
9. Centrifuge at 14,000×*g* at 4°C for 10 min.
10. Take clear supernatant (immunoprecipitate if necessary).
11. Make two sets of samples, one with sample buffer (no βME) and the other with 5% βME. Incubate samples at 37°C for 10–15 min (*see* **Note 3**).
12. Run 4–15% or 5% (depending on the protein mass) SDS-PAGE.
13. Western blot with anti-CFTR antibody (or look for CFTR-interacting partners using specific antibodies; *see* **Section 3.4**).
14. Representative data are shown in **Fig. 17.1** (also *see* (36)).

3.4. CFTR:NHERF Stoichiometry in Apical Plasma Membrane

1. Culture and polarize epithelial cells (Calu-3 or HT29-CL19A) on permeable support (24-mm-diameter Transwell in six-well plates) until they form tight junction (usually takes 10–15 days).

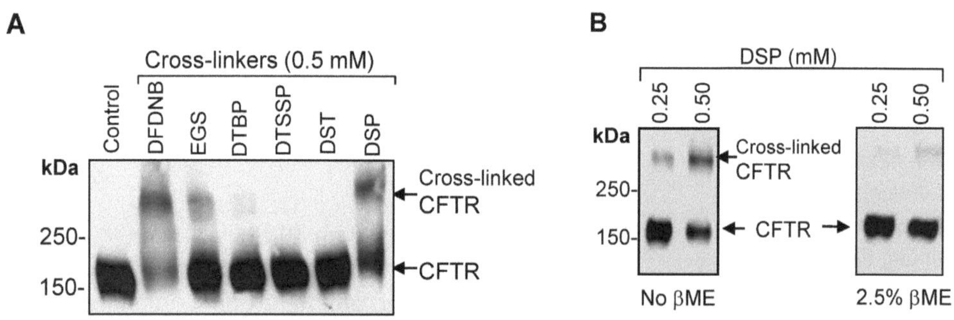

Fig. 17.1. CFTR exists as a higher order complex in plasma membrane through cross-linking. (**a**) Calu-3 cells were cross-linked as described in the text. The cells were lysed in RIPA buffer and blotted for CFTR (R1104). (**b**) Calu-3 cells cross-linked with DSP were lysed in RIPA buffer, then 50 μg of total proteins were solubilized with sample buffer in the absence (*left*) or the presence (*right*) of 2.5% β-mercaptoethanol (βME) before immunoblotting for CFTR (R1104). (Reproduced from (36) with permission from American Society for Biochemistry and Molecular Biology.)

2. Wash cells twice with prewarmed PBS-C/M.
3. Transfer the Transwell to new, clean six-well plates and wash cells once with prewarmed PBS-C/M.
4. Cross-link cells at both sides (apical/basolateral) with 1 mM prewarmed DSP (dissolved in DMSO and made fresh in prewarmed PBS-C/M) for 10 min at 37°C.
5. Wash cells twice with chilled PBS-C/M on ice.
6. Surface biotinylate the cells only at the apical surface with 0.5 mg/ml sulfo-NHS-LC-biotin (water soluble and made fresh in PBS-C/M), 500 μl for each Transwell (3 ml for six Transwell inserts). Keep the plate on ice, wrap with aluminum foil, and incubate at 4°C for 60 min.
7. Stop the reaction by adding 1–2 ml chilled TBS to the apical surface of cells.
8. Scrape off the cells from the Transwell very carefully with buffer A (*see* **Section 2.2, step 11**), total volume less than 10 ml for six Transwell inserts; pool cells into clean 15-ml BD Falcon tube.
9. Spin the cell suspension in the centrifuge at 800×*g* for 5 min at 4°C.
10. Discard the supernatant and transfer the cell pellet into homogenizer (7 ml capacity) with buffer B (*see* **Section 2.2, step 12**). Keep the total volume to less than 5 ml. Homogenize the cells twice for 20 strokes on ice.
11. Spin the cell homogenate at 800×*g* for 5 min at 4°C. Collect the supernatant (postnuclear supernatant, PNS) and resuspend PNS with buffer B to make total volume of 6 ml.
12. Overlay the above-made 6 ml PNS over 6 ml of 1.16 M sucrose cushion in buffer B. Balance and spin at 100,000×*g* for 1 h at 4°C using SW41 rotor (Beckman).
13. Collect the broad band at the homogenate and sucrose cushion interface (plasma membrane, about 1–2 ml) into a clean 1.5- or 2.0-ml microcentrifuge tube (try to keep less than 1.5 ml). Add 100 μl streptavidin agarose beads and mix at 4°C for 45–60 min (*see* **Note 4**).
14. Spin at 1,200×*g* for 1 min.
15. Wash the beads twice with buffer A.
16. Elute the protein with 500 μl RIPA buffer containing 2 mM regular biotin [D(+)-biotin, ACROS, made as 2.4 mg/5 ml in RIPA buffer] plus protease inhibitors, and mix at 4°C for 5 min. Spin at 1,200×*g* for 1 min and collect the supernatant. Repeat the elution step and pool the supernatant.

17. Into the supernatant add anti-NBD1-R IgG cross-linked with protein A/G beads (*see* **Note 5**). Mix at 4°C overnight.
18. Spin down the beads at 1,200×*g* for 1 min and collect the supernatant (to check the unbound CFTR and its interacting partners later, if necessary).
19. Wash the beads extensively three times with buffer A (*see* **Note 6**).
20. Elute the co-immunoprecipitated proteins from beads with 15 μl sample buffer (+2.5% βME).
21. Resolve the eluted proteins on 10% SDS-PAGE (*see* **Note 7**).
22. On the same gel, load a wide range of known amounts of purified $CFTR_{his10}$ as a standard to quantitate CFTR, purified GST–NHERF1–PDZ2 as a standard to quantitate the co-immunoprecipitated NHERF1, and purified GST–NHERF2 as a standard to quantitate the co-immunoprecipitated NHERF2.
23. Western blot using anti-CFTR (*see* **Note 8**) and anti-NHERF1 or anti-NHERF2 antibodies. Representative data are shown in **Fig. 17.2** (also *see* (36)).
24. To analyze and identify other CFTR-interacting partners that are co-precipitated with CFTR, two-dimensional gel electrophoresis can be performed to confirm the known co-immunoprecipitated proteins (*see* **Note 9**), or mass spectroscopy analysis can also be performed to identify unknown binding partners (*see* **Note 10**).

3.5. In Vitro CFTR-Containing Macromolecular Complex Assembly (CFTR–NHERF2–LPA_2 Complex)

1. Into 200 μl of lysis buffer (PBS–0.2% Triton X-100 + protease inhibitors), add MBP–CFTR-C tail (a.a. 1454–1480) fusion protein (1 μM) immobilized on amylose beads (20 μl) (*see* **Note 11**).
2. Add various amounts of purified GST–NHERF2 fusion protein and mix at 22°C for 2 h.
3. During this time, prepare the cell lysates. Lyse the HEK293 parental cells transiently transfected with Flag- LPA_2 via Lipofectamine 2000 (five 60-mm dishes were used); use 500 μl lysis buffer for each dish (*see* **Note 12**).
4. Wash the complex once with lysis buffer.
5. Add the above-prepared cell lysates to the beads and gently mix at 4°C for 3 h or overnight.
6. Wash the beads three times with lysis buffer.
7. Elute the proteins using sample buffer (+ βME).
8. Incubate in 37°C water bath for 10–15 min and spin at 5,000×*g* for 30 s to precipitate the beads.

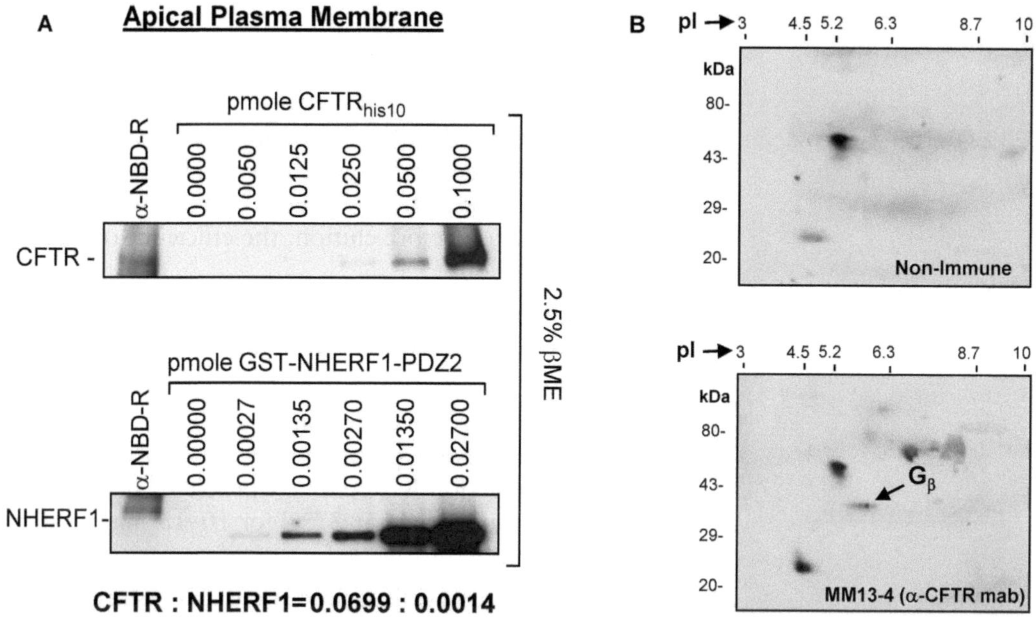

Fig. 17.2. Stoichiometry of CFTR:NHERF1 in the complex. (**a**) Polarized Calu-3 cells were cross-linked with 1 mM DSP and then apically biotinylated with sulfo-NHS-LC-biotin. The plasma membrane was isolated, and the apical plasma membrane was captured using streptavidin agarose beads and then subjected to co-immunoprecipitation using anti-NBD-R IgG. The immunoprecipitated complex was treated with 2.5% βME to dissociate the cross-linked complex and dissolved on 10% SDS-PAGE. Purified $CFTR_{his10}$ was used as a standard to quantitate CFTR (*upper panel*), and GST–PDZ2 of NHERF1 was used as a standard to quantitate the co-immunoprecipitated NHERF1 (*bottom panel*). (**b**) Calu-3 cells were cross-linked with 1 mM DSP, lysed in RIPA buffer, and subjected to co-immunoprecipitation using mouse anti-CFTR antibody (MM13-4; *bottom panel*) or normal mouse IgG (*upper panel*). The samples were eluted and subjected to 2D gel electrophoresis (Bio-Rad). IEF (p*I* 3–10) was performed in the first dimension, and SDS-PAGE was performed in a 10% polyacrylamide gel in the second dimension and blotted with affinity-purified rabbit G_β IgG. (Reproduced from (36) with permission from American Society for Biochemistry and Molecular Biology.)

9. Load as much eluate as possible onto 4–15% gel.
10. Western blot with anti-Flag mouse antibody.
11. Representative data are shown in **Fig. 17.3** (also *see* (22)).

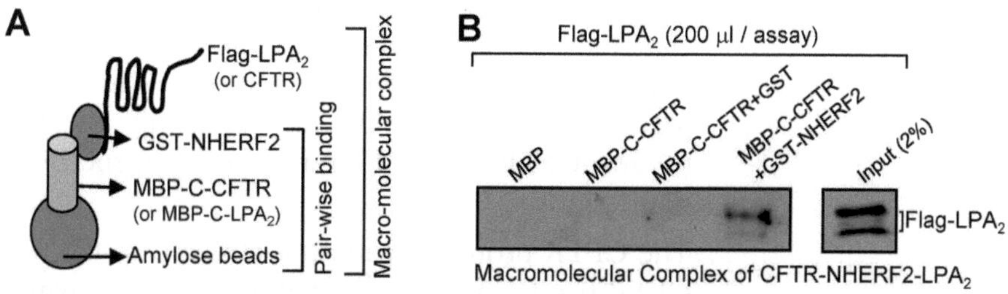

Fig. 17.3. LPA_2 forms a macromolecular complex with CFTR mediated through NHERF2. (**a**) A pictorial representation of the macromolecular complex assay. (**b**) A macromolecular complex of MBP–CFTR-C, GST–NHERF2, and Flag-tagged LPA_2 that is assembled in vitro. (Reproduced from (22) with permission from Rockefeller University Press.)

4. Notes

1. It is important that the pH of the elution buffer be adjusted to 8.0 after adding reduced glutathione. The pH can be as low as 3.0 after the addition of reduced glutathione. If the pH is not adjusted before elution, the efficiency of elution will drastically reduce.
2. If using membrane preparation, one could directly add Tris–glycine to a final concentration of 100 mM to quench the reaction.
3. It is strongly recommended not to boil the CFTR-containing complex samples prepared for Western blotting as CFTR aggregation is a common problem. Instead, the samples should be heated at 37°C for 10–15 min prior to loading the gel.
4. To make fresh streptavidin agarose beads (50% slurry), gently tap the stock beads in the bottle (ImmunoPure® immobilized streptavidin; Pierce); take 200 μl and mark the volume on the tube wall; and spin, discard the supernatant, and wash twice with PBS. Then add PBS to the marked volume level (50% slurry) to working concentration.
5. Cross-link anti-CFTR IgG to protein A/G agarose beads. Incubate CFTR monoclonal or polyclonal antibodies (1.0 μg) with 20 μl of protein A/G agarose beads (Santa Cruz Biotech, Santa Cruz, CA) on ice for at least 1 h and gently tap the mixture every 10 min. Wash the beads bound with IgG twice with 1 ml of 0.1 M *N*-ethyl morpholine (NEM; pH 7.5) buffer. Cross-link anti-CFTR IgG to protein A/G beads using 10 mM dimethyl pimelimidate (DMP; Pierce) in 0.5 ml NEM buffer and mix at 22°C for 30 min. Stop the cross-linking reaction by washing the beads with 1 ml of 100 mM Tris–base (pH 8.0) or TBS buffer. Then the anti-CFTR IgG cross-linked to the protein A/G agarose beads is ready for the subsequent co-immunoprecipitation procedure.
6. When co-immunoprecipitating cross-linked CFTR-containing complex, the use of 0.5 M urea in the wash buffer facilitates the complete removal of non-cross-linked partners, without significantly affecting CFTR binding to anti-CFTR IgG. This reduces non-specific binding significantly.
7. The CFTR protein is run on a 10% gel so that the mature CFTR band can be detected as a sharp band, which can be quantitated by densitometry.

8. If immunoblotting for CFTR, anti-CFTR IgG from a different host origin must be used; use a monoclonal antibody (if polyclonal CFTR antibody is cross-linked on the beads) or a polyclonal antibody (if monoclonal CFTR antibody is cross-linked on the beads) raised against CFTR. Heavy- or light-chain contamination is thereby minimized using this method of coupling.
9. Two-dimensional gel electrophoresis can be performed to confirm the known co-immunoprecipitated proteins according to manufacturer's instruction (such as Bio-Rad). In brief, cross-link Calu-3 or HT29-CL19A epithelial cells with 1 mM DSP as described in **Section 3.3** and then lyse the cells with RIPA buffer. Immunoprecipitate CFTR with mouse anti-CFTR antibody (MM13-4) or normal mouse IgG immobilized on protein A/G agarose beads (Santa Cruz) through constant mixing at 4°C overnight. Rehydrate 7-cm IPG strips with 2D Protein MW Marker Mix (Pierce) or 150 μl CFTR proteins extracted with sequential extraction reagent II (8 M urea, 4% CHAPS, 40 mM Tris, 0.2% Bio-Lyte 3/10) supplemented with 2 mM TBP at 20°C for 12–16 h. Perform isoelectric focusing (IEF) at 20°C in an IEF tray by using the following program: 250 V for 15 min, linear ramp, S3 = 4,000 V until 20,000 vhs is reached. Equilibrate the strips for 10 min in a solution containing 6 M urea, 3% SDS, 375 mM Tris–HCl (pH 8.6), 30% (v/v) glycerol, and 2% (w/v) DTT. Perform a second equilibration step for another 10 min in the same solution containing 3% (w/v) iodoacetamide instead of DTT. Separate the proteins in the strip in a 10% polyacrylamide gel and immunoblot with specific affinity-purified antibodies (such as anti-G_β IgG or anti-syntaxin-1A IgG). Stain molecular marker gel with GelCode Blue Stain Reagent (Pierce) and acquire and analyze the images with Quantity One (Bio-Rad).
10. Mass spectrometry analysis can also be performed to identify unknown binding partners. In brief, cross-link the cells (HEK293 stably overexpressing Flag-CFTR; or Calu-3 or HT29-CL19A cells expressing endogenous CFTR). Purify Flag-CFTR from HEK293 cells by using anti-Flag M2 affinity gel (EZview Red ANTI-FLAG M2; Sigma), or co-immunoprecipitate CFTR from Calu-3 (or HT29-CL19A) cells. Run SDS-PAGE and stain the gel with Coomassie blue. Send the respective bands for mass spectrometry analysis to identify the interacting proteins. Using this approach, we identified several scaffolding proteins HSP70 and HSP90 as interacting partners, which are co-immunoprecipitated with CFTR.

11. Alternatively, purified His-S-CFTR-C tail (a.a. 1400–1480) fusion protein can also be used. Briefly, add 50 μl of S-protein agarose (Novagen) into 200 μl of lysis buffer (PBS–0.2% Triton X-100 + protease inhibitors). Add 50 μg of His-S-CFTR-C tail and mix at 22°C for 1 h. Spin at 1,200×*g* and wash three times with lysis buffer.
12. Alternatively, use purified Flag-LPA_2 at this step instead of the cell lysates, which also contain other components.

Acknowledgments

We thank Dr David Armbruster for critically reading the manuscript and Ms. Feng Zhou for formatting the references. This work was supported by National Institute of Diabetes and Digestive and Kidney Diseases grants DK058545 and DK074996 (to A.P.N.), and American Heart Association (Midwest Affiliate) Beginning-grant-in-aid #0765185B (to C.L.).

References

1. Quinton, P. M. (1983) Chloride impermeability in cystic fibrosis. *Nature* **301**, 421–422.
2. Anderson, M. P., Gregory, R. J., Thompson, S., Souza, D. W., Paul, S., Mulligan, R. C., et al. (1991) Demonstration that CFTR is a chloride channel by alteration of its anion selectivity. *Science* **253**, 202–205.
3. Bear, C. E., Li, C. H., Kartner, N., Bridges, R. J., Jensen, T. J., Ramjeesingh, M., et al. (1992) Purification and functional reconstitution of the cystic fibrosis transmembrane conductance regulator (CFTR). *Cell* **68**, 809–818.
4. Welsh, M. J., Tsui, L. -C., Boat, T. F., and Beaudet, A. L. (1995) Cystic fibrosis, in (Scriver, C., Beaudet, A. L., Sly, W. S., Valle, D. (eds)) *The Metabolic and Molecular Basis of Inherited Diseases: Membrane Transport Systems.* McGraw-Hill, New York, NY, pp. 3799–3876.
5. Li, C., and Naren, A. P. (2005) Macromolecular complexes of cystic fibrosis transmembrane conductance regulator and its interacting partners. *Pharmacol. Ther.* **108**, 208–223.
6. Chao, A. C., de Sauvage, F. J., Dong, Y. J., Wagner, J. A., Goeddel, D. V., and Gardner, P. (1994) Activation of intestinal CFTR Cl- channel by heat-stable enterotoxin and guanylin via cAMP-dependent protein kinase. *EMBO J.* **13**, 1065–1072.
7. Dean, M., Rzhetsky, A., and Allikmets, R. (2001) The human ATP-binding cassette (ABC) transporter superfamily. *Genome Res.* **11**, 1156–1166.
8. Riordan, J. R., Rommens, J. M., Kerem, B., Alon, N., Rozmahel, R., Grzelczak, Z., et al. (1989) Identification of the cystic fibrosis gene: cloning and characterization of complementary DNA. *Science* **245**, 1066–1073.
9. Guggino, W. B., and Stanton, B. A. (2006) New insights into cystic fibrosis: molecular switches that regulate CFTR. *Nat. Rev. Mol. Cell Biol.* 7, 426–436.
10. Knowles, M. R., Stutts, M. J., Spock, A., Fischer, N., Gatzy, J. T., and Boucher, R. C. (1983) Abnormal ion permeation through cystic fibrosis respiratory epithelium. *Science* **221**, 1067–1070.
11. Gabriel, S. E., Clarke, L. L., Boucher, R. C., and Stutts, M. J. (1993) CFTR and outwardly rectifying chloride channels are distinct proteins with a regulatory relationship. *Nature* **363**, 263–268.
12. McNicholas, C. M., Guggino, W. B., Schwiebert, E. M., Hebert, S. C., Giebisch, G., and Egan, M. E. (1996) Sensitivity

of a renal K^+ channel (Romk2) to the inhibitory sulfonylurea compound glibenclamide is enhanced by coexpression with the ATP-binding cassette transporter cystic fibrosis transmembrane regulator. *Proc. Natl. Acad. Sci. USA* **93**, 8083–8088.
13. Kunzelmann, K., Mall, M., Briel, M., Hipper, A., Nitschke, R., Ricken, S., et al. (1997) The cystic fibrosis transmembrane conductance regulator attenuates the endogenous $Ca2^+$ activated Cl^- conductance of *Xenopus* oocytes. *Pflugers Arch.* **435**, 178–181.
14. Schreiber, R., Nitschke, R., Greger, R., and Kunzelmann, K. (1999) The cystic fibrosis transmembrane conductance regulator activates aquaporin 3 in airway epithelial cells. *J. Biol. Chem.* **274**, 11811–11816.
15. Lee, M. G., Wigley, W. C., Zeng, W., Noel, L. E., Marino, C. R., Thomas, P. J., et al. (1999) Regulation of Cl^-/ $HCO3^-$ exchange by cystic fibrosis transmembrane conductance regulator expressed in NIH 3T3 and HEK 293 cells. *J. Biol. Chem.* **274**, 3414–3421.
16. Shumaker, H., Amlal, H., Frizzell, R., Ulrich, C. D., and Soleimani, M. (1999) CFTR drives Na^+-nHCO(3)(−) cotransport in pancreatic duct cells: a basis for defective $HCO3^-$ secretion in CF. *Am. J. Physiol. Cell Physiol.* **276**, C16–C25.
17. Ahn, W., Kim, K. H., Lee, J. A., Kim, J. Y., Choi, J. Y., Moe, O. W., et al. (2001) Regulatory interaction between the cystic fibrosis transmembrane conductance regulator and $HCO3^-$ salvage mechanisms in model systems and the mouse pancreatic duct. *J. Biol. Chem.* **276**, 17236–17243.
18. Sugita, M., Yue, Y., and Foskett, J. K. (1998) CFTR Cl^- channel and CFTR-associated ATP channel: distinct pores regulated by common gates. *EMBO J.* **17**, 898–908.
19. Naren, A. P., Nelson, D. J., Xie, W., Jovov, B., Tousson, A., Pevsner, J., et al. (1997) Regulation of CFTR chloride channels by syntaxin and Munc 18 isoforms. *Nature* **390**, 302–305.
20. Naren, A. P., Anke, D., Cormet-Boyaka, E., Boyaka, P. N., McGhee, J. R., Zhou, W., et al.(1999) Syntaxin 1A is expressed in airway epithelial cells where it modulates CFTR Cl^- currents. *J. Clin. Invest.* **105**, 377–386.
21. Naren, A. P., Cobb, B., Li, C., Roy, K., Nelson, D., Heda, G. D., et al. (2003) A macromolecular complex of beta 2 adrenergic receptor, CFTR, and ezrin/radixin/moesin-binding phosphoprotein 50 is regulated by PKA. *Proc. Natl. Acad. Sci. USA* **100**, 342–346.
22. Li, C., Dandridge, K. S., Di, A., Marrs, K. L., Harris, E. L., Roy, K., et al. (2005) Lysophosphatidic acid inhibits cholera toxin-induced secretory diarrhea through CFTR-dependent protein interactions. *J. Exp. Med.* **202**, 975–986.
23. Li, C., Krishnamurthy, P. C., Penmatsa, H., Marrs, K. L., Wang, X. Q., Zaccolo, M. J., et al. (2007) Spatiotemporal coupling of cAMP transporter to CFTR chloride channel function in the gut epithelia. *Cell* **131**, 940–951.
24. Li, C., Schuetz, J. D., and Naren, A. P. (2010) Tobacco carcinogen NNK Transporter MRP2 Regulates CFTR Function in lung epithelia: implications for lung cancer. *Cancer Lett.* **292**, 246–253.
25. Fanning, A. S. and Anderson, J. M. (1999) Protein modules as organizers of membrane structure. *Curr. Opin. Cell Biol.* **11**, 432–439.
26. Harris, B. Z. and Lim, W. A. (2001) Mechanism and role of PDZ domains in signaling complex assembly. *J. Cell Sci.* **114**, 3219–3231.
27. Li, C. and Naren, A. P. (2010) CFTR chloride channel in the apical compartments: spatiotemporal coupling to its interacting partners. *Integr. Biol.* **2**, 161–177.
28. Hall, R. A., Ostedgaard, L. S., Premont, R. T., Blitzer, J. T., Rahman, N., Welsh, M. J., et al. (1998) A C-terminal motif found in the beta2-adrenergic receptor, P2Y1 receptor and cystic fibrosis transmembrane conductance regulator determines binding to the Na^+/H^+ exchanger regulatory factor family of PDZ proteins. *Proc. Natl. Acad. Sci. USA* **95**, 8496–8501.
29. Short, D. B., Trotter, K. W., Reczek, D., Kreda, S. M., Bretscher, A., Boucher, R. C., et al. (1998) An apical PDZ protein anchors the cystic fibrosis transmembrane conductance regulator to the cytoskeleton. *J. Biol. Chem.* **273**, 19797–19801.
30. Wang, S., Yue, H., Derin, R. B., Guggino, W. B., and Li, M. (2000) Accessory protein facilitated CFTR-CFTR interaction, a molecular mechanism to potentiate the chloride channel activity. *Cell* **103**, 169–179.
31. Sun, F., Hug, M. J., Lewarchik, C. M., Yun, C. H., Bradbury, N. A., and Frizzell, R. A. (2000) E3KARP mediates the association of ezrin and protein kinase A with the cystic fibrosis transmembrane conductance regulator in airway cells. *J. Biol. Chem.* **275**, 29539–29546.
32. Cheng, J., Moyer, B. D., Milewski, M., Loffing, J., Ikeda, M., Mickle, J. E., et al. (2002) A Golgi-associated PDZ domain pro-

tein modulates cystic fibrosis transmembrane regulator plasma membrane expression. *J. Biol. Chem.* **277**, 3520–3529.

33. Scott, R. O., Thelin, W. R., and Milgram, S. L. (2002) A novel PDZ protein regulates the activity of guanylyl cyclase C, the heat-stable enterotoxin receptor. *J. Biol. Chem.* **277**, 22934–22941.
34. Lee, J. H., Richter, W., Namkung, W., Kim, K. H., Kim, E., Conti, M., et al. (2007) Dynamic regulation of cystic fibrosis transmembrane conductance regulator by competitive interactions of molecular adaptors. *J. Biol. Chem.* **282**, 10414–10422.
35. Naren, A. P. (2002) Methods for the study of intermolecular and intramolecular interactions regulating CFTR function. *Methods Mol. Med.* **70**, 175–186.
36. Li, C., Roy, K., Dandridge, K., and Naren, A. P. (2004) Molecular assembly of cystic fibrosis transmembrane conductance regulator in plasma membrane. *J. Biol. Chem* **279**, 24673–24684.

Chapter 18

Methods to Monitor Cell Surface Expression and Endocytic Trafficking of CFTR in Polarized Epithelial Cells

Jennifer M. Bomberger, William B. Guggino, and Bruce A. Stanton

Abstract

Cystic fibrosis transmembrane conductance regulator (CFTR)-mediated chloride secretion is critical to maintaining airway surface hydration and efficient mucociliary clearance in the upper airways. Mutations in CFTR in cystic fibrosis lead to reduced expression of functional CFTR channels at the apical plasma membrane of the airway epithelium, leading to dehydration of the airway surface liquid and diminished mucociliary clearance. Cell surface CFTR is modulated by changes in CFTR endocytosis and recycling, effectively altering the cell surface abundance of the channel. This chapter examines current methods employed to measure the cell surface expression of CFTR, as well as methods to monitor CFTR movement through the endocytic pathway.

Key words: Cystic fibrosis, cystic fibrosis transmembrane conductance regulator, endocytosis, recycling, intracellular trafficking.

1. Introduction

The number of CFTR channels in the apical plasma membrane of polarized epithelial cells – and thus, the rate of transepithelial Cl secretion – is determined in part by regulating the endocytic trafficking of CFTR (1). Endocytic trafficking is the process of sequestration and internalization of cargo proteins from the plasma membrane into endocytic vesicles, called endosomes, trafficking of endosomes among intracellular organelles, and then recycling of endosomes back to the plasma membrane, or delivery of endosomes to lysosomes where cargo proteins are degraded (2). In general, endocytosed proteins are delivered to

M.D. Amaral, K. Kunzelmann (eds.), *Cystic Fibrosis*, Methods in Molecular Biology 741,
DOI 10.1007/978-1-61779-117-8_18, © Springer Science+Business Media, LLC 2011

early endosomes and either recycle back to the plasma membrane via recycling endosomes or move progressively from multivesicular bodies to late endosomes and to lysosomes where cargo is degraded. A fascinating variety of proteins regulate the endocytic trafficking of cargo proteins, including Rab GTPases, SNAREs, PDZ domain-containing proteins, myosin motors, numerous lipids including phosphoinositide-P (3) and phosphoinositide-P_2 (3, 5), and a host of other regulatory proteins (1, 2).

In this chapter, we will discuss methods to detect and quantify the apical membrane abundance of CFTR and follow the intracellular trafficking of CFTR through the endocytic pathway. Cell surface biotinylation methods will be discussed as an effective measure of apical membrane CFTR abundance (3, 4). This chapter will also present an OptiPrep gradient fractionation method to separate subcellular compartments and a cell surface biotinylation-based endocytosis and recycling assay (4). These methods provide the ability to quantify the trafficking of CFTR through the endocytic pathway, as well as the ability to measure the effect of a particular treatment on CFTR trafficking through this pathway.

2. Materials

All reagents were purchased from Sigma-Aldrich, unless noted otherwise. Ezrin antibody was purchased from BD Biosciences (San Jose, CA), CFTR antibody (clone 596) from University of North Carolina Cystic Fibrosis Center (funded by the Cystic Fibrosis Foundation), NHS-LC-biotin (Cat. # 21335) from Thermo Scientific (Waltham, MA), and streptavidin agarose beads (Cat. # 20349) from Thermo Scientific (Waltham, MA). Phosphate buffered saline (PBS, 500 ml bottle) was purchased premade from Invitrogen (Carlsbad, CA). Permeable membrane supports were purchased from Corning (Costar 24-mm Transwell support, 0.4 μm pore, Cat. # 3412; Corning, Inc., Corning, NY).

2.1. Buffers

(a) Dulbecco's PBS/Mg/Ca, pH 7.0 (PBS/Mg/Ca):
1 ml of 0.5 M $MgCl_2$
0.1 ml of 0.5 M $CaCl_2$

(b) Lysis buffer (LB), pH 8.2:
25 mM HEPES, pH 8.0
1% (v/v) Triton X-100
10% (v/v) glycerol

(c) LB + protease inhibitor (LB[C]):
One complete protease inhibitor tablet (Roche, Cat. # 1697498)

50 ml lysis buffer

(d) Loading sample buffer (LSB):
Laemmli buffer (Bio-Rad Laboratories, Hercules, CA)

90 mM DTT

(e) Homogenization buffer
0.25 M sucrose

78 mM KCl

4 mM $MgCl_2$

8.4 mM $CaCl_2$

10 mM EGTA

50 mM HEPES–NaOH, pH 7.0

One complete protease inhibitor tablet (Roche, Cat. # 1697498)/ 50 ml of buffer

(f) Working solution diluent
78 mM KCl

4 mM $MgCl_2$

8.4 mM $CaCl_2$

10 mM EGTA

50 mM HEPES–NaOH, pH 7.0

(g) Glutathione solution, pH 8.6 (GSH; Sigma, Cat. # G6529), in deionized water:
50 mM GSH

75 mM NaCl

1 mM $MgCl_2$

0.1 mM $CaCl_2$

Add just before use:

80 mM NaOH

10% FBS

*The NaOH neutralizes the carboxyl group and deprotonates half the cysteine residues in glutathione. It is strongly buffered at the pK_a of this cysteine, which is pH 8.6.

3. Methods

3.1. Cell Surface CFTR

1. Culture human airway epithelial cells on permeable membrane supports at air–liquid interface to polarize cells and perform desired treatments.

- 24-mm Transwell permeable membrane support/treatment.

2. Remove all fluid by placing the filters at an angle to allow draining of the fluid to one side.
3. Wash wells with cold PBS/Mg/Ca, pH 8.2, three times, each wash for 2 min (*see* **Note 1**).
4. Incubate with 1 ml of NHS-LC-biotin (in PBS/Mg/Ca, pH 8.2; 1 mg/ml) on the apical side of the membrane support in the dark for 60 min at 4°C (*see* **Note 2**).
5. Wash wells with cold PBS/Mg/Ca, pH 8.2, three times, each wash for 2 min.
6. Add 300 μl of LB[C] to each well.
7. Incubate in the dark for 15 min shaking vigorously on an orbital shaker at 4°C.
8. Scrape cells from filter with a rubber policeman and collect in a 1.5-ml Eppendorf tube.
9. Homogenize each sample with a pipette tip and spin at 14,000 × *g* for 10 min at 4°C.
10. Add 50 μl of sample buffer (LSB) to 30 μl of supernatant and place sample at 85°C for 5 min (whole cell lysate (WCL) sample).
11. Prepare 100 μl aliquots of 50% streptavidin agarose beads and aspirate all fluid.
12. Wash with 1 ml of PBS/Mg/Ca twice, pelleting the beads with a pulse spin between the washes.
13. Wash with 1 ml LB[C] once (to equilibrate the beads before adding the cell lysates); suction dry the beads (*see* **Note 3**).
14. Incubate the remaining supernatants with washed streptavidin beads (bring the volume up to 1.0 ml with LB[C]) rotating in the dark for at least 2 h or overnight at 4°C.
15. Wash beads with 1 ml LB three times, each wash for 2 min, pulse spin the beads between washes, and suction dry the fluid after the last wash.
16. Incubate beads with 80 μl LSB at 85°C for 5 min.
17. Pulse spin the beads.
18. Collect the supernatant in 1.5-ml Eppendorf tubes and place sample at –20°C until ready to perform Western blot analysis.
19. Load samples on 7.5% Tris–HCl ready gels (Bio-Rad Laboratories, Hercules, CA) and run at 120 mV.

20. Transfer onto polyvinylidene fluoride (PVDF) membrane in cold room for 1.5–2 h at 95 mV.
21. Incubate membranes in 5% milk in TBS+0.1% Tween 20 blocking buffer at room temperature for 1 h.
22. Perform Western blot analysis with both WCL and biotinylation reaction samples, probing blots overnight with 1:1000 CFTR monoclonal antibody (clone 596) and 1:1000 ezrin monoclonal antibody (loading control) in 5% bovine serum albumin (BSA) in PBS+0.1% Tween 20 at 4°C (*see* **Note 4**). Goat anti-mouse secondary antibody conjugated to horseradish peroxidase (1:3000) in 5% milk in TBS+0.1% Tween 20 is used for detection.

3.2. CFTR Trafficking Through Intracellular Compartments Utilizing OptiPrep Gradients

Protocol adapted from Biemesderfer D, et al. (2002) AJP Renal 282:F785-94(6). Please *see* **Note 5**:

1. Culture human airway epithelial cells on permeable membrane supports at air–liquid interface to polarize cells and perform desired treatments:
   - 24-mm or (1) 100-mm Transwell permeable membrane support/treatment.
2. Prepare OptiPrep gradient:
   a. Add 1.9 ml volume of 20% OptiPrep in working solution diluent to the bottom of a 4.4-ml ultracentrifuge tube.
   b. Add 1.9 ml of 5% OptiPrep in working solution diluent on top of the 20% layer (with peristaltic pump).
   c. Allow continuous gradient to form over 3–4 h at room temperature (or overnight at 4°C) or use gradient maker to generate continuous gradient.
3. Remove all fluid by placing the filters at an angle to allow draining of the fluid to one side.
4. Wash filters with cold PBS/Mg/Ca, pH 8.2, three times, each wash for 2 min (*see* **Note 1**).
5. Incubate with 1 ml of NHS-LC-biotin (in PBS/Mg/Ca, pH 8.2; 1 mg/ml) in the dark for 60 min at 4°C.
6. Wash wells with cold PBS/Mg/Ca, pH 8.2, three times, each wash for 2 min (*see* **Note 2**).
7. Lyse cells on filters with 200 μl/well of 1% Triton X-100 in homogenization buffer.
8. Scrape the filters and pass through a 22-gauge, 3–in. needle 20 times.
9. Spin lysates at 1,500×*g* for 8 min.
10. Transfer 0.5 ml of the supernatant to a TH-660 ultracentrifuge tube (polyallomer), overlaying continuous

OptiPrep gradient (with p200, 100 μl at a time *very gently*!!).

11. After overlaying prepared lysates, centrifuge gradients for 18 h at 100,000×*g* in TH-660 swing-bucket rotor in Sorvall Ultra Pro 80 ultracentrifuge.
12. Analyze the gradient in 0.25 ml fractions by WB analysis (18 fractions total; last fraction contains plasma membrane pellet).
13. Add 50 μl of sample buffer to 30 μl of supernatant and place at 85°C for 5 min (whole cell lysate (WCL) sample).
14. Prepare 100 μl aliquots of 50% streptavidin agarose beads for each fraction and aspirate all fluid.
15. Wash with 1 ml of PBS/Mg/Ca twice, pelleting the beads with a pulse spin between the washes.
16. Wash with 1 ml LB[C] once [to equilibrate the beads before adding the cell lysates]; suction dry the beads (*see* **Note 3**).
17. Incubate the remaining supernatants from each fraction of the gradient with washed streptavidin beads (bring the volume up to 1.0 ml with LB[C]) rotating in the dark for at least 2 h or overnight at 4°C.
18. Wash beads with 1 ml LB three times, each wash for 2 min, pulse spin the beads between washes, and suction dry the fluid after the last wash.
19. Incubate beads with 80 μl LSB at 85°C for 5 min.
20. Pulse spin the beads.
21. Collect the supernatant in 1.5-ml Eppendorf tubes and place at –20°C until ready to perform Western blot analysis.
22. Load samples on 7.5% Tris–HCl ready gels (Bio-Rad) and run at 120 mV.
23. Transfer onto PVDF membrane in cold room for 1.5–2 h at 95 mV.
24. Incubate membranes in 5% milk in TBS+0.1% Tween 20 blocking buffer at room temperature for 1 h.
25. Perform Western blot analysis with both WCL and biotinylation reaction samples, probing blots overnight with 1:1000 CFTR monoclonal antibody (clone 596) and 1:1000 ezrin monoclonal antibody (loading control) in 5% bovine serum albumin (BSA) in PBS+0.1% Tween 20 at 4°C (*see* **Notes 4** and **6**). Goat anti-mouse secondary antibody conjugated to horseradish peroxidase (1:3000) in 5% milk in TBS+0.1% Tween 20 is used for detection.

26. Intracellular compartment location in the gradient is detected by Western blot analysis, probing with antibodies specific for each compartment.
    a. Plasma membrane (fraction 18): Na/K ATPase, gp135 (BD Biosciences, San Jose, CA);
    b. Endosome (fractions 9–13): Rab5a (Santa Cruz Biotechnology, Santa Cruz, CA);
    c. Lysosome (fractions 5–9): LAMP-1 (BD Biosciences, San Jose, CA).

3.3. CFTR Endocytosis and Recycling Assays

Culture human airway epithelial cells on permeable membrane supports at air–liquid interface to polarize cells. Plates A–D (*see* below) are needed for a recycling assay, but only plates A–C are needed if endocytosis is being measured.

*(1) 24-mm Transwell permeable membrane support/ treatment.

3.3.1. Prepare the Previous Night

1. PBS/Mg/Ca, pH 8.2, at 37°C.
2. PBS/Mg/Ca, pH 8.2, at 4°C.
3. PBS/Mg/Ca, pH 8.6, at 4°C.
4. LB[C] at 4°C.
5. Deionized water at 4°C.

see* **Note 7.

3.3.2. Day of thc Experiment

Use warm PBS/Mg/Ca at 37°C to fill wells of six well plates as needed for endocytosis and recycling assays. Place these plates in the 37°C incubator that will be used for the warming during the assay.

3.3.3. Biotinylation Reaction

1. Perform desired treatments on cultured human airway epithelial cells.
2. Place filters on ice (*see* **Note 8**).
3. Wash the apical and basolateral sides of filters with ice-cold PBS/Mg/Ca, pH 8.2, three times, each wash for 2 min (*see* **Notes 9** and **10**).
4. Incubate with 1.0 ml of 1 mg/ml NHS-S-S-biotin in PBS/Mg/Ca, pH 8.2, buffer on the apical side, 1.5 ml PBS/Mg/Ca, pH 8.2, on the basolateral side in the dark in the cold room for 60 min (*see* **Note 9**).
5. Wash with PBS/Mg/Ca, pH 8.2, three times, each wash for 2 min.
6. Leave PBS/Mg/Ca, pH 8.2, on all filters.
7. Arrange filters into plates that will receive the same treatment in the endocytosis/recycling assays as indicated in **Table 18.1** (*see* **Note 11**).

Table 18.1
Arrangement of filters in plates for the endocytosis/recycling assays

	Plate A	Plate B	Plate C	Plate D
Number of filters	2–3	2–3	2–3	2–3
Biotinylation	+	+	+	+
1st Warming			+ 5 min	+ 5 min
1st GSH		+	+	+
2nd Warming				+5 min
2nd GSH				+

3.3.4. Endocytic Assay

8. Leave plates A and B in the cold room.
9. Place plates C and D on ice and bring the plates on ice close to the 37°C incubator (used for endocytosis and recycling time points).
10. Pour off cold PBS/Mg/Ca and put filters in wells of warm PBS/Mg/Ca, pH 8.2, at 30 s intervals. Incubate at 37°C for 5 min. *Raising the temperature to 37° C will induce endocytosis.*
11. At 5 min, put filters in six-well plates containing ice-cold PBS/Mg/Ca, pH 8.2, on ice (keep the same timing as in the initiation of endocytosis, this will mean staggering by 30 s). *This step will terminate endocytosis* (*see* **Note 12**).
12. Bring plates C and D on ice back to the cold room.
13. Remove all PBS/Mg/Ca from plates A to D.
14. Incubate plates B–D with 1.0 ml of glutathione (GSH) solution, pH 8.6, on the apical side and 1.5 ml PBS/Mg/Ca, pH 8.6, on the basolateral side, in the cold room in the dark five times, each time for 15 min (don't need to change the PBS on the basolateral side) (make enough GSH solution for just endocytosis washes, *see* **Note 13**).
15. At the same time, incubate plate A with PBS/Mg/Ca, pH 8.6 (*see* **Note 14**).
16. After GSH incubation is finished, wash plates B and C with PBS/Mg/Ca, pH 8.6, three times, each wash for 2 min.
17. Wash plate D with PBS/Mg/Ca, pH 8.2, three times, each wash for 2 min.
18. Leave plates A–C in the cold room.

3.3.5. Recycling Assay

19. Subject the remaining plate (D) to a second warming for 5 min (plate D), staggering each filter by 30 s, as above for endocytosis protocol (*see* **Note 15**). *This incubation at 37°C allows endocytosed CFTR to recycle.*
20. Put the filters in ice-cold PBS/Mg/Ca, pH 8.2, and wash with PBS/Mg/Ca, pH 8.2, three times, each wash for 2 min. *This step terminates recycling.*
21. Incubate plate D with freshly made glutathione (GSH) solution, pH 8.6, in the dark three times, each GSH treatment for 15 min (*see* **Note 13**) at 4°C.
22. At the same time, incubate plates A–C with PBS/Mg/Ca, pH 8.6.
23. Remove all fluid by placing the plates at an angle to allow draining of the fluid to one side.
24. Add 300 μl LB[C] to each filter.
25. Incubate in the dark at 4°C for 15 min by shaking vigorously on an orbital shaker.
26. Scrape the cells from filter with a rubber policeman and collect in a 1.5-ml Eppendorf tube.
27. Homogenize each sample with a pipette tip and spin at 14,000×*g* for 10 min at 4°C.
28. Add 50 μl of sample buffer to 30 μl of supernatant and put at 85°C for 5 min (whole cell lysate (WCL) sample).
29. Prepare 100 μl aliquots of 50% streptavidin agarose beads and aspirate all fluid.
30. Wash with 1 ml of PBS/Mg/Ca twice, pelleting the beads with a pulse spin between the washes.
31. Wash with 1 ml LB[C] once (to equilibrate the beads before adding the cell lysates); suction dry the beads (*see* **Note 3**).
32. Incubate the remaining supernatants with washed streptavidin agarose beads (bring the volume up to 1.0 ml with LB[C]) rotating in the dark for at least 2 h or overnight at 4°C.
33. Wash beads with 1 ml LB three times, each wash for 2 min, pulse spin the beads between washes, and suction dry the fluid after the last wash.
34. Incubate beads with 80 μl LSB at 85°C for 5 min.
35. Pulse spin the beads.
36. Collect the supernatant in 1.5-ml Eppendorf tubes and place at −20°C until ready to perform Western blot analysis.

37. Load samples on 7.5% Tris–HCl ready gels (Bio-Rad Laboratories, Hercules, CA) and run at 120 mV.
38. Transfer onto PVDF membrane in cold room for 1.5–2 h at 95 mV.
39. Incubate membranes in 5% milk in TBS+0.1% Tween 20 blocking buffer at room temperature for 1 h.
40. Perform Western blot analysis with both WCL and biotinylation reaction samples, probing blots overnight with 1:1000 CFTR monoclonal antibody (clone 596) and 1:1000 ezrin monoclonal antibody (loading control) in 5% bovine serum albumin (BSA) in PBS+0.1% Tween 20 at 4°C (*see* **Note 4**). Goat anti-mouse secondary antibody conjugated to horseradish peroxidase (1:3000) in 5% milk in TBS+0.1% Tween 20 is used for detection.

3.3.6. Analysis of Data

41. Biotinylated CFTR is quantitated and normalized for WCL CFTR or ezrin abundance (*see* **Note 4**).
42. Samples from plate A are set as the control biotinylated signal (set to 100%) (**Fig. 18.1**).
43. GSH cleavage efficiency is examined by percentage of plate A biotinylated CFTR signal found in plate B (*see* **Note 16, Fig. 18.1**):
    a. GSH cleavage efficiency: ((100–5)/100)100 = 95%.

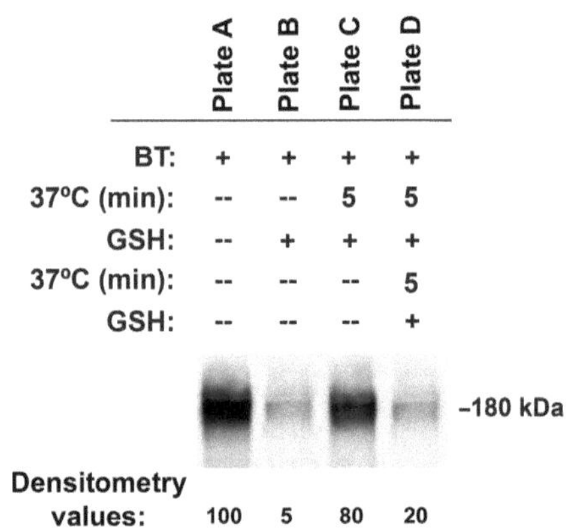

Fig. 18.1. The endocytic recycling of CFTR. Polarized CFBE41o- cells were grown on 24-mm Transwell permeable membrane supports for 7 days. *A*, Endocytosis and recycling experiments were performed as described in text and detailed in figure. *B*, Representative blots from endocytic and recycling assays. Cells from all *four lanes* were cooled to 4°C and biotinylated. The amount of biotinylated CFTR remaining in the plasma membrane after GSH treatment at 4°C (*lane 2*) was subtracted from the amount of CFTR remaining biotinylated after warming to 37°C and GSH treatment (*lane 3*) to determine the amount of endocytosed CFTR. Cells from lane 3 were then warmed at 37°C to allow recycling of endocytosed CFTR before a second GSH treatment. CFTR recycling was calculated as the difference between the amount of biotinylated CFTR after the first (*lane 3*) and second (*lane 4*) GSH treatments.

44. Endocytosis of CFTR is calculated by subtracting the biotinylated CFTR signal from plate C from the signal of GSH-cleaved biotinylated CFTR in plate B. This number is expressed as the percentage of total biotinylated CFTR in plate A:
    a. Endocytosis of CFTR: 80–5 = 75;
    b. Percentage of total CFTR endocytosed: (75/100)100 = 75%.
45. Recycled CFTR is the fraction of the biotinylated CFTR signal from plate D of the endocytosed CFTR calculation from step 42. This number is then expressed as the percentage of endocytosed CFTR that recycles:
    a. Recycling of CFTR: (20/75)100 = 26.67;
    b. Percentage of endocytosed CFTR recycled: 100–26.67 = 73.33.
46. The results of the experiment depicted in **Fig. 18.1** are as follows:
    a. GSH cleavage efficiency is 95%.
    b. The percentage of total biotinylated CFTR that endocytosed in 5 min is 75%.
    c. The percentage of endocytosed CFTR that recycled in 5 min is 73.33%.

4. Notes

1. The biotinylation labeling efficiency has been optimized for pH 8.2 of the PBS/Mg/Ca used in the labeling reaction. Other pH of PBS/Mg/Ca will work, but pH 8.2 is the most effective at labeling cell surface proteins.
2. Gently washing cells before and after biotinylation procedure, as well as strict adherence to temperatures called for in protocol, will yield most reliable cell surface CFTR measures. This will also limit inappropriate biotinylation of intracellular CFTR proteins.
3. When aspirating the streptavidin agarose beads dry, use a 1-in., 27-gauge syringe needle with suction. The 27-gauge needle will remove all liquid, but not aspirate the beads.
4. Cell surface CFTR abundance can be normalized to total CFTR expressed in the WCL or to ezrin in the WCL sample. Both can be effective loading controls, given that the treatments being assessed do not change the expression of either WCL CFTR or ezrin. In our experience, many treat-

ments alter actin expression in the cell lysate, while ezrin abundance remains quite constant. Therefore, we chose to normalize protein abundance in our samples to ezrin abundance.

5. This method enables the tracking of a cell surface protein through the endocytic pathway. By biotinylating cell surface proteins before treatments are applied, you can track the movement of a particular protein (i.e., CFTR) that begins the time course at the cell surface and analyze how different treatments alter the endocytic trafficking of that protein.
6. CFTR abundance in each fraction is represented as a percentage of total CFTR in all fractions.
7. All steps are done on ice or in the cold room, unless noted otherwise. Maintaining cold temperature, except during endocytosis or recycling time points, is absolutely critical in obtaining accurate measures of CFTR trafficking in this assay.
8. All treatments within the experiment are performed in duplicate or triplicate.
9. Check the pH of the various PBS/Mg/Ca solutions on the day of the experiment to make sure they are correct. An incorrect pH of the PBS/Mg/Ca will reduce the efficiency of the biotin labeling reaction, thus increasing the noise in the experiment.
10. Gently washing cells before and after biotinylation procedure, as well as strict adherence to temperatures called for in protocol, will yield most reliable cell surface CFTR measures. This will also limit inappropriate biotinylation of intracellular CFTR proteins. Be sure to use *NHS-S-S biotin* in this protocol to allow cleavage by GSH.
11. Arranging the filters in six-well plates (plates A–D), according to the condition during the endocytosis/recycling assay, is incredibly helpful during the endocytosis and recycling time points of the assay. Be sure to label plates carefully, detailing which well received which treatment.
12. The endocytosis and recycling time points are the most critical steps to strictly adhere to the temperatures called for in the protocol. Using large volumes of PBS/Mg/Ca for the washes ensures rapid temperature changes during time points. Previous experiments have been performed in CFBE41o- cells to determine that CFTR endocytosis is linear between 1 and 5 min. Performing this assay in a new cell type would require a time course to determine at which time points the endocytosis of CFTR is linear and

suitable for the assay. Because endocytosed CFTR recycles rapidly, time points longer than ~5 min measure a composite of endocytosis and recycling back to the plasma membrane.

13. For best results with GSH cleavage of biotin, strictly adhere to the pH recommended in the protocol and make GSH just before use in each step.

14. Sequester plate A during the GSH washes, so GSH is not inadvertently added to plate A. This is the control that all samples will be compared to during analysis. If the biotin is cleaved from this plate, there is no control and the experiment is lost.

15. Previous experiments have been performed in CFBE41o- cells to determine that CFTR recycling is linear at 2.5 and 5 min. Performing this assay in a new cell type would require a time course to determine at which time points the recycling of CFTR is linear and suitable for the assay.

16. GSH treatment (plate B) must achieve 85% cleavage of NHS-S-S-biotin from control filters (plate A) to be considered a successful experiment. Lesser cleavage makes interpretation and quantitation of results quite difficult (5).

References

1. Guggino, W. B., and Stanton, B. A. (2006) New insights into cystic fibrosis: Molecular switches that regulate CFTR. *Nat. Rev. Mol. Cell. Biol.* 7, 426–436.
2. Gruenberg, J., and van der Goot, F. G. (2006) Mechanisms of pathogen entry through the endosomal compartments. *Nat. Rev. Mol. Cell. Biol.* 7, 495–504.
3. Swiatecka-Urban, A., Boyd, C., Coutermarsh, B., Karlson, K. H., Barnaby, R., Aschenbrenner, L., et al. (2004) Myosin VI regulates endocytosis of the cystic fibrosis transmembrane conductance regulator. *J. Biol. Chem.* **279**, 38025–38031.
4. Bomberger, J. M., Barnaby, R. L., and Stanton, B. A. (2009) The deubiquitinating enzyme USP10 regulates the post-endocytic sorting of cystic fibrosis transmembrane conductance regulator in airway epithelial cells. *J. Biol. Chem.* **284**, 18778–18789.
5. Swiatecka-Urban, A., Talebian, L., Kanno, E., Moreau-Marquis, S., Coutermarsh, B., Hansen, K., et al. (2007) Myosin VB is required for trafficking of CFTR in RAB11A-specific apical recycling endosomes in polarized human airway epithelial cells. *J. Biol. Chem.* **282**, 23725–23736.
6. Biemesderfer, D., Mentone, S. A., Mooseker, M., and Hasson, T. (2002) Expression of myosin VI within the early endocytic pathway in adult and developing proximal tubules. *Am. J. Physiol. Renal Physiol.* **282**, F785–F794.

Chapter 19

Segmental and Subcellular Distribution of CFTR in the Kidney

François Jouret, Pierre J. Courtoy, and Olivier Devuyst

Abstract

Besides its location at the plasma membrane, CFTR is present in intracellular vesicles along both the exocytic and the endocytic pathways. *Immunostaining and subcellular fractionation studies* of mouse kidney demonstrate that CFTR is located in endosomes of the cells lining the terminal part of the proximal tubule (PT). The PT cells efficiently reabsorb the ultrafiltered low molecular weight (LMW) proteins by apical endocytosis involving the multiligand receptors megalin and cubilin. The progression from early endosomes to lysosomes depends on the integrity of the cytoskeleton, as well as on vesicular acidification. The latter is mediated by the vacuolar H^+-ATPase (V-ATPase) and requires an anionic conductance to dissipate the transmembrane potential gradient. CFTR might ensure such chloride conductance, thereby participating to endosomal acidification and protein uptake by PT cells. *Immunostaining with well-characterized antibodies* shows that CFTR is located in the terminal segment of PT, where it co-distributes with megalin and cubilin. *Subcellular fractionation* of total mouse kidneys through Percoll gradients demonstrates the co-localization of CFTR with the V-ATPase and early endosome markers including the Cl^-/H^+ exchanger, ClC-5, and the small GTPase, Rab5a. *Deglycosylation studies and immunoblotting* show a distinct glycosylation pattern for CFTR in mouse kidney and lung. The segmental and subcellular distribution of CFTR in mouse kidney supports a role for CFTR in PT receptor-mediated endocytosis of ultrafiltered LMW proteins.

Key words: Cystic fibrosis, CFTR, ClC-5, receptor-mediated endocytosis, megalin, cubilin, endosomal acidification, kidney, proximal tubule cells, low molecular weight protein, antigen retrieval, immunostaining, analytical subcellular fractionation, Percoll gradients.

1. Introduction

A significant amount of albumin and low molecular weight (LMW) plasma proteins is continuously filtered through the glomeruli, to be reabsorbed by proximal tubule (PT) cells (1). By

M.D. Amaral, K. Kunzelmann (eds.), *Cystic Fibrosis*, Methods in Molecular Biology 741,
DOI 10.1007/978-1-61779-117-8_19,

definition, LMW proteins are characterized by a molecular mass lower than that of albumin (69 kDa). Most filtered LMW proteins are reabsorbed and metabolized by PT cells, and the human urine is virtually devoid of plasma proteins under physiological conditions. This massive uptake of proteins from the primitive urine accounts for as much as 80% of the total metabolic clearance of small proteins and peptides and plays a key role in hormone and vitamin homeostasis (for a review, see (2)).

The uptake of LMW proteins by PT cells essentially involves receptor-mediated endocytosis. Clathrin-mediated endocytosis represents the predominant pathway for protein uptake across the apical membrane of PT cells, with an endocytic pathway consisting of five main interrelated compartments: (i) microvilli and clathrin-coated pits, (ii) early endosomes, (iii) dense apical tubules responsible for apical recycling, (iv) late endosomes, and (v) lysosomes (3). The process essentially requires two multiligand receptors, megalin and cubilin, that are expressed at the brush border of PT cells (2). Ligand binding and interactions between both receptors induce their internalization into coated vesicles and their subsequent delivery to endosomes and lysosomes for ligand processing and receptor degradation or recycling (**Fig. 19.1**). Receptor-mediated endocytosis of albumin depends on the integrity of the actin cytoskeleton and the microtubules (4), whereas progression along the endocytic apparatus requires a sustained vesicular acidification from early to late endosomes and finally to lysosomes (5, 6). In PT cells, the endosomal acidification is driven by the electrogenic vacuolar H^+-ATPase. The translocation of H^+ from the cytoplasm into the endosomes generates a transmembrane electrical potential ($\Delta\Psi$) resulting in a rapid inhibition of V-ATPase activity. Thus, in order to ensure progressive vesicular acidification, either anions have to enter vesicles or cations have to leave. In most cases, vesicular acidification seems dependent on a parallel Cl^- conductance (7, 8). Furthermore, the intravesicular Cl^- concentration itself could directly affect the V-ATPase activity (9) as well as the vesicle recycling independently of its effect on pH (6).

Besides its location at the plasma membrane, CFTR is distributed in intracellular organelles along the endocytic and secretory pathways, in which it might act as a pH regulator by importing Cl^- in parallel to H^+ accumulation (10). Mutant epithelial cells derived from CF patients exhibit no cAMP-dependent regulation of endocytosis and exocytosis, unless transfected with cDNA encoding wild-type CFTR (11). Incubation of freshly isolated nasal polyps from CF patients harboring the F508del mutation with 3-(2,4-dinitroanilino)-3′-amino-*N*-methyldipropylamine (DAMP), used as a semiquantitative marker of vesicular acidification, showed that DAMP accumulation was significantly lowered in specific biosynthetic compartments, i.e.,

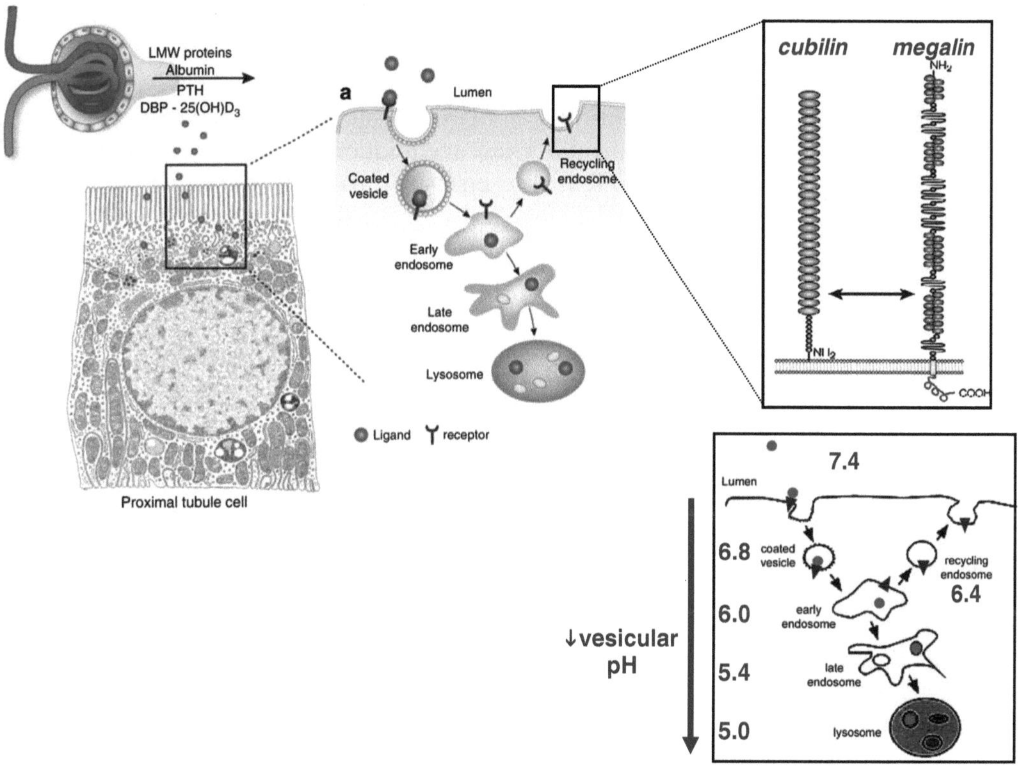

Fig. 19.1. **Reabsorption of low molecular weight proteins by proximal tubule cells.** Albumin and low molecular weight (LMW) proteins that are naturally filtered by the glomerulus into the primary urine are endocytosed by PT cells via the megalin/cubilin receptor pathway. Following internalization in coated vesicles, the receptor–ligand complexes progress along the endocytic pathway. The endosomes undergo a progressive acidification that results in the dissociation of the receptor–ligand complexes, with megalin and cubilin (*inset*) being recycled to the apical membrane, whereas the ligand is directed to lysosomes for degradation. Modified from (18).

trans-Golgi and pre-lysosomal organelles (12). Moreover, the monitoring of membrane potential in a light microsomal fraction from CF and non-CF epithelial cells showed that acidification is limited in CF cells by a high $\Delta\Psi$ resulting from insufficient Cl^- counterion conductance. In turn, defective acidification may induce lysosomal enzyme deficiencies and abnormal trafficking and processing of newly synthesized polypeptides in cells lacking CFTR (10). However, the role of CFTR in regulating organelle pH remains controversial, with hyper- rather than hypo-acidification suggested to occur in CF respiratory epithelial cells. Indeed, cell ratiometric imaging with luminally exposed pH-sensitive green fluorescent protein has demonstrated that CFTR decreases the pH of endosomal organelles because of a loss of CFTR inhibitory effects on Na^+ transport and a defect in cyclic guanosine 3,5-monophosphate signaling cascade (13). In addition, recycling of transferrin receptor is impaired in CFTR mutant lung epithelial cells, with possible functional consequences at the plasma membrane and within endosomal compartments (14).

This section focuses on the segmental and subcellular distribution of CFTR in the epithelial cells lining the PT of mouse kidney using immunostaining following antigen retrieval, as well as immunoblotting and analytical subcellular fractionation through Percoll gradients. These techniques defined the distribution and role of CFTR in the endocytic pathway operating in PT cells. Further biochemical and functional investigations performed on CFTR-deficient mouse models and in CF patients have confirmed the role of CFTR in the uptake of ultrafiltered LMW proteins by the mammalian kidney (15).

2. Materials

2.1. Antigen Retrieval and Immunoperoxidase Labeling Procedures with Paraffin-Embedded Serial Sections of Mouse Kidney

2.1.1. Formaldehyde Solution

1. Phosphate buffer (0.2 M, pH 7.4):
   (a) Solution A: dilute 22.7 g Na_2HPO_4 anhydrous (Sigma S3397, Sigma-Aldrich, St. Louis, MO) in 800 ml of double distilled water (DDW)
   (b) Solution B: dilute 6.2 g KH_2PO_4 (Sigma P9791) in 250 ml DDW
   (c) Titrate the pH of solution A up to 7.4 by adding solution B
   (d) Level it up to 1 l with DDW
2. Dilute 4 g paraformaldehyde in phosphate buffer (0.2 M, pH 7.4)
3. Make fresh as required
4. Wear a mask when working with formaldehyde powder

2.1.2. Citrate Buffer

1. Mix in 1 l of DDW:
   (a) Citric acid $C_6H_8O_7$ H_2O (Merck 244, Overijse, Belgium): 3.77 g
   (b) Sodium citrate $C_6H_5Na_3O_7$ $2H_2O$ (Merck 1.06448.0500): 25.12 g
2. Store the solution (1 M, pH 5.8) as aliquots at –20°C for up to 3 months
3. Make fresh the final solution (0.01 M), as required

2.1.3. Ethanol Solutions at Distinct Concentrations (Dilute with DDW)

Dilute ethanol with DDW into decreasing concentrations: 100–96–80–70–50–30%.

2.1.4. Methanol-H_2O_2 (0.3 %) Solution

1. Add 2 ml H_2O_2 (Sigma H1009, stable at 4°C for up to 1 month) to 198 ml methanol
2. Make it fresh as required

2.1.5. TRIS Solution (1 M, pH 7.4)

1. Mix in 2 l of DDW
   (a) TRIZMA base (Sigma T6066): 12.2 g
   (b) NaCl: 50 g
   (c) HCl 32%: 8.75 ml
2. Titrate up to pH 7.4

2.1.6. TRIS-Tween 0.02 %

1. Add 160 μl of Tween-20 (Sigma P1379) to 800 ml TRIS solution

2.1.7. TRIS-Bovine Serum Albumin (BSA) 2 %

1. Add 2 g of BSA (Sigma A-7638) to 100 ml TRIS solution

2.1.8. ABC Vectastain Elite (Vector Laboratories, Orton Southgate, Peterborough, UK)

2.1.9. 3-Amino-9-Ethylcarbazole (AEC) Reagent Kit (Vector Laboratories)

2.2. Analytical Subcellular Fractionation and Immunoblotting

2.2.1. Anesthetic Drugs

1. Rompun® (40 μg/g body weight; stock 2%; Bayer, Brussels, Belgium)
2. Anesketin® (20 μg/g body weight; Eurovet, AD Bladel, The Netherlands)

2.2.2. SIPPI Solution

1. Sucrose (Sigma S7903) 0.25 M
2. Imidazole (Sigma I-0125) buffer 3 mM, pH 7.4
3. Protease inhibitors (Roche, Brussels, Belgium): 1 pellet/50 ml

4. Phosphatase inhibitors (sodium orthovanadate 2 mM, Acros Organics, Geel, Belgium; NaF 10 mM, Merck)

2.2.3. Percoll (Sigma P1644)

2.2.4. Sample Buffer (5x)

1. Mix in 50 ml of DDW:
   (a) SDS (Lauryl sulfate, Invitrogen 15525-017, Merelbeke, Belgium): 3.75 g
   (b) Glycerol (Sigma G8773): 15 ml
   (c) Bromophenol blue 0.1% (Sigma B8026): 2 ml
   (d) TRIS (Bio-Rad 161-0719) 1 M, pH 6.8: 2.5 ml
2. Keep at 4°C (to avoid SDS precipitation)

2.2.5. Fairbanks Buffer (20x)

1. Mix in 1 l of DDW
2. TRIZMA base (Sigma T6066): 48.19 g
3. Sodium acetate: 16.41 g (Sigma S3272)
4. Na-EDTA: 7.44 g (Sigma E5513)
5. Titrate to pH 7.4 with acetic acid
6. Make it fresh as required by diluting 20 times with distilled water

2.2.6. Block Buffer

1. Mix in 800 ml of DDW
   (a) Na_3PO_4 (Aldrich 342483) (0.5 M, pH 7.4): 80 ml
   (b) NaCl 5 M: 24 ml
   (c) Tween-20 (Sigma P1379): 8 ml

2.2.7. Milk Block Buffer

1. Dilute 2 g milk powder 5% in 40 ml Block buffer

3. Methods

3.1. Antigen Retrieval and Immunoperoxidase Labeling Procedures with Paraffin-Embedded Serial Sections of Mouse Kidney

3.1.1. Paraffin Removal and Rehydration

1. Paraffin removal: immerse the slides into xylene for 4 min.
2. Rehydration: immerse the slides for 3 min into ethanol solutions of decreasing concentration (100–96–80–70–50–30%). Rinse for 5 min in DDW.

3.1.2. Antigen Retrieval (See Note 1)

1. Immerse the slides into citrate buffer pre-warmed to 97°C for 75 min.
2. Let the slides in solution cool down at room temperature for 20 min.
3. Rinse the slides with DDW for 5 min and prepare the methanol-H_2O_2 (0.3%) solution.

3.1.3. Inhibition of Endogenous Peroxidase

1. Immerse the slides into methanol-H_2O_2 (0.3%) solution at room temperature for 30 min.
2. Rinse the slides with TRIS solution (2 × 10 min).

3.1.4. Block of Unspecific Immunoreactive Sites (See Note 2)

1. Prepare the blocking solution by diluting 75 μl blocking serum (non-immune serum of same species as primary or secondary antibodies) into 5 ml TRIS solution. Vortex and keep it on ice.
2. Dry the slides individually with paper and/or aspiration.
3. Delineate the tissue section with the hydrophobic pen (5 mm far from the sample).
4. Place the slide on a support in a humid chamber.
5. Drop 150 μl blocking serum on tissue samples.
6. Incubation time: 20 min.

3.1.5. Incubation with Primary Antibodies (See Note 3)

1. Dilute the primary antibodies in an Eppendorf with TRIS-BSA 2% solution. Keep it on ice.
   (a) Affinity-purified rabbit polyclonal antibodies (MD1314) against the C-terminus of rodent CFTR (MD1314, Dr. C.R. Marino, VA Medical Center, University of Tennessee, Memphis, TN): 1/500;
   (b) Rabbit polyclonal antibodies against the water channel, AQP1 (Chemicon, Temecula, CA): 1/400.
2. Aspirate the blocking serum and drop the solution with primary antibodies on tissue samples.
3. Incubation time: 45 min.
4. Save the primary antibodies for future experiments.
5. Rinse with TRIS-Tween (2 × 5 min) and TRIS (5 min).

3.1.6. Incubation with Secondary Biotinylated Antibodies

1. Mix in an Eppendorf 5 ml TRIS solution, 75 μl blocking serum, and 25 μl secondary biotinylated antibodies (Vector Laboratories, Brussels, Belgium; final concentration: 1/200). Vortex and keep it on ice.
2. Prepare the slides as described in **Section 3.1.4**.
3. Drop 150 μl of the solution with secondary antibodies on tissue samples.

4. Incubation time: 45 min.
5. Rinse with TRIS-Tween (2 × 5 min) and TRIS (5 min).

3.1.7. Incubation with Avidin-Coupled Peroxidase

1. Dilute the avidin DH/biotinylated horseradish peroxidase H macromolecular complex (Vectastain Elite ABC kit PK6100, Vector Laboratories) in TRIS solution (5 ml).
2. Prepare the slides as described in **Section 3.1.4**.
3. Drop 150 μl of the ABC solution on tissue samples.
4. Incubation time: 45 min.
5. Rinse with TRIS (3 × 5 min).

3.1.8. Revelation Using the 3-Amino-9-Ethylcarbazole (AEC) Reagent Kit (Vector Laboratories, SK4200)

1. Immediately before use, prepare the substrate solution according to the manufacturer's recommendations:
   (a) Add 2 drops of the Buffer Stock solution to 1 ml distilled water;
   (b) Add 3 drops of the AEC Stock solution and mix;
   (c) Add 2 drops of the hydrogen peroxide solution and mix.
2. Prepare the slides as described in **Section 3.1.4**.
3. Drop 150 μl of the final AEC solution on tissue samples.
4. Incubation time: 15 min.
5. Rinse with distilled water (3 × 5 min).

3.1.9. Mounting of Slides (See Note 4)

1. Aspire the liquid completely from the slide and mount them with glycerol-enriched water.
2. Leave the slide on a flat surface for the next 24 h before viewing.

3.1.10. Imaging Procedure

1. Use a Leica DMR coupled to a Leica DC300 digital camera (Leica, Heerbrugg, Switzerland) (**Fig. 19.2**)

3.2. Analytical Subcellular Fractionation and Immunoblotting Procedures

3.2.1. Tissue Sampling (See Note 5)

1. Measure the mouse body weight.
2. Induce anesthesia by intraperitoneal injection of Rompun® (40 μg/g body weight; stock 2%; Bayer, Brussels, Belgium) and Anesketin® (20 μg/g body weight; Eurovet, AD Bladel, The Netherlands).
3. Inject ^{125}I-β_2-microglobulin (M4890, Sigma-Aldrich) in the periorbital plexus (typically >1,000 cpm/ng and >95% trichloroacetic acid precipitable; ~600 ng radioligand per

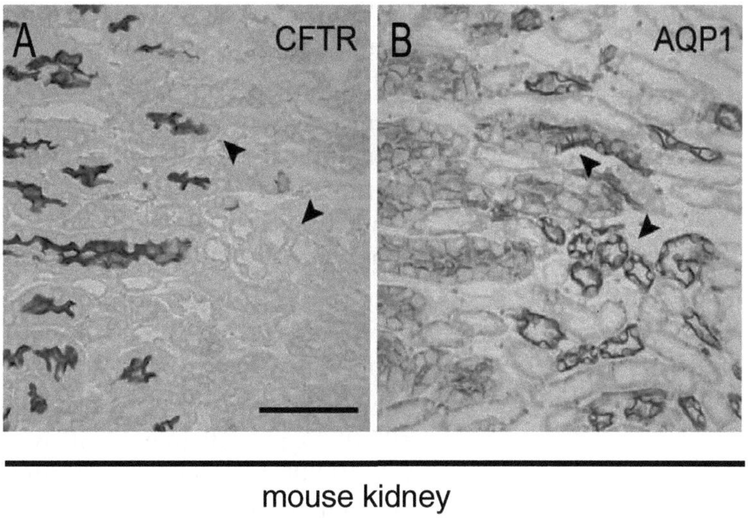

Fig. 19.2. **Segmental distribution of CFTR along the mouse nephron.** Immunoperoxidase labeling for CFTR (**a**) and AQP1 (**b**) was performed on serial sections (5 μm) of mouse *Cftr*$^{+/+}$ kidneys. The high signal for CFTR at the cortico-medullary junction, combined with the segmental co-localization of CFTR and AQP1, indicates that CFTR is particularly abundant in the apical area of the distal S3 segment of PT, just before the transition with the descending thin limb (**a** and **b**, *arrowheads*). Bar: 100 μm.

gram body weight injected in a maximal volume of 150 μl; the exact dose is calculated by weighing the syringe before and after injection).

4. Perform laparotomy, expose kidneys and *vena cava inferior*. Section the vein.
5. Collect a small sample of blood with a heparinized tuberculin syringe for further analysis.
6. Flood with PBS kept at 37°C until no blood efflux can be seen (~20 s).
7. Excise exsanguinated kidneys, section the hile, and remove kidney capsule.
8. From this point, all subsequent steps are performed at 4°C.
9. Weigh kidneys in ice-cold SIPPI.
10. If fractionation is combined with autoradiography, ~1/3 of one kidney is fixed by immersion in cold, 4% (w/v) freshly prepared formaldehyde overnight, followed by rinsing in cold PBS and paraffin embedding.

3.2.2. Homogenization and Differential Sedimentation

1. Mince kidneys and homogenize in SIPPI with three to five strokes of a Potter–Elvehjem tissue homogenizer (B1804, Thomas Scientific, Swedesboro, NJ).

2. Perform a first low-speed sedimentation at 10,000×*g* × 10 min (Jouan centrifuge; 2,070 rpm, 4°C) and collect the first low-speed supernatant.
3. Extract again the low-speed pellet by rehomogenization using three strokes of the Potter–Elvehjem homogenizer and centrifuge again at 10,000×*g* × 10 min; the final pellet, denoted nuclear fraction ("N"), corresponds to nuclei, cell debris, and insoluble extracellular matrix.
4. Pool low-speed supernatants as "post-nuclear supernatant" (referred to as "MPLS") to a final volume of ~8 ml; save 1 ml for further analysis.
5. Submit the remaining 7 ml to high-speed centrifugation at 100,000×*g* × 60 min (Ti50 rotor, Beckman, Palo Alto, CA; 40,000 rpm), using acceleration and brake (Optima LE-80 K ultracentrifuge, Beckman).
6. The high-speed supernatant (~6.5 ml), denoted fraction "S," corresponds to the cytosol; the high-speed pellet corresponds to post-nuclear particles (referred to as "MLP" fraction). Resuspend this MLP fraction with a tigette in ~2 ml of SIPPI and further homogenize with a Dounce (loose pestle). One milliliter is used for further analysis by density gradient centrifugation, and the remainder is saved for further analysis.

3.2.3. Density Gradient Centrifugation (See Note 6)

1. Verify that organelles are well homogenized as individual particles by evidence of Brownian motion under phase contrast microscopy.
2. Mix 1 ml of post-nuclear particles with 7 ml of Percoll at 16% (v/v) in a #355630 centrifuge tube (Beckman); the heterogeneity (polydispersity) of Percoll particles will ensure a self-generating gradient upon centrifugation (in this case, close to linearity).
3. Inject 250 μl of pure Percoll below this mixture using a syringe equipped with a long needle, as cushion.
4. Resolve subcellular particles in this self-forming gradient by centrifugation at 60,000×*g* × 30 min (30,000 rpm in the Ti50 rotor).
5. Withdraw the brake shortly before the end of centrifugation, when speed declines to ~1,000 rpm.
6. Collect 10 fractions (of ~800 μl each) in pre-weighed empty tubes, starting by aspiration of the bottom of the tube.
7. Weigh filled tubes and determine the fraction weight by the difference.
8. Determine density refractometry (Refractometer Abbé, Bellingham and Stanley). The exact volume of each fraction is given by the ratio of weight to density.

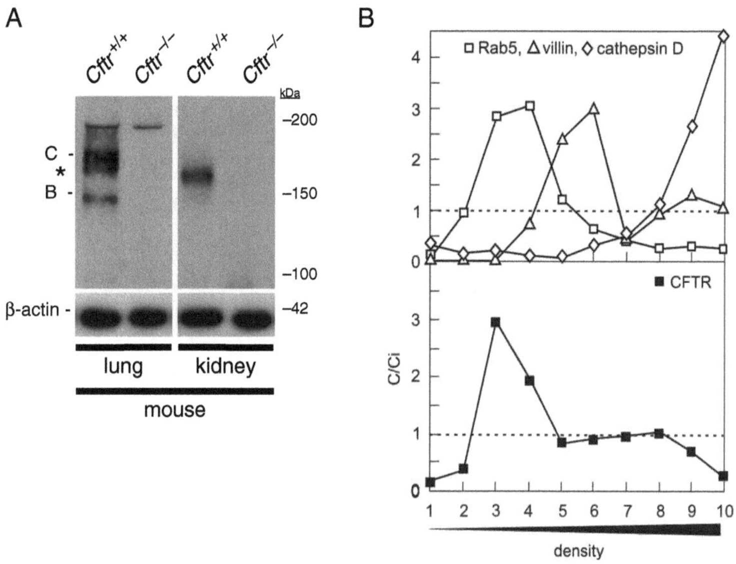

Fig. 19.3. **Immunoblotting and density distribution of CFTR in mouse kidney homogenates using Percoll gradient.** (**a**) Representative immunoblotting for CFTR in lung and kidney from *Cftr*$^{+/+}$ and *Cftr*$^{-/-}$ mice. Membrane extracts (30 μg/lane) were run on 5% PAGE and transferred to nitrocellulose. The blot was probed with MD1314 anti-CFTR antibodies (1:500) and, after stripping, β-actin (1:10,000). In lung, both B- (150 kDa) and C-bands (180 kDa) are present, whereas, in kidney, CFTR is detected as a single large band at approximately 160 kDa (*asterisk*). In both tissues, immunoreactive bands for CFTR are absent in *Cftr*$^{-/-}$ extracts. (**b**) Distributions after centrifugation are presented by comparison with the initial concentration as C/Ci (*broken line*), where values >1 reflect organelle enrichment and values <1 reflect organelle depletion. The *upper panel* indicates the resolution of endosomal peak (Rab5a), brush border (villin), and lysosomes (mature cathepsin D). The *lower panel* indicates that CFTR peaks at the position of endosomes, is not enriched at the position of the brush border, and is depleted at the position of lysosomes. The shape of the gradient is given by the density as indicated below. Whereas the positions of endosomes and lysosomes are constant, the position of the brush border varies according to slight variations of the shape of the Percoll gradient (for additional information, see (15, 19–20)).

3.2.4. Distribution Analysis (See Note 7)

1. Count radioactivity (e.g., Minaxi Auto Gamma 5,000 series, Gamma counter, Packard) in dilutions corresponding to 5 μl of injection or 10 μl of blood, in 100 μl of differential sedimentation fractions (nuclear fraction, post-nuclear supernatant, post-nuclear particles, and high-speed supernatant) and 250 μl for each fraction of the Percoll gradient.
2. Probe fractions by immunoblotting for organelle markers (**Fig. 19.3**).

3.2.5. Immunoblotting

1. *Handling of the samples* (*see* **Note 8**)
   (a) Aliquot each fraction obtained through the Percoll gradient (from #1 to #10) and add sample buffer as 4/1 (v/v).
   (b) Heat the samples at 60°C for 12 min.

(c) Place 10 μl of each sample in individual pits at the top of 0.1 × 9 × 6 cm SDS 5%-polyacrylamide gel (PAGE) slabs.

2. *Migration of the samples through the SDS-PAGE* (*see* **Note 9**)
   (a) Start the migration with a potential difference of 100 V for 10 min.
   (b) Increase the potential to 200 V once the samples have fully entered the gel. Keep it for at least 40 min.
3. *Transfer of the samples from the SDS-PAGE to the nitrocellulose membrane* (*see* **Note 10**)
   (a) Immerse the SDS-PAGE and the nitrocellulose membrane between two fiber pads in Fairbanks. Cool the solution down to 4°C by setting ice pack in the container.
   (b) Turn it on, with a current of 250 mA for 60 min (electroblotting).
   (c) Remove the membrane from the SDS-PAGE and identify the molecular weight standards with a blue pen.
   (d) Wash the membrane with distilled water.
4. *Block of aspecific immunoreactive sites*
   (a) Incubate the membrane with Milk Block buffer for 30 min.
5. *Incubation with primary antibodies* (*see* **Note 11**)
   (a) Dilute the primary antibodies in Block buffer 2% BSA:
      - Affinity-purified rabbit polyclonal antibodies (MD1314) against the C-terminus of rodent CFTR (Dr. C.R. Marino): 1/1,500;
      - Rabbit polyclonal antibodies against Rab5a (KAP-GP006, Stressgen): 1/5000;
      - Rabbit polyclonal antibodies against villin (Dr. D. Louvard and S. Robine, Institut Curie, Paris, France): 1/10,000;
      - Goat polyclonal antibodies against mature cathepsin D (C-20, SC6486, Santa Cruz Biotechnology): 1/2,000.
   (b) Remove the Milk Block buffer.
   (c) Wash the membrane with Block buffer for 5 min.
   (d) Incubate the membrane overnight at 4°C with primary antibodies.
6. *Incubation with secondary antibodies*
   (a) Save the primary antibodies for future experiments.
   (b) Rinse with Block buffer for 15 min (2×) and 5 min (2×).

(c) Incubate the nitrocellulose membrane with secondary antibodies (dilution: 1/1,500 in Milk Block) at room temperature for 60 min.

7. ***Chemiluminescence detection***

   (a) Wash the membrane with Block buffer for 15 min (2×) and 5 min (2×).

   (b) Incubate the nitrocellulose membrane with Pierce ECL solution (Thermo Fisher Scientific, Erembodegem, Belgium).

   (c) Dry the membrane and expose to X-ray film for 1–5 min (**Fig. 19.3**)

4. Notes

1. Make sure that citrate buffer has been pre-warmed to 97°C in a water bath. Do not use a microwave oven to warm your solutions and slides because of the lack of homogeneity in the heating. Plunging the container filled with citrate buffer allows a homogenous and straight heating (up to 97°C).
2. Do not touch tissue samples during manipulations. Tissue samples may not dry. Thus, manipulate the slides one by one and leave the others in TRIS solution (or in the humid chamber). Make sure that the blocking serum covers the entire surface which has been delineated by the hydropho bic pen.
3. Make sure that primary antibodies have been correctly thawed before starting the procedure. Prepare enough solution to cover each circled area with ~150 μl, but retrieve precious antibodies after use. Take advantage of each rinsing period to prepare the next solutions.
4. AEC produces a red reaction product. Slides developed with AEC must be mounted in a water solution since the reaction product is soluble in organic solvents. Monitor (by eye) the incubation time, which may vary from 10 to 30 min.
5. Keep a sample from each animal in order to confirm genotype. For example, cut the tip of mouse tail, identify it, and freeze it in an individual plastic bag.
6. The verification that organelles are well homogenized by evidencing Brownian motion of individual particles under phase contrast microscopy is essential to exclude aggregation.
7. When interpreting data, remember that (i) distributions must be validated by recovery (sum of all fractions =

starting material ± 20% max) and resolution (separation between peaks) and (ii) separation is proof, co-distribution may also reflect aggregation (16).

8. Use specific loading tip to place each sample into the defined lane at the top of the gel. Be careful not to contaminate adjacent fractions when loading. One empty lane is advised between MLP and gradient fractions.
9. Check the correct migration of the colored molecular weight standards in order to avoid loss of target proteins going out of the gel.
10. Check transfer efficiency by incubating the nitrocellulose membrane with Ponceau Red dye (Sigma) for 1 min: sample smear should rapidly appear.
11. When characterizing the position of lysosomes in Percoll gradients by probing the fractions by immunoblotting, do *not* rely on LAMP-1, which is associated with both lysosomes and low-density endosomes. Prefer the distribution of mature cathepsin D. Alternatively assay for *N*-acetyl-β-hexosaminidase activity, which is *not* inhibited by protease and phosphatase inhibitors.

Acknowledgments

The authors thank Y. Cnops, Th. Lac, and P. Van der Smissen for excellent technical assistance. The *Cftr* mice were kindly provided by H. R. De Jonge (Erasmus University Medical Center, Rotterdam, The Netherlands) and the anti-CFTR antibody MD1314 by C.R. Marino (University of Tennessee, Memphis, TN).

P. Courtoy wishes to thank G. Dom, M. Leruth, B. Marien, and F. N'Kuli for patiently adapting to mouse kidney the analytical subcellular fractionation procedure originally developed for rat liver (17). These studies were supported by the Belgian agencies FNRS and FRSM, the "Fondation Alphonse and Jean Forton," Concerted Research Actions, an Inter-university Attraction Pole (IUAP P6/05), the DIANE project (Communauté Française de Belgique), and the EUNEFRON (FP7, GA#201590) program of the European Community.

References

1. Birn, H., and Christensen, E. I. (2006) Renal albumin absorption in physiology and pathology. *Kidney Int.* **69**, 440–449.
2. Christensen, E. I., and Birn, H. (2002) Megalin and cubilin: multifunctional endocytic receptors. *Nat. Rev. Mol. Cell. Biol.* **3**, 256–266.
3. Conner, S. D., and Schmid, S. L. (2003) Regulated portals of entry into the cell. *Nature* **422**, 37–44.

4. Gekle, M. (2005) Renal tubule albumin transport. *Annu. Rev. Physiol.* **67**, 573–594.
5. Shi, L. B., Fushimi, K., Bae, H. R., and Verkman, A. S. (1991) Heterogeneity in ATP-dependent acidification in endocytic vesicles from kidney proximal tubule. Measurement of pH in individual endocytic vesicles in a cell-free system. *Biophys. J.* **59**, 1208–1217.
6. Faundez, V., and Hartzell, H. C. (2004) Intracellular chloride channels: determinants of function in the endosomal pathway. *Sci. STKE* **233**, re8.
7. Jentsch, T. J. (2008) CLC chloride channels and transporters: from genes to protein structure, pathology and physiology. *Crit. Rev. Biochem. Mol. Biol.* **43**, 3–36.
8. Devuyst, O., and Guggino, W. B. (2002) Chloride channels in the kidney: lessons learned from knockout animals. *Am. J. Physiol. Renal Physiol.* **283**, F1176–F1191.
9. Moriyama, Y., and Nelson, N. (1987) The purified ATPase from chromaffin granule membranes is an anion-dependent proton pump. *J. Biol. Chem.* **262**, 9175–9180.
10. Bradbury, N. A. (1999) Intracellular CFTR: localization and function. *Physiol. Rev.* **79**, S175–S191.
11. Bradbury, N. A., Jilling, T., Berta, G., Sorscher, E. J., Bridges, R. J., and Kirk, K. L. (1992) Regulation of plasma membrane recycling by CFTR. *Science* **256**, 530–532.
12. Barasch, J., Kiss, B., Prince, A., Saiman, L., Gruenert, D., and Al-Awqati, Q. (1991) Defective acidification of intracellular organelles in cystic fibrosis. *Nature* **352**, 70–73.
13. Poschet, J. F., Skidmore, J., Boucher, J. C., Firoved, A. M., Van Dyke, R. W, and Deretic, V. (2002) Hyperacidification of cellubrevin endocytic compartments and defective endosomal recycling in cystic fibrosis respiratory epithelial cells. *J. Biol. Chem.* **277**, 13959–13965.
14. Poschet, J. F., Fazio, J. A., Timmins, G. S., Ornatowski, W., Perkett, E., Delgado, M., et al. (2006) Endosomal hyperacidification in cystic fibrosis is due to defective nitric oxide-cyclic GMP signalling cascade. *EMBO Rep.* **7**, 553–559.
15. Jouret, F., Bernard, A., Hermans, C., Dom, G., Terryn, S., Leal, T., et al. (2007) Cystic fibrosis is associated with a defect in apical receptor-mediated endocytosis in mouse and human kidney. *J. Am. Soc. Nephrol.* **18**, 707–718.
16. Beaufay, H., and Amar-Costesec, A. (1976) Cell fractionation techniques. In (Korn, E. D., ed.) *Methods in Membrane Biology*, vol. 6. Plenum Press, New York, NY, pp. 1–100.
17. Courtoy, P. J. (1993) Analytical subcellular fractionation of endosomal compartments in rat hepatocytes. In (Bergeron, J. J. M., Harris, J. R., eds) *Subcellular Biochemistry: Endocytic Components: Identification and Characterization*, vol. 19. Plenum Press, New York, NY, pp. 29–68.
18. Devuyst, O., and Pirson, Y. (2007) Genetics of hypercalciuric stone forming diseases. *Kidney Int.* **72**, 1065–1072.
19. Draye, J.-P., Courtoy, P. J., Quintart, J., and Baudhuin, P. (1987) Relations between plasma membrane and lysosomal membrane. 2. Quantitative evaluation of plasma membrane marker enzymes in the lysosomes. *Eur. J. Biochem.* **170**, 405–411.
20. Christensen, E. I., Devuyst, O., Dom, G., Nielsen, R., Van der Smissen, P., Verroust, P., et al. (2003) Loss of chloride channel ClC-5 impairs endocytosis by defective trafficking of megalin and cubilin in kidney proximal tubules. *Proc. Natl. Acad. Sci. USA* **100**, 8472–8477.

Chapter 20

Endocytic Sorting of CFTR Variants Monitored by Single-Cell Fluorescence Ratiometric Image Analysis (FRIA) in Living Cells

Herve Barrière, Pirjo Apaja, Tsukasa Okiyoneda, and Gergely L. Lukacs

Abstract

The wild-type CFTR channel undergoes constitutive internalization and recycling at the plasma membrane. This process is initiated by the recognition of the Tyr- and di-Leu-based endocytic motifs of CFTR by the AP-2 adaptor complex, leading to the formation of clathrin-coated vesicles and the channel delivery to sorting/recycling endosomes. Accumulating evidence suggests that conformationally defective mutant CFTRs (e.g. rescued F508del and glycosylation-deficient channel) are unstable at the plasma membrane and undergo augmented ubiquitination in post-Golgi compartments. Ubiquitination conceivably accounts for the metabolic instability at cell surface by provoking accelerated internalization, as well as rerouting the channel from recycling towards lysosomal degradation. We developed an in vivo fluorescence ratiometric image analysis (FRIA) that in concert with genetic manipulation can be utilized to establish the post-endocytic fate and sorting determinants of mutant CFTRs.

Key words: CF mutations, conformational defect, endosomal sorting, recycling, lysosomal targeting, ubiquitin-binding protein, plasma membrane, ESCRT, vesicular pH, siRNA.

1. Introduction

1.1. Endocytic Membrane Trafficking: An Overview

Endocytosis is critical in preserving homeostasis at the cellular, organ and organism level by regulating cell surface receptor density, cell polarity and motility; providing nutrient uptake; as well as antigen presentation just to mention a few examples (1). Endocytosis entails the cellular uptake of macromolecules

M.D. Amaral, K. Kunzelmann (eds.), *Cystic Fibrosis*, Methods in Molecular Biology 741,
DOI 10.1007/978-1-61779-117-8_20, © Springer Science+Business Media, LLC 2011

(e.g. hormones, nutrients and viruses) from the extracellular space as well as polypeptides and lipids from the plasma membrane (1). Trafficking pathways of incoming cargo molecules, regardless of their specific entry route, seem to converge at early endosomes (1, 2). Subsequent maturation of early endosomes coincides with progressive acidification by V-ATPases and formation of the tubular endosomal network (TEN), one of the critical structures to accomplish endocytic cargo sorting (1, 3).

The biochemical and functional subcompartmentalization of the TEN in concert with adaptor and coat protein assembly at the cytoplasmic surface, defined by multiple interactions between sorting signal(s) and oligomeric adaptors with binding surfaces for coat proteins, sorting signals and phospholipid membrane, facilitates the concentration and packaging of transmembrane cargo molecules (4). Three major destinations have been delineated from the TEN (1, 5). Membrane proteins can be recycled back to the plasma membrane either by bulk flow or by signal-dependent recycling pathway (4, 6, 7). Cargo molecules could also be routed to late endosome/lysosome (e.g. Lamp1 and Lamp2) and lysosome-like organelle, relying on a variety of lysosomal sorting signals (e.g. Tyr-, di-Leu- or ubiquitin-based motifs) (8, 9). The third destination is represented by the trans-Golgi network (TGN) (e.g. TGN38 and CI-MPR) (10, 11) and mediated by retrograde transport, utilizing acidic cluster, Phe-, Trp- or Pro-rich motifs (4, 12).

1.2. Endocytic Sorting of CFTR

It has been recognized that constitutive, clathrin-dependent internalization of wt CFTR relies on the recognition of tyrosine- and di-leucine-based endocytic motifs by the heterotetrameric clathrin adaptor, the AP-2 complex (13, 14). This association is a prerequisite for CFTR concentration in invaginated plasma membrane patches and recruitment of the clathrin coat (clathrin-coated pits, CCP) that culminates in the fission of clathrin-coated vesicles (CCV) in a dynamin-mediated process. Interfering with AP-2 binding to CFTR, as well as with dynamin or Rab5 function, prevented CFTR internalization (14, 15).

Considering the channel internalization (3–4%/min) and limited translational rate (16–18), targeting of endocytosed CFTR back to the cell surface by the endosomal sorting machinery is a prerequisite to preserve its slow metabolic turnover in post-Golgi compartments ($t_{1/2}$ ~14–18 h) and avoid premature degradation (2, 17, 19). Since CFTR undergoes numerous internalization and exocytic cycles, even modest inhibition of recycling could lead to intracellular retention and concomitant destabilization of the cell surface pool, as exemplified by the cellular phenotype of conformationally destabilized mutant CFTRs (2). In accord with these considerations, wt CFTR is recycled with high efficiency via

Rab-11-positive recycling endosomes to the cell surface, utilizing an Rme1-dependent vesicular transport mechanism (15, 19). In contrast, partially unfolded mutant CFTRs are subjected to ubiquitination at a presently unidentified location in post-Golgi compartments and recognized by ubiquitin-dependent endosomal sorting machinery (ESCRT0-III; (2)). While physical association with F508del-CFTR has been detected, the functional consequence of ESCRT interaction with CFTR remains poorly defined. Here we describe a method to determine not only the post-endocytic fate but also the functional relevance of endocytic adaptors to interorganellar transport based on vesicular pH (pH_v) measurements of internalized CFTR-containing transport vesicles.

1.3. Determination of CFTR Localization in Endo-lysosomal Compartment by Vesicular pH Measurements

Since the pH_v of sorting endosome, recycling endosome, late endosome/MVB, lysosome and the trans-Golgi network (TGN) has been relatively well defined (1), the pH_v of CFTR-containing transport vesicles could be taken as an indicator of the channel localization. The pH_v is determined by single-cell fluorescence ratiometric image analysis (FRIA). The FRIA technique was originally described for lysosomal pH determination following the labelling of lysosomal compartment with the fluid-phase marker dextran, conjugated to the pH-sensitive fluorescein isothiocyanate (FITC) (20).

Here we summarize the FRIA developed in order to determine the destination and sorting kinetics of CFTRs after synchronized internalization of the channel in complex with FITC-labelled Ab (**Section 3.1**). This approach is recommended to define the destination and interorganellar transport kinetics of the CFTR. If the limited plasma membrane density of the cargo precludes the sufficient labelling of endocytic compartments by synchronized internalization, continuous Ab capture is used to increase the sensitivity of the assay, as described in **Section 3.2**. The authors used these methods to uncover endosomal sorting pathways of multiple cargo molecules, including CFTR variants (21, 22). Determination of the fluorescence intensity ratio as a function of vesicular pH provides the in situ calibration for FRIA experiments as described in **Section 3.3**. The application of FRIA to determine the functional relevance of ubiquitin-binding ESCRT adaptors is described in **Section 3.4**. Considering that cell-specific variations may occur in the steady-state pH_v of organelles, pH_v measurements of recycling endosomes and lysosomes are included in **Section 3.5**. Finally, a brief description of immunolocalization experiments is included to validate the results obtained by FRIA (**Section 3.6**).

2. Materials

2.1. Monitoring Endocytic Trafficking of CFTR by Fluorescence Ratiometric Image Analysis (FRIA) of Vesicular pH

2.1.1. Cell Culture Medium

Use the appropriate bicarbonate-containing medium (e.g. Dulbecco's modified Eagle's medium (DMEM) for HeLa cells or DMEM/F12 for BHK cells) supplemented with 10% or 5% FBS, respectively (Invitrogen) for culturing the cells in a CO_2 incubator. Sodium bicarbonate- and phenol red-free medium, containing 15 mM HEPES and 5% bovine serum (BS), is used for incubating the cells on ice. Medium should be stored at 4°C.

PBS++: Phosphate-buffered saline supplemented with 1 mM $CaCl_2$, 0.1 mM $MgCl_2$, 0.5% BSA, bovine serum albumin. Store at 4°C.

2.1.2. CFTR Labelling

1. Anti-HA antibody (1:500 dilution equivalent to 10 μg/ml, MMS-101R, Covance)
2. FITC-conjugated goat anti-mouse secondary Fab (Jackson ImmunoResearch Laboratories)

2.1.3. Instrumentation

1. Tissue culture incubator at 37°C with 5% CO_2
2. Inverted microscope equipped for fluorescence ratio imaging (**Note 1**)
3. 6-well culture plates (Falcon #353046)
4. Glass coverslip 25 mm with standard #1 or #1.5 thickness
5. Perfusion chamber (MSC-TD, Warner Instruments, Inc.)

2.2. Multi-point In Situ pH Calibration

1. 10 mg/ml nigericin (Sigma, #N-7143) in ethanol. Store at –20°C.
2. 10 mg/ml monensin (Sigma, # M-5273) in ethanol. Store at –20°C.
3. K^+-rich buffer for in situ pH calibration: 10 mM NaCl, 135 mM KCl, 10 mM glucose, 1 mM $CaCl_2$, 0.1 mM $MgCl_2$, 20 mM MES for pH $\leq$5.5, 20 mM HEPES for pH >5.5. Adjust pH with KOH and store at 4°C.
4. NaKH solution: 140 mM NaCl, 5 mM KCl, 10 mM HEPES, 10 mM glucose, 1 mM $CaCl_2$, 0.1 mM $MgCl_2$. Adjust the pH to 7.3 and store at 4°C.

2.3. FRIA to Assess the Role of ESCRT Component in the Endocytic Sorting of CFTR

1. HeLa cell lines stably expressing the reverse tetracyclin transactivator and the Hrs-specific shRNAmir plasmid (pTRIPZ, OpenBiosystems) (*see* **Section 3.4.1**)

2.4. Measuring the pH of Recycling Endosomes and Lysosomes

1. FITC-transferrin (Tf) (Molecular Probes, Inc.)
2. Holotransferrin (#T-0665, Sigma)
3. Albumin chicken (ovalbumin) (#A-2153, Sigma)
4. FITC-dextran (M.W.: 10 kDa anionic, #D1822 Molecular Probes, Inc.)
5. Dextran (M.W.: 68.8 kDa, #D4876 Sigma)

2.5. Immunocolocalization of Internalized CFTR with Organellar Markers

1. Paraformaldehyde 4%: Add 1 g PFA to 20 ml PBS and heat to 65°C to dissolve. Add 750 μl 1 M sucrose and make up the volume to 25 ml with PBS. Filter and store the solution in the dark at –20°C up to 2 weeks
2. TRITC-conjugated goat anti-mouse Fab (1:500 dilution, Jackson ImmunoResearch Laboratories, West Grove, PA, USA)
3. FITC-Tf (Molecular Probes, Inc.), FITC-dextran (M.W.: 10 kDa anionic, Molecular Probes, Inc.)
4. Mounting medium (Vectashield H-1200, Vector Laboratories, Burlingame, CA)
5. Laser confocal fluorescence microscope (e.g. LSM 510 Carl Zeiss)

3. Methods

To monitor the post-endocytic trafficking, CFTR variants with the 3HA-tag in the fourth extracellular loop were expressed heterologously (e.g. BHK, HeLa and CFBE (2, 22, 23)). Labelling of CFTR-3HA with primary anti-HA IgG and FITC-conjugated secondary Fab by Ab capture in vivo enabled to determine the luminal pH of endocytic vesicles harbouring the CFTR channel (2, 22, 23).

3.1. Monitoring Synchronized Endocytic Trafficking of CFTR by Fluorescence Ratiometric Image Analysis (FRIA) of Vesicular pH

This method illustrates the distinct post-endocytic sorting of the wt and rescued (r)F508del-CFTR following synchronized internalization. First, the anti-HA primary and FITC-conjugated secondary Fab were bound to CFTR-3HA expressing BHK cells on ice. Then internalization was initiated by raising the temperature to 37°C for 0–60 min, followed by FRIA using an inverted epifluorescence microscope. Cells were illuminated alternatively with 495 and 440 nm fluorescent light and the (PFA) emitted

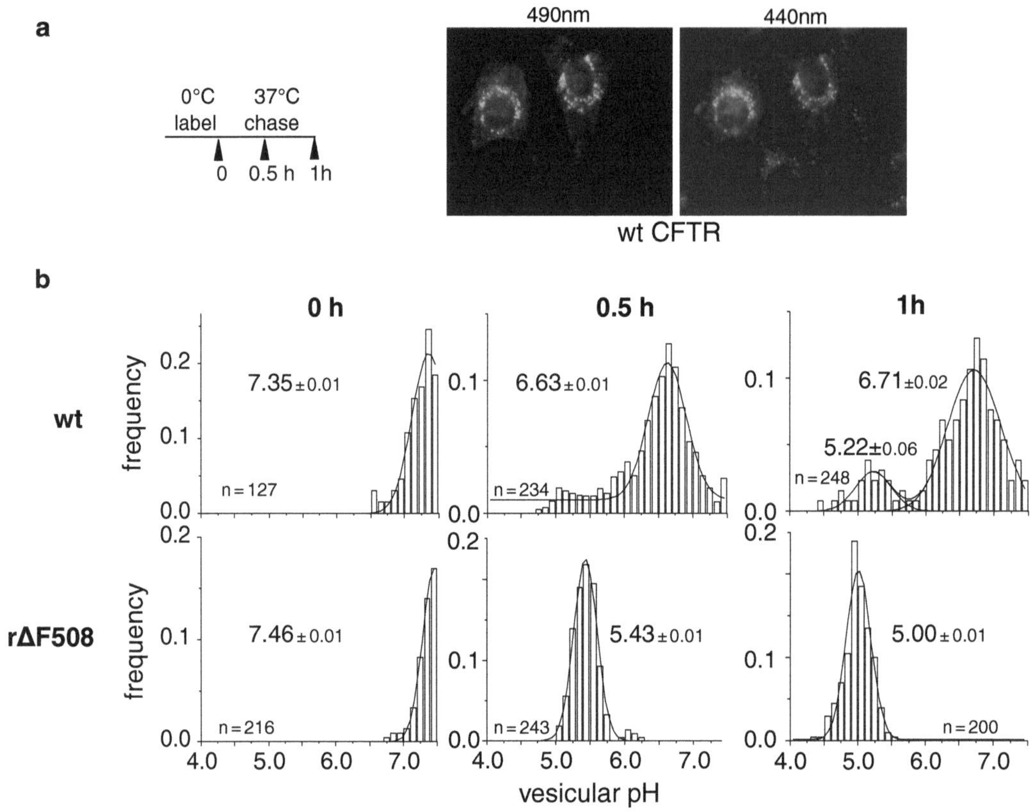

Fig. 20.1. Monitoring the wt and rF508del-CFTR-3HA post-endocytic sorting by vesicular pH (pH_V) measurement using the FRIA. (**a**) Anti-HA antibody and FITC-conjugated secondary Fab were bound to CFTR-expressing BHK cells for 1 h at 0°C. Then the temperature was raised to 37°C for 0, 0.5 or 1 h, and the pH_V was measured by FRIA. Representative fluorescent micrographs of wt CFTR-containing vesicles at 490 (pH-sensitive) and 450 nm (pH-insensitive) excitation wavelengths expressed in BHK cells after 30 min chase. (**b**) The lysosomal delivery kinetics of rF508del-CFTR. Data are expressed as frequency of pH_V and means (±SEM) pH_V of the major endosomal population. The number of vesicles analysed in a single experiment is indicated.

fluorescence was detected at 535 nm with a cooled CCD camera (**Fig. 20.1**). Since FITC fluorescence at 495 nm excitation, but not at 440 nm, is sensitive to pH, normalization ensures that the fluorescence light intensity ratio ($495_{nm}/440_{nm}$) is largely pH-dependent and independent of the dye concentration (24).

3.1.1. Cell Preparation

1. Seed BHK cells stably expressing CFTR-3HA (2, 23) on sterile glass coverslips at least 24 h before the experiment. Use 6-well tissue culture plates and 2 ml DMEM/F12 supplemented with 5% v/v FBS. Prepare non-transfected cells to verify that the non-specific fluorescent signal is negligible. By the time of the FRIA, cells should be at 60–70% confluence.

3.1.2. Labelling with the pH-Sensitive Probe

1. Rinse the cells twice with 2 ml ice-cold medium (bicarbonate-free DMEM/F12) gently to avoid cell loss.
2. Bind the primary anti-HA antibody (1:400–800 dilution) in 0.8 ml bicarbonate-free DMEM/F12 containing 5% v/v bovine serum (BS) for 1 h on ice (**Note 2**).
3. Rinse the cells with 2 ml ice-cold bicarbonate-free DMEM/F12 supplemented with 5% (v/v) BS three times.
4. Bind FITC-conjugated goat anti-mouse Fab (1:500 dilution) in 0.8 ml bicarbonate-free DMEM/F12 supplemented with 5% v/v BS on ice.
5. Rinse the cells with 2 ml ice-cold bicarbonate-free DMEM/F12 three times.

3.1.3. Internalization

1. CFTR endocytosis is induced by the addition of 2 ml pre-warmed DMEM/F12 supplemented with bicarbonate and 5% v/v FBS and by transferring the plate into the tissue culture incubator (37°C) for the desired time.
2. Terminate the internalization by rinsing the cells with 2 ml ice-cold PBS++ solution and placing the coverslip in 35 mm tissue culture dish on ice in 2 ml NaKH solution.

3.1.4. Acquisition of Fluorescent Ratio Images

1. Mount the coverslip in the perfusion chamber and add 0.8 ml of NaKH solution (25°C). Place the chamber in the thermostated coverslip holder pre-warmed to 25°C. The microscope objective temperature should be maintained at 25°C with a dedicated heater.
2. Acquire image pairs at 495 and 440 nm excitation wavelengths by selecting at least 10–15 areas on the coverslip. This step should be performed in a timely manner to avoid significant cargo processing (**Note 3**).

3.1.5. Single-Point In Situ pH Calibration

After completing image acquisition, single-point calibration is performed to verify that the microscope optical characteristics correspond to that observed during the multi-point calibration.

1. Aspirate the NaKH solution and add 0.8 ml of freshly prepared K^+-rich medium containing 10 μM nigericin and 10 μM monensin (pH = 6.5, 25°C).
2. To ensure that vesicular H^+ concentration is equilibrated with the extracellular medium pH, replace the K^+-rich medium (0.8 ml) supplemented with nigericin and monensin once more (**Note 4**).
3. Record the fluorescence ratio. If the fluorescence ratio is different from that observed by the multi-point calibration technique, the system has to be recalibrated as described in **Section 3.3**.

3.1.6. Vesicular pH Analysis

1. Set up the MetaFluor program to obtain the average fluorescence intensity values of selected regions of interest (ROIs) at 495 and 440 nm excitation wavelengths in an Excel table. The average fluorescence intensity represents the integrated fluorescence intensity divided by the area of the ROI (**Note 1**).
2. Select all of the ROIs corresponding to labelled vesicles in the first cell (**Note 5**).
   In the same cells select three cytoplasmic ROIs that are free of labelled vesicles. These ROIs with comparable size to that of selected ROIs in the previous step will serve to calculate the background fluorescence.
3. Acquire the mean fluorescence intensity value of ROIs for all cells repeating steps 1 and 2.
   The Excel file contains the mean fluorescence intensity value for each ROI at 495 and 440 nm excitation wavelengths and the background signal for each cell. Calculate the mean background fluorescence intensity at 495 and 440 nm excitation wavelengths for each cell. Subtract the mean background fluorescence values from the mean fluorescence intensity of each ROI at 495 and 440 nm excitation wavelengths to obtain the specific fluorescent signal.
4. Calculate the mean fluorescence intensity ratio for each ROI by dividing the background subtracted mean fluorescence intensity at 495 and 440 nm. Based on the multi-point calibration curve (*see* **Section 3.1**), the fluorescence ratio values of ROIs are converted to pH_V values.
5. Frequency distributions of pH_V values are plotted by the Origin 7.0 software using single- or multi-component Gaussian distribution (**Fig. 20.1b**). The mean pH_V is calculated for the individual peak. Partitioning of cargo molecule into various organelles can be estimated based on the fractional distribution of vesicles in the individual peak relative to the total number of vesicles.

3.2. Monitoring Endocytic Trafficking of CFTR by Continuous Antibody Capture and FRIA

If the steady-state expression of the mutant CFTR (e.g. low temperature rF508del-CFTR) at the cell surface is insufficient for synchronized labelling and endocytosis (**Section 3.1**), association of Ab with a larger cohort of channels could be achieved by continuous labelling in the presence of extracellular primary anti-HA and FITC-labelled secondary Fab at 37°C. This 0.5–1 h labelling usually provides sufficient signal followed by 0–2 h chase at 37°C. Although the temporal resolution of this assay is reduced as compared to that described in **Section 3.1**, the lysosomal targeting of F508del and the glycosylation-deficient CFTR and the highly efficient recycling of the wt form were readily demonstrated (2, 22, 23). The assay could be used in both stably and transiently transfected cells. The detailed methodology, including cell preparation, imaging and data analysis, is similar to that described in **Section 3.1** except the labelling step of CFTR.

3.2.1. Labelling CFTR with pH-Sensitive Probe

1. Incubate the cells on individual coverslip with anti-HA antibody and FITC-conjugated goat anti-mouse Fab for 30–60 min in 1 ml cell medium supplemented with FBS at 37°C in tissue culture incubator. The usual antibody dilution is decreased due to the loss of respective antibody affinity (1/100–500) when they are complexed simultaneously.
2. Thoroughly wash away the extracellular antibodies with 2 ml PBS++ at room temperature (RT) and resume the incubation of cells in 2 ml cell medium + FBS for 0–200 min at 37°C in the tissue culture incubator.

3.3. Multi-point In Situ pH Calibration

To calibrate the fluorescence ratio values as a function of pH_v, FRIA was performed after clamping the luminal pH of intracellular organelles loaded with primary Ab and FITC-conjugated secondary Fab. To optimize signal-to-noise ratio, calibration was usually, but not exclusively, performed on cells expressing cargo molecule that was retained intracellularly (e.g. rF508del-CFTR). If the cargo is recycled with high efficiency, plasma membrane-bound Abs should be removed by acid washes (**Note 6**). Following the loading of intracellular vesicles with FITC-conjugated Fab, the luminal pH of intracellular compartments was clamped to the extracellular pH (pH_e) in the presence of monensin and nigericin, ionophores that mediate H^+/Na^+ and H^+/K^+ exchange (25, 26). Multi-point calibration curve was obtained by conducting FRIA at various pH_e in the range of 7.4–4.5. The theoretical basis of this method has been previously described (24). For each pH_e value, ~200–300 vesicles are determined and the mean pH_v is calculated, based on single-peak Gaussian distribution of pH_v (**Fig. 20.2a–b**). Considering that the pH sensitivity of FITC is reduced at pH < 5.4 (pK_a ~ 6.4), the methodology at pH_v < 5.4 can be validated using a mixture of Oregon Green-dextran (70%) and FITC-dextran (30%) (**Note** 7).

3.3.1. Cell Preparation

See **Section 3.1.1**.

3.3.2. Preparation of Calibration Solutions

1. Prepare 50 ml aliquots of K^+-rich medium and adjust the pH to 4.5, 5.0, 5.5, 6.0, 6.3, 6.6, 6.9, 7.2 and 7.4. Add nigericin (10 μM) and monensin (10 μM) from 10 mM stocks before the experiment. The buffer composition of the calibration medium should be changed according to its final pH. Use 20 mM MES and 20 mM HEPES for medium with

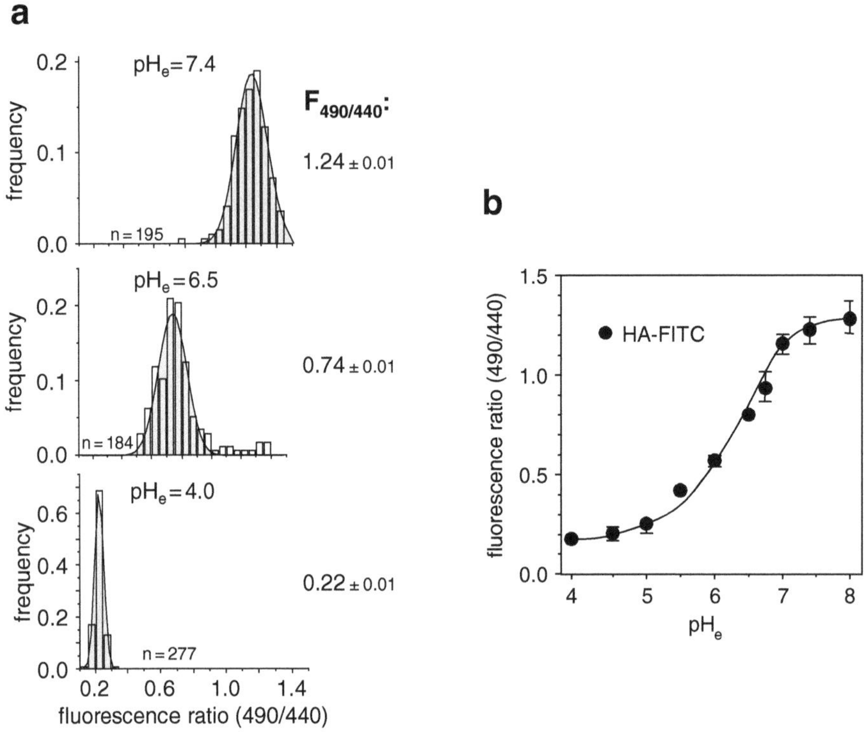

Fig. 20.2. In situ calibration of the FRIA. (**a**) Distributions of fluorescence ratios of intracellular vesicles after clamping the intracellular space at the indicated extracellular pH (pHe) in the presence of monensin and nigericin. Anti-HA primary Ab and FITC-conjugated secondary Fab were complexed with CFTR and chased for 30 min before FRIA as described in **Section 3.3**. (**b**) Calibration curve using CFTRwt-3HA in BHK cells. Internalization of Ab was performed as described in **Section 3.1**. Data were obtained on indicated number of vesicles on 15 fields (means ± SEM).

pH ≤ 5.5 and pH > 5.5, respectively. The medium pH should be adjusted with 1 M KOH at 25°C and filter sterilized. Do not store buffers longer than 4 weeks at 4°C and check the medium pH prior to use at 25°C.

3.3.3. Labelling CFTR with pH-Sensitive Probe

1. Internalize anti-HA primary IgG and FITC-conjugated secondary Fab in complex with CFTR-3HA as described in **Section 3.1**. The internalization time could be extended to increase the fluorescence signal-to-noise ratio.
2. Wash the cells three times with 2 ml PBS++ at RT.

3.3.4. Acquisition of Fluorescence Ratiometric Images

1. Place the coverslips in the perfusion chamber and add 0.8 ml K^+-rich calibration medium containing 10 μM nigericin and 10 μM monensin at 25°C.
2. Incubate for 1–2 min and replace the medium to facilitate fast equilibration of the intracellular and extracellular pH (identical volume as step 4). Wait for an additional 2–3 min and proceed with image acquisition by selecting 10–20 areas on the coverslip (**Note 8**).

3.3.5. In Situ Calibration of Fluorescence Ratio Values as a Function of pH_v

Calculation of the intracellular vesicle pH is based on the relationship between fluorescence ratio and pH_v values, established by the in situ multi-point calibration technique (**Fig. 20.2**).

1. The fluorescence ratios of intracellular vesicles clamped to pH 4.5–7.4 are fitted by non-linear regression analysis according to a modified version of the Henderson–Hasselbalch equation, as described originally (24):

$$pH_i = pK_a - \log_{10}\left(\frac{R_{max} - R_i}{R_i - R_{min}}\right),$$

where R_i is the fluorescence ratio $(I_{495\,nm}/I_{440\,nm})$ after background subtraction; R_{max} and R_{min} are the asymptotes of minimum and maximum ratio values at highly acidic and alkaline pH, respectively. The apparent dissociation constant of FITC is indicated by pK_a, and pH_i is the intracellular pH. Rearranging the equation for defining R yields (27)

$$R_i = \frac{R_{min} + R_{max}10^{(pH_i - pK_a)}}{10^{(pH_i - pK_a)} + 1}$$

2. Based on measured ratio values at different pH, the R_{max} and R_{min} values were iterated by the Prism 4® (GraphPad software, San Diego, CA, USA) software. The pH_v of CFTR-containing vesicles was calculated by Excel using extrapolated constants and the calculated R value.

3.4. Using FRIA to Assess the Role of ESCRT in the Endocytic Sorting of CFTR

The cell surface density of plasma membrane receptors and transporters is regulated by signal-dependent ubiquitination and coupled downregulation via the endo-lysosomal-associated degradation (ELAD) (21, 28). A similar paradigm was proposed for the rapid retrieval of rescued (r)F508del and glycosylation-deficient CFTR from the cell surface with the distinction that the destabilized channel downregulation is initiated by partial unfolding (2, 22). Association of the Ub-binding endosomal sorting complex components (e.g. Hrs, STAM and TSG101) with the rF508del-CFTR has been documented (2). Here FRIA was used to assess whether Hrs binding has any functional role in the lysosomal delivery of the rF508del-CFTR by monitoring the post-endocytic membrane trafficking of the internalized channel in Hrs-depleted cells (**Fig. 20.3**).

3.4.1. Cell Preparation

1. To achieve Hrs downregulation, the HeLa cells were stably transfected with pTRIPZ lentivirus expressing microRNA-adapted short hairpin RNA (shRNAMir, Open Biosystem) containing 30miR for Hrs sequence (V2THS_36954). The pTRIPZ is an inducible bicistronic vector containing the tetracycline-inducible promoter-driven shRNA and

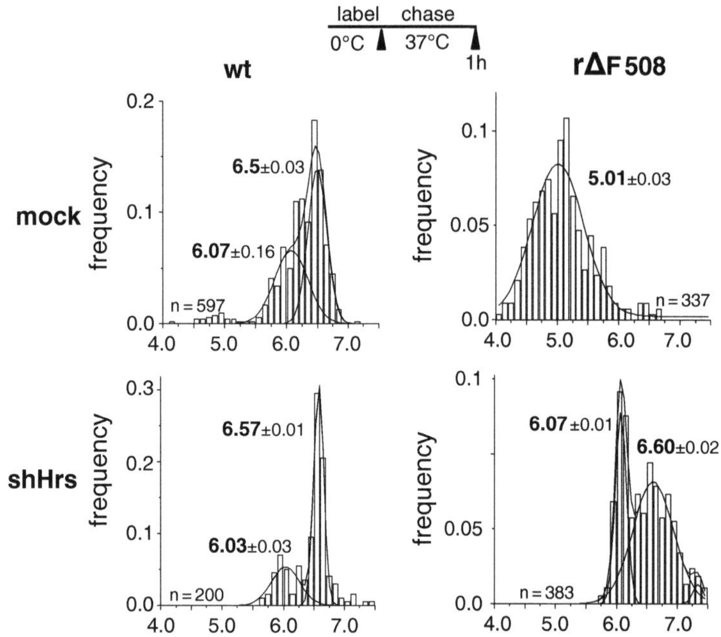

Fig. 20.3. Hrs knockdown impedes the rF508del-CFTR delivery into lysosomes. Post-endocytic targeting of internalized CFTRs was monitored by vesicular pH (pH_V) measurement on HeLa cells transiently expressing the indicated CFTR variant as described in **Section 3.5**. Anti-HA antibody and FITC-conjugated secondary Fab were bound for 1 h at 0°C to HeLa-expressing shHrs, as well as the wt or rF508del-CFTR. Cells were chased for 1 h at 37° C prior to FRIA. Data were obtained on indicated number of vesicles on 10–15 fields (means ± SEM). The mean pH_V of the subpopulations is depicted.

the turbo red fluorescent protein (TurboRFP). The cells were selected in the presence of 5 μg/ml puromycin, and the expression of shRNA was verified inducing the cells with 500 ng/ml doxycycline for 24 h and checking the TurboRFP fluorescence marking the inducible shRNA expression. Immunoblotting showed that doxycycline (500 ng/ml) treatment for 5 days reduced the cellular Hrs expression level by 75% (data not shown). After 3 days of doxycycline induction, HeLa cells were transiently transfected with wt or F508del-CFTR-3HA using Fugene (Roche) according to the instructions of the manufacturer. On the fourth day the cells were seeded on glass coverslips and incubated for an additional 24–36 h at 26°C in the presence of doxycycline to rescue the F508del-CFTR processing defect.

3.4.2. CFTR Labelling, FRIA, Calibration and Data Analysis

These steps are performed as described in **Section 3.1**. **Figure 20.3** illustrates that the lysosomal delivery of internalized rF508del-CFTR-3HA was significantly delayed in Hrs-depleted, but not in parental, cells (**Note 9**).

3.5. Measuring the pH of Recycling Endosomes and Lysosomes

To confine the internalized CFTR localization to specific endocytic organelles based on pH_V determination, determination of the luminal pH of early recycling endosomes, lysosomes and TGN is recommended using organelle-specific markers. Here, the labelling of recycling endosomes and lysosomes for FRIA is described (21, 23, 29). Since approximately 80% of the cellular transferrin receptor (TfR) pool is confined to recycling endosomes in steady state (1, 23), FITC-Tf was used to monitor the pH of recycling endosomes. Selective labelling of the lysosomal compartment was achieved by the fluid-phase marker, FITC-dextran (30). Following the FITC-dextran uptake, cells were incubated in dextran-free medium to ensure that early and late endosomes were cleared of fluorophores. Colocalization of FITC-dextran loaded lysosomes with Lamp1 can validate the specificity of the dextran labelling (21, 28, 31). Following the labelling of recycling endosomes and lysosomes, FRIA, image acquisition, calibration and data analysis were performed as described in **Sections 3.1** and **3.3**.

3.5.1. Labelling of Recycling Endosomes with FITC-Tf

1. Deplete endogenous Tf by incubating cells in 2 ml serum-free, bicarbonate-containing DMEM for 45 min at 37°C in the tissue culture incubator.
2. Load the cells in 1 ml serum-free DMEM containing 5–15 μg/ml FITC-Tf and bicarbonate for 1 h at 37°C in the tissue culture incubator.
3. Transfer the cells on ice and rinse the cells four times with 1 mg/ml ovalbumin and 0.1 mg/ml holotransferrin containing 2 ml bicarbonate-free DMEM with 5% v/v BS.

3.5.2. Lysosomes Labelling with FITC-Dextran

1. Incubate cells with 50 μg/ml FITC-dextran overnight in 2 ml DMEM in the tissue culture incubator at 37°C. Filter-sterilize the dextran solution (0.22 μm disposable sterile filter unit) to avoid contamination of cells.
2. Rinse the cells three times with 2 ml PBS++.
3. Incubate the cells in 2 ml DMEM containing 10% FBS and 100 μg/ml dextran for 3 h in the tissue culture incubator at 37°C.

3.5.3. CFTR Labelling, FRIA, Calibration and Data Analysis

These steps can be performed as described in **Section 3.1**.

3.6. Immunocolocalization of Internalized CFTR with Organellar Markers

Subcellular distribution of internalized CFTR, determined by FRIA, should be validated by colocalization studies using organellar markers. To this end internalized CFTR is labelled with the Ab capture assay as described for FRIA experiment (**Section 3.2**). Although recycling endosomes and lysosomes could be labelled with fluorophore-conjugated Tf and dextran, respectively (21, 23), these organelles could also be visualized by organelle-specific antibodies, e.g. TfR or rab11 (recycling endosomes), Lamp1, Lamp2 and CD63 (MVB/lysosomes) and TGN46 or giantin (TGN) that are available commercially.

3.6.1. Labelling Internalized CFTR by Ab Capture

1. Internalize the anti-HA primary and secondary Abs complexed with cargo molecule of interest as described in **Section 3.2**. The use of secondary TRITC- or Cy3-conjugated Fab is recommended to minimize photobleaching. If mouse primary Ab is only available for organelle identification, CFTR immunostaining should be performed using goat anti-HA Ab (#A190-107P/F, Bethyl, Montgomery, TX, USA).
2. The loading protocol for recycling endosomes and lysosomes with TRITC-Tf and TRITC-dextran has been described (21, 23, 29). It is possible to label two different cargoes simultaneously. For example, during the 45 min TRITC-Tf (5 μg/ml) loading period, CFTR labelling was carried out with anti-HA Ab.
3. Incubate the cells in 2 ml Ab-free medium for 30 min or as performed in the FRIA experiment (**Note 10**).
4. Wash the cells twice with 2 ml ice-cold PBS++.
5. Fix the cells in 1 ml PBS++ containing 4% PFA for 10 min at RT.
6. Wash the cells three times (5 min each) with 2 ml PBS++ solution, once with 0.1 M glycine containing PBS++ to quench the PFA.
7. Mount the cells in mounting medium.
8. Collect single optical sections with laser confocal fluorescence microscope (21, 23).
9. The extent of colocalization can be analysed quantitatively by using an appropriate software program (e.g. Volocity®, PerkinElmer or Imaris®, Bitplane).

4. Notes

1. The FRIA measurement could be performed on a fluorescence microscope (e.g. Zeiss Axiovert 100 TV) equipped with an excitation filter wheel and high-sensitivity cooled CCD camera. Our microscope had the following configuration: Planachromat objective (63× NA 1.4, Carl Zeiss MicroImaging, Inc.); excitation filters, D495/10

and D440/20; emission filter, D535/25 (these filters are included in the filter set for ratiometric analysis of BCECF by Chroma. Inc.) incorporated into the Lambda 10-2 (Sutter Instrument) filter wheel; X-Cite 120 fluorescence illumination system (EXFO) allowing the adjustment of the Xe-lamp intensity and Hamamatsu ORCA-ER CCD camera. The temperature was maintained by a thermostated coverslip holder (Bipolar temperature controller, TC-202, Med Systems Corp., Greenvale, NY) and objective heater (TempControl mini, Carl Zeiss MicroImaging, Inc.). Data acquisition and analysis were performed by MetaFluor® (MDS Analytical Technologies) Imaging System and OriginPro7® (OriginLab® Corporation) software run on a PC computer.

2. Optimize the antibody concentration to maximize the fluorescence signal and minimize the background fluorescence. This could be achieved by using serial dilutions of the primary and secondary Abs on transfected and non-transfected cells in pilot studies in concert with quantitative fluorescence video image analysis.
3. It is advised that the first coverslip is used to adjust the exposure time, the camera gain and the fluorescence light intensity and/or the lamp intensity to avoid photobleaching and saturation of the CCD camera. This is particularly important when cargo molecules partition between lysosomes and recycling endosomes in the same experiment.
4. The equilibration time required for clamping the intracellular pH to 6.5 may vary according to the vesicles and cell analysed. Therefore it is important to ascertain that the fluorescence ratio reached a steady-state value by repeated image acquisition during an ~5 min time period.
5. Use the image obtained at 495 nm excitation wavelength for the selection since the signal-to-noise ratio is better at 495 than at 440 nm. Identify as many vesicles as possible. Usually we avoid analysing vesicles residing in close proximity to the plasma membrane.
6. Stripping of cell surface Ab could be accomplished by incubating the cells in 1 ml ice-cold medium at pH 2.5 for 2 min (0.2 M acetic acid, 0.2 M NaCl, adjust to pH 2.5 with NaOH), washing with 1.5 ml ice-cold PBS++ twice and then incubating the cells for 3 min in 1 ml cold Recovery buffer (150 mM NaCl, 20 mM HEPES, 1 mM $CaCl_2$, 5 mM KCl, 0.1 mM $MgCl_2$, adjust to pH 7.4 with NaOH). These steps should be repeated three to four times at least.
7. The combination of dyes increases the pH sensitivity at acid pH, since the pK_a of Oregon Green is ~4.7 (32). The

Oregon Green/FITC-dextran loading protocol provided similar lysosomal pH_v values to that obtained with FITC-dextran alone, suggesting that the extrapolating procedure for $pH_v < 5.4$ in the presence of FITC alone is fairly reliable (21).

8. It is critical to use identical or very similar acquisition parameters, including exposure time, light intensities and camera gain, during the calibration and the FRIA experiment. If the emitted fluorescence light intensities are either below or above the detection limit, adjust the illumination light intensity, camera gain and/or exposure time appropriately.
9. To monitor the non-specific effect of Hrs downregulation, it is recommended to determine the lysosomal delivery kinetics of various lysosomal cargoes (e.g. Lamp1, Lamp2 and CD63 and the fluid-phase marker dextran). This would rule out non-specific effects as described previously (22).
10. Due to the rapid recycling and extracellular dissociation of the FITC-Tf from the Tf-receptor, incubation of cells at 37°C should be avoided in the absence of labelled Tf. To accomplish this goal, the chase of labelled CFTR is performed in the presence of fluorophore-conjugated Tf.

References

1. Mukherjee, S., Ghosh, R., and Maxfield, F. (1997) Endocytosis. *Physiol. Rev.* **77**, 759–803.
2. Sharma, M., Pampinella, F., Nemes, C., Benharouga, M., So, J., Du, K., et al. (2004) Misfolding diverts CFTR from recycling to degradation: quality control at early endosomes. *J. Cell Biol.* **164**, 923–933.
3. Sun-Wada, G. H., Wada, Y., and Futai, M. (2004) Diverse and essential roles of mammalian vacuolar-type proton pump ATPase: toward the physiological understanding of inside acidic compartments. *Biochim. Biophys. Acta* **1658**, 106–114.
4. Bonifacino, J. S., and Traub, L. M. (2003) Signals for sorting of transmembrane proteins to endosomes and lysosomes. *Annu. Rev. Biochem.* **72**, 395–447.
5. Katzmann, D. J., Odorizzi, G., and Emr, S. D. (2002) Receptor downregulation and multivesicular-body sorting. *Nat. Rev. Mol. Cell Biol.* **3**, 893–905.
6. Maxfield, F. R., and McGraw, T. E. (2004) Endocytic recycling. *Nat. Rev. Mol. Cell Biol.* **5**, 121–132.
7. von Zastrow, M., and Sorkin, A. (2007) Signaling on the endocytic pathway. *Curr. Opin. Cell Biol.* **19**, 436–445.
8. Janvier, K., and Bonifacino, J. S. (2005) Role of the endocytic machinery in the sorting of lysosome-associated membrane proteins. *Mol. Biol. Cell* **16**, 4231–4242.
9. Marks, M. S., Woodruff, L., Ohno, H., and Bonifacino, J. S. (1996) Protein targeting by tyrosine- and di-leucine-based signals: evidence for distinct saturable components. *J. Cell Biol.* **135**, 341–354.
10. Ghosh, P., Dahms, N. M., and Kornfeld, S. (2003) Mannose 6-phosphate receptors: new twists in the tale. *Nat. Rev. Mol. Cell Biol.* **4**, 202–212.
11. Humphrey, J. S., Peters, P. J., Yuan, L. C., and Bonifacino, J. S. (1993) Localization of TGN38 to the trans-Golgi network: involvement of a cytoplasmic tyrosine-containing sequence. *J. Cell Biol.* **120**, 1123–1135.
12. Bonifacino, J. S., and Rojas, R. (2006) Retrograde transport from endosomes to the trans-Golgi network. *Nat. Rev. Mol. Cell Biol.* **7**, 568–579.

13. Lukacs, G. L., Segal, G., Kartner, N., Grinstein, S., and Zhang, F. (1997) Constitutive internalization of cystic fibrosis transmembrane conductance regulator occurs via clathrin-dependent endocytosis and is regulated by protein phosphorylation. *Biochem. J.* **328**, 353–361.
14. Weixel, K. M., and Bradbury, N. A. (2001) Mu 2 binding directs the cystic fibrosis transmembrane conductance regulator to the clathrin-mediated endocytic pathway. *J. Biol. Chem.* **276**, 46251–46259.
15. Gentzsch, M., Chang, X. B., Cui, L., Wu, Y., Ozols, V. V., Choudhury, A., et al. (2004) Endocytic trafficking routes of wild type and DeltaF508 cystic fibrosis transmembrane conductance regulator. *Mol. Biol. Cell* **15**, 2684–2696.
16. Prince, L. S., Peter, K., Hatton, S. R., Zaliauskiene, L., Cotlin, L. F., Clancy, J. P., et al. (1999) Efficient endocytosis of the cystic fibrosis transmembrane conductance regulator requires a tyrosine-based signal. *J. Biol. Chem.* **274**, 3602–3609.
17. Swiatecka-Urban, A., Duhaime, M., Coutermarsh, B., Karlson, K. H., Collawn, J., Milewski, M., et al. (2002) PDZ domain interaction controls the endocytic recycling of the cystic fibrosis transmembrane conductance regulator. *J. Biol. Chem.* **277**, 40099–40105.
18. Swiatecka-Urban, A., Boyd, C., Coutermarsh, B., Karlson, K. H., Barnaby, R., Aschenbrenner, L., et al. (2004) Myosin VI regulates endocytosis of the cystic fibrosis transmembrane conductance regulator. *J. Biol. Chem.* **279**, 38025–38031.
19. Picciano, J. A., Ameen, N., Grant, B. D., and Bradbury, N. A. (2003) Rme-1 regulates the recycling of the cystic fibrosis transmembrane conductance regulator. *Am. J. Physiol. Cell Physiol.* **285**, C1009–C1018.
20. Ohkuma, S., and Poole, B. (1978) Fluorescence probe measurement of the intralysosomal pH in living cells and the perturbation of pH by various agents. *Proc. Natl. Acad. Sci. USA* **75**, 3327–3331.
21. Barriere, H., Nemes, C., Du, K., and Lukacs, G. L. (2007) Plasticity of poly-ubiquitin recognition as lysosomal targeting signals by the endosomal sorting machinery. *Mol. Biol. Cell* **18**, 3952–3965.
22. Glozman, R., Okiyoneda, T., Mulvihill, C. M., Rini, J. M., Barriere, H., and Lukacs, G. L. (2009) N-glycans are direct determinants of CFTR folding and stability in secretory and endocytic membrane traffic. *J. Cell Biol.* **184**, 847–862.
23. Barriere, H., Bagdany, M., Bossard, F., Okiyoneda, T., Wojewodka, G., Gruenert, D., et al. (2009) Revisiting the role of cystic fibrosis transmembrane conductance regulator and counterion permeability in the pH regulation of endocytic organelles. *Mol. Biol. Cell* **20**, 3125–3141.
24. Geisow, M. J. (1984) Fluorescein conjugates as indicators of subcellular pH. A critical evaluation. *Exp. Cell Res.* **150**, 29–35.
25. Harold, F. M., and Baarda, J. R. (1968) Effects of nigericin and monactin on cation permeability of Streptococcus faecalis and metabolic capacities of potassium-depleted cells. *J. Bacteriol.* **95**, 816–823.
26. Tartakoff, A., Vassalli, P., and Detraz, M. (1978) Comparative studies of intracellular transport of secretory proteins. *J. Cell Biol.* **79**, 694–707.
27. Erdahl, W. L., Chapman, C. J., Taylor, R. W., and Pfeiffer, D. R. (1995) Effects of pH conditions on Ca2+ transport catalyzed by ionophores A23187, 4-BrA23187, and ionomycin suggest problems with common applications of these compounds in biological systems. *Biophys. J.* **69**, 2350–2363.
28. Kumar, K. G., Barriere, H., Carbone, C. J., Liu, J., Swaminathan, G., Xu, P., et al. (2007) Site-specific ubiquitination exposes a linear motif to promote interferon-alpha receptor endocytosis. *J. Cell Biol.* **179**, 935–950.
29. Barriere, H., and Lukacs, G. L. (2008) Analysis of endocytic trafficking by single-cell fluorescence ratio imaging. *Curr. Protoc. Cell. Biol.* Ch. 15, Unit 15 13.1–13.21.
30. Lencer, W. I., Weyer, P., Verkman, A. S., Ausiello, D. A., and Brown, D. (1990) FITC-dextran as a probe for endosome function and localization in kidney. *Am. J. Physiol.* **258**, C309–C317.
31. Falcon-Perez, J. M., Nazarian, R., Sabatti, C., and Dell'Angelica, E. C. (2005) Distribution and dynamics of Lamp1-containing endocytic organelles in fibroblasts deficient in BLOC-3. *J. Cell Sci.* **118**, 5243–5255.
32. Delmotte, C., and Delmas, A. (1999) Synthesis and fluorescence properties of Oregon Green 514 labeled peptides. *Bioorg. Med. Chem. Lett.* **9**, 2989–2994.

Section IV

CFTR Structure

Chapter 21

Introduction to Section IV: Biophysical Methods to Approach CFTR Structure

Juan L. Mendoza, André Schmidt, and Philip J. Thomas

Abstract

Inefficient folding of CFTR into a functional three-dimensional structure is the basic pathophysiologic mechanism leading to most cases of cystic fibrosis. Knowledge of the structure of CFTR and placement of these mutations into a structural context would provide information key for developing targeted therapeutic approaches for cystic fibrosis. As a large polytopic membrane protein containing disordered regions, intact CFTR has been refractory to efforts to solve a high-resolution structure using X-ray crystallography. The following chapters summarize current efforts to circumvent these obstacles by utilizing NMR, electron microscopy, and computational methodologies and by development of experimental models of the relevant domains of CFTR.

Key words: CFTR structure, NMR, EM, crystallography, spectroscopy.

Mutations in the cystic fibrosis transmembrane conductance regulator (CFTR) lead to the development of cystic fibrosis (CF), one of the most common, fatal autosomal-recessive diseases (1, 2). CFTR is a large membrane protein composed of at least five individual domains: two nucleotide-binding domains (NBDs), two transmembrane domains (TMDs), and a regulatory domain (RD) (**Fig. 21.1**). The NBDs and TMDs are common to the ABC transporter supergene family, of which CFTR is a member of the C subfamily (ABCC7). These domains (3, 4) allow CFTR to mediate chloride conductance (5–7) and regulate the activity of several other critical transport systems in the apical membrane of epithelial cells (8–11). Detailed structural information at a variety of resolutions is critical for understanding how the protein performs these functions. The presence of disease-causing mutations in the CFTR gene leads to an absence of one or more of these activities. Such loss-of-function effects can arise from one or more of several distinct mechanisms including direct effects on

M.D. Amaral, K. Kunzelmann (eds.), *Cystic Fibrosis*, Methods in Molecular Biology 741,
DOI 10.1007/978-1-61779-117-8_21, © Springer Science+Business Media, LLC 2011

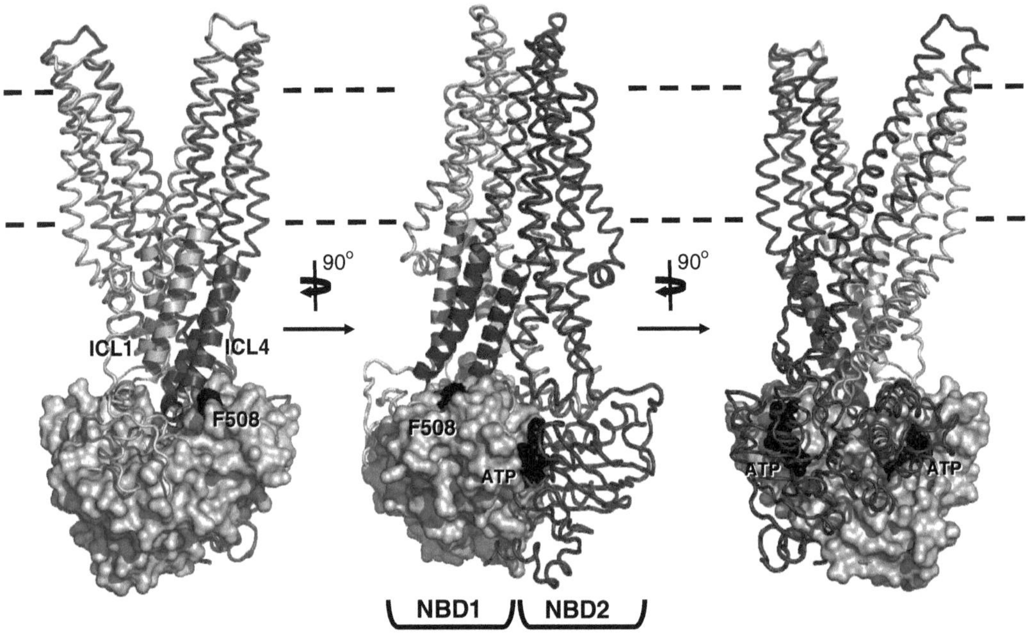

Fig. 21.1. **Three views of a model of CFTR** sans the R domain, which is largely disordered. The model was produced using the crystal structures of CFTR-NBD1 and the structures of related ABC transporters as previously described (3). In all views, NBD1 is shown with a *gray surface*, ICL1 as a *gray cartoon ribbon*, ICL4 as a *charcoal cartoon ribbon*, F508 as a *black surface*, ATP as a *black space-fill*, and NBD2 and the rest of the TMDs as a *cartoon line*. The views are all from the perspective of the plane of the membrane (*dotted line* indicates approximate position of the interfacial portion of the membrane) and are rotated by 90° relative to each other on the indicated axis. The image, produced with pymol, highlights the position of F508 on the surface of NBD1 at the interface with ICL4, the two ATP molecules sandwiched between NBD1 and NBD2 that correspond to the open state of the channel, and predicted domain swap between the TMDs where ICL1 and ICL4 form a unit that interacts with NBD1.

channel function (12–14), effects on regulation (15), or effects that cause aberrant folding (16, 17) and trafficking (18) or a combination of these. Whereas the primary sequence of a protein contains the information required for achieving a functional, native conformation, it is not surprising that defective CFTR folding is the most common of the mechanisms leading to dysfunction (16, 17). Again, structural information can provide critical insight into the molecular pathogenesis of these mutations and the means to counter the aberrant steps.

Information about the structure of the CFTR molecule can be generated at several different levels of detail. First, biochemical and immunochemical methods can reveal the presence of post-translational modifications that reflect the enzymes CFTR has come in contact with and, thus, its history in a cell. The cell has its own intricate methods for distinguishing and sorting aberrant protein molecules from those that continue on to a functional native structure, which are reflected in these changes (19–21). This information indicates, at an extremely reliable, albeit gross level, whether or not CFTR has folded into a native structure. These approaches are covered in great detail in a number of other chapters within **Section III** of this book. At the next level of detail, studies of full-length CFTR can provide information about the state of individual domains by combining limited proteolysis and electrophoretic separation with identification of domains using antibodies with known CFTR epitopes. In this manner, the effects of specific mutations on domains can be assessed by comparisons to the wild-type protein (22–24). Low-resolution approaches have greatly informed our understanding of the structure and function of CFTR and the molecular pathology of many of the disease-causing mutations. However, a desire to understand function and dysfunction at a structural level motivates the difficult goal of determining higher resolution structures of CFTR and its domains that are summarized in the next four chapters.

The structure of full-length CFTR at a resolution that allows for determining the relative apposition of the domains can be elucidated experimentally using incisive biophysical approaches such as electron microscopy and electron crystallography as described in **Chapter 22** by Ford et al. (22, 25, 26). These approaches require significant amounts of purified full-length CFTR and are sample preparation, data collection, and computationally intensive. The structures produced to date provide information about the identity of domains in the structure and changes in their relationship that correlate with alterations in nucleotide content and phosphorylation state, two parameters known to regulate the activity of CFTR. These methods hold great promise for the future in that resolution in the single digit Ångstrom level can be achieved and the presence of disordered regions in CFTR does not interfere as much as they might in the case of X-ray crystallography.

While full-length CFTR has proven refractory to X-ray crystallography to date, structures of other members of the ABC transporter family have been solved to high resolution utilizing this approach (27–29). While these homologues lack some important features of CFTR, for example, the R-domain and regulatory insertion (RI) and regulatory extension (RE) within NBD1, they share the four fundamental domains and, can thus, act as a starting point for producing structural models of CFTR. This approach, described in **Chapter 23** by Serohijos et al., can provide molecular models useful for formulating specific hypotheses for experimental testing (3, 30–33). More sophisticated computational approaches that calculate the folding trajectories of CFTR-NBD1 have been developed and utilized to identify differences between wild-type and F508del and residues important in these differences (33). This work points the way to novel therapeutic interventions by small molecules to circumvent the differences in the mutant and wild-type folding.

An ultimate goal remains, however, the solution of high-resolution structures of the intact CFTR and mutants thereof in a variety of states that define the functional and pathogenic mechanisms. In particular, structures in the low Ångstrom resolution range will be required to reveal the conformation of the side chains as would be required for defining the binding mode of CFTR ligands. Also, information about the structural dynamics is also likely to be key and will come from NMR, as discussed in **Chapter 25** by Kanelis et al., and related experiments. A dissect and build approach has been utilized in the absence of technology to produce and analyze the full-length CFTR at this resolution at the present time. The assumption underlying this operation is that the domains of CFTR can be isolated as independent units that retain structure and at least partial function. This dissection has proven valid for the case of the NBDs and the R-domain. The second half of the operation is to build by recombining the high-resolution information garnered from the component domains, perhaps as directed by electron microscopy results.

To date, high-resolution structures have been produced for the NBD1 domains from murine and human CFTR (34–37) and human NBD2 (in fusion with a portion of the related bacterial NBD, MalK) (***pdb: 3GD7***). These structures have provided important insight into the fold of the CFTR NBDs, the details of how they interact with nucleotide ligands, and the position of the critical F508 residue and other positions mutated in CF (35). The B-factors for these structures point to increased dynamics of particular regions when specific mutations or phosphorylations are introduced (36). Methods for producing and characterizing these domains are presented in **Chapters 23**, **24**, and **25**. **Chapter 24** focuses on the history of development of systems for producing CFTR-NBD1 as an illustrative example.

Dynamical changes in the conformation of CFTR are important at a variety of levels. Changes in conformation and in the relative orientation of the domains define the mechano-chemical reaction cycle of gating. Order–disorder transitions and conformational rearrangements underlie control of these domain rearrangements and, thus, the mechanisms by which nucleotide binding and hydrolysis and CFTR phosphorylation regulate the activity of the channel (38, 39). Folding is by definition the dynamic changes in conformation that occur as the native state is assembled. Where static structural information is difficult, dynamic structural information requires temporal information about the structure over many different timescales. **Chapter 25**, by Kanelis et al., summarizes the use of NMR spectroscopy to address many of the critical questions about the regulation of CFTR and the effects of mutations on the dynamics of the domains.

Structural information relevant to the function and dysfunction of CFTR forms the basis of a rational approach to therapeutic discovery and development. However, CFTR is an integral membrane protein that is produced in cells in low abundance creating significant obstacles to structural studies. Moreover, it contains significant regions of disorder even when it is in its native state – disorder that is central to its function, but that impedes many structural experiments – obviating a need for information about the dynamics of these structures. Finally, in several cases, including the prevalent F508del mutation, the mutant protein does not fold efficiently into the final structure. Since many of these disease-causing folding mutants retain at least partial function when they are induced to fold in vitro or in cell culture systems (40, 41), a critical challenge is to produce structural information relevant to these partially folded or misfolded states. Computational methods have a key advantage for directing work in this difficult area. The following chapters provide a primer on current experimental and computational methods for structural work on full-length CFTR, its domains, and the dynamical states central to folding and function. Understanding the structural details of function and the folding process may not only provide fundamental knowledge but also have practical application in the development of future treatments for the disease.

Acknowledgments

The authors are grateful for the support provided by the NIH-NIDDK, Welch Foundation, and the CF Foundation for much of the work summarized. Also we would like to thank the many investigators that have contributed to these studies and our thinking regarding the utility of structural approaches including the authors of **Chapters 22**, **23**, and **25**, the members of the CFTR folding consortium, the SGX-CFFT joint research committee, Chad Brautigam, Hanoch Senderowitz, Martin Mense, and former members of the laboratory at UT Southwestern, including Bao-He Qu, Elizabeth Strickland, Michael Dorwart, Patrick Thibodeau, John Richardson, Jarod Watson, and Emmanuel Caspa.

References

1. Cutting, G. R. (1993) Spectrum of mutations in cystic fibrosis. *J. Bioenerg. Biomembr.* **25**, 7–10.
2. Riordan, J. R., Rommens, J. M., Kerem, B., Alon, N., Rozmahel, R., Grzelczak, Z., et al. (1989) Identification of the cystic fibrosis gene: Cloning and characterization of complementary DNA. *Science* **245**, 1066–1073.
3. Mendoza, J. L., and Thomas, P. J. (2007) Building an understanding of cystic fibrosis on the foundation of ABC transporter structures. *J. Bioenerg. Biomembr.* **39**, 499–505.

4. Riordan, J. R. (2008) CFTR function and prospects for therapy. *Annu. Rev. Biochem.* 77, 701–726.
5. Choi, J. Y., Joo, N. S., Krouse, M. E., Wu, J. V., Robbins, R. C., Ianowski, J. P., et al. (2007) Synergistic airway gland mucus secretion in response to vasoactive intestinal peptide and carbachol is lost in cystic fibrosis. *J. Clin. Invest.* **117**, 3118–3127.
6. Devor, D. C., Bridges, R. J., and Pilewski, J. M. (2000) Pharmacological modulation of ion transport across wild-type and DeltaF508 CFTR-expressing human bronchial epithelia. *Am. J. Physiol.* **279**, C461–479.
7. Quinton, P. M., and Reddy, M. M. (1992) Control of CFTR chloride conductance by ATP levels through non-hydrolytic binding. *Nature* **360**, 79–81.
8. Ko, S. B., Zeng, W., Dorwart, M. R., Luo, X., Kim, K. H., Millen, L., et al. (2004) Gating of CFTR by the STAS domain of SLC26 transporters. *Nat. Cell. Biol.* **6**, 343–350.
9. Kunzelmann, K., Kiser, G. L., Schreiber, R., and Riordan, J. R. (1997) Inhibition of epithelial Na+ currents by intracellular domains of the cystic fibrosis transmembrane conductance regulator. *FEBS Lett.* **400**, 341–344.
10. Mall, M., Bleich, M., Kuehr, J., Brandis, M., Greger, R., and Kunzelmann, K. (1999) CFTR-mediated inhibition of epithelial Na^+ conductance in human colon is defective in cystic fibrosis. *Am. J. Physiol.* **277**, G709–716.
11. Schreiber, R., Hopf, A., Mall, M., Greger, R., and Kunzelmann, K. (1999) The first-nucleotide binding domain of the cystic-fibrosis transmembrane conductance regulator is important for inhibition of the epithelial Na^+ channel. *Proc. Natl. Acad. Sci. USA* **96**, 5310–5315.
12. Linsdell, P., Zheng, S. X., and Hanrahan, J. W. (1998) Non-pore lining amino acid side chains influence anion selectivity of the human CFTR Cl^- channel expressed in mammalian cell lines. *J. Physiol.* **512**, 1–16.
13. McCarty, N. A. (2000) Permeation through the CFTR chloride channel. *J. Exp. Biol.* **203**, 1947–1962.
14. Sheppard, D. N., Rich, D. P., Ostedgaard, L. S., Gregory, R. J., Smith, A. E., and Welsh, M. J. (1993) Mutations in CFTR associated with mild-disease-form Cl^- channels with altered pore properties. *Nature* **362**, 160–164.
15. Fulmer, S. B., Schwiebert, E. M., Morales, M. M., Guggino, W. B., and Cutting, G. R. (1995) Two cystic fibrosis transmembrane conductance regulator mutations have different effects on both pulmonary phenotype and regulation of outwardly rectified chloride currents. *Proc. Natl. Acad. Sci. USA* **92**, 6832–6836.
16. Qu, B. H., Strickland, E., and Thomas, P. J. (1997) Cystic fibrosis: A disease of altered protein folding. *J. Bioenerg. Biomembr.* **29**, 483–490.
17. Thomas, P. J., Ko, Y. H., and Pedersen, P. L. (1992) Altered protein folding may be the molecular basis of most cases of cystic fibrosis. *FEBS Lett.* **312**, 7–9.
18. Gregory, R. J., Rich, D. P., Cheng, S. H., Souza, D. W., Paul, S., Manavalan, P., et al. (1991) Maturation and function of cystic fibrosis transmembrane conductance regulator variants bearing mutations in putative nucleotide-binding domains 1 and 2. *Mol. Cell. Biol.* **11**, 3886–3893.
19. Hutt, D. M., Herman, D., Rodrigues, A. P., Noel, S., Pilewski, J. M., Matteson, J., et al. (2010) Reduced histone deacetylase 7 activity restores function to misfolded CFTR in cystic fibrosis. *Nat. Chem. Biol.* **6**, 25–33.
20. Wang, X., Venable, J., LaPointe, P., Hutt, D. M., Koulov, A. V., Coppinger, J., et al. (2006) Hsp90 cochaperone Aha1 downregulation rescues misfolding of CFTR in cystic fibrosis. *Cell* **127**, 803–815.
21. Younger, J. M., Fan, C. Y., Chen, L., Rosser, M. F., Patterson, C., and Cyr, D. M. (2005) Cystic fibrosis transmembrane conductance regulator as a model substrate to study endoplasmic reticulum protein quality control in mammalian cells. *Methods Mol. Biol.* **301**, 293–303.
22. Awayn, N. H., Rosenberg, M. F., Kamis, A. B., Aleksandrov, L. A., Riordan, J. R., and Ford, R. C. (2005) Crystallographic and single-particle analyses of native- and nucleotide-bound forms of the cystic fibrosis transmembrane conductance regulator (CFTR) protein. *Biochem. Soc. Trans.* **33**, 996–999.
23. Kleizen, B., van Vlijmen, T., de Jonge, H. R., and Braakman, I. (2005) Folding of CFTR is predominantly cotranslational. *Mol. Cell* **20**, 277–287.
24. Cui, L., Aleksandrov, L., Chang, X. B., Hou, Y. X., He, L., Hegedus, T., et al. (2007) Domain interdependence in the biosynthetic assembly of CFTR. *J. Mol. Biol.* **365**, 981–994.
25. Zhang, L., Aleksandrov, L. A., Zhao, Z., Birtley, J. R., Riordan, J. R., and Ford, R. C. (2009) Architecture of the cystic fibrosis transmembrane conductance regulator protein and structural changes associated with

phosphorylation and nucleotide binding. *J. Struct. Biol.* **167**, 242–251.
26. Rosenberg, M. F., Kamis, A. B., Aleksandrov, L. A., Ford, R. C., and Riordan, J. R. (2004) Purification and crystallization of the cystic fibrosis transmembrane conductance regulator (CFTR). *J. Biol. Chem.* **279**, 39051–39057.
27. Aller, S. G., Yu, J., Ward, A., Weng, Y., Chittaboina, S., Zhuo, R., et al. (2009) Structure of P-glycoprotein reveals a molecular basis for poly-specific drug binding. *Science* **323**, 1718–1722.
28. Dawson, R. J., and Locher, K. P. (2006) Structure of a bacterial multidrug ABC transporter. *Nature* **443**, 180–185.
29. Locher, K. P., Lee, A. T., and Rees, D. C. (2002) The E. coli BtuCD structure: A framework for ABC transporter architecture and mechanism. *Science* **296**, 1091–1098.
30. Huang, S. Y., Bolser, D., Liu, H. Y., Hwang, T. C., and Zou, X. (2009) Molecular modeling of the heterodimer of human CFTR's nucleotide-binding domains using a protein-protein docking approach. *J. Mol. Graph.* **27**, 822–828.
31. Moran, O. (2007) Model of the cAMP activation of chloride transport by CFTR channel and the mechanism of potentiators. *J. Theor. Biol.* **262**, 73–79.
32. Mornon, J. P., Lehn, P., and Callebaut, I. (2009) Molecular models of the open and closed states of the whole human CFTR protein. *Cell. Mol. Life Sci.* **66**, 3469–3486.
33. Serohijos, A. W., Hegedus, T., Aleksandrov, A. A., He, L., Cui, L., Dokholyan, N. V., et al. (2008) Phenylalanine-508 mediates a cytoplasmic-membrane domain contact in the CFTR 3D structure crucial to assembly and channel function. *Proc. Natl. Acad. Sci. USA* **105**, 3256–3261.
34. Atwell, S., Brouillette, C. G., Conners, K., Emtage, S., Gheyi, T., Guggino, W. B., et al. (2010) Structures of a minimal human CFTR first nucleotide-binding domain as a monomer, head-to-tail homodimer, and pathogenic mutant. *Protein Eng. Des. Sel.* **23**, 375–384.
35. Lewis, H. A., Buchanan, S. G., Burley, S. K., Conners, K., Dickey, M., Dorwart, M., et al. (2004) Structure of nucleotide-binding domain 1 of the cystic fibrosis transmembrane conductance regulator. *EMBO J.* **23**, 282–293.
36. Lewis, H. A., Wang, C., Zhao, X., Hamuro, Y., Conners, K., Kearins, M. C., et al. (2010) Structure and dynamics of NBD1 from CFTR characterized using crystallography and hydrogen/deuterium exchange mass spectrometry. *J. Mol. Biol.* **396**, 406–430.
37. Thibodeau, P. H., Brautigam, C. A., Machius, M., and Thomas, P. J. (2005) Side chain and backbone contributions of Phe508 to CFTR folding. *Nat. Struct. Mol. Biol.* **12**, 10–16.
38. Baker, J. M., Hudson, R. P., Kanelis, V., Choy, W. Y., Thibodeau, P. H., Thomas, P. J., et al. (2007) CFTR regulatory region interacts with NBD1 predominantly via multiple transient helices. *Nat. Struct. Mol. Biol.* **14**, 738–745.
39. Kanelis, V., Hudson, R. P., Thibodeau, P. H., Thomas, P. J., and Forman-Kay, J. D. (2010) NMR evidence for differential phosphorylation-dependent interactions in WT and DeltaF508 CFTR. *EMBO J.* **29**, 263–277.
40. Brown, C. R., Hong-Brown, L. Q., Biwersi, J., Verkman, A. S., and Welch, W. J. (1996) Chemical chaperones correct the mutant phenotype of the delta F508 cystic fibrosis transmembrane conductance regulator protein. *Cell Stress Chaperones* **1**, 117–125.
41. Denning, G. M., Anderson, M. P., Amara, J. F., Marshall, J., Smith, A. E., and Welsh, M. J. (1992) Processing of mutant cystic fibrosis transmembrane conductance regulator is temperature-sensitive. *Nature* **358**, 761–764.

Chapter 22

CFTR Three-Dimensional Structure

Robert C. Ford, James Birtley, Mark F. Rosenberg, and Liang Zhang

Abstract

CFTR is a member of the ATP-binding cassette family of membrane proteins. This is one of the best characterised membrane protein families in terms of structure and function. CFTR operates as an ion channel, unlike nearly all other family members which are active transporters. Here, we discuss methods that have allowed such data to be obtained for CFTR.

Key words: CFTR, cystic fibrosis, structure, ion channel, membrane protein, electron microscopy, electron crystallography.

1. Introduction: The ABC Family of Membrane Proteins and What Is Known About Their Structure

CFTR is a membrane protein and a member of one of the largest families of membrane proteins – the ATP binding cassette protein (ABC) family. This family of proteins are active transporters of substances across a membrane, using ATP to power the transport (1). Somewhat unusually, CFTR is an ion channel, rather than an active transporter, and hence has been subject to different evolutionary pressures compared to the rest of the family for the past ~400 Myr (2, 3). CFTR orthologues are found in animals thought to have emerged after this evolutionary time point, and sharks probably represent the most primitive extant species to carry the CFTR protein. In contrast, ABC proteins in general probably evolved very early in the development of life, and are present in archaebacteria onwards, with many different ABC protein functions evolving within living cells (1). Sequencing of

M.D. Amaral, K. Kunzelmann (eds.), *Cystic Fibrosis*, Methods in Molecular Biology 741, DOI 10.1007/978-1-61779-117-8_22,

genomes of bacteria and higher organisms has shown not only that the ABC family is one of the most commonly represented but also that a plenitude of ABC proteins is associated with hard graft. Autotrophs such as plants and cyanobacteria have >100 of these proteins in their cells, whereas parasites survive with rather few (only 13 ABC proteins in the malaria-causing parasite *Plasmodium falciparum*).

It is not our intention in this chapter to provide a detailed review of ABC protein structure nor what is known about the relationship between structure and function in this family. We point the reader to recent reviews that have addressed these issues (1, 4), as well as other chapters within this book. It suffices to say for the present exercise that CFTR is likely to share a similar structural fold to that displayed by three of the eight ABC proteins for which structural models have been obtained by X-ray crystallography (5–16). These are (in order of their elucidation) Sav1866 (6, 7), MsbA (15) and P-glycoprotein (5). All three are thought to function as efflux pumps, with a diverse range of potential allocrites (transport substrates). All three have the typical four core domains of ABC proteins, i.e. two cytoplasmic nucleotide-binding domains and two transmembrane domains. The cytoplasmic domains share a common structure across the ABC family (as far as we know), whereas the transmembrane domains are more diverse (three completely different folds have been identified so far) (1, 4). However, Sav1866, MsbA, and P-glycoprotein (and probably CFTR) show the same transmembrane domain fold, with six membrane-spanning α-helices per domain. CFTR, as mentioned above, is not a pump, but a channel, and hence it has specialisations that are encoded by its primary structure (amino acid sequence). The most obvious specialisation is the so-called R-region (or R-domain), an ~200 amino acid insertion between the first ATP-binding domain and the second transmembrane domain. Phosphorylation of this domain is associated with control of CFTR channel activity (2, 3). However, CFTR is also differentiated from the rest of the ABC family by its short regulatory insertion in NBD1 as well as a C-terminal region containing a PDZ-binding motif (2, 3). Amino acid residues in the TMDs have also been identified as probably involved in forming the transmembrane chloride channel (*see* other chapters in this book).

Here we focus our attention on structural methods that have given data for full-length CFTR (**Sections 3.1**, **3.2**, **3.3** and **3.4**) and also on a method which could provide such data for the complete protein (**Section 3.5**). Other chapters in this book cover structural methods that have given rise to data for CFTR domains (*see* Chapters 24 and 25).

2. Materials

2.1. Conventional EM: Equipment Required

Carbon-coated EM grids (these are most conveniently purchased from a range of suppliers).

A glow-discharge apparatus (most EM suites will have one, but at a pinch, a plasma cleaner coupled to a rotary vacuum pump should be OK).

Transmission electron microscope (usually operated as a central facility in most universities and charged out at an hourly rate to both internal and external users).

Images will usually be collected using a *digital recording device* (a charge-coupled device or CCD), and hence can be transferred straight to image analysis software (*see* later section). Usually a 2000 × 2000 pixel device is sufficient for negatively stained specimens.

Sometimes, images are still recorded on film and here the negatives need to be scanned by a *high-resolution scanner*. These scanners are now very cheap.

2.2. Cryo-EM: Equipment Required

Transmission electron microscope, ideally with a Field Emission Gun (FEG) electron source operating at 200 kV acceleration voltage or greater and with a cryo-stage capable of reaching temperatures <100 K (there are still rather few universities and research institutes with such equipment, due to cost and infrastructure requirements). *Rapid freezing device* (the FEI 'Vitrobot' is a good example). For image capture, a *CCD camera* of 4,000 × 4,000 pixels or better is ideally needed. Alternatively, film must be used which is slow and does not allow the instant appraisal of the quality of the images and specimen that a CCD camera does.

3. Methods

3.1. Conventional Transmission Electron Microscopy (TEM) of Detergent-Solubilised Membrane Proteins, Including CFTR

TEM provides a method for examining the structure of purified membrane proteins (17). The advantages and disadvantages of the technique are summarised in **Table 22.1**. Probably the biggest advantage is that only tiny amounts of purified protein are required for preliminary studies. By preparing glow-discharged EM grids (where the carbon-support film is made hydrophilic using an electrical discharge) physisorption of the protein to the grid surface is possible. Because protein is greatly concentrated at

Table 22.1
Advantages and disadvantages of electron microscopy for structural biology of membrane proteins

Advantages	Disadvantages
Non-crystalline specimens are OK	High vacuum in microscope – dehydration
Small amounts of protein are OK	Very thin specimens are required
Images contain phases (no phase problem)	Image distortions must usually be corrected
Structural data can be obtained rapidly	Significant expertise/training required
Proteins can be studied in solution at the instant they were frozen	Resolution is usually limited, preventing tracing of the polypeptide chain
Proteins and their domains can be stained and specifically labelled prior to imaging	Weak scattering of electrons by the protein atoms themselves
No upper size limitation for protein complexes	Lower size limit of ~100 kD for single particle methodology
Electrons interact strongly with matter – individual proteins can be imaged	Electron beam damage to the sample must be minimised

the surface of such glow-discharged grids, starting concentrations as low as ~10 μg/ml can be employed, and 1–3 μl of liquid is sufficient to cover the surface of the grid. Hence ~10 ng protein is sufficient to obtain some preliminary information about the protein of choice and may even allow the generation of a rough 3D structure. Moreover, since the protein tends to be strongly bound to the surface of the glow-discharged grid, it is possible to wash the grid surface to remove buffer salts and other unwanted solutes and to stain the attached protein using a heavy atom solution such as 2–4% w/v uranyl acetate. Here the protein is surrounded by a very thin, glass-like cast of heavy atoms that strongly scatter electrons (hence providing high-contrast images) as well as providing some resistance to distortions caused by the harsh conditions in the microscope (high vacuum and high electron flux). Since membrane proteins (and CFTR in particular) are difficult to express and purify, one is often left with vanishingly small yields of protein at the end of an arduous purification procedure. Under such circumstances, then, EM offers a lifeline to the scientist keen to learn something about the structure of the protein (17–20).

Experience required: Most users can prepare glow-discharged grids and load them with protein after a few attempts. Usually an EM facility technician will provide this training. Operation of a transmission electron microscope, however, is a much more demanding skill and may require several hours of one-to-one training before a novice will be allowed to go solo. Hence EM facilities often offer the hire of a skilled operator to collect images. It is important, however, to have the person who has purified the protein present during data collection to give advice and feedback during data collection.

3.2. Cryo-electron Microscopy of Detergent-Solubilised Membrane Proteins, Including CFTR

Over the last few decades, proteins have increasingly been studied using transmission electron microscopy in the absence of a heavy atom stain (21). The clear advantage here is that one is studying the true structure of the protein rather than heavy atoms surrounding the protein, and in principle, there is no limit on resolution imposed by the graininess of the stain (22, 23). Since such specimens are unprotected in the electron microscope, measures need to be taken to avoid dehydration by the high vacuum and damage to the protein by the electron beam. Two measures are taken: (i) The specimen is rapidly frozen to liquid nitrogen temperatures and maintained at this temperature in the microscope. This has two beneficial effects: First the surrounding frozen water does not sublime away in the high vacuum (provided the temperature is maintained below ~110 K), and hence the specimen remains hydrated (21). Second, the low temperature reduces the effects of electron beam damage to some degree (24). (ii) The microscope is operated in 'low dose' mode. In this mode all search operations are carried out at low magnification/low dose. All focussing adjustments are carried out at high magnification, but on an area adjacent to the region of interest, hence avoiding any damage at this stage. The actual exposure at high magnification is taken with minimal electron dose (usually a single 0.5 or 1 s exposure).

As the relatively light atoms present in proteins scatter electrons weakly, unstained protein provides weakly contrasted images compared to negatively stained protein. Moreover the atoms in the frozen water surrounding the protein and the underlying carbon-support film of the grid scatter electrons almost as well as the protein atoms, and hence images of unstained proteins tend to be very noisy. The restriction on electron dose (*see* above) makes this situation worse. A few strategies help in this respect: (i) Usually images are recorded at strong underfocus where the phase contrast will be good. (ii) The surrounding water layer is kept to the minimal thickness possible and ideally images will be recorded for protein molecules in a water layer that is spanning a micron-sized hole in the carbon-support film (hence avoiding the background scattering of carbon atoms). We will see an example of such a layer of water with CFTR molecules embedded in it. The layer becomes so thin at the centre of the hole that CFTR molecules are actually excluded from the centre, suggesting that it is of the order of 10–15 nm thick.

Going about a cryo-EM experiment: Cryo-EM can also be performed on detergent-solubilised protein with the same continuous carbon-coated grids that can be purchased very cheaply (about 1 UK£ per grid). The grids may be glow discharged to increase the protein concentration at the surface, and washed as before, allowing for relatively little consumption of protein. Ideally, however, one will instead employ holey carbon grids (i.e. where the carbon film is perforated by micron-sized holes) so that contrast can be increased. The cost for such grids is about 10× higher. With these grids, glow discharging may also be attempted, but it is unlikely to significantly increase the protein concentration in the frozen water trapped in the holes of the grid. Hence for cryo-EM, if at all possible, it is best to have the concentration of the protein in the range of 0.5–4 mg ml^{-1}. One is able to calculate the optimal concentration of your protein using simple calculations based on the diameter of the holes (e.g. 1–2 μm), the expected ice thickness in the hole (0.1–0.02 μm) and the minimal number of protein molecules per hole needed to make structural analysis practical (typically 50–200). For CFTR, we have employed concentrations around 1–4 mg ml^{-1}. Note that at this concentration, aggregation is a problem for the DDM-solubilised protein. By exchanging into another detergent (lysophosphatidylglycerol – LPG), it was possible to achieve higher protein concentrations. Since one still needs 1–3 μl of protein per grid, then cryo-EM will consume considerably more protein than conventional EM.

Freezing: The sample is mostly blotted away using filter paper, leaving behind a rapidly thinning layer of liquid. After a few seconds of blotting (determined by trial and error), the grid is immediately plunged into a bath of liquid ethane that is surrounded by liquid nitrogen (21). Ethane is a much better conductor of heat than nitrogen and allows the water surrounding the protein on the grid to be frozen in milliseconds, too fast to allow water crystal formation. The vitreous form of ice that is produced is essential for successful imaging (as crystalline ice will diffract the electrons). The thickness of the frozen water layer is determined by many factors (humidity, blotting time, viscosity, solutes), and hence a certain amount of trial and error is needed at the start of a cryo-EM project. If the water layer is too thick, then at the worst no electrons penetrate the sample or at the best the contrast is too low. If the blotting is too long, then no water layer will be present, the holes in the grid will be empty and the protein attached to the carbon layer will probably be dehydrated. Fortunately, there are usually gradients of vitreous ice thickness across a frozen grid, and hence one stands a reasonable chance of finding 'good' areas, even where most of the grid is obscured by thick ice. As soon as the grid is frozen, great care must be taken during subsequent transfers into the specimen holder and then the microscope to minimise contact with air, as water vapour will condense on the grid, causing contamination. Small hexagonal ice crystals on the surface of the grid are an indication of this problem, although minor contamination with <5% surface coverage can usually be tolerated. Minimising air flow around a specimen preparation area will help to reduce this contamination.

Experience required: Training in specimen preparation and transfer of the grid into the specimen holder is usually easy and may only need a few hours of one-to-one training. However, transfer of the specimen holder into the microscope is very tricky, and the potential for expensive damage to the microscope is high. This usually means that extensive training and monitoring are needed before a trainee is allowed to carry out this task alone. The potential for running up impressive repair bills also means that operation of the microscope will normally be done by a specialist with only some input from the non-expert user. However, the sheer expense of these microscopes means that there is currently a strong impetus towards automation of their operation and of data collection so that the equipment can be run as efficiently as possible – i.e. almost 24 h a day. Hopefully, it will be possible in the future to deliver samples to a facility and then interact remotely with the experiment, while image data are downloaded to a local computer.

3.3. Image Processing and 3D Reconstruction (Structure Generation)

A common misconception regarding transmission EM data for single particles is that one is observing the surface of the particle. This probably arises because we are used to looking at everyday 3D objects in this way, with our own eyes, i.e. processing the light photons bouncing off the surface of 3D objects using the amazing networks of neurons in our brains. In the transmission electron microscope, however, we are viewing the electrons that are transmitted *through* the 3D objects rather than those that bounce off them. This means that we are seeing *projections* of the 3D objects. It is as though we lived in a world where everything was translucent: imagine a scuba diver looking up at a fluther of jellyfish passing across the rays of the sun. Thus image processing and 3D reconstruction using EM data work by calculating the relationships between different projections of the same 3D object.

The complex protocols for single particle image processing and 3D reconstruction can be broken down into steps:

(i) Particle selection from the EM images that have been recorded.

(ii) Correction for microscope-induced distortions of the images of the particles.

(iii) Pre-processing to remove particles that are outliers from the data set.

(iv) Classification of the raw particles so that similar views (projections) of the protein are gathered together.

(v) Iterative alignment of particles within each class (rotational and translational alignment) so that an average can be generated for each projection class.

(vi) Estimation of the likely angular relationships between the various projection classes.

(vii) 'Reprojection' of each class average along the path determined in the previous step so that a preliminary, virtual 3D density map can be generated.

(viii) Refinement of the preliminary 3D structure by repeating steps (iv) to (viii), but using regularly spaced views (projections) of the preliminary and then subsequent 3D structures for classifying the raw particles.

(ix) Testing and interpretation of the refined 3D structure.

Some of these steps can be carried out in a semi-automated fashion, but there is presently no software package that automatically generates a 3D structure starting from a set of EM images. It is possible that in 5–10 years time such software will exist. Presently, there must be some user input at each step, although refinement of the structure (viii) usually occurs with minimal input from the user. Steps (i) and (ii) currently require considerable input from the operator. Most image-processing software packages are able to do some automated selection of particles, but this generally involves some initial setting up of parameters and training of the auto-selector by manually picking some particles. Moreover, once automated particle selection has taken place, the selected particles must be scrutinised and any obvious mistaken selections deleted.

3.4. Electron Crystallography

3.4.1. Two-Dimensional Crystallisation

There are two main ways to generate 2D crystals: (a) Reconstitution using dialysis, dilution or the use of an adsorptive matrix to remove detergent is the most commonly employed for membrane proteins. (b) Surface crystallisation using chelation, the use of a lipid monolayer and by using precipitating agents commonly used in the generation of 3D crystals have also been employed, and this has proven successful for the generation of 2D crystals of both soluble and membrane proteins such as CFTR. We will focus on this area alone for reasons of space.

3.4.2. Surface Crystallisation: Precipitation

One of the main difficulties in generating 2D crystals using surface methods is the poor reproducibility of 2D crystallisation experiments, which could be caused by changes in the purified protein preparations as well as microscopic variations of the surface properties. In our group we have managed to improve the reproducibility of generating CFTR 2D crystals (to 90% in some cases) by using chemicals normally used for precipitating proteins in X-ray crystallography. Manfred Auer and Werner Kühlbrandt in Germany originally pioneered this technique more than 10 years ago where the crystals grow at a grid surface/water interface to initiate protein/protein contacts (25–27). We adapted this for CFTR and other membrane proteins such as P-glycoprotein (28, 29).

The main advantage of this technique is the very small amounts of protein used which can be advantageous for membrane proteins that are difficult to express like CFTR. One can readily check for 2D crystals by negative-stain TEM but the crystals need to be generated each time for collecting higher resolution data by cryo-electron microscopy. Another caveat is that the crystals must grow all over the grid surface and be readily distinguishable because when collecting high-resolution data with cryo-electron microscopy one cannot inspect the crystals before recording images because this will destroy the crystals. Fortunately, we have overcome both these difficult prerequisites for CFTR (**Fig. 22.1**).

The experimental setup resembles a conventional hanging drop vapour diffusion experiment commonly used in X-ray crystallography, except that a carbon-coated electron microscope grid covers the drop surface (**Fig. 22.2**). A mix of CFTR with ammonium sulphate, polyethylene glycol (4,000–6,000), *N*-dodecyl-β-D-maltoside is used to form the CFTR crystals. As Manfred Auer has found, the thickness of the electron microscope (EM) grid is an important factor influencing the number of crystals found on

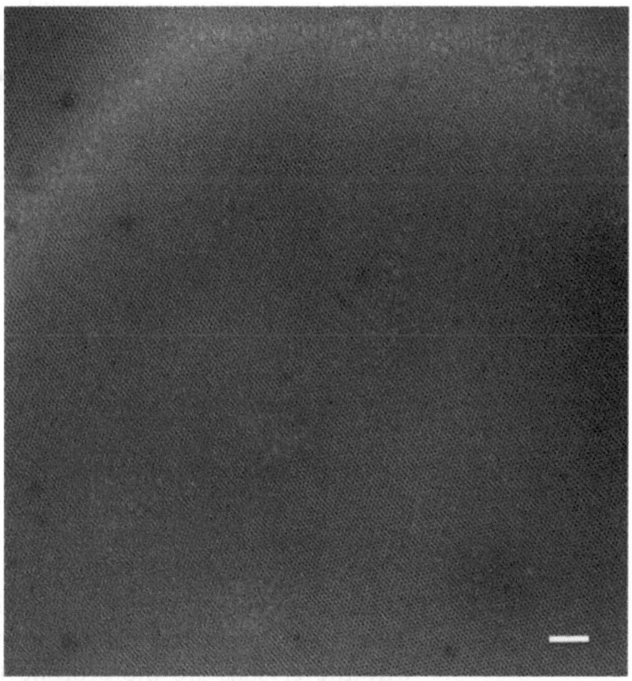

Fig. 22.1. CFTR 2D crystals grown by the precipitation technique. The *scale bar* corresponds to 75 nm.

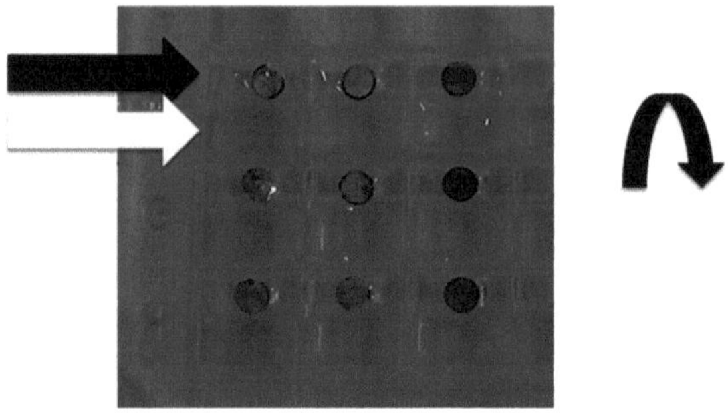

Fig. 22.2. Crystallisation plate with grids placed in the sitting drop wells. The *black arrow* points to the gold (first two columns from the *left*) or molybdenum (last column on the *right*)/carbon grids in contact with CFTR and 'precipitation mix' containing PEG 4000, ammonium sulphate, *N*-β-D dodecyl-maltoside in Tris buffer. The *white arrow* points to the reservoir well containing 1 M $MgCl_2$ which drives the concentration of the protein and precipitant solution via water diffusion through the vapour phase. This system is sealed with plastic film.

a grid. The use of gold-coated copper electron microscope grids is advantageous because they are thinner than conventional grids enabling a closer contact between the carbon film and the drop surface. The hydrophobic nature of the carbon surface does not appear to affect crystal formation, and CFTR 2D crystals grow equally well on hydrophobic carbon films compared with those made hydrophilic by glow discharging in air. For CFTR, the 2D crystals take approximately 17 h to grow at 4°C using very small amounts of protein (50 ng). Shorter incubation times produce smaller crystals, and longer incubation periods increase the risk of multi-layer formation (i.e. thin 3D crystals) which is usually undesirable for electron crystallography.

Micrographs of 2D crystals grown using this method routinely yield structural data to 6 Å in-plane resolution after correction for lattice distortions. Recently, however, CFTR crystals have been produced which show structural data extending to 4 Å resolution using a highly purified batch of protein (unpublished data).

Unlike most other 2D crystals of membrane proteins, the surface 2D crystals do not necessarily contain a lipid bilayer, but more typically consist of crystalline arrays of detergent–protein micelles. Therefore, these 2D crystals are more akin to 3D crystals of membrane proteins. This was shown from the 3D structure of the plasma membrane H^+ ATPase at 8 Å resolution which revealed that the crystals consisted of tightly packed ATPase hexamers, each surrounded by a toroidal micelle of the detergent dodecyl-β-D-maltoside (26). The lack of a lipid bilayer explains why the crystals are more prone to disruption by the interfacial forces, which occur when they are transferred onto electron microscope grids. For this 2D crystals of CFTR are grown directly on the surface of the carbon EM grid, as it avoided the fragmentation of the crystals.

The mechanism of crystal formation is thought to be that the protein molecules diffuse freely in solution and adsorb to the carbon film. The rate of adsorption of the molecules onto the carbon surface is higher than the rate of desorption, as the monomers can accumulate at the interface. The monomers then possibly diffuse along the carbon surface and accumulate into a close-packed array. Crystallisation on the carbon film was more reproducible for CFTR and easier to control than on an air–water interface. As the reproducibility of crystallisation experiments often depends on stable crystal nucleii, the carbon film seems to have a favourable effect in protecting the nucleii from disintegrating, as well as providing an interface at which molecules accumulate and rearrange (25).

3.4.3. 3D Crystallisation and X-Ray Crystallography

X-ray diffraction is still the method of choice for yielding atomic resolution structural information about proteins. Attempts may already have taken place in order to achieve 3D crystals of full-length CFTR, but as evidenced by the lack of a publication all have no doubt ended in failure. Progress towards a structural understanding of isolated fragments of CFTR using X-ray diffraction has been achieved. The crystal structure of isolated mouse NBD1 and in complex with nucleotide analogues has been published (30, 31). The mouse NBD2 crystal structure has also been solved and the atomic coordinates have now been deposited in the Protein Data Bank. The last four residues of CFTR (1477–1480, DTRL) were fused to the Na^+/H^+ exchange regulator factor and the structure solved using X-ray diffraction (32).

NMR spectroscopy has also been beneficial in terms of gaining structural insights into the R region of CFTR. An isolated R region was analysed alone and with the addition of NBD1 (33). This gave residue-level information regarding R region interactions and dynamics. Part of the structure of the N-terminal tail of CFTR (residues 30–63) has also been analysed using NMR spectroscopy (34). Descriptions of methods for studying isolated CFTR domains are available in other chapters of this book.

3.4.4. Potential Strategies to Crystallise Difficult Membrane Proteins Such As CFTR

Recent advances in the crystallisation of eukaryotic membrane proteins are summarised below.

(a) T4-lysozyme insertion: The β-2 adrenergic receptor crystallised upon insertion of the T4-lysozyme protein into the third intracellular loop of the protein (35). T4-lysozyme is a stable and readily crystallised protein and its insertion into this loop region gave additional surface area with which to form essential crystal contacts. T4-lysozyme could also be useful for the crystallisation of CFTR. The third extracellular loop of CFTR is believed to be floppy and deletion of some of it and insertion of T4-lysozyme may give the protein new properties with which to crystallise.

(b) Antibody-mediated crystallisation: Another way of enhancing the crystallisation properties of proteins is to add antibody fragments. Like T4-lysozyme, some antibody fragments can readily crystallise (e.g. FAB fragments) in isolation. When fused or added individually to proteins they can bind to and stabilise flexible regions and also provide additional surface area with which to form crystal contacts and space for the detergent micelle. The first example of a membrane protein being crystallised in the presence of an antibody fragment was the cytochrome c oxidase from *P. denitrificans*, the Fv fragments being involved in all crystal contacts (36). Such an approach could be necessary for CFTR structure determination.

(c) Creation of thermostable proteins: The β-1 adrenergic receptor was only crystallised upon the creation of a thermostable form. Alanine scanning mutagenesis was used as the basis of preferentially selecting amino acids sites that when changed gave increased receptor stability. The final optimised protein contained six point mutations that led to an apparent increase in the melting temperature of the protein by 21°C (37).

(d) Testing of orthologues: There is absolutely no guarantee that human CFTR is the optimal choice in the animal kingdom with respect to expression, purification, stability and yield – let alone its ability to crystallise. For these reasons it is advisable to test CFTR proteins from other species (orthologues). It could also be relatively straightforward to screen these orthologues and test their expression, stability and yield. A recent high-throughput approach in this regard fuses the membrane protein of interest to green fluorescent protein (GFP) (38). Quite simply, the assumption is that if your protein folds properly and is trafficked to the membrane then your cell will be fluorescent (38).

CFTR orthologues could be cloned into suitable expression vectors and heterologous expression and purification trials undertaken in the yeasts *Pichia pastoris* (39), *Saccharomyces cerevisiae* (38) and the baculovirus/insect cell system (40). A phylogenetic tree of CFTR orthologues is shown in **Fig. 22.3**. The tree implies that CFTR found in present-day fish species is relatively divergent from other species, which is of interest from a functional perspective as well as offering the prospect of different physico-chemical properties for expression, purification and crystallisation.

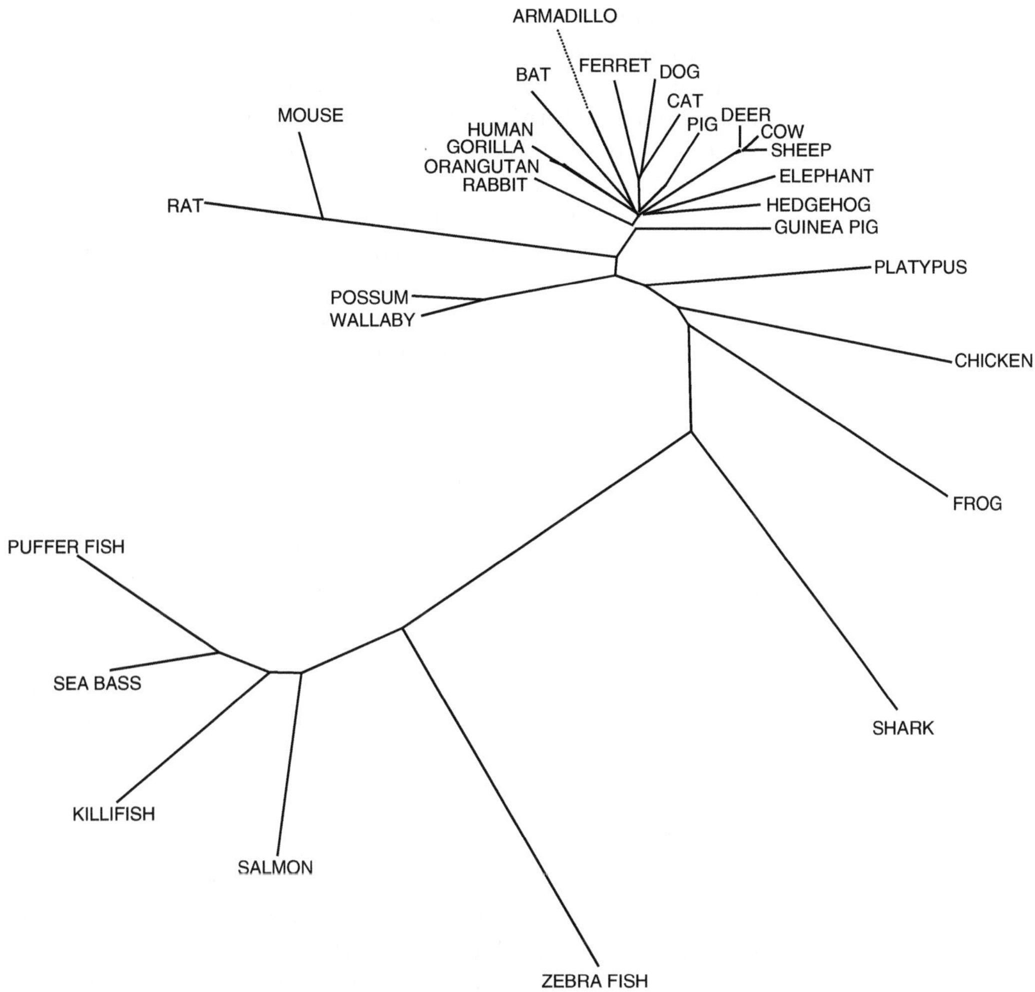

Fig. 22.3. Phylogenetic tree showing potential relationships between CFTR sequences from various animal species.

4. Notes

1. *Software required*. There are several very good image-processing packages for single particle approaches, and some being better than others, it is often a good idea to have alternative packages available. Generally these packages run best on Linux or Mac workstations, although some are Windows compatible. EMAN, authored by Steve Ludtke, does an excellent job, is easy to install and is extremely well documented with help files (41–43). The package lacks a good 3D visualisation component, so it is recommended that a separate piece of software is obtained for this purpose. We have found that Chimera fulfils these needs (44). SPIDER, which has a long pedigree and has been authored and developed by Joachim Frank and Michael Radermacher, is

slightly more hands-on than EMAN and requires a little more time to get to grips with (45). The package allows considerable scope for the operator to develop routines and commands and to program new algorithms. New users are probably best advised to begin with the EMAN package and to approach an existing user for some advice and for checking that they are making sensible choices for parameters input into the package.

2. *Electron crystallography software.* Images of 2D crystals can be recorded on photographic film (with subsequent digitisation) or on CCD cameras. The resulting 2D image data sets may contain high-resolution information covered by very high levels of noise. This is especially the case for cryo-electron microscopy images of 2D crystals because the electron dosage levels are usually and necessarily quite low. Computer image processing can be applied to extract the structural information from the recorded images. Richard Henderson at the Medical Research Council (MRC) in UK and co-workers developed a powerful suite of programs for this purpose, which is available as the MRC-LMB software suite (46). The MRC programs are a collection of programs, mostly written in Fortran-77, which perform image processing and data merging of several crystals. The basic algorithm for the processing of one image consists of determining the 2D crystal distortions that might be present in one image and correcting these by computer image 'crystal unbending'. This proceeds by calculating a correlation map between the whole crystal area and a small reference area of the crystal. Correlation peaks in the map occur at the position of each unit cell, and hence can be used to identify lateral distortions in crystal lattice. These can then be corrected and a distortion-corrected image is produced. After a few repeats of the procedure, the final corrected image is Fourier transformed (i.e. a frequency representation of the image is obtained), and for every reciprocal lattice point, values for amplitudes and phases are determined. These structure factors can then be used to regenerate the real-space structural data relatively free of the noise that contaminated it in the original EM image. The phase component of the structure factors is especially important as these, when combined, determine the shape of the molecule. The structure factors are also corrected for the effect of the electron microscope's contrast transfer function (distortions caused by phase contrast). After all these processes, a projection map of one or more unit cells of the 2D crystal structure is often generated. If data from several different images are available, these can also be merged into one common data set, which in the case of several non-tilted images will then give a more reliable, or better resolved, projection map of the crystal structure. More significantly, though, data from tilted 2D crystals can be merged with data from untilted crystals to give a 3D data set, which eventually will lead to a full 3D reconstruction of the membrane protein structure (47). The resolution of such a

3D reconstruction will usually be asymmetric – typically it will be better resolved in the crystal plane than perpendicular to it. This is because it is impossible to tilt the 2D crystals beyond about 70° in the microscope (the grid bars start to impinge on the image). This restriction means that there is a missing cone of structure factors in the 3D data which gives rise to the anisotropic resolution described above.

An interesting development for 2D crystal image processing is the IPLT software package, which can also be used for processing electron diffraction images (48). However, a new piece of software developed by Henning Stahlberg, Bryant Gipson and co-workers shows tremendous promise for processing 2D images (49, 50). This software suite (2dx) is available under the GNU General Public License at http://2dx.org and runs on MacOSX and Linux. It is also anticipated that IPLT might be incorporated into 2dx in the near future. 2dx is essentially a graphics user interface (GUI) frontage written in C++ for Richard Henderson's MRC programs but is more user friendly. The central component of this software is 2dx_image, which allows the partly automated processing of one 2D crystal image mainly by lattice unbending. The GUI helps the user through the different processing steps, assists in the choice of processing parameters and provides graphical and commented feedback on the processing results. 2dx_image also contains several functions and independent programs to assist the user, streamline the processing and allow automation – as in the case of the automatic lattice determination for 2D crystal images. 2dx_image also contains a module for Maximum Likelihood processing of data from one 2D crystal image, and for a cross-correlation-based single particle processing of the 2D crystal unit cell images (47).

As part of 2dx a new program called 2dx_merge assists the user in the management of a 2D crystal image-processing project and facilitates the merging of the data from multiple images. 2dx-merge (like 2dx-image) allows the user to edit scripts, change and save parameters and view images and log file outputs at different information content levels (49). In the case of untilted images, an average projection structure can be generated and when the images are tilted a 3D density map can be generated. The merged data set can be used as a reference to re-process all images in an iterative manner until convergence is reached, which usually improves the resolution of the final 3D reconstruction (51).

Acknowledgements

We are extremely grateful to our collaborators at the University of North Carolina (Chapel Hill) led by Professor John Riordan. Without their advice, information, resources and protein, we would not have delved into the CFTR structural world. The authors acknowledge the financial support of the Cystic Fibrosis Foundation (USA).

References

1. Rees, D. C., Johnson, E., and Lewinson, O. (2009) ABC transporters: The power to change. *Nat. Rev. Mol. Cell Biol.* **10**, 218–227.
2. Riordan, J. R. (2008) CFTR function and prospects for therapy. *Annu. Rev. Biochem.* 77, 701–726.
3. Riordan, J. R., Rommens, J. M., Kerem, B., Alon, N., Rozmahel, R., Grzelczak, Z., et al. (1989) Identification of the cystic fibrosis gene: Cloning and characterization of complementary DNA. *Science* **245**, 1066–1073.
4. Kos, V., and Ford, R. C. (2009) The ATP-binding cassette family: A structural perspective. *Cell. Mol. Life Sci.* **66**, 3111–3126.
5. Aller, S. G., Yu, J., Ward, A., Weng, Y., Chittaboina, S., Zhuo, R., et al. (2009) Structure of P-glycoprotein reveals a molecular basis for poly-specific drug binding. *Science* **323**, 1718–1722.
6. Dawson, R. J., and Locher, K. P. (2006) Structure of a bacterial multidrug ABC transporter. *Nature* **443**, 180–185.
7. Dawson, R. J., and Locher, K. P. (2007) Structure of the multidrug ABC transporter Sav1866 from *Staphylococcus aureus* in complex with AMP-PNP. *FEBS Lett.* **581**, 935–938.
8. Hollenstein, K., Frei, D. C., and Locher, K. P. (2007) Structure of an ABC transporter in complex with its binding protein. *Nature* **446**, 213–216.
9. Locher, K. P. (2004) Structure and mechanism of ABC transporters. *Curr. Opin. Struct. Biol.* **14**, 426–431.
10. Locher, K. P., Lee, A. T., and Rees, D. C. (2002) The *E. coli* BtuCD structure: A framework for ABC transporter architecture and mechanism. *Science* **296**, 1091–1098.
11. McDevitt, C. A., Shintre, C. A., Grossmann, J. G., Pollock, N. L., Prince, S. M., Callaghan, R., et al. (2008) Structural insights into P-glycoprotein (ABCB1) by small angle X-ray scattering and electron crystallography. *FEBS Lett.* **582**, 2950–2956.
12. Oldham, M. L., Davidson, A. L., and Chen, J. (2008) Structural insights into ABC transporter mechanism. *Curr. Opin. Struct. Biol.* **18**, 726–733.
13. Oldham, M. L., Khare, D., Quiocho, F. A., Davidson, A. L., and Chen, J. (2007) Crystal structure of a catalytic intermediate of the maltose transporter. *Nature* **450**, 515–521.
14. Pinkett, H. W., Lee, A. T., Lum, P., Locher, K. P., and Rees, D. C. (2007) An inward-facing conformation of a putative metal-chelate-type ABC transporter. *Science* **315**, 373–377.
15. Ward, A., Reyes, C. L., Yu, J., Roth, C. B., and Chang, G. (2007) Flexibility in the ABC transporter MsbA: Alternating access with a twist. *Proc. Natl. Acad. Sci. USA* **104**, 19005–19010.
16. Kadaba, N. S., Kaiser, J. T., Johnson, E., Lee, A., and Rees, D. C. (2008) The high-affinity E. coli methionine ABC transporter: Structure and allosteric regulation. *Science* **321**, 250–253.
17. Holzenburg, A., Wilson, F. H., Finbow, M. E., and Ford, R. C. (1992) Structural investigations of membrane proteins: The versatility of electron microscopy. *Biochem. Soc. Trans.* **20**, 591–597.
18. Bremer, A., Henn, C., Engel, A., Baumeister, W., and Aebi, U. (1992) Has negative staining still a place in biomacromolecular electron microscopy? *Ultramicroscopy* **46**, 85–111.
19. Brenner, S., and Horne, R. W. (1959) A negative staining method for high resolution electron microscopy of viruses. *Biochim. Biophys. Acta* **34**, 103–110.
20. Harris, J. R., and Holzenburg, A. (1995) Human erythrocyte catalase: 2-D crystal nucleation and production of multiple crystal forms. *J. Struct. Biol.* **115**, 102–112.
21. Dubochet, J., Adrian, M., Chang, J. J., Homo, J. C., Lepault, J., McDowall, A. W., et al. (1988) Cryo-electron microscopy of vitrified specimens. *Q. Rev. Biophys.* **21**, 129–228.
22. Henderson, R. (1995) The potential and limitations of neutrons, electrons and X-rays for atomic resolution microscopy of unstained biological molecules. *Q. Rev. Biophys.* **28**, 171–193.
23. Henderson, R. (2004) Realizing the potential of electron cryo-microscopy. *Q. Rev. Biophys.* **37**, 3–13.
24. Knapek, E., and Dubochet, J. (1980) Beam damage to organic material is considerably reduced in cryo-electron microscopy. *J. Mol. Biol.* **141**, 147–161.

25. Auer, M., Scarborough, G. A., and Kuhlbrandt, W. (1999) Surface crystallisation of the plasma membrane H+-ATPase on a carbon support film for electron crystallography. *J. Mol. Biol.* **287**, 961–968.
26. Auer, M., Scarborough, G. A., and Kuhlbrandt, W. (1998) Three-dimensional map of the plasma membrane H^+-ATPase in the open conformation. *Nature* **392**, 840–843.
27. Auer, M., Madden, D. R., Kuhlbrandt, W., and Scarborough, G. A. (1998) Structure of the neurospora plasma membrane H+-ATPase at 8 angstrom resolution. *Biophys. J.* **74**, A43–A43.
28. Rosenberg, M. F., Callaghan, R., Modok, S., Higgins, C. F., and Ford, R. C. (2005) Three-dimensional structure of P-glycoprotein – The transmembrane regions adopt an asymmetric configuration in the nucleotide-bound state. *J. Biol. Chem.* **280**, 2857–2862.
29. Rosenberg, M. F., Kamis, A. B., Aleksandrov, L. A., Ford, R. C., and Riordan, J. R. (2004) Purification and crystallization of the cystic fibrosis transmembrane conductance regulator (CFTR). *J. Biol. Chem.* **279**, 39051–39057.
30. Lewis, H. A., Buchanan, S. G., Burley, S. K., Conners, K., Dickey, M., Dorwart, M. et al (2004) Structure of nucleotide-binding domain 1 of the cystic fibrosis transmembrane conductance regulator. *EMBO J.* **23**, 282–293.
31. Lewis, H. A., Zhao, X., Wang, C., Sauder, J. M., Rooney, I., Noland, B. W., et al. (2005) Impact of the deltaF508 mutation in first nucleotide-binding domain of human cystic fibrosis transmembrane conductance regulator on domain folding and structure. *J. Biol. Chem.* **280**, 1346–1353.
32. Karthikeyan, S., Leung, T., Birrane, G., Webster, G., and Ladias, J. A. (2001) Crystal structure of the PDZ1 domain of human Na(+)/H(+) exchanger regulatory factor provides insights into the mechanism of carboxyl-terminal leucine recognition by class I PDZ domains. *J. Mol. Biol.* **308**, 963–973.
33. Baker, J. M., Hudson, R. P., Kanelis, V., Choy, W. Y., Thibodeau, P. H., Thomas, P. J., et al. (2007) CFTR regulatory region interacts with NBD1 predominantly via multiple transient helices. *Nat. Struct. Mol. Biol.* **14**, 738–745.
34. Cormet-Boyaka, E., Jablonsky, M., Naren, A. P., Jackson, P. L., Muccio, D. D., and Kirk, K. L. (2004) Rescuing cystic fibrosis transmembrane conductance regulator (CFTR)-processing mutants by transcomplementation. *Proc. Natl. Acad. Sci. USA* **101**, 8221–8226.
35. Rosenbaum, D. M., Cherezov, V., Hanson, M. A., Rasmussen, S. G., Thian, F. S., Kobilka, T. S., et al. (2007) GPCR engineering yields high-resolution structural insights into beta2-adrenergic receptor function. *Science* **318**, 1266–1273.
36. Ostermeier, C., Iwata, S., Ludwig, B., and Michel, H. (1995) Fv fragment-mediated crystallization of the membrane protein bacterial cytochrome c oxidase. *Nat. Struct. Biol.* **2**, 842–846.
37. Tate, C. G., and Schertler, G. F. (2009) Engineering G protein-coupled receptors to facilitate their structure determination. *Curr. Opin. Struct. Biol.* **19**, 386–395.
38. Drew, D., Newstead, S., Sonoda, Y., Kim, H., von Heijne, G., and Iwata, S. (2008) GFP-based optimization scheme for the overexpression and purification of eukaryotic membrane proteins in *Saccharomyces cerevisiae*. *Nat. Protoc.* **3**, 784–798.
39. Chloupkova, M., Pickert, A., Lee, J. Y., Souza, S., Trinh, Y. T., Connelly, S. M., et al. (2007) Expression of 25 human ABC transporters in the yeast *Pichia pastoris* and characterization of the purified ABCC3 ATPase activity. *Biochemistry* **46**, 7992–8003.
40. Eifler, N., Duckely, M., Sumanovski, L. T., Egan, T. M., Oksche, A., Konopka, J. B., et al. (2007) Functional expression of mammalian receptors and membrane channels in different cells. *J. Struct. Biol.* **159**, 179–193.
41. Ludtke, S. J., Baldwin, P. R., and Chiu, W. (1999) EMAN: Semi-automated software for high-resolution single-particle reconstructions. *J. Struct. Biol.* **128**, 82–97.
42. Ludtke, S. J., Jakana, J., Song, J. L., Chuang, D. T., and Chiu, W. (2001) A 11.5 A single particle reconstruction of GroEL using EMAN. *J. Mol. Biol.* **314**, 253–262.
43. Ludtke, S. J., Chen, D. H., Song, J. L., Chuang, D. T., and Chiu, W. (2004) Seeing GroEL at 6 A resolution by single particle electron cryomicroscopy. *Structure* **12**, 1129–1136.
44. Pettersen, E. F., Goddard, T. D., Huang, C. C., Couch, G. S., Greenblatt, D. M., Meng, E. C., et al. (2004) UCSF Chimera – a visualization system for exploratory research and analysis. *J. Comput. Chem.* **25**, 1605–1612.
45. Frank, J., Radermacher, M., Penczek, P., Zhu, J., Li, Y., Ladjadj, M., et al. (1996) SPIDER and WEB: Processing and visualization of images in 3D electron microscopy and related fields. *J. Struct. Biol.* **116**, 190–199.

46. Crowther, R. A., Henderson, R., and Smith, J. M. (1996) MRC image processing programs. *J. Struct. Biol.* **116**, 9–16.
47. Zeng, X., Gipson, B., Zheng, Z. Y., Renault, L., and Stahlberg, H. (2007) Automatic lattice determination for two-dimensional crystal images. *J. Struct. Biol.* **160**, 353–361.
48. Philippsen, A., Schenk, A. D., Stahlberg, H., and Engel, A. (2003) Iplt-image processing library and toolkit for the electron microscopy community. *J. Struct. Biol.* **144**, 4–12.
49. Gipson, B., Zeng, X., Zhang, Z. Y., and Stahlberg, H. (2007) 2dx – User-friendly image processing for 2D crystals. *J. Struct. Biol.* **157**, 64–72.
50. Gipson, B., Zeng, X., and Stahlberg, H. (2007) 2dx_merge: Data management and merging for 2D crystal images. *J. Struct. Biol.* **160**, 375–384.
51. Kunji, E. R. S., von Gronau, S., Oesterhelt, D., and Henderson, R. (2000) The three-dimensional structure of halorhodopsin to 5 angstrom by electron crystallography: A new unbending procedure for two-dimensional crystals by using a global reference structure. *Proc. Natl. Acad. Sci. USA* **97**, 4637–4642.

Chapter 23

Molecular Modeling Tools and Approaches for CFTR and Cystic Fibrosis

Adrian W.R. Serohijos, Patrick H. Thibodeau, and Nikolay V. Dokholyan

Abstract

Cystic fibrosis is a multi-faceted disease resulting from the dysfunction of the CFTR channel. Understanding the structural basis of channel function and the structural origin of the defect is imperative in the development of therapeutic strategies. Here, we describe molecular modeling tools that, in conjunction with complementary experimental tools, lead to significant findings on CFTR channel function and on the effect of the pathogenic mutant F508del.

Key words: Cystic fibrosis, CFTR, ABC proteins, molecular modeling, homology modeling, discrete molecular dynamics, protein stability estimations.

1. Introduction

Because of the significance of understanding CFTR function and the CF disease, solving the crystal structure of the full-length CFTR has been a Holy Grail in the field since the discovery of the CF gene (1), but still remains elusive. In the absence of an experimentally determined structure for the whole protein, structural models of the protein, albeit at lower resolution and accuracy, guide functional and experimental investigations. Modeling efforts already lead to insights and discoveries such as the identification of the molecular interface-mediated Phe508 and other deleterious mutations and the misfolding and aberrant folding kinetics of NBD1. Models for the folding and structure of CFTR have been experimentally tested using a variety of biochemical, functional, and cell biological approaches. The results of thesc assays both inform and experimentally test models of CFTR

M.D. Amaral, K. Kunzelmann (eds.), *Cystic Fibrosis*, Methods in Molecular Biology 741,
DOI 10.1007/978-1-61779-117-8_23, © Springer Science+Business Media, LLC 2011

structure and folding. While these data, and the models generated and refined with them, are of relatively low resolution, they are informative for experimental design and interpretation and facilitate the generation of new hypotheses.

1.1. Modeling of the CFTR Structure

There is a strong incentive to model the structure of the CFTR protein, and ABC proteins in general, because of the available experimental structures that can serve as reasonable templates for comparative modeling. The goal is to build a model of reasonable accuracy that will enable detailed understanding of the CFTR function and the defect at the molecular level. From structural models of the complete CFTR derived from recently experimentally determined structures of ABC transporters, we found that Phe508 in NBD1 interacts with the second membrane-spanning domain through the fourth cytoplasmic loop (CL4) (2). This interface was predicted (and subsequently experimentally verified) to be perturbed upon Phe508 deletion. Other interfaces between the membrane and the cytoplasmic region that were predicted by the model have been validated experimentally (3).

1.2. Investigation of NBD1 Folding Kinetics Using Molecular Dynamics Simulations

Protein folding is the process by which the nascent chain eventually assumes its native three-dimensional structure. It is a broad experimental and theoretical scientific discipline and the reader is referred to numerous excellent reviews for a broader introduction (4, 5). Here, we focus on the folding of NBD1 primarily because of the misfolding defect induced by the Phe508 deletion. It has been found experimentally that the deletion of the Phe508 backbone may shift a fraction of the nascent NBD1s of the CFTR-F508del off the wild-type folding pathway, causing misfolding and eventual rapid degradation of the protein (6–8). Solubilizing and rescue mutations both in the wild type and F508del background have also been shown to attenuate the folding kinetics of NBD1 (9). Thus, there is a need for understanding the detailed structural origin of the perturbed kinetics in NBD1. Using molecular dynamics simulations and simplified protein models, we identified putative metastable folding intermediates and the folding pathways of the wild type and mutant NBD1. We likewise reproduced the experimentally observed difference in folding kinetics. Moreover, from the structures of the intermediate states, we found that this difference in kinetics could be attributed to the conformation of specific loop regions in NBD1.

2. Materials

In modeling the CFTR structure, we used the Sav1866 crystal structure as the template for the transmembrane domains. To eliminate clashes, short molecular dynamics simulation was performed on the model structure using discrete molecular dynamics DMD (http://dokhlab.unc.edu/tools/ifold/) (*see* below for details). DMD was likewise used in investigating the folding kinetics of NBD1. Apart from molecular dynamics simulations, all other computing may be performed in a standard desktop computer.

3. Methods

3.1. Modeling the CFTR Structure

The basic protocol for homology modeling involves constructing a structural model of protein of unknown structure (the target protein) by copying the coordinates of a related protein of known experimental structure (the template protein) (**Fig. 23.1a**).

Several servers automatically perform homology modeling of single-domain cytosolic proteins without human interventions. However, modeling of multi-domain transmembrane proteins such as CFTR is more nuanced. We outline below the procedure for modeling the structure of CFTR and other transmembrane proteins.

3.1.1. Choosing a Template

The most crucial step in homology modeling is choosing the template structure since it sets the upper bound for the accuracy of the model; choosing an unrelated protein as template leads to an altogether wrong model. In general, proteins sharing sequence identity of ~25% or greater will obey the same overall topology, although members of more ubiquitous protein families can exhibit lower sequence identity. In searching for homologs, several servers are available; most notable is the 3DJURY meta-server, which combines the results of independent servers that each implement different homology search algorithms, thus increasing the accuracy of the prediction (10).

CFTR consists of two nucleotide-binding domains (NBD1 and NBD2), two membrane-spanning domains (MSD1 and MSD2), and a regulatory region (R domain) (**Fig. 23.1b**). The two nucleotide-binding domains follow the canonical folds of the NBDs in ABC transporters. In fact, several structures of NBD1 already exist (11, 12), which subsequently inspired the construction of homology model for NBD2 (13). A putative model of the R domain was also derived from ab initio folding (3). Thus, the outstanding task for modeling the complete CFTR structure was building the membrane-spanning domains and determining the quaternary organization of the protein.

Threading the sequences CFTR MSDs did not result in statistically significant hits to any known protein structure because there were few known structures of ABC proteins. Also, the sequences of the membrane-spanning regions of ABC proteins are

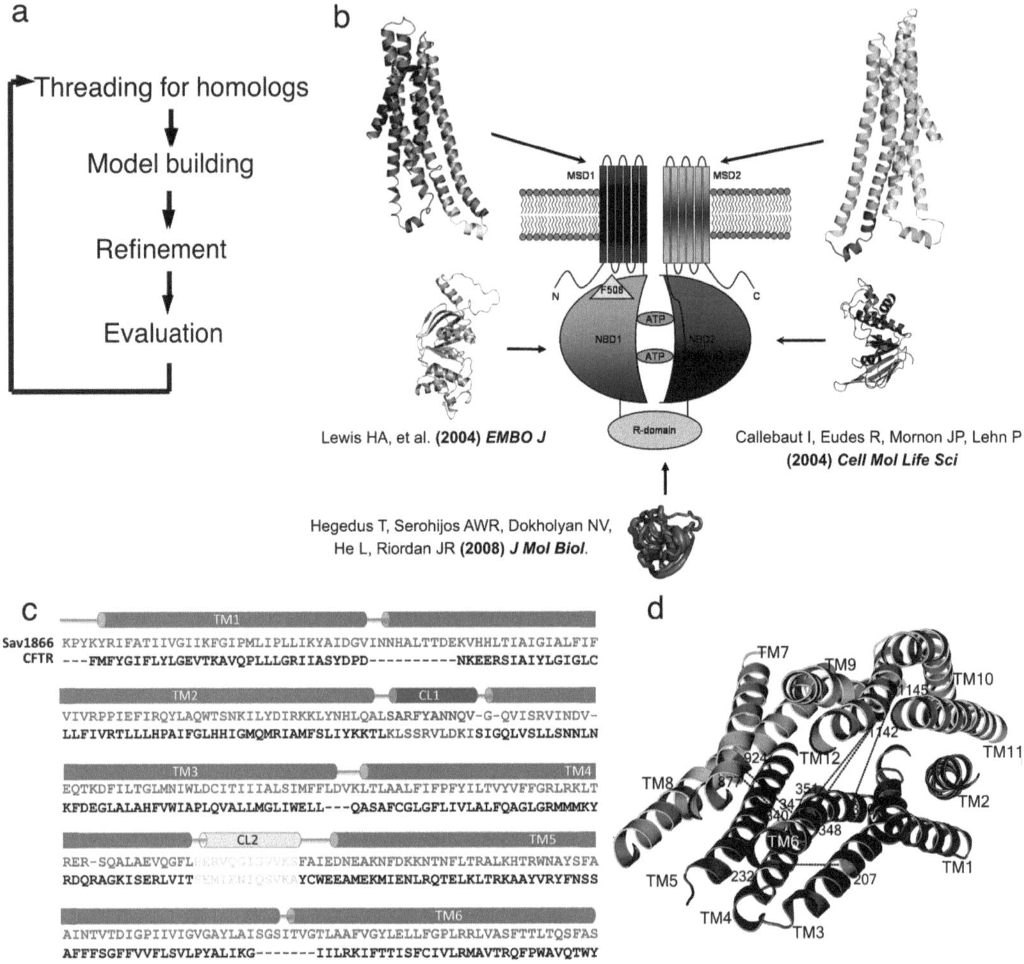

Fig. 23.1. (**a**) Homology modeling. To construct a model, the sequence of the protein of unknown structure is mapped to the sequence of the protein with known structure. The mapping optimizes the alignment of conserved residue regions. An all-atom model is then constructed by copying the backbone topology (and when possible, the rotameric states of the side chains) of the known structure. The model structure is refined using molecular dynamic simulations. The quality of the model structure is then evaluated for correct geometry and sterics. (**b**) CFTR domains. Prior to the modeling of the full CFTR structure (2, 43), there were existing model structures of the cytoplasmic domains: NBD1 from X-ray crystallography (11, 12), NBD2 from homology modeling (13), and R-domain from ab initio protein folding (44). (**c**) Alignment between CFTR and Sav1866 MSD. Alignment between the membrane-spanning domains was guided by the boundaries of putative membrane-embedded regions of each transmembrane helix and by the conserved coupling loops (CLs). (**d**) Experimental constraints. The model is evaluated as to whether it satisfies known data such as those derived from cross-linking experiments and accessibility studies.

not strictly conserved, even between those known to share similar topologies such as Sav1866, PgP, and MsbA (14–18). Nonetheless, several reasons suggest the bacterial multi-drug transporter Sav1866 (14) as a reasonable starting point for modeling the CFTR MSDs. Both CFTR and Sav1866 contain 12 transmembrane helices that are of similar length, indicating that CFTR and Sav1866 are of equal distance from the membrane-plane.

3.1.2. Model Construction

In our CFTR model construction, the starting point is an alignment of the sequences of the template and target proteins (Sav1866 and CFTR, respectively) (**Fig. 23.1c**). The alignment of Sav1866 and CFTR was dictated by the position of their corresponding membrane-embedded regions and the conserved coupling helices in the intracellular loops (**Fig. 23.1c**). The membrane-embedded regions of the Sav1866 helices were identified from the PDB_TM database (19), whereas the approximate locations of CFTR TM helices were defined using the results from glycosylation site insertion studies (20) and the HMMTOP transmembrane prediction server (www.enzim.hu/hmmtop) (21). In practice, major sources of error in this step can come from insertions (i.e., sequences in the target sequence that do not have a corresponding structure in the template) and deletions (i.e., regions in the template structure without a corresponding sequence in the target). Several models must be constructed from various possible alignments and validated against known experimental data (*see* below).

Using the alignment as input, structural models can be constructed using commercially available homology modeling tools such as the Homology suite of INSIGHTII (Accelrys, Inc.) or homology modeling servers such as HOMER (http://protein.cribi.unipd.it/homer/). The MSD models of CFTR were constructed in the Homology suite of INSIGHTII.

To arrive at the quaternary structure of CFTR, the MSDs and NBDs were superimposed with the corresponding domains in Sav1866 (**Fig. 23.1b**). To eliminate any major steric clashes, a short MD simulation was performed where the protein backbone is constrained in the neighborhood of the model structure. We used the discrete molecular dynamics (DMD), a fast sampling algorithm, and the Medusa force field (22, 23) (*see* **Section 4** for more detailed description of DMD). We likewise optimized the rotameric states of the side chains using Medusa (23–25).

3.1.3. Model Validation

A homology model needs to be evaluated for its geometry and sterics. An excellent tool used primarily to evaluate experimental protein structures is Molprobity (26), a server that determines all-atom contacts and unusual backbone and side chain conformations by identifying Ramachandran and rotamer outliers. The second set of validation entails examining whether the model agrees with known experimental data on specific structural features. For example, residue pairs known to be cross-linked or form a salt-bridge or a hydrogen bond should have a conformation that favors the formation of these interactions. Residues known to be accessible to MTS reagents using SCAM (substituted cysteine accessibility mutagenesis) are expected to face the pore region (**Fig. 23.1d**). The CFTR model we constructed was evaluated against these experimental constraints (**Fig. 23.1d**). Expectedly, since neither the experiment nor the model is perfect, there may be contentious data points and model features. These specific contentious points and other model features could then be validated or resolved with further experiments.

The primary utility of structural models is that they allow for positing specific features that could be tested experimentally. For example, the CFTR model predicted a cross-over of the two CFTR MSDs, similar to that in Sav1866. This cross-over predicted that the Phe508 in NBD1 interacts with CL4 of MSD2, as subsequently validated by cross-linking experiments and functional experiments (2). Other inter-domain interfaces in CFTR model have also been verified (3).

It must be noted that while the protocol is described linearly, the modeling and validation is a recursive process – additional experiments increase the accuracy of the model, and more accurate models lead to better experiments. Since the publication of the CFTR computational model, several of its features have been explored by other groups.

3.2. Folding Simulations of NBD1

Single domain proteins of approximately ~100 residues or less have been successfully folded using traditional molecular dynamics with protein models that use physical force fields and all-atom models of proteins (27, 28). Several successful folding trajectories have been reported for these small proteins. However, elucidating the CFTR NBD1 kinetics and folding pathways is intractable for traditional methodologies because the domain is large (~200 residues long). More importantly, folding is a stochastic event and determining the dominant pathways requires multiple folding simulations to acquire significant statistics. However, using discrete molecular dynamics and simplified protein models surmounts this difficulty.

3.2.1. Folding Simulations

The two major components of molecular dynamics are the system (protein model and their interactions) and the engine (calculator of the system evolution). Accessing longer time scales for MD simulations entails simplifying the protein model by using fewer atoms or simplifying the description of the interaction potentials between the various atoms. We apply both simplifications to the NBD1 folding problem.

3.2.1.1. Simplified Models of Proteins

Several simplified models have been developed by various groups through the years elucidating important aspects of various protein folding problems (29) (*see* **Note 1**). Obviously, the type of model depends on the specific phenomena under consideration. In our experience, the following protein model can recapitulate the difference in folding kinetics of wild type and mutant NBD1: glycines are represented as three beads (–N, Cα, C′); aromatic residues phenylalanine, tyrosine, tryptophan, and histidine by five beads (–N, Cα, C′, Cβ, Cγ); and all other residues by four beads (–N, Cα, C′, Cβ) (30, 31). This simplified protein model maintains important features of the protein such as side chain packing and has been successfully employed in studying protein aggregation (31). The bonded interactions exist between pairs of atoms that are consecutive, next-nearest neighbors under angular constraints and atoms linked by dihedral interaction.

To model the long-range interaction between atoms in the model, we also used a structure-based potential, called the Go-model, where particles that are within a predefined distance (typically less than 4.5 Å) in the native structure are assigned an attractive potential, and zero otherwise. Since the Go-potential is structure based, we needed the native structure of the protein to infer the non-native and native interactions for the long-range interaction. We used the following structures for wild type and mutant NBD1s: wild type (PDB ID: 2BBO), F508del (PDB ID: 1XMJ), and F508A (PDB ID: 1XMI) (*see* **Note 2**). The F508A mutant has been shown to exhibit intermediate folding defects compared to F508del (7), and thus is an interesting control for the folding simulations.

3.2.1.2. Discrete Molecular Dynamics

The calculation of the system's governing state equations in MD drives the evolution of the system. In traditional MD, the interactions are usually defined by continuous potentials, and the system evolution involves the time integration of Newton's laws to obtain. On the other hand, in discrete molecular dynamics (DMD), the potentials are discretized, maintaining only the significant features of the interactions (29). Since the potentials in DMD are discretized, all atoms move at constant velocity unless they encounter a collision with other particles or a discrete step in the potential function. Because atoms move at constant velocity between collision events, the system is essentially updated only during collisions. This algorithm allows for the rapid update of the systems state. In the limit of sufficiently large number of steps, DMD becomes equivalent to the traditional MD based on Newtonian dynamics. Simulations of using DMD can be performed using the iFold server (http://dokhlab.unc.edu/tools/ifold/) (32).

3.2.2. Simulation Protocol

Using the simplified models described above, in our previous studies, we performed folding simulations for each NBD1-WT, NBD1-F508del, and NBD1-F508A. Starting from fully unfolded chains, the temperature of the system is progressively reduced to allow NBD1 to fold to its native structure. Folding simulations proceeded until a time $t_{\max}$, which is chosen to be longer than the typical folding time of the protein (33). For a particular trajectory, a structure is considered folded when (1) its energy is less than or

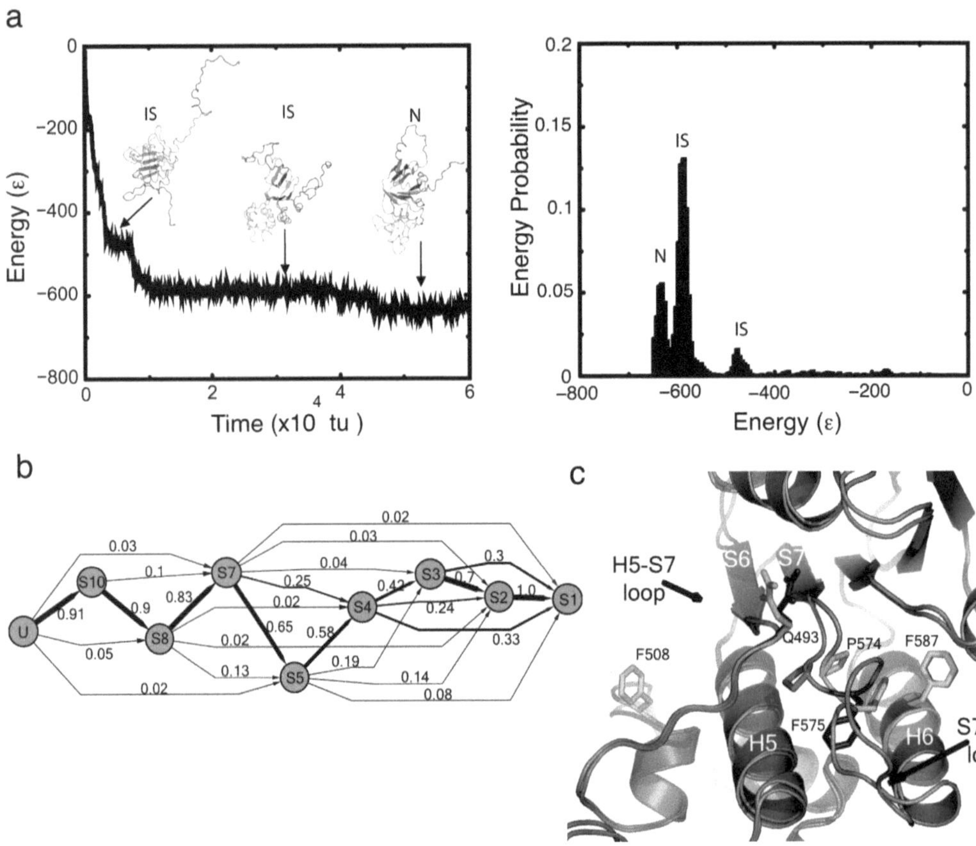

Fig. 23.2. (**a**) Folding trajectory of NBD1. Annealing simulations are performed to facilitate folding of NBD1. Shown is a representative time evolution of energy starting from the unfolded to the native (N) state. As the protein proceeds toward its native state, it goes through metastable folding intermediate states (IS), which are observed as peaks in the energy probability distribution. (**b**) Folding pathways. Probability of kinetic transitions between intermediate states of wild-type NBD1. The probability of exiting a state is normalized to 1 and the thickness is rendered proportional to the probability. (**c**) Contacts in NBD1-WT that perturbed in the F508A and F508del mutants. Difference between average contact frequencies of structures within intermediate states shows malformed contacts in NBD1–F508del (*light gray*) compared to NBD1-WT (*black*). These identified malformed contacts in the mutants are critical determinants of NBD1 folding kinetics. In particular, P574 interacts with Q493 in wild type but not in the mutant. Also, F575 interacts with F587 in mutant but not in wild type. Redesigning these contacts to their wild-type interactions in the F508del background can potentially rescue F508del–NBD1.

equal to the energy of the native state (2), its structure is within 2.5 Å RMSD (root-mean-square deviation) from the native state, and (3) the secondary structural elements possess correct topological wiring. Shown in **Fig. 23.2a** is a typical folding trajectory that reached a folding structure within t_{max}. As the protein folds toward the native state, it proceeds through metastable folding intermediates.

3.2.3. Analysis

1. Folding probability. Addresses the question of whether there is intrinsic folding difference between the wild type and the mutant NBD1s, as suggested by experiments. We calculated

the folding probability defined as the ratio of the number of trials that successfully folded to the native state and the total number of folding trials. Assuming that the folding simulation is a Bernoulli process with a binary outcome, folded or unfolded, one can estimate the error associated with the folding probability as $\sigma^2 = p(1-p)/n$, where p is the probability of folding and n is the total number of folding simulations. We found that at the given $t_{\max}$, wild type exhibited higher folding probability than the F508del, and F508A folding probability is intermediate to that of wild type and F508del.

2. Intermediate states. The intermediate states can be inferred from the folding trajectory. Using the energy as the reaction coordinate, we first calculated the normalized energy distribution, then fitted a sum of multiple Gaussian curves $\sum_i a_i \exp[(x-b_i)^2/c_i^2]$, where a_i, b_i, and c_i are height, center, and standard deviation of the ith Gaussian curve, respectively. Each Gaussian curve represents a putative folding intermediate. By comparing the intermediate states of the wild type and mutant, one can then determine if some intermediate states are specific only to either wild type or mutant.
3. Folding pathways. Once the putative folding intermediates are identified, one can then map the sequence of folding events by estimating the transition probabilities between intermediate states. The probability of transition between any two given states is proportional to the number of trajectories that exhibited the transition. The sum of the probabilities emanating from a given state is normalized to 1, which physically means that the system always exits from its current intermediate state (and assuming that backward transitions are ignored). Shown in **Fig. 23.2b** are the estimated transition probabilities for the set of simulations on NBD1-WT constructs. Since the transition probabilities represent independent conditional probabilities, the probability of a pathway is the product of the probabilities of traced edges, and the dominant pathways are the traced edges with the highest probability. The dominant pathways of various NBD1 constructs can then illustrate if the folding pathways for the wild type and NBD1 are distinct and which states are unique to each construct.
4. Structural characterization of intermediate states. Since energy as defined in the simplified models is not the exact reaction coordinate, there will be degeneracy in the structures populating our identified intermediate states. To identify the dominant structural features of a coordinate, the ensemble of structures can be clustered according to their

pairwise RMSD. Alternatively, one can calculate the contact frequency between all residue pairs to determine the persistent contacts in the structural ensemble. Using these analyses on our simulations of NBD1, we found that specific loop regions in NBD1 can be potential determinants of its folding kinetics (**Fig. 23.2c**).

3.3. Experimental Evaluation of CFTR Models

The functional and structural characterization of NBD1, apart from other CFTR domains, follows from observations of the ABC transporter protein family. Within the ABC transporter family of proteins, the cytosolic NBDs are highly conserved across single- and multi-cell organisms (35, 36). While mammalian ABC transporters are most often encoded as multi-domain proteins on one or two polypeptides, many bacterial ABC transporters are encoded as multiple single-domain polypeptides that assemble post-translationally to form a functional transporter (37). As such, the sequence of mammalian NBDs, while fused to other ABC domains, may also fold autonomously and respond independently to mutation.

The cloning of CFTR and identification of the F508del mutation first implicated a role of NBD1 in CF pathophysiology. To better understand the detailed molecular mechanisms associated with the F508del mutation, further, more refined biophysical analyses were needed. As the bacterial ABC transport systems suggested that the NBDs could fold and function autonomously, the isolated NBD domain was produced to evaluate the impact of the F508del mutation on its folding and function (6, 11, 12, 38). These data could then be correlated with the trafficking and function of the full-length CFTR protein. Importantly, the isolation of this domain has greatly simplified biochemical experimentation and has allowed for solution-based studies otherwise untenable with a transmembrane protein. In addition, the development of NBD1 reagents and accessibility to milligram quantities of soluble, highly purified NBD1 protein have facilitated new studies on NBD1 folding, stability, and function.

3.3.1. NBD1 Production

Methods for the production of large quantities of CFTR NBD1 were initially generated by Structural GenomiX (SGX) working with Cystic Fibrosis Foundation Therapeutics (11). From these efforts, multiple NBD1 structures have been solved from *Mus musculus* and *Homo sapiens*. Though domain boundaries and specific site mutations have been engineered for both species, expression and purification of soluble NBD1 follow similarly for the murine and human NBDs.

Expression and purification follow standard techniques for recombinant protein production in *Escherichia coli* and are based on the methods presented in Refs. (7, 11). The initial expression and purification of murine NBD1 utilized a fusion strategy, with the NBD1 sequence fused, in frame, to a His_6-Smt3 tag (39). This Smt3-NBD1 protein is expressed using the pET T7 protein expression system in BL21(DE3) *E. coli*. Clonal cultures are started and grown overnight to inoculate expression cultures. Expression cultures are grown to induction at 37°C with constant agitation and antibiotic selection. At induction, the cultures are shifted to low temperature for expression (between 15 and 20°C, depending on species and mutational background). Protein expression is then induced by addition of IPTG, triggering expression of the T7 RNA polymerase and the T7-regulated Smt3-NBD1 fusion protein. Protein is expressed for 12–16 h under these conditions.

Cells from the expression culture are harvested by centrifugation and lysed by sonication or French press. The lysates are clarified by centrifugation prior to purification. NBD1 protein is found in both the supernatant and the insoluble fractions after centrifugation and the relative quantities of NBD found in either pool vary with NBD1 construct, species, and mutational background (quantity of soluble mouse wild-type NBD1 > mouse F508del-NBD1 $\approx$ human wild-type NBD1 > human F508del-NBD1) (7, 9, 11). The soluble fraction of NBD1 protein is bound to Ni-NTA resin in either column or batch format. The protein is washed and eluted with increasing concentrations of imidazole and eluted fractions containing the partially purified NBD1 are collected.

Following initial purification, the His_6-Smt3 fusion is cleaved using Ulp1 protease. The Ulp1 protease recognizes the specific tertiary structure of the Smt3 protein and cleaves at the junction between the Smt3 and NBD1 proteins. This cleavage is highly efficient, resulting in no non-specific cleavage or breakdown of the NBD1 protein. The resulting fragments are then partially separated by gel filtration chromatography and the residual His_6-Smt3 protein is removed by a second Ni-NTA chromatography step. As the NBD1 protein no longer contains a His_6-tag, it remains unbound and can be separated from its fusion partner. The resulting protein can then be concentrated and frozen prior to use. Using these techniques, milligram quantities of protein can be produced and concentrated to multiple milligrams per milliliter concentrations, sufficient for both structural and biochemical studies.

3.3.2. Evaluation of NBD Properties

Classic protein folding studies have relied on biochemical experiments to quantify both kinetic and thermodynamic parameters associated with various folding and unfolding transitions in model proteins (28). These model proteins are usually small, highly soluble, single-domain proteins and folding studies are run under idealized in vitro conditions. Quantification of thermodynamic and kinetic parameters is often limited to these small proteins as protein solubility and reversibility of the folding/unfolding reaction are often confounded by aggregation in more complicated protein folds (those with re-entrant sequences and high contact order). Further, these analyses are often modeled as two state, in part due to the difficulty in isolating and measuring intermediates, and as a means of simplifying the data analyses.

3.3.2.1. Kinetic Analyses of NBD1 Folding

Early studies of CFTR folding suggested that the F508del mutation resulted in a conformational arrest of CFTR in an intermediate state due to alterations in the kinetics of folding (40, 41). Based on the rationale for studying NBD in isolation described previously, kinetic analyses of NBD1 folding and unfolding were undertaken to ascertain the impact of mutation in this domain.

The analysis of NBD1 folding kinetics has been studied using two different kinetic methods. First, rapid mixing, or stop-flow, kinetic experiments have been performed to assess the rates of folding and unfolding of purified NBD1 (12). These experiments are completed by measuring an intrinsic spectral parameter of the purified protein as it is rapidly mixed in or out of the denaturant. These experiments are generally performed under conditions where the folding reaction is reversible and the product of the reaction is a single structural state. The spectral data from these experiments are fit to generate one or more discrete rate constants and can be used to characterize individual steps in a folding/unfolding pathway.

Second, "kinetic partitioning" experiments have been used to evaluate the relative rates of multiple pathways. These experiments are performed under conditions where competing pathways promote the formation of multiple structural species that can be separated from one another (i.e., folded and aggregated protein) (6). The relative quantities of the two separable species can then be used to assess the relative rates of the competing pathways (**Fig. 23.3a**). These experiments generally do not provide discrete rate parameters, but instead describe the overall efficiency of the reactions under evaluation.

Studies with NBD1 have suggested that the global parameters of protein folding and unfolding are unaffected by the F508del mutation. That is to say, in stop flow and rapid mixing experiments, there is no obvious change in the rate constants of folding and unfolding as a function of the F508del mutation. The aggregate folding and unfolding do not appear to be impacted by the mutation under conditions that promote protein folding (12). In contrast, under conditions where both folding and aggregation can occur, the F508del mutation impacts the formation of folded, soluble protein. Specifically, when folding reaction temperature is used as a variable to manipulate the multiple folding and aggregation pathways, the F508del protein produces less soluble protein than the wild-type NBD1. Specifically, as temperature increases

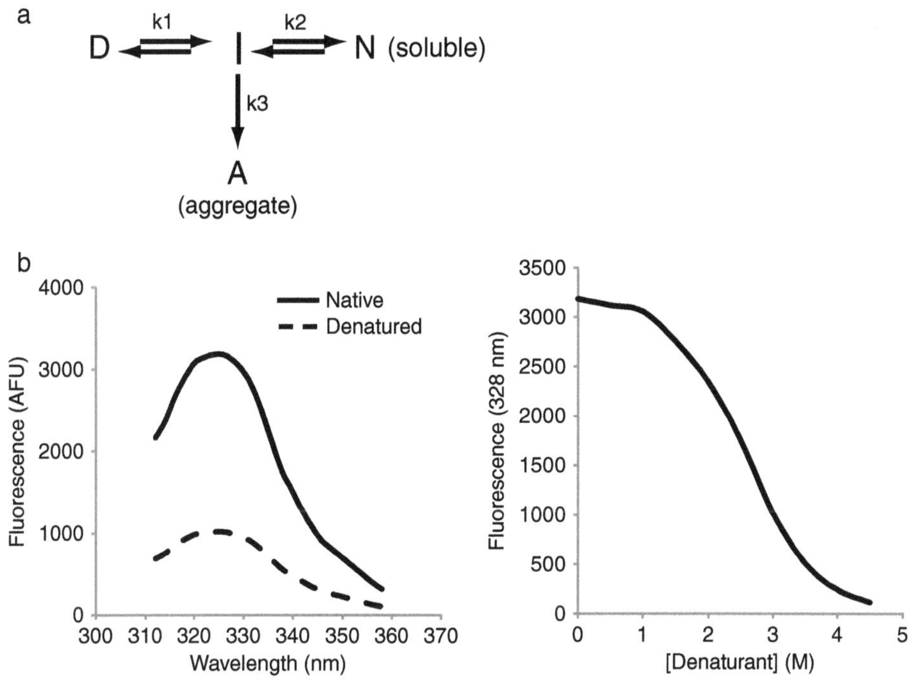

Fig. 23.3. (**a**) Simplified kinetic model for partitioning experiments. A four-state model is shown illustrating the concept behind the kinetic partitioning experiments. Denatured protein (D) is refolded under conditions where both the native state (N) and an off-pathway state (A) can be populated. The kinetic competition between k_2 and k_3 will result in portioning between the off-pathway, aggregated state, and the soluble, native state. For CFTR NBD1, the competing processes that result in the native and off-pathway states compete and are impacted by the F508del mutation (6, 42). Transition to the off-pathway aggregate is assumed to be irreversible; reverse rates are omitted for clarity. (**b**) Thermodynamic characterization in vitro. The concentration dependence of changes in biochemical parameters can be used to assess thermodynamic properties of a purified protein. Fluorescence of the native and denatured states of purified NBD protein can be monitored as a function of titration with chemical denaturant, *left*. The denaturant dependence of the transition from native to denatured, *right*, can be used to assess apparent thermodynamic parameters of the folding and unfolding transitions.

the amount of soluble F508del-NBD decreases relative to the amount of soluble wild-type NBD1 (6). From these experiments it is not possible to know exactly what steps are impacted by the F508del mutation; however, the decrease in soluble NBD1 production is consistent with local alteration of the NBD1 structure and/or alteration to its folding and aggregation pathways.

3.3.2.2. Thermodynamic Analyses of NBD1

The second critical parameter in defining the reaction pathway for protein folding is the thermodynamic stability of the various structural states. Again, protein folding pathways are generally assumed to be two-state, though examples of metastable intermediates and multi-state reactions have been reported in the literature (28). The difference in energy between any two states (i.e., folded and unfolded, folded and intermediate) can be measured and, as in other chemical reactions, this difference in energy is the driving force for the reaction.

As with the kinetic studies described above, characterization of thermodynamic properties is often based on monitoring a spectral property of the experimental protein (fluorescence, secondary structure). The experimental sample is incubated with denaturant or heated and solution-based studies completed. For rigorous thermodynamic parameters to be calculated, the reaction must be reversible and show no hysteresis (that is to say, it must be the same in the forward and reverse directions). However, relative stability – sensitivities to perturbations by heat and/or temperature – can also be informative and does not require reaction reversibility.

Initial studies on NBD1 stability relied on the folding and unfolding of model NBD1 proteins and suggested that the stability of the fold was not sensitive to the F508del mutation (**Fig. 23.3b**) (6, 7, 12). That is to say, the F508del mutation had no significant impact on the stability of the native state relative to the wild-type protein (42). However, emerging evidence suggests that the NBD proteins undergo multiple structural transitions in their denaturation and that these transitions may be sensitive to the F508del mutation. Significantly, and consistent with prior studies, complete folding and unfolding show similar relative stabilities; however, transition through one or more intermediate states appears to be impacted by the F508del mutation. Thus, the native–denatured states transition appears to be similar in the wild type and F508del proteins, though individual transitions between the (1) native and intermediate and (2) intermediate and denatured states appear sensitive to the F508del mutation. Further experimental characterization of these structural alterations is necessary to fully elucidate the impact of the F508del mutation on domain stability.

4. Notes

1. Apart from the details and accuracy of the protein model or of the MD algorithm, most if not all of MD simulations of protein folding aim to recapitulate the folding of the protein in vitro. While the complete CFTR in vitro is known to fold co-translationally in vivo with the aid of chaperones (34), this effect is not included in the modeling just described. Folding simulations of NBD1 using MD investigate the intrinsic folding properties of the domain as dictated by the physico-chemical nature of the polypeptide chain. However, focusing on NBD1, both MD simulations and experimental refolding experiments already show that Phe508 deletion can impair the intrinsic folding pathway of the protein.

2. The use of the structure-based potential effectively smoothens the folding landscape of the protein and shortens the search time for the native structure to within computationally tractable realm. Since the structural information of the native structure is used as input in the modeling, it is necessary that crystal structures of the native structure be known a priori. For the case of CFTR NBD1, while there are several structures of wild type and mutants, most of these contain solubilizing and rescue mutations, which have been shown experimentally to affect the folding properties of the whole protein. In the absence of pure wild-type NBD1 and F508del, one may argue that the folding rescue effects of the accompanying mutants are embedded in the simulation and that any observation already reflects rescue effects of the protein. Nonetheless, to address this issue, we choose structures of wild type and mutant NBD1 that contain the same background of solubilizing mutations such that any observed difference in the folding properties from the simulations can be attributed to the presence or absence of the Phe508 residue.

Acknowledgments

The authors would like to thank Drs. J. R. Riordan, A. L. Aleksandrov, L. Cui, L. He, F. Ding, and T. Hegedus. We also acknowledge the support of the Cystic Fibrosis Foundation.

References

1. Riordan, J. R., Rommens, J. M., Kerem, B. S., Alon, N., Rozmahel, R., Grzelczak, Z., et al. (1989) Identification of the cystic-fibrosis gene – cloning and characterization of complementary-DNA. *Science* **245**, 1066–1072.
2. Serohijos, A. W., Hegedus, T., Aleksandrov, A. A., He, L., Cui, L., Dokholyan, N. V., et al. (2008) Phenylalanine-508 mediates a cytoplasmic-membrane domain contact in the CFTR 3D structure crucial to assembly and channel function. *Proc. Natl. Acad. Sci. USA* **105**, 3256–3261.
3. He, L., Aleksandrov, A. A., Serohijos, A. W., Hegedus, T., Aleksandrov, L. A., Cui, L., et al. (2008) Multiple membrane-cytoplasmic domain contacts in the cystic fibrosis transmembrane conductance regulator (CFTR) mediate regulation of channel gating. *J. Biol. Chem.* **283**, 26383–26390.
4. Shakhnovich, E. (2006) Protein folding thermodynamics and dynamics: where physics, chemistry, and biology meet. *Chem. Rev.* **106**, 1559–1588.
5. Bowie, J. U. (2005) Solving the membrane protein folding problem. *Nature* **438**, 581–589.
6. Qu, B. H., Strickland, E. H., and Thomas, P. J. (1997) Cystic fibrosis: a disease of altered protein folding. *J. Bioenerg. Biomembr.* **29**, 483–490.
7. Thibodeau, P. H., Brautigam, C. A., Machius, M., and Thomas, P. J. (2005) Side chain and backbone contributions of Phe508 to CFTR folding. *Nat. Struct. Mol. Biol.* **12**, 10–16.

8. Cyr, D. M. (2005) Arrest of CFTRDeltaF508 folding. *Nat. Struct. Mol. Biol.* **12**, 2–3.
9. Pissarra, L. S., Farinha, C. M., Xu, Z., Schmidt, A., Thibodeau, P. H., Cai, Z., et al. (2008) Solubilizing mutations used to crystallize one CFTR domain attenuate the trafficking and channel defects caused by the major cystic fibrosis mutation. *Chem. Biol.* **15**, 62–69.
10. Ginalski, K., and Rychlewski, L. (2003) Detection of reliable and unexpected protein fold predictions using 3D-Jury. *Nucleic Acids Res.* **31**, 3291–3292.
11. Lewis, H. A., Buchanan, S. G., Burley, S. K., Conners, K., Dickey, M., Dorwart, M., et al. (2004) Structure of nucleotide-binding domain 1 of the cystic fibrosis transmembrane conductance regulator. *EMBO J.* **23**, 282–293.
12. Lewis, H. A., Zhao, X., Wang, C., Sauder, J. M., Rooney, I., Noland, B. W., et al. (2005) Impact of the Delta F508 mutation in first nucleotide-binding domain of human cystic fibrosis transmembrane conductance regulator on domain folding and structure. *J. Biol. Chem.* **280**, 1346–1353.
13. Callebaut, I., Eudes, R., Mornon, J. P., and Lehn, P. (2004) Nucleotide-binding domains of human cystic fibrosis transmembrane conductance regulator: detailed sequence analysis and three-dimensional modeling of the heterodimer. *Cell. Mol. Life Sci.* **61**, 230–242.
14. Dawson, R. J. P., and Locher, K. P. (2006) Structure of a bacterial multidrug ABC transporter. *Nature* **443**, 180–185.
15. Hollenstein, K., Dawson, R. J. P., and Locher, K. P. (2007) Structure and mechanism of ABC transporter proteins. *Curr. Opin. Struct. Biol.* **17**, 412–418.
16. Hollenstein, K., Frei, D. C., and Locher, K. P. (2007) Structure of an ABC transporter in complex with its binding protein. *Nature* **446**, 213–216.
17. Pinkett, H. W., Lee, A. T., Lum, P., Locher, K. P., and Rees, D. C. (2007) An inward-facing conformation of a putative metal-chelate-type ABC transporter. *Science* **315**, 373–377.
18. Ward, A., Reyes, C. L., Yu, J., Roth, C. B., and Chang, G. (2007) Flexibility in the ABC transporter MsbA: alternating access with a twist. *Proc. Natl. Acad. Sci. USA* **14**, 19005–19010.
19. Tusnady, G. E., Dosztanyi, Z., and Simon, I. (2005) PDB_TM: selection and membrane localization of transmembrane proteins in the protein data bank. *Nucleic Acids Res.* **33**, D275–D278.
20. Chang, X. B., Hou, Y. X., Jensen, T. J., and Riordan, J. R. (1994) Mapping of cystic-fibrosis transmembrane conductance regulator membrane topology by glycosylation site insertion. *J. Biol. Chem.* **269**, 18572–18575.
21. Tusnady, G. E., and Simon, I. (2001) The HMMTOP transmembrane topology prediction server. *Bioinformatics* **17**, 849–850.
22. Ding, F., and Dokholyan, N. V. (2006) Emergence of protein fold families through rational design. *PloS Comput. Biol.* **2**, 725–733.
23. Ding, F., Tsao, D., Nie, H., and Dokholyan, N. V. (2008) Ab initio folding of proteins with all-atom discrete molecular dynamics. *Structure* **16**, 1010–1018.
24. Yin, S., Ding, F., and Dokholyan, N. V. (2007) Modeling backbone flexibility improves protein stability estimation. *Structure* **15**, 1567–1576.
25. Yin, S., Ding, F., and Dokholyan, N. V. (2007) Eris: an automated estimator of protein stability. *Nat. Methods* **4**, 466–467.
26. Davis, I. W., Leaver-Fay, A., Chen, V. B., Block, J. N., Kapral, G. J., Wang, X., et al. (2007) MolProbity: all-atom contacts and structure validation for proteins and nucleic acids. *Nucleic Acids Res.* **35**, W375–W383.
27. Dill, K. A., Ozkan, S. B., Shell, M. S., and Weikl, T. R. (2008) The protein folding problem. *Annu. Rev. Biophys.* **37**, 289–316.
28. Chen, Y., Ding, F., Nie, H., Serohijos, A. W., Sharma, S., Wilcox, K. C., et al. (2008) Protein folding: then and now. *Arch. Biochem. Biophys.* **469**, 4–19.
29. Ding, F., and Dokholyan, N. V. (2005) Simple but predictive protein models. *Trends Biotechnol.* **23**, 450–455.
30. Serohijos, A. W., Hegedus, T., Riordan, J. R., and Dokholyan, N. V. (2008) Diminished self-chaperoning activity of the DeltaF508 mutant of CFTR results in protein misfolding. *PLoS Comput. Biol.* **4**, e1000008.
31. Khare, S., Ding, F., and Dokholyan, N. V. (2003) Hybrid molecular dynamics studies on Cu,Zn superoxide dismutase reveal topologically important residues. *Abstr. Pap. Am. Chem. Soc.* **225**, U704–U704.
32. Sharma, S., Ding, F., Nie, H., Watson, D., Unnithan, A., Lopp, J., et al. (2006) iFold: a platform for interactive folding simulations of proteins. *Bioinformatics* **22**, 2693–2694.
33. Hubner, I. A., Shimada, J., and Shakhnovich, E. I. (2004) Commitment and nucleation in the protein G transition state. *J. Mol. Biol.* **336**, 745–761.

34. Goldberg, A. L. (2003) Protein degradation and protection against misfolded or damaged proteins. *Nature* **426**, 895–899.
35. Davidson, A. L., and Chen, J. (2004) ATP-binding cassette transporters in bacteria. *Annu. Rev. Biochem.* **73**, 241–268.
36. Dean, M., Rzhetsky, A., and Allikmets, R. (2001) The human ATP-binding cassette (ABC) transporter superfamily. *Genome Res.* **11**, 1156–1166.
37. Wilken, S., Schmees, G., and Schneider, E. (1996) A putative helical domain in the MalK subunit of the ATP-binding-cassette transport system for maltose of Salmonella typhimurium (MalFGK2) is crucial for interaction with MalF and MalG. A study using the LacK protein of Agrobacterium radiobacter as a tool. *Mol. Microbiol.* **22**, 655–666.
38. Strickland, E., Qu, B. H., Millen, L., and Thomas, P. J. (1997) The molecular chaperone Hsc70 assists the in vitro folding of the N-terminal nucleotide-binding domain of the cystic fibrosis transmembrane conductance regulator. *J. Biol. Chem.* **272**, 25421–25424.
39. Mossessova, E., and Lima, C. D. (2000) Ulp1-SUMO crystal structure and genetic analysis reveal conserved interactions and a regulatory element essential for cell growth in yeast. *Mol. Cell* **5**, 865–876.
40. Cheng, S. H., Gregory, R. J., Marshall, J., Paul, S., Souza, D. W., White, G. A., et al. (1990) Defective intracellular transport and processing of CFTR is the molecular basis of most cystic fibrosis. *Cell* **63**, 827–834.
41. Lukacs, G. L., Mohamed, A., Kartner, N., Chang, X. B., Riordan, J. R., and Grinstein, S. (1994) Conformational maturation of CFTR but not its mutant counterpart (delta F508) occurs in the endoplasmic reticulum and requires ATP. *EMBO J.* **13**, 6076–6086.
42. Richardson, J. M., Thibodeau, P. H., Watson, J., and Thomas, P. J. (2007) Identification of a non-native state of NBD1 that is affected by ΔF508. *Pediatr. Pulmonol. Suppl.* **30**, 1.
43. Mendoza, J. L., and Thomas, P. J. (2007) Building an understanding of cystic fibrosis on the foundation of ABC transporter structures. *J. Bioenerg. Biomembr.* **39**, 499–505.
44. Hegedus, T., Serohijos, A. W., Dokholyan, N. V., He, L., and Riordan, J. R. (2008) Computational studies reveal phosphorylation dependent changes in the unstructured R domain of CFTR. *J. Mol. Biol.* **378**, 1052–1063.

Chapter 24

Biochemical and Biophysical Approaches to Probe CFTR Structure

André Schmidt, Juan L. Mendoza, and Philip J. Thomas

Abstract

The cystic fibrosis transmembrane regulator (CFTR) is a multi-domain integral membrane protein central to epithelial fluid secretion (*see* Chapter 21). Its activity is defective in the recessive genetic disease cystic fibrosis (CF). The most common CF-causing mutation is F508del in the first nucleotide binding domain (NBD1) of CFTR. This mutation is found on at least one allele of more than 90% of all CF patients. It is known to interfere with the trafficking/maturation of CFTR through the secretory pathway, leading to a loss-of-function at the plasma membrane. Notably, correction of the trafficking defect by addition of intragenic second-site suppressor mutations, or the alteration of bulk solvent conditions, such as by reducing the temperature or adding osmolytes, leads to appearance of functional channels at the membrane – thus, the rescued F508del-CFTR retains measurable function. High-resolution structural models of NBD1 from X-ray crystallographic data indicate that F508 is exposed on the surface of the domain in a position predicted by homologous ABC transporter structures to lie at the interface with the intracellular loops (ICLs) connecting the transmembrane spans. Determining the relative impact of the F508del mutation directly on NBD1 folding or on steps of domain assembly or both domain folding and assembly requires methods for evaluating the structure and stability of the isolated domain.

Key words: CFTR structure, CFTR folding, stability, NBD1, spectroscopy.

1. Introduction

1.1. Polytopic Membrane Protein Folding

The maturation of polytopic multi-domain membrane proteins is a complex process which often requires the proper folding and assembly of individual domains to form a functional complex (1, 2). These processes may be tightly coupled and occur simultaneously or may proceed in a hierarchical fashion. In addition, the processes may proceed in either a co- or post-translational

M.D. Amaral, K. Kunzelmann (eds.), *Cystic Fibrosis*, Methods in Molecular Biology 741,
DOI 10.1007/978-1-61779-117-8_24, © Springer Science+Business Media, LLC 2011

manner. The unique nature of these proteins often requires chaperone systems to promote the proper interactions both within and across multiple protein domains and within multiple solvent phases (3, 4). Perturbations that alter the structures of the individual domains or that alter the interactions of these multidomain complexes are recognized by the cellular quality control machines which ultimately target a newly synthesized protein for maturation or degradation (5, 6). The recognition of these mutations is dependent on two principal components: the physical alteration(s) to the nascent polypeptide chain and the necessary cellular components which recognize these changes. These two things are interrelated, but distinct, and the understanding of both of these findings is necessary for the comprehensive appreciation of the biosynthetic processes of complex, polytopic membrane proteins. Here we summarize methods developed to study the structure and stability of the NBD1 of CFTR.

1.2. Membrane Protein Misfolding in CF

Studies of the CFTR, the 1480 amino acid protein whose loss-of-function results in CF, and the most common disease-causing mutation, a deletion of phenylalanine 508 (F508del), have provided insight into the cellular systems that promote the proper folding of membrane proteins (7). CFTR (ABCC7) is a member of the ABC transporter family of proteins and is composed of five distinct domains: two transmembrane domains, TMD1 and TMD2; two nucleotide binding domains, NBD1 and NBD2; and a regulatory region or domain, RD, unique to CFTR. The F508del mutation is located in the cytoplasmic NBD1 at a putative interface between the NBD and the TMDs (*see* Chapter 21, **Fig. 21.1**) (8). This single amino acid deletion results in the loss of mature CFTR, resident at the plasma membrane (9), as the immature protein is arrested in a conformationally intermediate state which is recognized by the cellular quality control machinery (10) and targeted for degradation by the ubiquitin-proteasome system (5, 6). The question is why does misfolding of the mutant CFTR occur and can it be corrected for therapeutic benefit?

Previous work has shown that the F508del-CFTR can be "rescued" by a variety of treatments including low-temperature protein expression (11), addition of osmolytes to cell culture medium (12, 13), alterations to cellular quality control systems (14–16), and by additional mutations within NBD1 (17–19). None of these manipulations is likely to be of therapeutic benefit. Moreover, while most attempts to rescue F508del-CFTR are likely non-specific, mediated through gross changes to protein–protein interactions and/or protein–solvent interactions, the identification of suppressor mutations indicates that the specific rescue of this folding defect is possible. A single mutation, R553Q, was first identified in a patient, homozygous for the

F508del allele, but having only a mild CF phenotype (20, 21). Subsequently, in a screen for suppressor mutations of the F508del defect, the original R553Q suppressor mutation was identified as were I539T, G550E, R553Q, and R555K (18, 19). These mutations, when introduced into an F508del background, promote trafficking, although with lower efficiency than the wild-type protein, and restored function at the plasma membrane. Understanding how these mutations and other intragenic suppressors correct folding should provide important insight into the normal folding process. For example, they may alter the properties of the NBD itself (*see* below), altering its folding and subsequent assembly with other CFTR domains, thereby rescuing trafficking. Alternatively, they may promote the interaction of CFTR domains, while leaving the biochemical and biophysical properties of the NBD unaltered. In this case, the stabilization of domain–domain interactions would then be largely responsible for the rescue of the F508del trafficking defect. Finally, these suppressors might also have little influence on the properties of the polypeptide in *cis*, but may alter the interaction of cellular quality control machinery with CFTR, thereby promoting CFTR trafficking in *trans* (17, 22). Finally, suppression of the F508del defect may be the result of a combination of these events with specific intradomain, interdomain, and cellular components.

1.3. Interaction of CFTR with Quality Control Proteins

Other recent studies have focused on a variety of chaperones and chaperone systems that are directly involved in facilitating the maturation of wild-type CFTR and the recognition of F508del-CFTR (23, 24). These chaperone systems include ER-luminal and cytoplasmic chaperones, as well as ER-resident membrane proteins, suggesting that a number of different CFTR domains may be monitored structurally during the biosynthetic process. Among these chaperones, the cytoplasmic proteins Hsc/p 40, 70, 90, and associated co-chaperones CHIP (16) and Aha1 (15) and the integral membrane protein Derlin have recently been shown to monitor and direct wild-type and F508del-CFTR for maturation or degradation (25–27), and it has been suggested that this happens fairly early in the biosynthetic process – perhaps before translation has been completed. It is not clear, however, which quality control interactions occur first, are most proximal to the folding defect, and are the committed off-pathway point of no return. Moreover, it is not clear which domains of CFTR are primarily impacted by the F508del mutation (28–30), which structural alterations are secondary (downstream) effects, and which domains in F508del-CFTR signal its ER-retention and subsequent degradation. All of these are essential, unanswered questions whose resolution will provide critical details about polytopic membrane protein folding and the molecular pathology of CF.

1.4. CFTR and ABC Transporter Structure

Both high- and low-resolution structural information is available for CFTR NBD1 (8, 31–34) and homologous ABC transporters (35–38), providing at least some insight into the structure and association of CFTR domains. Some structures of homologous bacterial transporter systems indicate that the F508 position is predicted to lie at the interface between the NBD and an intracellular loop of the TMDs, likely ICL4 (36). This interface is predicted to couple the energy of ATP binding and hydrolysis in the NBDs to the transport or channel activity of the TMDs and provide the specificity for the TMD–NBD interaction in systems encoded by multiple polypeptides. The structures of CFTR NBD1 show that the F508 side chain is surface exposed in the isolated domain and that the chemical and physical characters of this position contribute directly to the characteristics of the putative TMD-NBD domain–domain interaction surface (8). Consistent with the relatively high surface exposure of the 508 side chain, NBD1 tolerates several non-conservative missense mutations with minimal structural changes, although full-length CFTR fails to fold when charged and bulky substitutions are made for the F508 side chain (34).

Several structures of F508del-NBD1 have also been solved (31, 33). Again, minimal changes to the protein backbone are evident, although local perturbations to the putative domain–domain interaction surface proximal to the F508 position are seen. The alterations noted in the static structures of the missense and F508del-NBDs and the sensitivity of full-length CFTR to charged and bulky substitutions at the 508 position led to models wherein appropriate NBD-TMD domain–domain associations were altered and this triggered the cellular response and degradation of the mutant proteins. However, it is interesting to note that many of the structures of F508del-NBD1, solved to date, include a variety of mutations introduced to increase soluble protein production and facilitate crystallization. These include known second-site suppressors of the F508del mutation and novel solubilizing mutations (17). The introduction of these additional mutations partially rescues the folding, trafficking, and function of F508del-CFTR, although they are not proximal to F508 nor do they contribute to the surface defined by the F508 side chain. This suggests that alterations to the surface of NBD1, at least those seen statically in the NBD1 crystal structures, are not the sole defect in F508del-CFTR maturation as F508del-CFTR can mature and function properly when additional mutations which do not directly alter or restore this physical domain–domain interaction surface are introduced into the protein sequence.

In addition, previous studies have demonstrated that the biochemical and biophysical properties of NBD1 are directly altered by the introduction of the F508del mutation (32, 34, 39). The soluble production of protein, both in vitro and in vivo, has been shown to be directly impacted by the F508del mutation, suggesting that NBD1 is directly impacted by this mutation. However, analyses of the soluble, native protein, have demonstrated that the wild-type and F508del-NBD proteins are similar with respect to their native state structures, suggesting that the primary effect of the mutation is not a dramatic alteration of native state conformation, but rather effects on the folding kinetics, stability and attendant changes in the dynamics of the domain. Recent NMR (39) and mass spectrometry (32) data are consistent with local changes in conformational dynamics of the mutant domain. The data presented below further highlight this point and strongly support the notion that the effects of the F508del mutation are first evident in the efficiency of folding and stability of NBD1 prior to its interaction with other domains of CFTR.

1.5. NBD1 Production

The dissect and build approach, which underlies the studies summarized above and the methods outlined below, requires the ability to produce significant amounts of highly purified, monodisperse NBD1 of sufficient stability to allow for characterization. This goal was not easily reached in spite of considerable effort, as the boundaries of the NBD1 were not necessarily obvious from the sequence and even domains with proper boundaries often have issues of stability since they did not evolve as independent biochemical entities.

The earliest attempts at production of NBD1 tended to rely on the position of exon boundaries to define extent of the domain (40–44). This assumption leads to the production and study of model domains that were in fact incomplete and thus had suboptimal properties, although they did retain the ability to bind nucleotide. The earliest systematic approach to assessment of the correct extent of NBD1 was undertaken by Dearborn and colleagues (44). These investigators suggested that the NBD1 was actually larger than had originally been assumed. Gadsby attempted to address this issue by determining the positions in CFTR that tolerated introduction of new N- and C- termini, that is, CFTR was produced as two complementing pieces and function was assessed (45). The tolerated position was suggested to define the N-terminal boundaries of NBD1. A team at Structural Genomix lead by Lewis and advised by the US CF foundation took a "brute force" approach in producing scores of constructs from a variety of species to identify well-behaved NBD1 (8). This effort ultimately led to the solution of the crystal structure of murine NBD1 (389-673). Interestingly, the structure included a disordered regulatory insertion between the first and the second β-strands. The insertion was the position where the new termini were tolerated in the Gadsby approach and corresponded to the start sites for the domain previously employed by several other groups, including our own. Notably, this insertion is also accessible to protease cleavage which has, in other cases, been employed to define the core of a domain in conjunction with mass spectrometry. In the case of CFTR this is misleading as it identifies the position of the insertion and not the domain boundaries, much as the complementation approach. In retrospect, it is worth noting that one of the earliest and simplest alignments of NBD1 homologues was remarkably accurate, but was not utilized for design of expression constructs (46). All of the methods outlined below utilize the boundaries of 389–673 as determined by Lewis (8).

2. Materials

2.1. Buffers and Reagents

Buffer L: 50 mM Tris, 500 mM NaCl, 100 mM L-arginine, 5 mM $MgCl_2$, 4 mM ATP, 2 mM DTT, 12.5% (v/v) glycerol, pH 7.6.

Buffer W: 20 mM Tris, 500 mM NaCl, 60 mM imidazole, 12.5% (v/v) glycerol, pH 7.6.

Buffer E: 20 mM Tris, 250 mM NaCl, 400 mM imidazole, 2 mM DTT, 12.5% (v/v) glycerol, pH 7.6.

Buffer S: 50 mM Tris–HCl, 150 mM NaCl, 5 mM $MgCl_2$, 2 mM ATP, 2 mM DTT, pH 7.6.

Buffer M: 50 mM Tris–HCl, 150 mM NaCl, 5 mM $MgCl_2$, 65 μM ATP, 65 μM DTT, pH 7.6.

Solution P: 3–4 M sodium acetate, pH 7.2–7.8.

2.2. Equipment

Protein purification chromatography is carried out with a Akta Prime (GE).

Circular dichroism (CD) measurements are carried out on a Jasco-810 spectrophotometer. Temperature was controlled by a six-position Peltier effect cell changer in 1 mm quartz cuvettes (Starna).

Fluorescence measurements were performed in 3 mm micro-volume quartz cuvettes using a Photon Technologies Incorporated spectrofluorometer with a Felix32 software package. Temperature was controlled with a Turret 400 Peltier effect cell holder from Quantum Northwest.

3. Methods

3.1. Purification of NBD1-CFTR

Purification of all variants of NBD1 (*see* **Notes 1** and **2**) is performed essentially as described before (8).

1. NBD1 cDNA is used as a template to amplify NBD1 residues 389–673, which was cloned into the pSMT3 expression vector (47).
2. The His_6-Smt3 tagged NBD1 fusion proteins are expressed in BL21 (DE3) codon-plus cells.
3. Bacterial cultures are grown to an OD (A_{600}) of 1.5–2 at 37°C.
4. Cultures are then shifted to 15°C after induction with 1 mM IPTG and allowed to express for 16 h.
5. Cells are harvested by centrifugation and lysed in Buffer L. Lysate is centrifuged to remove insoluble matter.
6. Soluble NBD1 is captured by immobilized metal affinity chromatography (IMAC) from lysate, then washed (with Buffer W) before elution (with Buffer E). Relevant fractions are concentrated.
7. Concentrate is separated by size-exclusion chromatography, and His_6-Smt3 tag is cleaved by His-tagged protease (47).
8. A second IMAC is done to remove any uncleaved His_6-Smt3 tagged NBD1 fusion protein and His-tagged protease.
9. A second size-exclusion chromatography is done, final eluate is concentrated (>7.5 mg/ml), and immediately frozen in liquid N_2, storage at –80°C, in Buffer S.

For an example of final concentrated protein preparation eluate, *see* **Fig. 24.1**a.

3.2. Crystallization of NBD1-CFTR

Murine NBD1 crystals were grown essentially as previously described (8).

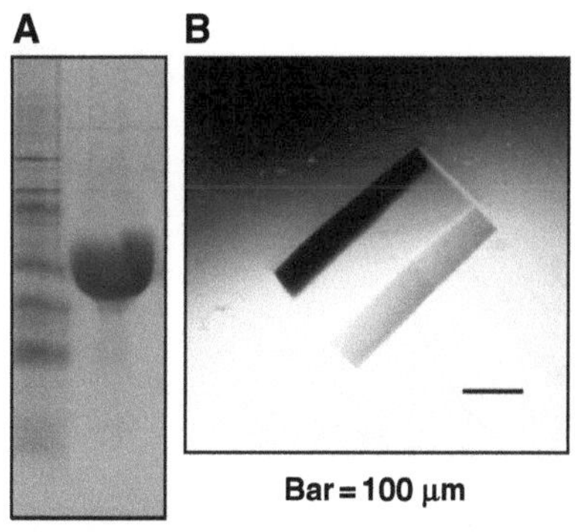

Fig. 24.1. Assessment of the homogeneity of NBD1 preparations. (**a**) Coomassie blue stained SDS-Page polyacrylamide gel of human WT-NBD1 (aa 389-673), *left lane marker*, *right lane* 50 μg of human WT-NBD1, indicating it is the predominant protein in the preparation (*see* **Section 3.1**). (**b**) Crystal of murine F508del-NBD1, with no further mutations (aa 389–673), again, suggestive of high homogeneity of preparation (*see* **Section 3.2**).

1. One microliter of purified protein (>7.5 mg/ml) in Buffer S was added to 1 μl of solution P at 4°C.
2. Crystals were allowed to form over a period of 1–3 days in a hanging drop conformation over a well containing 1 ml of solution P at 4°C.

For an example of murine F508del-NBD1 crystal with no further mutations, *see* **Fig. 24.1b**.

3.3. Circular Dichroism (CD)

1. Measured values for the ellipticity Θ (in mdeg) are converted into the molar ellipticity per amino acid residue [Θ] (deg cm^2 $dmol^{-1}$), with the following formula:

$$[\Theta] = \frac{\Theta}{(10nCl)}$$

where l is the optical path length of the cell (in cm), C is the molar concentration of protein (in mol/l), and n is the number of residues for the proteins used.

2. All CD experiments were preformed in Buffer M. The spectra were corrected by subtracting the signal of the Buffer M. Concentration of protein was 6 μM.

For an example of CD signal of native human NBD1, *see* **Fig. 24.2a**.

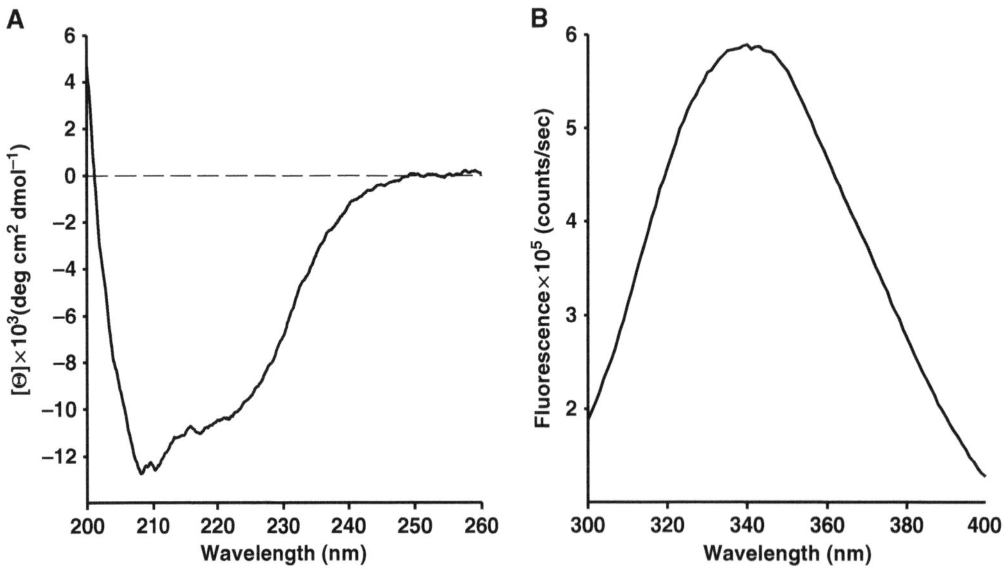

Fig. 24.2. Characterization of purified human WT-NBD1 (aa 389–673) structure. (**a**) Measurement of circular dichroism (ellipticity, Θ) of far-UV spectra reveals secondary and tertiary structure of native protein (*see* **Section 3.3**). (**b**) Fluorescence emission scan (300–400 nm), excitation wavelength is 280 nm, peak is at 343 nm (*see* **Section 3.4**).

3.4. Fluorescence Spectra

1. Emission spectra from 300 to 400 nm with excitation at 280 nm were taken at 4°C, to maintain the native fold of protein.
2. All fluorescence experiments were carried out in Buffer M, protein concentration was 1 μM.

For an example of fluorescence spectrum of native human NBD1, *see* **Fig. 24.2b**.

3.5. Thermal Denaturation of NBD1-CFTR

Thermal denaturation was measured by monitoring turbidity (aggregation) at 300 nm of 5 μM NBD1-CFTR in Buffer M (see (48)) in the presence or absence of putative ligands (*see* **Note 3**). As an example, when saturating concentrations of ATP (e.g., 2 mM) are present in the Buffer M, murine F508-NBD1 T_M shifts by ~8°C (48).

1. Turbidity was measured every 0.5°C, rate of temperature increase was 0.5°C/min.
2. Melting temperature (T_M) was determined by taking the second derivative.

For an example of thermal melt of human NBD1 in Buffer M, *see* **Fig. 24.3**.

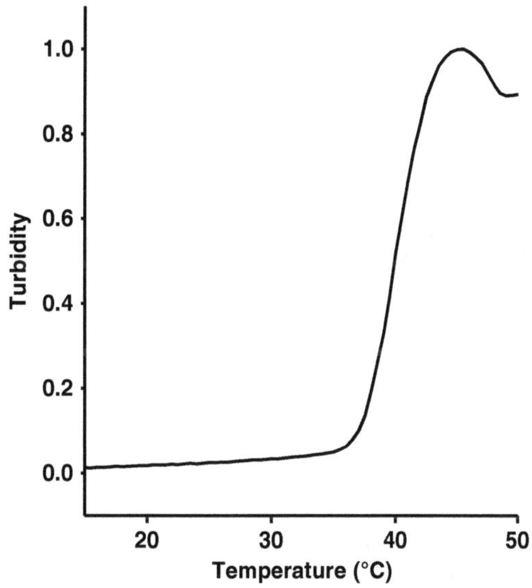

Fig. 24.3. Thermal denaturation of human WT-NBD1 (aa 389–673): Trace is from a representative experiment: Relative turbidity as a function of temperature of human WT-NBD1 in Buffer M (*see* **Section 3.5**).

4. Notes

1. For purification of any variant of human NBD1, it is critical not to freeze the bacterial pellet, i.e., the purification must always be immediately made from fresh material, ensuring that working temperature is constantly 4°C.

2. Amount of soluble Smt3-NBD1 fusion protein in bacterial cell lysates correlates well with intrinsic stability and solubility dissimilarity between different NBD1 variants (e.g., human, murine, F508del, so-called solubilizing mutations, and other second-site mutations), as measured by CD, fluorescence, T_M, and other methods.
3. For thermal melt experiments, it is critical to dilute the stock protein (in Buffer S) into Buffer M already containing putative ligands at 4°C. This is especially important when using human NBD1, as different variants are more or less sensitive to changes in buffer and temperature. Hence great care should be taken, so as to ensure native state of the protein, for performing experiments.

References

1. Kleizen, B., and Braakman, I. (2004) Protein folding and quality control in the endoplasmic reticulum. *Curr. Opin. Cell Biol.* **16**, 343–349.
2. Zhang, F., Kartner, N., and Lukacs, G. L. (1998) Limited proteolysis as a probe for arrested conformational maturation of delta F508 CFTR. *Nat. Struct. Biol.* **5**, 180–183.
3. Amaral, M. D. (2006) Therapy through chaperones: sense or antisense? Cystic fibrosis as a model disease. *J. Inherit. Metab. Dis.* **29**, 477–487.
4. Wigley, W. C., Corboy, M. J., Cutler, T. D., Thibodeau, P. H., Oldan, J., Lee, M. G., et al. (2002) A protein sequence that can encode native structure by disfavoring alternate conformations. *Nat. Struct. Biol.* **9**, 381–388.
5. Jensen, T. J., Loo, M. A., Pind, S., Williams, D. B., Goldberg, A. L., and Riordan, J. R. (1995) Multiple proteolytic systems, including the proteasome, contribute to CFTR processing. *Cell* **83**, 129–135.
6. Ward, C. L., Omura, S., and Kopito, R. R. (1995) Degradation of CFTR by the ubiquitin-proteasome pathway. *Cell* **83**, 121–127.
7. Mendoza, J. L., and Thomas, P. J. (2007) Building an understanding of cystic fibrosis on the foundation of ABC transporter structures. *J. Bioenerg. Biomembr.* **39**, 499–505.
8. Lewis, H. A., Buchanan, S. G., Burley, S. K., Conners, K., Dickey, M., Dorwart, M., et al. (2004) Structure of nucleotide-binding domain 1 of the cystic fibrosis transmembrane conductance regulator. *EMBO J.* **23**, 282–293.
9. Cheng, S. H., Gregory, R. J., Marshall, J., Paul, S., Souza, D. W., White, G. A., et al. (1990) Defective intracellular transport and processing of CFTR is the molecular basis of most cystic fibrosis. *Cell* **63**, 827–834.
10. Yang, Y., Janich, S., Cohn, J. A., and Wilson, J. M. (1993) The common variant of cystic fibrosis transmembrane conductance regulator is recognized by hsp70 and degraded in a pre-Golgi nonlysosomal compartment. *Proc. Natl. Acad. Sci. USA* **90**, 9480–9484.
11. Denning, G. M., Anderson, M. P., Amara, J. F., Marshall, J., Smith, A. E., and Welsh, M. J. (1992) Processing of mutant cystic fibrosis transmembrane conductance regulator is temperature-sensitive. *Nature* **358**, 761–764.
12. Brown, C. R., Hong-Brown, L. Q., Biwersi, J., Verkman, A. S., and Welch, W. J. (1996) Chemical chaperones correct the mutant phenotype of the delta F508 cystic fibrosis transmembrane conductance regulator protein. *Cell Stress Chaperones* **1**, 117–125.
13. Zhang, X. M., Wang, X. T., Yue, H., Leung, S. W., Thibodeau, P. H., Thomas, P. J., et al. (2003) Organic solutes rescue the functional defect in delta F508 cystic fibrosis transmembrane conductance regulator. *J. Biol. Chem.* **278**, 51232–51242.
14. Meacham, G. C., Lu, Z., King, S., Sorscher, E., Tousson, A., and Cyr, D. M. (1999) The Hdj-2/Hsc70 chaperone pair facilitates early steps in CFTR biogenesis. *EMBO J.* **18**, 1492–1505.
15. Wang, X., Venable, J., LaPointe, P., Hutt, D. M., Koulov, A. V., Coppinger, J., et al. (2006) Hsp90 cochaperone Aha1 downregulation rescues misfolding of CFTR in cystic fibrosis. *Cell* **127**, 803–815.

16. Younger, J. M., Ren, H. Y., Chen, L., Fan, C. Y., Fields, A., Patterson, C., et al. (2004) A foldable CFTR{Delta}F508 biogenic intermediate accumulates upon inhibition of the Hsc70-CHIP E3 ubiquitin ligase. *J. Biol. Chem.* **167**, 1075–1085.
17. Pissarra, L. S., Farinha, C. M., Xu, Z., Schmidt, A., Thibodeau, P. H., Cai, Z., et al. (2008) Solubilizing mutations used to crystallize one CFTR domain attenuate the trafficking and channel defects caused by the major cystic fibrosis mutation. *Chem. Biol.* **15**, 62–69.
18. Teem, J. L., Berger, H. A., Ostedgaard, L. S., Rich, D. P., Tsui, L. C., and Welsh, M. J. (1993) Identification of revertants for the cystic fibrosis delta F508 mutation using STE6-CFTR chimeras in yeast. *Cell* **73**, 335–346.
19. Teem, J. L., Carson, M. R., and Welsh, M. J. (1996) Mutation of R555 in CFTR-delta F508 enhances function and partially corrects defective processing. *Recept. Channels* **4**, 63–72.
20. Dork, T., Wulbrand, U., Richter, T., Neumann, T., Wolfes, H., Wulf, B., et al. (1991) Cystic fibrosis with three mutations in the cystic fibrosis transmembrane conductance regulator gene. *Hum. Genet.* **87**, 441–446.
21. Dork, T., Wulbrand, U., Steinkamp, G., and Tummler, B. (1992) Mild course of cystic fibrosis associated with heterozygosity for infrequent mutations in the first nucleotide-binding fold of CFTR. *Acta Paediatr.* **81**, 82–83.
22. Roxo-Rosa, M., Xu, Z., Schmidt, A., Neto, M., Cai, Z., Soares, C. M., et al. (2006) Revertant mutants G550E and 4RK rescue cystic fibrosis mutants in the first nucleotide-binding domain of CFTR by different mechanisms. *Proc. Natl. Acad. Sci. USA* **103**, 17891–17896.
23. Farinha, C. M., and Amaral, M. D. (2005) Most F508del-CFTR is targeted to degradation at an early folding checkpoint and independently of calnexin. *Mol. Cell. Biol.* **25**, 5242–5252.
24. Rosser, M. F., Grove, D. E., Chen, L., and Cyr, D. M. (2008) Assembly and misassembly of cystic fibrosis transmembrane conductance regulator: folding defects caused by deletion of F508 occur before and after the calnexin-dependent association of membrane spanning domain (MSD) 1 and MSD2. *Mol. Biol. Cell* **19**, 4570–4579.
25. Gnann, A., Riordan, J. R., and Wolf, D. H. (2004) Cystic fibrosis transmembrane conductance regulator degradation depends on the lectins Htm1p/EDEM and the Cdc48 protein complex in yeast. *Mol. Biol. Cell* **15**, 4125–4135.
26. Younger, J. M., Chen, L., Ren, H. Y., Rosser, M. F., Turnbull, E. L., Fan, C. Y., et al. (2006) Sequential quality-control checkpoints triage misfolded cystic fibrosis transmembrane conductance regulator. *Cell* **126**, 571–582.
27. Schmidt, B. Z., Watts, R. J., Aridor, M., and Frizzell, R. A. (2009) Cysteine string protein promotes proteasomal degradation of the cystic fibrosis transmembrane conductance regulator (CFTR) by increasing its interaction with the C terminus of Hsp70-interacting protein and promoting CFTR ubiquitylation. *J. Biol. Chem.* **284**, 4168–4178.
28. Du, K., Sharma, M., and Lukacs, G. L. (2005) The DeltaF508 cystic fibrosis mutation impairs domain-domain interactions and arrests post-translational folding of CFTR. *Nat. Struct. Biol.* **12**, 17–25.
29. Cui, L., Aleksandrov, L., Chang, X. B., Hou, Y. X., He, L., Hegedus, T., et al. (2007) Domain interdependence in the biosynthetic assembly of CFTR. *J. Mol. Biol.* **365**, 981–994.
30. Kleizen, B., van Vlijmen, T., de Jonge, H. R., and Braakman, I. (2005) Folding of CFTR is predominantly cotranslational. *Mol. Cell* **20**, 277–287.
31. Atwell, S., Brouillette, C. G., Conners, K., Emtage, S., Gheyi, T., Guggino, W. B., et al. (2010) Structures of a minimal human CFTR first nucleotide-binding domain as a monomer, head-to-tail homodimer, and pathogenic mutant. *Protein Eng. Des. Sel.* **23**, 375–384.
32. Lewis, H. A., Wang, C., Zhao, X., Hamuro, Y., Conners, K., Kearins, M. C., et al. (2010) Structure and dynamics of NBD1 from CFTR characterized using crystallography and hydrogen/deuterium exchange mass spectrometry. *J. Mol. Biol.* **396**, 406–430.
33. Lewis, H. A., Zhao, X., Wang, C., Sauder, J. M., Rooney, I., Noland, B. W., et al. (2005) Impact of the deltaF508 mutation in first nucleotide-binding domain of human cystic fibrosis transmembrane conductance regulator on domain folding and structure. *J. Biol. Chem.* **280**, 1346–1353.
34. Thibodeau, P. H., Brautigam, C. A., Machius, M., and Thomas, P. J. (2005) Side chain and backbone contributions of Phe508 to CFTR folding. *Nat. Struct. Mol. Biol.* **12**, 10–16.
35. Aller, S. G., Yu, J., Ward, A., Weng, Y., Chittaboina, S., Zhuo, R., et al. (2009) Structure of P-glycoprotein reveals a molecular basis

for poly-specific drug binding. *Science* **323**, 1718–1722.
36. Dawson, R. J., and Locher, K. P. (2006) Structure of a bacterial multidrug ABC transporter. *Nature* **443**, 180–185.
37. Locher, K. P., Lee, A. T., and Rees, D. C. (2002) The E. coli BtuCD structure: a framework for ABC transporter architecture and mechanism. *Science* **296**, 1091–1098.
38. Reyes, C. L., and Chang, G. (2005) Lipopolysaccharide stabilizes the crystal packing of the ABC transporter MsbA. *Acta Crystallogr.* **61**, 655–658.
39. Kanelis, V., Hudson, R. P., Thibodeau, P. H., Thomas, P. J., and Forman-Kay, J. D. (2010) NMR evidence for differential phosphorylation-dependent interactions in WT and DeltaF508 CFTR. *EMBO J.* **29**, 263–277.
40. Hartman, J., Huang, Z., Rado, T. A., Peng, S., Jilling, T., Muccio, D. D., et al. (1992) Recombinant synthesis, purification, and nucleotide binding characteristics of the first nucleotide binding domain of the cystic fibrosis gene product. *J. Biol. Chem.* **267**, 6455–6458.
41. Ko, Y. H., Thomas, P. J., Delannoy, M. R., and Pedersen, P. L. (1993) The cystic fibrosis transmembrane conductance regulator. Overexpression, purification, and characterization of wild type and delta F508 mutant forms of the first nucleotide binding fold in fusion with the maltose-binding protein. *J. Biol. Chem.* **268**, 24330–24338.
42. Neville, D. C., Rozanas, C. R., Tulk, B. M., Townsend, R. R., and Verkman, A. S. (1998) Expression and characterization of the NBD1-R domain region of CFTR: evidence for subunit-subunit interactions. *Biochemistry* **37**, 2401–2409.
43. Qu, B. H., and Thomas, P. J. (1996) Alteration of the cystic fibrosis transmembrane conductance regulator folding pathway. *J. Biol. Chem.* **271**, 7261–7264.
44. Yike, I., Ye, J., Zhang, Y., Manavalan, P., Gerken, T. A., and Dearborn, D. G. (1996) A recombinant peptide model of the first nucleotide-binding fold of the cystic fibrosis transmembrane conductance regulator: comparison of wild-type and delta F508 mutant forms. *Protein Sci.* **5**, 89–97.
45. Chan, K. W., Csanady, L., Seto-Young, D., Nairn, A. C., and Gadsby, D. C. (2000) Severed molecules functionally define the boundaries of the cystic fibrosis transmembrane conductance regulator's NH(2)-terminal nucleotide binding domain. *J. General Phys.* **116**, 163–180.
46. Gibson, A. L., Wagner, L. M., Collins, F. S., and Oxender, D. L. (1991) A bacterial system for investigating transport effects of cystic fibrosis-associated mutations. *Science* **254**, 109–111.
47. Mossessova, E., and Lima, C. D. (2000) Ulp1-SUMO crystal structure and genetic analysis reveal conserved interactions and a regulatory element essential for cell growth in yeast. *Mol. Cell* **5**, 865–876.
48. Hutt, D. M., Herman, D., Rodrigues, A. P., Noel, S., Pilewski, J. M., Matteson, J., et al. (2010) Reduced histone deacetylase 7 activity restores function to misfolded CFTR in cystic fibrosis. *Nat. Chem. Biol.* **6**, 25–33.

Chapter 25

NMR Spectroscopy to Study the Dynamics and Interactions of CFTR

Voula Kanelis, P. Andrew Chong, and Julie D. Forman-Kay

Abstract

The cystic fibrosis transmembrane conductance regulator (CFTR) is a multi-domain membrane chloride channel whose activity is regulated by ATP at two nucleotide-binding domains (NBD1 and NBD2) and by phosphorylation of the regulatory (R) region. The NBDs and the R region have functionally relevant motions that are critical for channel gating. Nuclear magnetic resonance (NMR) spectroscopy is a highly useful technique for obtaining information on the structure and interactions of CFTR and is extremely powerful for probing dynamics. NMR approaches for studying CFTR are reviewed, using our previous NBD1 and the R region results to provide examples. These NMR data are yielding insights into the dynamic properties and interactions that facilitate normal CFTR regulation as well as pathological effects of mutations, including the most common disease mutant, deletion of F508 in NBD1.

Key words: Dynamics, NBDs, R region, protein disorder, protein interactions.

1. Introduction

1.1. Domain Organization of CFTR

Cystic fibrosis (CF) is caused by mutations in the gene encoding the cystic fibrosis transmembrane conductance regulator (CFTR) (1), a 1480-residue integral membrane protein which functions as a chloride channel (2, 3). As a member of the ATP-binding cassette (ABC) superfamily of proteins, CFTR is formed by two repeats each containing a membrane spanning domain (MSD) followed by a cytosolic nucleotide-binding domain (NBD) (**Fig. 25.1**) (4). The most common and a severe CF-causing mutation is deletion of F508 (F508del) in NBD1. A large disordered regulatory (R) region, which contains multiple sites for

M.D. Amaral, K. Kunzelmann (eds.), *Cystic Fibrosis*, Methods in Molecular Biology 741,
DOI 10.1007/978-1-61779-117-8_25, © Springer Science+Business Media, LLC 2011

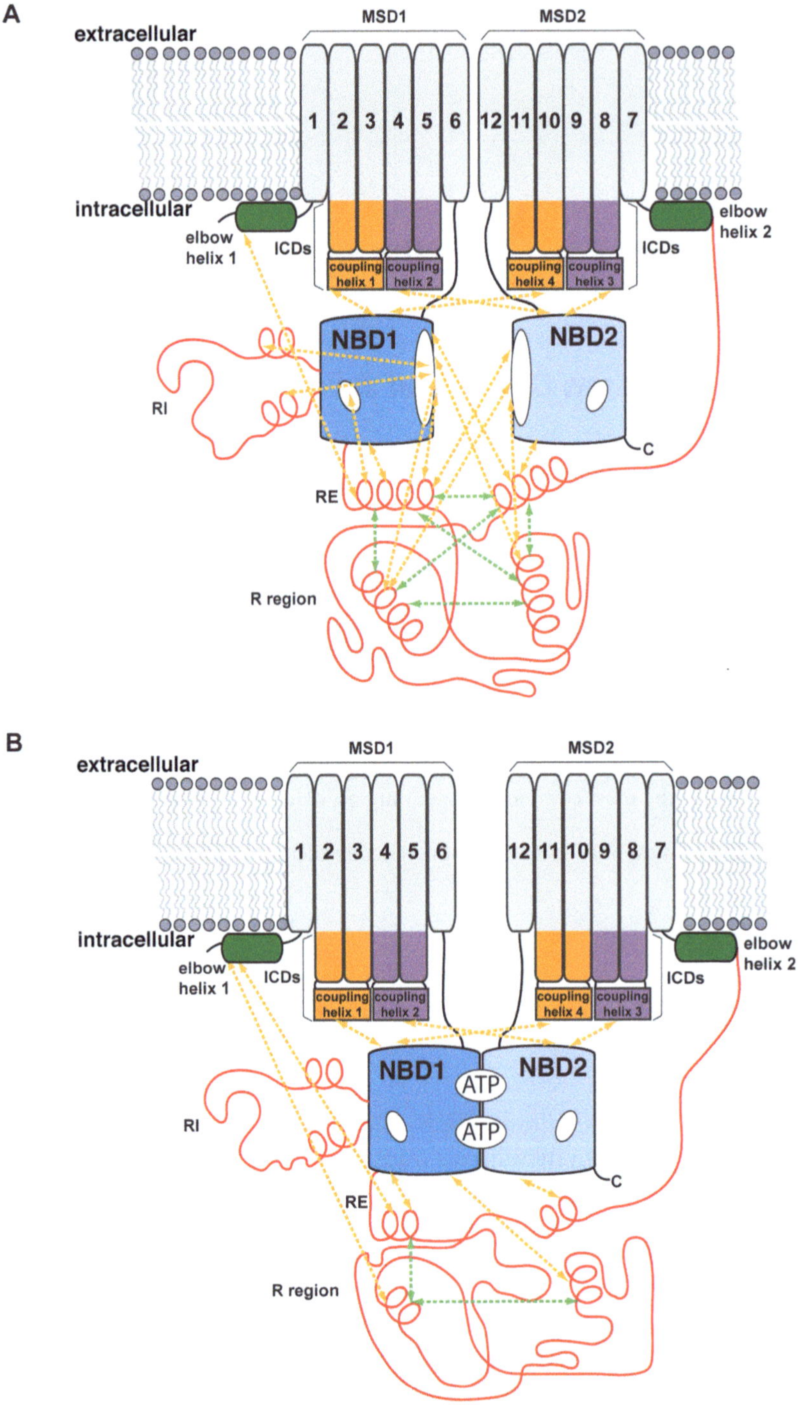

Fig. 25.1. Domain organization of CFTR in (**a**) non-phosphorylated and (**b**) phosphorylated states (adapted from (20)). CFTR contains two membrane spanning domains (MSD1 and MSD2) each formed from six transmembrane helices (*grey rectangles*), two nucleotide-binding domains (NBD1 and NBD2, *blue boxes*), and the intrinsically disordered regulatory (R) region. The RI contains one phosphorylation site, while the R region has a total of nine phosphorylation sites in human CFTR (not shown). The R region and RI in NBD1 are shown as *red curves* to illustrate their disordered states. Binding sites for the RI and R region on NBD1 and NBD2 are shown as *white ovals* in (**a**). Amphipathic helices parallel

phosphorylation by protein kinase A (PKA) and protein kinase C (PKC) and is unique to CFTR (2, 5–9), connects NBD1 and MSD2. Intracellular domains (ICDs) are formed by helical extensions of the transmembrane helices and their connecting loops. Short segments in the connecting loops, known as coupling helices, contact the NBDs (10).

Structural information on CFTR is derived from electron microscopy data on full-length CFTR (11–13), high-resolution crystal structures of the isolated NBD1 (14–17) and NBD2 (18), and NMR spectroscopy on NBD1 (19), the disordered R region (20), and transmembrane helical segments (21). CFTR NBD1 contains a regulatory insertion (RI) with a single PKA phosphorylation site (22). The RI links the first two strands of the β-sheet subdomain and is composed of two short α-helices separated by a disordered linker, most of which is not observed in the various crystal structures (14–16). As disordered phosphorylated segments, the R region and the RI can be considered as comprising the phosphoregulatory elements of CFTR. Most of the NBD1 constructs that have been crystallized also contain the first ~30 residues of the R region at their C-termini, which form the regulatory extension (RE) (14–16), which we call NBD1-RE. Dimeric NBD structures from other ABC transporters show the two NBDs in a "head-to-tail" association with two ATP molecules bound in the NBD dimer interface (17, 23–25). In the CFTR NBD1-RE crystal structures, the RI and RE phosphoregulatory elements interact with the NBD1 core in a manner postulated to sterically prevent NBD heterodimer formation (14–16). Importantly, the RI and RE adopt different orientations in the different NBD1-RE crystal structures (14, 15), implying that they are highly mobile and can dissociate from NBD1 to enable heterodimerization in full-length CFTR.

Each of the components of CFTR has internal dynamics and almost certainly moves with respect to other components during

Fig. 25.1. (continued) to the membrane are located N-terminal to MSD1 and MSD2 (elbow helix 1 and elbow helix 2, respectively, *green rectangles*). The transmembrane helices extend into the cytoplasm and together with residues N-terminal to the NBDs form the intracellular domains (ICDs) (78, 97, 98). Short, irregular helical linkers or coupling helices connect the long helical segments of the ICDs and interact with the NBDs. The long helical segments and coupling helices of the ICDs are colored according to their predicted interactions with the NBDs based on crystal structures of Sav1866 (10, 74), MsbA (75), and P-glycoprotein (73). Coupling helices 1 and 4 are predicted to bind NBD1 and are colored *orange*. Coupling helices 2 and 3 are predicted to bind NBD2 and are colored *purple*. Multiple interactions within helical segments of the R region, many of which are disrupted upon phosphorylation, are shown by *green arrows*. *Yellow arrows* illustrate identified and putative interactions between different parts of CFTR that are in many cases also phosphorylation-dependent. For example, phosphorylation of the RI and the R region disrupts interactions with NBD1 (19, 20) and phosphorylation of the R region enhances interactions with elbow helix 1 (108). ATP binding at the NBDs results in the formation of an NBD1/NBD2 heterodimer with two ATP molecules bound in the interface (**b**). Phosphorylation of the R region and RI and dimerization of the NBDs lead to channel opening.

the gating cycle. The NBDs are enzymes requiring substrate binding and conformational transitions for catalysis. Dynamics in CFTR may involve motions of conserved catalytic residues and motions of subdomains in the individual NBDs during catalysis and upon dimerization. Of note, NMR studies of the NBD from the bacterial ABC transporter MJ1267 demonstrated changes in dynamics in the α-helical subdomain 30 Å away from the ATP binding site upon nucleotide binding (26). Changes in interdomain interactions are also expected, such as those between NBDs and coupling helices, between NBDs and R region, and between the MSDs to open and close the channel pore. From homology models, the α-helical subdomain in CFTR NBD1 interacts with coupling helix 4 in structures of full-length transporters and therefore may link allosteric changes in the NBDs to the membrane domains. Further, multiple regions of CFTR are disordered including the R region and RI in NBD1, regions of the ICDs, and the N- and C-terminal tails based on homology modeling and computational prediction (27). It is likely that changes in interactions involving these disordered regions play a role in the gating cycle.

In order to probe the structure and dynamics of these domains of CFTR and their interactions, we have performed NMR studies on the isolated NBD1 (19) and R region (20), and some of their complexes. The NMR methods employed in these studies are reviewed in the following sections, with particular emphasis on methods useful for studying functionally relevant dynamics of CFTR.

1.2. Introduction to NMR and Its Applicability for Studies of CFTR

Protein structures can be determined by NMR, X-ray crystallography, and electron microscopy, leading to predominantly static images of proteins. NMR, in addition, enables studies of protein dynamics at atomic-level resolution on timescales from picoseconds to days. Relevant dynamics include slower motions of subdomains and domains required for catalysis and gating of the channel as described above, as well as faster, more subtle backbone and side chain conformational interconversions that effect folding and interaction energetics. NMR can also provide structural insight into transiently populated conformations in catalytic cycles (28), including those involved in CFTR gating (29, 30), and into dynamic modes of binding, such as those between the R region and NBD1 (20). Indeed, NMR is a critical tool for studying disordered proteins, like the R region, providing detailed information on the structures of the interconverting conformers (31, 32). Protein–ligand interaction NMR experiments enable measurement of binding affinities, identification of ligand-binding pockets and studies of allosteric changes in response to ligand binding. NMR can also be used to study the effect of post-translational modifications like phosphorylation on the conformation and dynamics of proteins (19, 20). Thus, NMR is a valuable tool for gaining insight into dynamic mechanisms of protein regulation.

NMR signals have two basic parameters, *frequency* and *relaxation rates*, both of which enable analysis of protein structure and dynamics (33). Signals from NMR-active nuclei (primarily the naturally abundant ^{1}H nucleus or proton and isotopically enriched ^{15}N and ^{13}C) resonate at specific frequencies (referred to as chemical shift), which are modulated by directly bonded atoms and chemical groups that are spatially close. For example, backbone nitrogen atoms of Gly residues in a protein will have similar, but not identical, frequencies because each Gly is in a different electronic environment. Thus, the chemical shift is a signature for a specific atom in the protein. In a simple one-dimensional (1D) NMR experiment, the intensity (height) and lineshape (sharp/broad) for the peak are easily observed (1D traces in **Fig. 25.2a**), providing information on the amount of protein and the relaxation properties (see below). Typical protein NMR utilizes 2D or 3D experiments that correlate the frequencies of atoms through bonds or through space, as well as providing resolution due to additional dimensions, analogous to separation of protein bands in 2D gel electrophoresis. For example, in a 2D ^{15}N–^{1}H correlation map, called the HSQC (34), the frequency of each amide proton is correlated with its directly bonded nitrogen, yielding a peak for every non-proline residue in the sequence with distinct chemical shifts (positions in the spectrum) reflecting their unique chemical environments (**Fig. 25.2b, c**). A contour plot clearly presents the peak positions, with intensity/lineshape represented by variable numbers and widths of contours. **Figure 25.2a** shows 1D traces through enlarged peaks from the 2D HSQC of WT NBD1-RE (**Fig. 25.2c**), illustrating the contours. Mapping each resonance frequency to a particular NMR-active nucleus (called resonance assignment) allows structural and dynamic data extracted from various spectra to be interpreted with atomic-level resolution.

The relaxation rates, which describe how quickly NMR signals disappear, are determined by the overall tumbling of the molecule in solution (related to molecular weight) and internal protein dynamics and can be quantified to extract information about protein mobility (33). Protein motion occurs on a range of timescales. Fast timescale dynamics (picosecond–nanosecond, ps–ns) involve rapid conversion between conformations separated by minimal energy barriers (i.e., side chain motions, movement of flexible loops, fast helix–coil transitions). Intermediate timescale dynamics (microsecond–millisecond, μs–ms) involve transitions between a ground state and one or more excited states separated by a higher energy barrier. Examples include domain reorientations and membrane channel opening. These intermediate

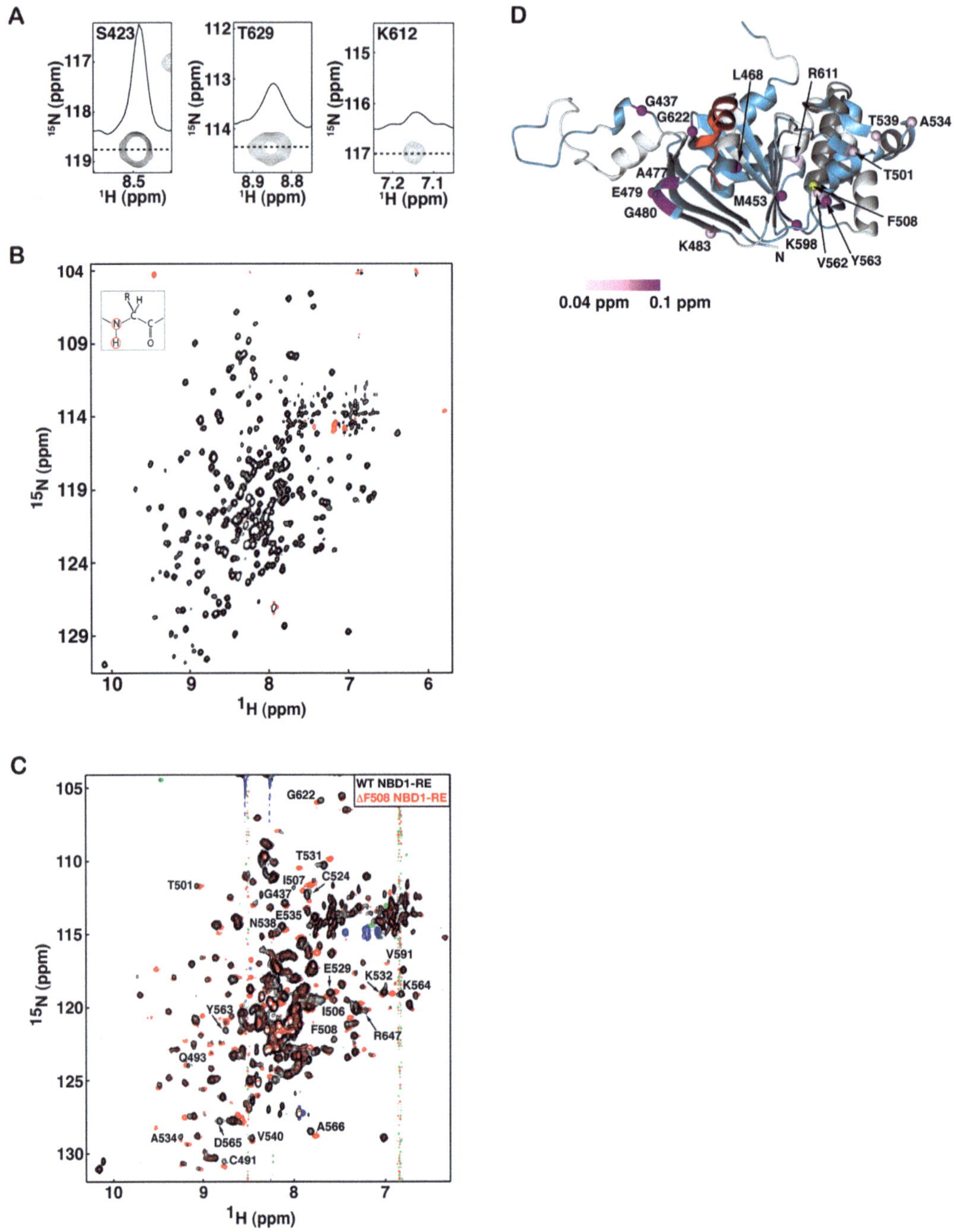

Fig. 25.2. NMR spectra of murine CFTR NBD1-RE. (**a**) Selected regions of the HSQC spectra of WT mNBD1-RE with peaks of different intensities and lineshapes. A trace through the approximate center of the peak is shown above each resonance, illustrating the lineshape. (**b**) HSQC spectrum of the G550E/R553M/R555K mutant NBD1-RE (398–673). Resonances of backbone nuclei, as well as those from side chain nuclei from Trp, Asn, and Gln residues, are colored in *black*. The *red* resonances in this spectrum are of opposite sign, caused by spectral aliasing, and are from side chain arginine $N_{\varepsilon}H_{\varepsilon}$ correlations and one backbone correlation. Approximately 250 backbone NH correlations are visible in this spectrum, which is consistent with the 280 expected correlations from non-proline residues and considering the significant overlap of RI and RE resonances. The *inset* shows a schematic diagram of an amino acid in a polypeptide,

processes impact the observed frequencies and lead to apparent relaxation losses. This relaxation loss can be quantified and used to measure the rate of exchange between the conformers and their populations (35), and even to determine the structures of low population excited states (28). Some processes, such as proline isomerization and protein folding, can occur on timescales of seconds or slower. Such slowly exchanging conformers give rise to separate signals in NMR experiments and can be characterized separately. Amide hydrogen exchange, which is used to probe slower timescale motions, can be quantified by using either hydrogen–deuterium exchange experiments that monitor the rate of exchange between amide protons ($^1H^N$) in the protein and solvent ^2H_2O (36) or by using experiments to measure (fast) magnetization transfer to $^1H^N$ from solvent ^1H_2O (37). Thus, NMR can probe protein conformational changes or interactions occurring on timescales from ps to days. Importantly, changes in chemical shift or dynamic parameters upon protein modification or ligand binding can provide valuable structural information about the effects of these perturbations.

2. Materials

2.1. Equipment and NMR Data Processing

High-field NMR spectrometers are required for optimal sensitivity and resolution (**Note 1**) in studies of protein structure, dynamics, and interactions. The work on CFTR reviewed below has been performed on Varian 500, 600, and 800 MHz spectrometers with triple resonance probes to enable NMR pulses on ^1H,

Fig. 25.2. (continued) highlighting the backbone N and H atoms that give rise to most of the peaks in the HSQC spectrum. (**c**) Comparison of HSQC spectra for WT and F508del NBD1-RE, with selected residues indicated. The spectrum of WT is shown in the foreground with resonances of backbone nuclei, as well as those from side chain nuclei from Trp, Asn, and Gln residues, in *black*. The *blue* resonances are from side chain arginine $^{15}N_\varepsilon{}^1H_\varepsilon$ correlations and one backbone correlation. The spectrum of F508del is shown in the background. Resonances colored *red* and *green* in the F508del spectrum correspond to those colored *black* and *blue* in the WT spectrum, respectively. Overall, the spectra of WT and F508del are very similar, with few differences in peak positions, indicating that WT- and F508del-NBD1 have the same overall structure. Differences in peak intensities (broadening), however, reflect distinct dynamic behavior. (**d**) Schematic ribbon diagram of the interaction between NBD1-RE and coupling helix 1 from a homology model based on Sav1866. The interacting peptide is in *red* and the NBD1-RE structure is colored *blue* for residues for which we have resonance assignments, *light grey* for those not assigned, and *dark grey* for those assigned in the G550E/R553M/R555K mutant but not transferable to WT NBD1-RE (19). The Cα atoms for residues that show chemical shift changes upon binding of coupling helix 1 in phospho-WT NBD1-RE and/or phospho-WT NBD1 are shown as *magenta* spheres. The Cα atom of Phe508, which does not show chemical shift changes upon addition of coupling helix 1, is highlighted in *yellow*. Chemical shifts observed with addition of coupling helix 1 reflect both binding of coupling helix 1 to the NBD1 surface and conformational changes in the protein, which may include displacement of the RI and RE from the NBD1 core (19). (This figure was first published in the *EMBO J.* 29, 263–277 (2010).)

^{15}N, and ^{13}C, facilitating experiments utilizing all three types of nuclei such as resonance assignment (see below). NMR data are processed and analyzed using various software packages (**Note 2**); we utilize nmrPipe/nmrDraw (38) and NMRView (39).

2.2. Samples for NMR Studies

2.2.1. Suitable Constructs

Extracting information on protein structure and dynamics using solution-state NMR generally requires soluble protein $\geq$100 μM. Since NMR lineshape is dependant on overall tumbling and thus molecular weight, there are significant size limitations; typical approaches are applicable to proteins up to ~40 kDa and state-of-the-art methods can provide detailed information on proteins or complexes up to ~100 kDa (40), with some exciting applications exploiting methyl resonances on complexes up to ~1 MDa (41, 42). Because of this, the modularity of proteins is often utilized to define individual domains or multi-domain fragments for NMR studies. It is critical that the boundaries chosen do not cut into any globular domains, preventing proper folding and leading to aggregation. The samples should be highly purified and homogenous, because the presence of multiple forms of the protein (i.e., different oligomerization or post-translational modifications) can greatly complicate the interpretation of NMR spectra. Soluble aggregation is also a problem because it decreases the overall molecular tumbling rate and concomitantly the intensity of the NMR signals. Obtaining soluble, pure, homogeneous samples can be particularly challenging for large, membrane proteins such as CFTR, even for cytoplasmic portions, due to their numerous intra- and inter-molecular regulatory interactions, which lead to the presence of aggregation-promoting hydrophobic patches. Note that different NMR experiments have different requirements for the quality of the NMR spectra. Resonance assignment and dynamics studies require high-quality NMR spectra with samples required to remain stable over several weeks, but interaction studies can frequently be accomplished with more poorly behaved samples. It is also possible to assign a well-behaved protein containing stabilizing amino acid substitutions or other modifications and then transfer the assignments to the more poorly behaved wild-type (WT) protein for interaction studies (19).

Defining fragments of CFTR and solution conditions that yield soluble, homogeneous samples has been a significant obstacle for NMR studies of CFTR. As full-length CFTR is currently not accessible to NMR due to its size and inability to produce concentrated protein samples, it is necessary to divide CFTR into soluble portions that are suitable for NMR. The modularity of CFTR allows its study, in part, as individual domains. A multifaceted approach for obtaining suitable samples involving refinement of domain boundaries, mutagenesis to introduce stabilizing or solubilizing amino acids, solubility screening of buffer conditions, and isotopic labeling strategies to simplify spectra is an ongoing process for biophysical studies of CFTR. NMR studies on CFTR MSDs have focused on interactions between two transmembrane segments using helix–loop–helix constructs comprising transmembrane helices 3 and 4 and the intervening extracellular loop (TM3/4) in micelles (21) that mimic the bilayer yielding particles that tumble rapidly enough to provide reasonable NMR lineshapes. With the available NMR resonance assignments of TM3/4 and through reconstitution of MSD1/2 with other helix–loop–helix constructs, the effects of CF-causing mutations on the structure of the MSDs can be probed. Work in our laboratory has focused on NBD1, NBD2, R region, and the coupling helices of the ICDs. As a disordered protein having a high fraction of charged residues, the R region was more easily amenable to solution NMR studies, once a better behaved construct containing the polymorphism F833L was identified (20). However, it has been more difficult to obtain suitable NBD1 (see below) and NBD2 constructs.

Much effort has gone into developing protein constructs for structural studies of NBD1, the site of F508 deletion. Domain boundaries, which can be defined using multiple sequence alignments and proteolysis experiments, affect protein solubility. Ideally, protein constructs should include all structural elements required for stability and exclude flexible regions N- and C-terminal to the domain, which sometimes reduce solubility. For NBD1, extensive empirical studies were necessary to identify suitable boundaries and mutations that improve solubility (14). Our recently published NMR studies used murine NBD1 (mNBD1) because of its enhanced solubility relative to human NBD1 (19). The solubility of mNBD1 is greatly improved by the inclusion of the RE (14), which transiently populates helical structures that interact with NBD1 (19, 20), and incorporation of the revertant mutations, G550E, R553M, and R555K (43–45), yielding an NBD1-RE construct that is sufficiently soluble for NMR assignment experiments. More recently it has been shown that the solubility of human NBD1 can be dramatically improved by deletion of the 30-residue RI (17). Alternatively, the protein can be modified to increase solubility by specific point mutations (F494N and to a lesser degree F429S and Q637R) without deleting the RI (46). **Table 25.1** lists suitable constructs of NBD1 for NMR studies. Buffer conditions for the mNBD1-RE sample were optimized using buffer screens (19). Mg/ATP (5 mM) and glycerol (2–4% v/v) both significantly stabilize the protein. Higher concentrations of glycerol and lower temperatures further stabilize the protein, but increase the viscosity of the solution, leading to

Table 25.1
List of preferred CFTR constructs for NMR studies

Construct	Boundaries	"Solubilizing" mutations
mNBD1-RE	389–673	G550E, R553M, R555K
hNBD1[a]	387–404, 437–646	None
hNBD1-RE[a]	387–404, 437–678	None
hNBD1-RE	389–678	F494N
hNBD1-RE	389–678	F429S, F494N, Q637R

[a]The RI (residues 405–436) have been deleted in these constructs.

slower molecular tumbling and decreased NMR signal intensities. Experiments were performed at 20°C, a balance between considerations of protein stability and optimal NMR conditions.

2.3. Buffer Conditions

For all proteins studied by NMR, buffer conditions need to be individually optimized to enhance solubility. Factors to test include pH, ionic strength, different buffers (i.e., sodium or potassium phosphate, Tris, HEPES, acetate) and salts, and additives such as glycerol, glycine, arginine, the combination of arginine and glutamate (47), and imidizole. Small ligands such as ATP/magnesium and drug-like compounds as well as protein interaction partners, either intra- or inter-molecular, can enhance the solubility by covering hydrophobic interaction surfaces and stabilizing the protein. Because of the enormous number of possible combinations it is advisable to screen many buffer conditions systematically using small volumes of protein (*see* **Section 3.1**). Details of the buffers we used for our NMR studies of NBD1 and the R region can be found in the corresponding publications (19, 20).

2.4. Isotope Labeling

NMR-active nuclei of relevance to proteins include ^{1}H, ^{2}H, ^{15}N, and ^{13}C (33). With the exception of ^{1}H, these isotopes have a low natural abundance and can be incorporated into protein samples by expressing the proteins in minimal media supplemented with isotopically enriched precursors using either *Escherichia coli* or *Pichia pastoris*. Uniform ^{15}N and ^{13}C labeling with minimal M9 media is straightforward and requires that the sole nitrogen (i.e., NH_4Cl) or carbon source (i.e., glucose) is fully enriched in the desired isotope. Specific labeling patterns (in an unlabeled background) can be achieved in *E. coli* by adding labeled amino acids or amino acid precursors (48, 49), as is done to obtain isotopically labeled methyls of Val and Leu residues. Specific labels reduce spectral complexity and facilitate assignment of signals to specific amino acids in the protein sequence. Selective incorporation of deuterium (^{2}H) into the protein removes pathways for signal relaxation and leads to a significant enhancement in signals derived from the remaining protons for large proteins (50).

3. Methods

NMR spectroscopy is a rich technique that is rapidly developing to address new challenges. There are many reviews of NMR approaches available (51–56). Here, rather than expound in detail the protocols for NMR spectroscopic experiments, our goal is to provide a guide for analysis and interpretation of NMR data, relevant to understanding CFTR structure, dynamics, and interactions. Initially, however, we provide a protocol for buffer condition optimization.

3.1. Buffer Screening Protocol

A simple screening protocol is the following:

1. Dilute a 100 μM protein solution into various test buffers in a 96-well plate, so that the final concentration of protein is 10 μM (**Note 3**).
2. Incubate the samples at increasing temperatures (i.e., room temperature, 30°C, 37°C, 45°C, 55°C) for 30 min to 1 h and subsequently observe the formation of visible aggregates using a light microscope (**Note 4**).
3. Solution conditions that minimize formation of visible aggregates can be further tested using a large molecular weight cutoff (i.e., 100 kDa, 500 μl Amicon Microcon) protein concentrators to distinguish between monomeric protein and soluble aggregates (57).
4. Solution conditions that are promising can then be used to prepare an NMR sample using ^{15}N-labeled protein for HSQC feasibility analysis (*see* below) (**Note 5**).

3.2. Heteronuclear Single Quantum Correlation (HSQC) Experiment

The HSQC (58) (*see* **Fig. 25.2b**) is typically used to assess the feasibility of using a particular protein construct and set of solution conditions (**Note 6**). This experiment is highly sensitive and can quickly demonstrate whether peaks are observed for all amide groups and whether their intensities are relatively homogeneous (note the lack of uniformity in **Fig. 25.2b**). Differential peak intensities imply μs–ms timescale motion. HSQCs can also be used to measure the temperature stability of protein samples and their stability over time, since NMR analysis may require experiments that take several days. The HSQC provides a simple and definitive test of whether a protein is folded or disordered. Stably folded proteins have a large dispersion of amide proton chemical shifts modulated by their specific environments, ranging from

6 to 10 ppm, as for the folded NBD1 seen in **Fig. 25.2b**. In disordered states, there is fast interconversion between highly distinct conformers so that, on average, all nuclei experience similar chemical environments. Disordered proteins have a much narrower dispersion with averaged amide proton chemical shifts over the ensemble that range from 8.0 to 8.8 ppm, as seen in spectra of the disordered R region (**Fig. 25.3a**). Importantly, the HSQC can also be used to monitor structural changes upon mutation or modification (*see* **Figs. 25.2c** and **25.3a**), dynamics, and ligand binding (*see* **Fig. 25.3c**). Provided that the NMR signals can be assigned, residue-level resolution is available by analyzing specific resonance changes in the HSQC.

3.3. NMR Resonance Assignment

NMR resonance assignment enables NMR structural, dynamic, and binding information to be interpreted at atomic- or residue-level resolution. Assignment involves mapping all resonances in a spectrum to specific NMR-active nuclei in the protein, including backbone (amide $^{1}H^{N}$ and ^{15}N, $^{13}C\alpha$, ^{13}C carbonyl) and side chain (^{1}H, ^{15}N, ^{13}C) resonances (**Note 7**). Methods for assigning chemical shifts for folded proteins the size of NBD1 are routine (51) but require well-behaved protein samples with uniform peak intensities. Proteins, like NBD1, with heterogeneous lineshapes due to dynamics, require case-specific isotope-labeling strategies, which must take into account bacterial amino acid metabolism (59). HSQC spectra recorded on samples specifically ^{15}N labeled on Leu residues, aromatic residues (Phe, Tyr, and Trp), or the combination of Gly, Ser, Asp, and Asn residues were used to assist in identification of residue type in order to achieve 70% assignment of the G550E, R553M, R555K mutant NBD1-RE, which were then transferred to the WT protein (19), as the level of uniformity of lineshapes was greater for the G550E, R553M, R555K mutant than either WT or F508del (compare **Fig. 25.2b, c**). This level of assignment, although not 100%, allowed residue-specific characterization of the protein. Additional site-specific information can be obtained using side chain resonances as probes. Protonated methyl groups in particular are highly sensitive, especially in a deuterated protein background. Recording spectra of a mutant protein containing a deletion of a particular methyl-containing side chain allows assignment of these methyl groups in highly dynamic or very large proteins.

Assignment of disordered proteins or regions of proteins is complicated by poor $^{1}H^{N}$ dispersion. Experiments relying on the greater dispersion of the ^{13}C-carbonyl are particularly useful and enabled assignment of the nearly 200-residue long disordered R region (20). Assignment is also often challenging in disordered regions due to broadening from partially stabilized structure (note that the non-phosphorylated R region assignment is missing resonances from 718 to 722) and repetitive sequences

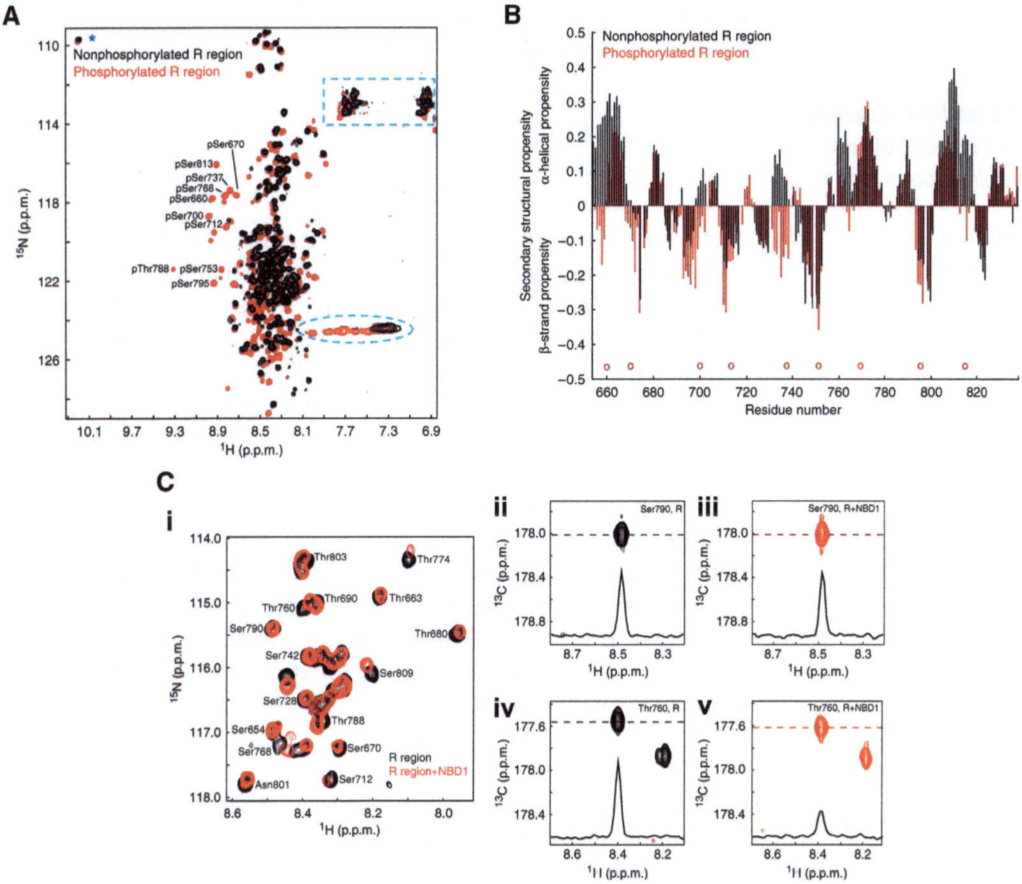

Fig. 25.3. NMR data for the human CFTR R region. (**a**) HSQC spectra of non-phosphorylated (*black peaks*) and phosphorylated (*red peaks*) R region are overlaid. The limited dispersion in $^1H^N$ chemical shift indicates that the R region is disordered. The *blue dashed box* highlights resonances of Asn and Gln side chain amide groups. The *blue dashed ellipse* marks resonances from Arg side chains. The peaks in the *top left hand corner* of the spectrum (marked with an *asterisk*) are from the side chain indole of a Trp residue. (**b**) SSP values of the non-phosphorylated and phosphorylated R region are plotted as a function of residue number. *Positive* SSP values reflect fractional helical structure for each residue, while *negative* SSP values reflect fractional β-structure. *Red circles* indicate phosphorylation sites. (**c**) Interaction of R region with murine NBD1. In this experiment, the R region is labeled with NMR-active nuclei (i.e., ^{15}N, ^{13}C), while the interaction partner (i.e., NBD1) is unlabeled and thus will be invisible in the NMR experiment. Addition of the unlabeled NBD1 to the labeled R region will cause chemical shift and lineshape changes in resonances of R region residues that bind NBD1 or that adopt different conformations. (i) Superposition of a selected region of the 2D ^{15}N–^1H correlation spectra of R region (*black peaks*) and R region bound to NBD1 (*red peaks*). Resonance assignments are given for resolved peaks. (ii–v) Slices through 3D HNCO experiments for the R region (ii, iv) and R region bound to NBD1 (iii, v). (The HNCO experiment correlates backbone $^1H^N$ and ^{15}N chemical shifts of a particular residue with the ^{13}C-carbonyl chemical shift of the previous residue.) Slices are taken at different ^{15}N chemical shifts, including (ii, iii) 115.36 ppm showing Ser 790 and (iv, v) 115.07 ppm showing Thr760. The resonance for Ser790 does not broaden or decrease intensity upon binding NBD1, indicating that Ser790 does not bind NDB1. In contrast, the intensity of Thr760 significantly decreases in the presence of NBD1, indicating that Thr760 is involved in direct interaction with NBD1 or is in contact with other residues in R region that bind NBD1. (This figure was first published in *Nat. Struct. Mol. Biol.* **14**, 738–745 (2007).)

that may arise in low-complexity disordered proteins (i.e., dibasic PKA sites) (**Note 8**).

3.4. NMR Approaches for Folded Proteins: Application to NBD1

3.4.1. Structure Determination

NMR can be used to determine the structures of proteins. Chemical shifts contain inherent secondary and tertiary structure information (60, 61), enabling structures of small proteins (<120 residues) to be determined with this information alone (62–64). Solving larger protein structures de novo by NMR requires more information, including inter-proton distance restraints from nuclear Overhauser effect (NOE) data (61, 65, 66), and is often time-consuming compared to X-ray crystallography. If a high-resolution crystal structure exists, NMR can be used to rapidly confirm that the same structure is maintained in the solution state using chemical shifts. In the presence of weakly aligning media (such as Pf1 phage solutions), where protein tumbling is partially restricted, residual dipolar couplings (RDCs) can also be measured (67, 68) to provide information on the relative orientations of inter-nuclear vectors. NMR structures can be solved solely based on RDCs for many different inter-nuclear vectors (69, 70). A smaller set of RDCs can be used to rapidly confirm that the solution structure is the same as the crystal structure or to identify changes in the relative orientation of secondary structural elements or subdomains (71) as might be observed in different states or conditions, such as comparisons of WT and F508del or phosphorylated and non-phosphorylated states of NBD1.

3.4.2. Monitoring Conformational Change and Interactions

Perturbation of chemical shifts and of lineshapes in HSQC spectra under various conditions is a rapid way to assess conformational changes due to changes in conditions, post-translational modifications, or mutations in a protein. For example, spectra of WT and F508del NBD1-RE have similar peak positions for most resonances (**Fig. 25.2c**), indicating that the mutation does not affect the overall fold of NBD1 (19). The small subset of peaks which do shift in this case allows one to pinpoint areas of the protein that are affected by the mutation. Phosphorylation of S422 in the RI and S659 and S670 in the RE results in many spectral changes, including the appearance of the downfield-shifted (high chemical shift value) amide proton peak for the phosphorylated S422 (19). Shifts are observed for residues on the surface of the NBD1 core that are close in space to the phosphorylation sites in some of the crystal structures. As noted in the introduction, the different orientations of the RI and RE in the crystal structures suggest that they are mobile. Notably, some of the chemical shift changes observed on phosphorylation of the RI and RE are identical to those observed when the mobile RE is removed, implying that phosphorylation of the RE interferes with interactions between the RE and the surface of the NBD1 core (19).

Chemical shift and lineshape changes can also provide critical information regarding binding of protein or small molecule partners. One area of focus in our group is probing the interactions of the coupling helices with the NBDs. Based on crystal structures of the bacterial exporters Sav1866 and MsbA, and the mammalian drug efflux pump P-glycoprotein (10, 72–75), NBD1 should interact with coupling helices 1 and 4 and NBD2 with coupling helices 2 and 3, although these interactions are likely correlated with specific NBD heterodimer conformations and nucleotide-binding states. Crosslinking studies have shown specific interactions of the coupling helices and the NBDs (76–78), with some coupling helices able to mediate interactions to both NBD1 and NBD2 (76), possibly representing different points in the CFTR gating cycle. Our NMR studies using chemical shift perturbation approaches indicate that binding of coupling helix 1 to WT but not F508del NBD1-RE is promoted by phosphorylation of the RI and RE (19), suggesting a molecular mechanism for one aspect of the impaired responsiveness to PKA stimulation (79). These chemical shift perturbations are consistent with the interface modeled based on other ABC transporter structures, as illustrated in **Fig. 25.2d**.

Another aspect of protein interactions of particular interest is characterization of binding of CF modulators including correctors and potentiators to CFTR. NMR is a powerful tool utilized by pharmaceutical companies in the drug discovery process due to its ability to identify even weak interactions ($K_d \sim$ mM), to map binding sites and to provide information on the structural and dynamic consequences of binding (80). Current studies in our laboratory have probed binding of such compounds to NBD1. It is important to mention that allosteric changes to the protein caused by binding (or modifications and mutations) can also affect chemical shifts and lineshapes. Thus, while these perturbations provide conclusive evidence for direct binding, they do not precisely localize binding pockets or sites of modification on the surface of a protein. For example, ligand binding can cause a subtle shift in protein conformation at sites that are distant from the binding pocket, resulting in additional chemical shift changes at these locations. (Note the scattering of chemical shift perturbations caused by binding of coupling helix 1 to NBD1 in **Fig. 25.2d**.) Binding pockets are more precisely localized using NOEs (51) or transfer of cross-saturation that results in signal losses specifically for residues at interfaces (81).

3.4.3. Quantifying Dynamic Processes

Fast ps–ns dynamics, such as certain backbone conformational transitions and side chain motions, can be quantified using relaxation experiments. Observation of low R_2 relaxation rates identifies residues that are flexible on this timescale. Using these approaches, we found that the RI and RE are mobile and flexible with respect to the core NBD1 (19). In cases of rapid interconversion between two discrete conformations, it is also possible to assess changes in the relative population of the two conformers because the observed chemical shift is a population-weighted average of the chemical shift for each state (35). Deviations of chemical shifts from structured values in the direction of random coil values also provide a measure of fast interconversion between folded and more disordered (higher energy intermediate or unfolded) states of a protein (82).

Interconversion between conformers on the slower μs–ms timescale, such as domain reorientation, which is the approximate time required to record the frequency of the atom during an NMR experiment, manifests as broadening of the peak and loss of peak intensity (*see* **Fig. 25.2a**). Unstable proteins, which undergo significant dynamic processes on the μs–ms timescale, have large-scale peak broadening and inhomogeneity in peak intensities. Both mouse and human NBD1 spectra exhibit broadening due to conformational exchange (**Fig. 25.2b**). Broadening in spectra of mNBD1-RE is likely caused by motions of the RI and RE, specifically binding to and releasing from the NBD1 core, as well as motion of the subdomains relative to each other as is often found in enzymes (19). Mapping broadened resonances to specific residues in NBD1 can pinpoint the location of the putative conformational exchange processes. The inhomogeneities in the peak intensities are related to (i) the locations of the dynamic processes and (ii) the magnitudes of the chemical shift differences between the resonances for the underlying states relative to the rates of the exchange processes. For some NBD1 residues, which are presumably near to the site experiencing conformational exchange, the peak broadening is severe enough to prevent observation and assignment. These NMR data suggest that NBD1 does not have a stable ground state conformation; rather it appears to be exchanging between two or more conformations. Biochemical evidence indicates that there are many single-point mutations in NBD1 with a profound effect on the function of CFTR and on the stability of isolated NBD1 in folding studies and is supportive of the complexity of the energy landscape of NBD1. NMR chemical shift dispersion methods have been designed to quantify broadening due to conformational exchange. Our laboratory is currently working on quantitative conformational exchange measurements of NBD1 in WT and mutant states (i.e., F508del) to provide insight into mechanisms by which F508del causes functional and processing defects in CFTR.

3.5. NMR Approaches for Disordered Proteins: Application to the R Region

NMR studies on the isolated regulatory (R) region of CFTR demonstrate that the R region is intrinsically disordered (20), consistent with prediction based on its unusual sequence composition (27, 83). Thus, we refer to this segment of CFTR as the R region rather than the R domain to reflect the lack of stable tertiary structure. The R region of CFTR contains multiple sites for phosphorylation (2, 5–9) and indeed most phosphorylation sites in proteins are located in disordered regions (84). In contrast to folded proteins, disordered proteins exist as an ensemble of rapidly interconverting conformers with wide variability in degree of compactness, secondary structure, and tertiary contacts (31). One function of disordered proteins is mediating multiple regulatory protein interactions (85), and "hub" proteins (those binding at least 10 partners) are significantly enriched in disorder (86). The R region has been implicated in interactions with many other portions of CFTR as well as other proteins, pointing to its functioning as a regulatory hub and consistent with its disordered nature. Upon binding its target proteins, the disordered protein may become ordered or retain significant mobility in the context of dynamic complexes involving transient interactions (87).

NMR is ideally suited for studying disordered states, which have structural heterogeneity and dynamics that make them inaccessible to study by X-ray crystallography. The rapid internal motion enhances the sensitivity of NMR experiments for disordered proteins compared to folded proteins of the same molecular weight. Even in the absence of stable structure, NMR resonance assignments provide site-specific information. Further, while X-ray crystallography and NMR spectroscopy can provide structural information on protein complexes in which the disordered protein becomes ordered upon binding, only NMR can provide site-specific information on highly dynamic or transient complexes.

3.5.1. Fluctuating Secondary Structure

As noted previously, the dispersion or range of backbone amide proton ($^1H^N$) chemical shifts provides a conclusive measure of the presence or absence of stable structure. The isolated R region exhibits poor dispersion of the backbone amide proton chemical shifts, which is diagnostic of a disordered protein (20) (**Fig. 25.3a**, compare to the folded NBD1 spectra in **Fig. 25.2b, c**). Deviations from random coil chemical shifts are sensitive to secondary structure, which in disordered proteins is only transient and fractionally populated (60, 88). The combination of different chemical shifts for a residue into a secondary structure propensity (SSP) score can be used to determine the fractional secondary structure for specific residues (88). SSP scores for the non-phosphorylated R region demonstrate multiple regions with α-helical propensity, which for most sites is decreased upon phosphorylation (20) (**Fig. 25.3b**).

3.5.2. Hydrodynamic Methods

The compactness of a protein is an important parameter for a disordered state since transient structure leads to compaction. NMR measurement of the translational diffusion coefficient in a magnetic field gradient (89) enables calculation of an ensemble-averaged hydrodynamic radius or R_h, which is also obtainable by size exclusion chromatography (90) (**Note 9**). Small-angle X-ray scattering (SAXS), in addition, provides hydrodynamic data in the form of distributions of heavy atom distances that are not ensemble averaged (91) (**Note 10**). Deviations from the hydrodynamic radius expected for a chemically denatured protein (89, 92) reflect tertiary contacts within the ensemble and are related to the proline content and net charge of the disordered region (93). Compactness is likely functionally significant and can modulate affinities for binding partners (94).

3.5.3. Distance from Spin Labels

Distance restraints can be measured using paramagnetic relaxation enhancements (PREs) to provide direct structural data about tertiary contacts within the ensemble (**Note 11**). Paramagnetic spin labels in the form of nitroxides are covalently linked to the protein of interest using disulfide bonds (**Note 12**). The interaction of an unpaired electron of the spin label causes significant signal broadening for nearby spins, even in transient states. The PRE between a proton and the spin label scales as r^{-6}, thereby allowing the transformation of relative intensities of $^1H^N$–^{15}N crosspeaks in HSQC spectra into distance restraints (95) between the paramagnetic site and an individual proton of up to 20–25 Å.

3.5.4. Protein Interactions

Chemical shift changes can be used to monitor inter-molecular interactions. For binding of a disordered protein that does not lead to its global folding, broadening of only interacting residues in the disordered protein is expected because the molecular tumbling rate decreases for bound residues but the whole protein does not order and tumble uniformly slowly. **Figure 25.3c** shows regions of the HSQC spectra for R region in the absence and presence of NBD1 (20). Changes in chemical shifts and/or intensities for R region resonances indicate either direct interaction of these residues with NBD1 or indirect structural or dynamic effects of binding. Interaction data for non-phosphorylated R region implicate multiple sites, with significant helical propensities, in binding NBD1. There is no increase in $^1H^N$ chemical shift dispersion and no uniform lineshape for resonances in the bound state as might be expected if the R region significantly ordered upon binding (**Note 13**). The data are highly suggestive of a dynamic complex involving transient helical stabilization of multiple segments of the R region on NBD1. Phosphorylation of R region reduces the helical propensity of most sites and reduces binding of NBD1 (20).

3.5.5. Structural Representations

NMR chemical shift, hydrodynamic, PRE, and RDC data (as well as SAXS data) for non-phosphorylated and phosphorylated R regions are currently being obtained in our laboratory to provide structural information that will enhance our understanding of the conformers present in the disordered state ensemble of R region and the mechanism by which R region interacts with binding partners. Collectively, these NMR probes of structure within disordered proteins enable us to restrain structure calculations in an ensemble-averaged manner and develop representations of the conformational ensembles of disordered proteins (**Note 14**) (96). Although computational modeling is important as detailed structural information on full-length CFTR is not available, published computational models of the isolated R region as an ensemble of distinct low-energy conformers (97) or of a folded R domain within full-length CFTR packed against the NBD1/NBD2 heterodimer (98) are not consistent with our NMR data. Secondary structure propensities for both models do not agree with that determined from experimental chemical shifts. Further, R region interactions in the full-length CFTR model do not account for experimental NBD1 interaction data (20). We are currently utilizing NMR data to develop ensemble representations consistent with experimental data for both the isolated R region in various phosphorylation states and its dynamic interactions with binding partners. We have calculated ensembles of other disordered proteins and their dynamic complexes (99, 100). Applying these new methods to dynamic R region complexes should provide significant insight into the molecular basis of regulation of CFTR channel function by the R region via its binding interactions.

4. Concluding Remarks

CFTR has multiple and various dynamic modes during the gating cycle that are critical for channel function and its regulation. NMR spectroscopy is ideally suited to studies of protein motion and interactions in CFTR, including those with CF modulators. Dynamic information can be obtained on a variety of timescales, and interactions can be probed for both stable and transient complexes, including those involving disordered proteins. Continuing NMR studies on the NBDs and R region and their complexes will yield insights into regulation of CFTR function in normal states and pathophysiology of CF.

5. Notes

1. Currently, 500–950 MHz NMR spectrometers are commercially available, having magnets at 11.7–22.3 Tesla. The nomenclature for naming the spectrometer is based on the frequency of the ^{1}H resonance in the given field strength. The higher the field strength, the faster the frequency of NMR resonances, the higher the resolution, and the greater the signal intensity. Due to the complexity of NMR spectra with resonances for each NMR-active nucleus in the sample, higher resolution enables information to be more easily extracted from NMR data. NMR, in general, is a low-sensitivity technique requiring signal averaging and sample concentrations of at least tens to hundreds of micromolar. Thus, higher fields are desirable.
2. NMR data are acquired as magnetization intensity as a function of time and are converted into intensity as a function of frequency, usually by Fourier transformation. Additional processing of data is utilized to enhance resolution, for instance. Software for automated analysis of processed NMR data to extract resonance assignments or structural restraints exists, but most proteins have less than ideal spectra requiring significant human intervention.
3. Since buffer optimization is needed to increase solubility, a first screen may be performed with overall lower concentration or with a lower initial concentration followed by less than tenfold dilution in the buffer of interest.
4. For less soluble proteins, lower temperatures and shorter times are required to observe visible aggregates.
5. NMR spectra are the ultimate test, as transiently formed soluble aggregates may pass through the light microscopy and filtration steps of the screening. In addition, monomeric protein that is unstable from a structural or dynamic perspective will have significant μs–ms timescale motions leading to broadening. Optimization of buffer conditions or introduction of specific point mutations to stabilize the protein in this regard can enable significant improvement of NMR spectra and increase the range of NMR studies that are feasible.
6. The appearance of the NMR spectrum is also dependent on the tumbling behavior of the molecule. Larger proteins or oligomers tumble more slowly and give rise to broader resonances. Qualitative or semi-quantitative lineshape analysis can be used to estimate the molecular weight by comparison with other proteins. NMR relaxation experiments can

be used to quantitatively determine a correlation time for overall tumbling that is related to molecular weight. The less spherical a protein or complex is, the more anisotropic the tumbling will be and the more heterogeneous the line-shapes. Again, NMR relaxation experiments can provide a quantitative determination of the anisotropy of rotational correlation in the form of a rotational diffusion tensor. These approaches can be used for multi-domain proteins to determine whether individual domains move together as a single particle or separately as beads on a string (101, 102).

7. Triple resonance assignment experiments make use of direct through-bond magnetization transfer (^{1}H to ^{15}N to ^{13}Cα to ^{13}C-carbonyl, etc.) between sequential residues to "walk" along the peptide backbone or between adjacent carbon atoms down a side chain.
8. *Cis/trans* proline peptide bond isomerization is facile in disordered regions, potentially yielding multiple resonances for the proline and residues immediately N- and C-terminal to it, further complicating assignment. In the R region, however, there was minimal evidence for duplicated resonances, possibly since its transient helical population destabilizes *cis* proline peptide bonds.
9. Dynamic light scattering can also be utilized for determination of R_h, although sufficient quantitative comparison of data with other methods (NMR, size exclusion chromatography) has not been performed to date.
10. Standard analyses of SAXS data to extract radius of gyration (R_g) or mean pair distribution function of heavy atom distances make assumptions about the protein being in a single dominant conformation and may not be appropriate for disordered proteins. The raw SAXS scattering curve contains all the information about the distribution of distances in the disordered ensemble and can be utilized directly in structural calculations of disordered states (96).
11. There are issues in interpretation of PRE values for highly dynamic proteins, such as disordered states, and various approaches have been utilized to address these issues. A semi-quantitative interpretation is often utilized to avoid over-interpretation (103).
12. The most commonly used of these nitroxide spin labels is MTSL (*S*-(2,2,5,5-tetramethyl-2,5-dihydro-1*H*-pyrrol-3-yl)methyl methanesulfonothioate). Other paramagnetic probes can also be employed, including Cu^{2+} bound to the N-terminal three-residue His-Xxx-Xxx ATCUN (amino terminal Cu^{2+} Ni^{2+}) motif (104). The ATCUN is best

utilized following a fusion tag that is cleaved revealing an unmodified N-terminal histidine able to coordinate Cu^{2+}. One issue with use of Cu^{2+} ATCUN is that coordination releases protons and changes the pH of the solution, requiring significant care in sample preparation. Another issue for all paramagnetic probes is non-specific interaction of the probe with the protein. Comparison of data in paramagnetic and diamagnetic states (oxidized and reduced nitroxide spin label or Cu^{2+} vs Ni^{2+} ATCUN) is the best control for this.

13. A plot of the ratio of the ^{1}H–^{15}N HSQC peak intensity for the disordered protein in the presence of a binding partner over the intensity in the free state as a function of residue is a valuable tool to analyze the effects of binding for a disordered protein. There will be a uniform value of 1 for all residues if there is no interaction. Relatively uniform values lower than 1 for all residues indicate folding upon binding, leading to tumbling of a particle containing both the disordered protein and its binding partner. If there is a dynamic complex with only a small portion of the disordered protein ordered in the complex or with transient interactions of different segments of the disordered protein, the plot of the ratios will have significant non-uniformity (ratios close to 1 represent segments with minimal interactions and regions with lower values represent more effects of interaction). This is the case for the R region (20).
14. Our computational approach for generating ensemble representations of disordered proteins consistent with a large amount of different experimental data is called ENSEMBLE. It utilizes a Monte Carlo algorithm to find the subset of a large input pool of conformers that best fit the data collectively. While unique ensembles are not possible, global structural features are reasonably well defined given adequate experimental restraints (96, 103, 105). Other methods exist, but utilize smaller subsets of data types (106, 107).

References

1. Rommens, J. M., Iannuzzi, M. C., Kerem, B., Drumm, M. L., Melmer, G., Dean, M., et al. (1989) Identification of the cystic fibrosis gene: chromosome walking and jumping. *Science* **245**, 1059–1065.
2. Kartner, N., Hanrahan, J. W., Jensen, T. J., Naismith, A. L., Sun, S. Z., Ackerley, C. A., et al. (1991) Expression of the cystic fibrosis gene in non-epithelial invertebrate cells produces a regulated anion conductance. *Cell* **64**, 681–691.
3. Bear, C. E., Li, C. H., Kartner, N., Bridges, R. J., Jensen, T. J., Ramjeesingh, M., et al. (1992) Purification and functional reconstitution of the cystic fibrosis transmembrane

conductance regulator (CFTR). *Cell* **68**, 809–818.
4. Dean, M., Rzhetsky, A., and Allikmets, R. (2001) The human ATP-binding cassette (ABC) transporter superfamily. *Genome Res.* **11**, 1156–1166.
5. Anderson, M. P., Rich, D. P., Gregory, R. J., Smith, A. E., and Welsh, M. J. (1991) Generation of cAMP-activated chloride currents by expression of CFTR. *Science* **251**, 679–682.
6. Cheng, S. H., Rich, D. P., Marshall, J., Gregory, R. J., Welsh, M. J., and Smith, A. E. (1991) Phosphorylation of the R domain by cAMP-dependent protein kinase regulates the CFTR chloride channel. *Cell* **66**, 1027–1036.
7. Ma, J., Tasch, J. E., Tao, T., Zhao, J., Xie, J., Drumm, M. L., et al. (1996) Phosphorylation-dependent block of cystic fibrosis transmembrane conductance regulator chloride channel by exogenous R domain protein. *J. Biol. Chem.* **271**, 7351–7356.
8. Picciotto, M. R., Cohn, J. A., Bertuzzi, G., Greengard, P., and Nairn, A. C. (1992) Phosphorylation of the cystic fibrosis transmembrane conductance regulator. *J. Biol. Chem.* **267**, 12742–12752.
9. Tabcharani, J. A., Chang, X. B., Riordan, J. R., and Hanrahan, J. W. (1991) Phosphorylation-regulated Cl- channel in CHO cells stably expressing the cystic fibrosis gene. *Nature* **352**, 628–631.
10. Dawson, R. J., and Locher, K. P. (2006) Structure of a bacterial multidrug ABC transporter. *Nature* **443**, 180–185.
11. Awayn, N. H., Rosenberg, M. F., Kamis, A. B., Aleksandrov, L. A., Riordan, J. R., and Ford, R. C. (2005) Crystallographic and single-particle analyses of native- and nucleotide-bound forms of the cystic fibrosis transmembrane conductance regulator (CFTR) protein. *Biochem. Soc. Trans.* **33**, 996–999.
12. Rosenberg, M. F., Kamis, A. B., Aleksandrov, L. A., Ford, R. C., and Riordan, J. R. (2004) Purification and crystallization of the cystic fibrosis transmembrane conductance regulator (CFTR). *J. Biol. Chem.* **279**, 39051–39057.
13. Zhang, L., Aleksandrov, L. A., Zhao, Z., Birtley, J. R., Riordan, J. R., and Ford, R. C. (2009) Architecture of the cystic fibrosis transmembrane conductance regulator protein and structural changes associated with phosphorylation and nucleotide binding. *J. Struct. Biol.* **167**, 242–251.
14. Lewis, H. A., Buchanan, S. G., Burley, S. K., Conners, K., Dickey, M., Dorwart, M., et al. (2004) Structure of nucleotide-binding domain 1 of the cystic fibrosis transmembrane conductance regulator. *EMBO J.* **23**, 282–293.
15. Lewis, H. A., Zhao, X., Wang, C., Sauder, J. M., Rooney, I., Noland, B. W., et al. (2005) Impact of the F508del mutation in first nucleotide-binding domain of human cystic fibrosis transmembrane conductance regulator on domain folding and structure. *J. Biol. Chem.* **280**, 1346–1353.
16. Thibodeau, P. H., Brautigam, C. A., Machius, M., and Thomas, P. J. (2005) Side chain and backbone contributions of Phe508 to CFTR folding. *Nat. Struct. Mol. Biol.* **12**, 10–16.
17. Atwell, S., Brouillette, C. G., Conners, K., Emtage, S., Gheyi, T., Guggino, W. B., et al. (2010) Structures of a minimal human CFTR first nucleotide-binding domain as a monomer, head-to-tail homodimer, and pathogenic mutant. *Protein Eng. Des. Sel.* **23**, 375–384.
18. Zhao, X., Conners, K., Emtage, S., Lu, F., and Atwell, S. (2008) The crystal structure of the second Nucleotide Binding Domain (NBD2) of CFTR suggests NBD2 subdomain movements are involved in channel opening. *Pediatr. Pulmonary* **43**, 205.
19. Kanelis, V., Hudson, R. P., Thibodeau, P. H., Thomas, P. J., and Forman-Kay, J. D. (2010) NMR evidence for differential phosphorylation-dependent interactions in WT and F508del-CFTR. *EMBO J.* **29**, 263–277.
20. Baker, J. M., Hudson, R. P., Kanelis, V., Choy, W. Y., Thibodeau, P. H., Thomas, P. J., et al. (2007) CFTR regulatory region interacts with NBD1 predominantly via multiple transient helices. *Nat. Struct. Mol. Biol.* **14**, 738–745.
21. Wehbi, H., Gasmi-Seabrook, G., Choi, M. Y., and Deber, C. M. (2008) Positional dependence of non-native polar mutations on folding of CFTR helical hairpins. *Biochim. Biophys. Acta* **1778**, 79–87.
22. Dahan, D., Evagelidis, A., Hanrahan, J. W., Hinkson, D. A., Jia, Y., Luo, J., et al. (2001) Regulation of the CFTR channel by phosphorylation. *Pflugers Arch.* **443**(Suppl 1), S92–96.
23. Smith, P. C., Karpowich, N., Millen, L., Moody, J. E., Rosen, J., Thomas, P. J., et al. (2002) ATP binding to the motor domain from an ABC transporter drives formation of a nucleotide sandwich dimer. *Mol. Cell* **10**, 139–149.
24. Verdon, G., Albers, S. V., van Oosterwijk, N., Dijkstra, B. W., Driessen, A. J., and Thun-

nissen, A. M. (2003) Formation of the productive ATP-Mg2+-bound dimer of GlcV, an ABC-ATPase from Sulfolobus solfataricus. *J. Mol. Biol.* **334**, 255–267.
25. Zaitseva, J., Oswald, C., Jumpertz, T., Jenewein, S., Wiedenmann, A., Holland, I. B., et al. (2006) A structural analysis of asymmetry required for catalytic activity of an ABC-ATPase domain dimer. *EMBO J.* **25**, 3432–3443.
26. Wang, C., Karpowich, N., Hunt, J. F., Rance, M., and Palmer, A. G. (2004) Dynamics of ATP-binding cassette contribute to allosteric control, nucleotide binding and energy transduction in ABC transporters. *J. Mol. Biol.* **342**, 525–537.
27. Li, X., Romero, P., Rani, M., Dunker, A. K., and Obradovic, Z. (1999) Predicting protein disorder for N-, C-, and internal regions. *Genome Inform. Ser. Workshop Genome Inform.* **10**, 30–40.
28. Vallurupalli, P., Hansen, D. F., and Kay, L. E. (2008) Structures of invisible, excited protein states by relaxation dispersion NMR spectroscopy. *Proc. Natl. Acad. Sci. USA* **105**, 11766–11771.
29. Cheung, J. C., Kim Chiaw, P., Pasyk, S., and Bear, C. E. (2008) Molecular basis for the ATPase activity of CFTR. *Arch. Biochem. Biophys.* **476**, 95–100.
30. Hwang, T. C., and Sheppard, D. N. (2009) Gating of the CFTR Cl- channel by ATP-driven nucleotide-binding domain dimerisation. *J. Physiol.* **587**, 2151–2161.
31. Eliezer, D. (2009) Biophysical characterization of intrinsically disordered proteins. *Curr. Opin. Struct. Biol.* **19**, 23–30.
32. Mittag, T., and Forman-Kay, J. D. (2007) Atomic-level characterization of disordered protein ensembles. *Curr. Opin. Struct. Biol.* **17**, 3–14.
33. Levitt, M. H. (2001) *Spin Dynamics: Basics of Nuclear Magnetic Resonance*, Wiley, Chichester.
34. Zhang, O., Kay, L. E., Olivier, J. P., and Forman-Kay, J. D. (1994) Backbone 1H and 15 N resonance assignments of the N-terminal SH3 domain of drk in folded and unfolded states using enhanced-sensitivity pulsed field gradient NMR techniques. *J. Biomol. NMR* **4**, 845–858.
35. Mulder, F. A., Mittermaier, A., Hon, B., Dahlquist, F. W., and Kay, L. E. (2001) Studying excited states of proteins by NMR spectroscopy. *Nat. Struct. Biol.* **8**, 932–935.
36. Krishna, M. M., Hoang, L., Lin, Y., and Englander, S. W. (2004) Hydrogen exchange methods to study protein folding. *Methods* **34**, 51–64.
37. Hwang, T. L., van Zijl, P. C., and Mori, S. (1998) Accurate quantitation of water-amide proton exchange rates using the phase-modulated CLEAN chemical exchange (CLEANEX-PM) approach with a Fast-HSQC (FHSQC) detection scheme. *J. Biomol. NMR* **11**, 221–226.
38. Delaglio, F., Grzesiek, S., Vuister, G. W., Zhu, G., Pfeifer, J., and Bax, A. (1995) NMRPipe: a multidimensional spectral processing system based on UNIX pipes. *J. Biomol. NMR* **6**, 277–293.
39. Johnson, B. A., and Blevins, R. A. (1994) NMRView: a computer program for the visualization and analysis of NMR data. *J. Biomol. NMR* **4**, 603–614.
40. Tugarinov, V., Hwang, P. M., and Kay, L. E. (2004) Nuclear magnetic resonance spectroscopy of high-molecular-weight proteins. *Annu. Rev. Biochem.* **73**, 107–146.
41. Sprangers, R., and Kay, L. E. (2007) Quantitative dynamics and binding studies of the 20S proteasome by NMR. *Nature* **445**, 618–622.
42. Sprangers, R., Velyvis, A., and Kay, L. E. (2007) Solution NMR of supramolecular complexes: providing new insights into function. *Nat. Methods* **4**, 697–703.
43. DeCarvalho, A. C., Gansheroff, L. J., and Teem, J. L. (2002) Mutations in the nucleotide binding domain 1 signature motif region rescue processing and functional defects of cystic fibrosis transmembrane conductance regulator F508del. *J. Biol. Chem.* **277**, 35896–35905.
44. Teem, J. L., Berger, H. A., Ostedgaard, L. S., Rich, D. P., Tsui, L. C., and Welsh, M. J. (1993) Identification of revertants for the cystic fibrosis F508del mutation using STE6-CFTR chimeras in yeast. *Cell* **73**, 335–346.
45. Teem, J. L., Carson, M. R., and Welsh, M. J. (1996) Mutation of R555 in CFTR-F508del enhances function and partially corrects defective processing. *Recept. Channels* **4**, 63–72.
46. Mulvihill, C. M., Rabeh, W. M., Di Bernardo, S., Bagdany, M., Du, K., and Lukacs, G. L. (2008) Characterization of wild-type and F508del NBD1 from CFTR with a single solubilization mutation. *Pediatr. Pulmonol.* **31**(Suppl.), 205.
47. Golovanov, A. P., Hautbergue, G. M., Wilson, S. A., and Lian, L. Y. (2004) A simple method for improving protein solubility and long-term stability. *J. Am. Chem. Soc.* **126**, 8933–8939.
48. Tugarinov, V., Kanelis, V., and Kay, L. E. (2006) Isotope labeling strategies for the study of high-molecular-weight proteins by

solution NMR spectroscopy. *Nat. Protoc.* **1**, 749–754.

49. Rosen, M. K., Gardner, K. H., Willis, R. C., Parris, W. E., Pawson, T., and Kay, L. E. (1996) Selective methyl group protonation of perdeuterated proteins. *J. Mol. Biol.* **263**, 627–636.
50. Gardner, K. H., and Kay, L. E. (1998) The use of 2H, 13C, 15N multidimensional NMR to study the structure and dynamics of proteins. *Annu. Rev. Biophys. Biomol. Struct.* **27**, 357–406.
51. Kanelis, V., Forman-Kay, J. D., and Kay, L. E. (2001) Multidimensional NMR methods for protein structure determination. *IUBMB Life* **52**, 291–302.
52. Kay, L. E. (2005) NMR studies of protein structure and dynamics. *J. Magn. Reson.* **173**, 193–207.
53. Sattler, M., Schleucher, J., and Griesinger, C. (1999) Heteronuclear multidimensional NMR experiments for the structure determination of proteins in solution employing pulsed field gradients. *Prog. NMR Spect.* **34**, 93–158.
54. Foster, M. P., McElroy, C. A., and Amero, C. D. (2007) Solution NMR of large molecules and assemblies. *Biochemistry (Mosc)* **46**, 331–340.
55. Grzesiek, S., and Sass, H. J. (2009) From biomolecular structure to functional understanding: new NMR developments narrow the gap. *Curr. Opin. Struct. Biol.* **19**, 585–595.
56. Baldwin, A. J., and Kay, L. E. (2009) NMR spectroscopy brings invisible protein states into focus. *Nat. Chem. Biol.* **5**, 808–814.
57. Richardson, J. M., Caspa, E., and Thomas, P. J. (2008) In vitro CFTR-NBD1-based folding assays for assessment of stabilizing ligands. *Pediatr. Pulmonol.* **31**(Suppl.), 202.
58. Pervushin, K., Riek, R., Wider, G., and Wuthrich, K. (1997) Attenuated T2 relaxation by mutual cancellation of dipole-dipole coupling and chemical shift anisotropy indicates an avenue to NMR structures of very large biological macromolecules in solution. *Proc. Natl. Acad. Sci. USA* **94**, 12366–12371.
59. Goto, N. K., and Kay, L. E. (2000) New developments in isotope labeling strategies for protein solution NMR spectroscopy. *Curr. Opin. Struct. Biol.* **10**, 585–592.
60. Wishart, D. S., and Sykes, B. D. (1994) Chemical shifts as a tool for structure determination. *Methods Enzymol.* **239**, 363–392.
61. Shen, Y., Delaglio, F., Cornilescu, G., and Bax, A. (2009) TALOS+: a hybrid method for predicting protein backbone torsion angles from NMR chemical shifts. *J. Biomol. NMR* **44**, 213–223.
62. Robustelli, P., Cavalli, A., Dobson, C. M., Vendruscolo, M., and Salvatella, X. (2009) Folding of small proteins by Monte Carlo simulations with chemical shift restraints without the use of molecular fragment replacement or structural homology. *J. Phys. Chem. B* **113**, 7890–7896.
63. Shen, Y., Lange, O., Delaglio, F., Rossi, P., Aramini, J. M., Liu, G., et al. (2008) Consistent blind protein structure generation from NMR chemical shift data. *Proc. Natl. Acad. Sci. USA* **105**, 4685–4690.
64. Cavalli, A., Salvatella, X., Dobson, C. M., and Vendruscolo, M. (2007) Protein structure determination from NMR chemical shifts. *Proc. Natl. Acad. Sci. USA* **104**, 9615–9620.
65. Lipsitz, R. S., and Tjandra, N. (2004) Residual dipolar couplings in NMR structure analysis. *Annu. Rev. Biophys. Biomol. Struct.* **33**, 387–413.
66. Nilges, M., Macias, M. J., O'Donoghue, S. I., and Oschkinat, H. (1997) Automated NOESY interpretation with ambiguous distance restraints: the refined NMR solution structure of the pleckstrin homology domain from beta-spectrin. *J. Mol. Biol.* **269**, 408–422.
67. Tjandra, N., and Bax, A. (1997) Direct measurement of distances and angles in biomolecules by NMR in a dilute liquid crystalline medium. *Science* **278**, 1111–1114.
68. Tolman, J. R., Flanagan, J. M., Kennedy, M. A., and Prestegard, J. H. (1995) Nuclear magnetic dipole interactions in field-oriented proteins: information for structure determination in solution. *Proc. Natl. Acad. Sci. USA* **92**, 9279–9283.
69. Hus, J. C., Marion, D., and Blackledge, M. (2001) Determination of protein backbone structure using only residual dipolar couplings. *J. Am. Chem. Soc.* **123**, 1541–1542.
70. Kontaxis, G., Delaglio, F., and Bax, A. (2005) Molecular fragment replacement approach to protein structure determination by chemical shift and dipolar homology database mining. *Methods Enzymol.* **394**, 42–78.
71. Skrynnikov, N. R., Goto, N. K., Yang, D., Choy, W. Y., Tolman, J. R., Mueller, G. A., et al. (2000) Orienting domains in proteins using dipolar couplings measured by liquid-state NMR: differences in solution and crystal forms of maltodextrin binding protein loaded with beta-cyclodextrin. *J. Mol. Biol.* **295**, 1265–1273.
72. Hollenstein, K., Frei, D. C., and Locher, K. P. (2007) Structure of an ABC transporter

in complex with its binding protein. *Nature* **446**, 213–216.
73. Aller, S. G., Yu, J., Ward, A., Weng, Y., Chittaboina, S., Zhuo, R., et al. (2009) Structure of P-glycoprotein reveals a molecular basis for poly-specific drug binding. *Science* **323**, 1718–1722.
74. Dawson, R. J., and Locher, K. P. (2007) Structure of the multidrug ABC transporter Sav1866 from Staphylococcus aureus in complex with AMP-PNP. *FEBS Lett.* **581**, 935–938.
75. Ward, A., Reyes, C. L., Yu, J., Roth, C. B., and Chang, G. (2007) Flexibility in the ABC transporter MsbA: alternating access with a twist. *Proc. Natl. Acad. Sci. USA* **104**, 19005–19010.
76. He, L., Aleksandrov, A. A., Serohijos, A. W., Hegedus, T., Aleksandrov, L. A., Cui, L., et al. (2008) Multiple membrane-cytoplasmic domain contacts in cftr mediate regulation of channel gating. *J. Biol. Chem.* **283**, 26383–26390.
77. Mendoza, J. L., and Thomas, P. J. (2007) Building an understanding of cystic fibrosis on the foundation of ABC transporter structures. *J. Bioenerg. Biomembr.* **39**, 499–505.
78. Serohijos, A. W., Hegedus, T., Aleksandrov, A. A., He, L., Cui, L., Dokholyan, N. V., et al. (2008) Phenylalanine-508 mediates a cytoplasmic-membrane domain contact in the CFTR 3D structure crucial to assembly and channel function. *Proc. Natl. Acad. Sci. USA* **105**, 3256–3261.
79. Wang, F., Zeltwanger, S., Hu, S., and Hwang, T. C. (2000) Deletion of phenylalanine 508 causes attenuated phosphorylation-dependent activation of CFTR chloride channels. *J. Physiol.* **524**(Pt 3), 637–648.
80. Pellecchia, M., Bertini, I., Cowburn, D., Dalvit, C., Giralt, E., Jahnke, W., et al. (2008) Perspectives on NMR in drug discovery: a technique comes of age. *Nat. Rev. Drug Discov* 7, 738–745.
81. Takahashi, H., Nakanishi, T., Kami, K., Arata, Y., and Shimada, I. (2000) A novel NMR method for determining the interfaces of large protein-protein complexes. *Nat. Struct. Biol.* 7, 220–223.
82. Berjanskii, M. V., and Wishart, D. S. (2008) Application of the random coil index to studying protein flexibility. *J. Biomol. NMR* **40**, 31–48.
83. Romero, P., Obradovic, Z., Li, X., Garner, E. C., Brown, C. J., and Dunker, A. K. (2001) Sequence complexity of disordered protein. *Proteins* **42**, 38–48.
84. Iakoucheva, L. M., Radivojac, P., Brown, C. J., O'Connor, T. R., Sikes, J. G., Obradovic, Z., et al. (2004) The importance of intrinsic disorder for protein phosphorylation. *Nucleic Acids Res.* **32**, 1037–1049.
85. Wright, P. E., and Dyson, H. J. (2009) Linking folding and binding. *Curr. Opin. Struct. Biol.* **19**, 31–38.
86. Dosztanyi, Z., Chen, J., Dunker, A. K., Simon, I., and Tompa, P. (2006) Disorder and sequence repeats in hub proteins and their implications for network evolution. *J. Proteome Res.* **5**, 2985–2995.
87. Mittag, T., Kay, L. E., and Forman-Kay, J. D. (2010) Protein dynamics and conformational disorder in molecular recognition. *J. Mol. Recognit* **23**, 105–116.
88. Marsh, J. A., Singh, V. K., Jia, Z., and Forman-Kay, J. D. (2006) Sensitivity of secondary structure propensities to sequence differences between alpha- and gamma-synuclein: implications for fibrillation. *Protein Sci.* **15**, 2795–2804.
89. Wilkins, D. K., Grimshaw, S. B., Receveur, V., Dobson, C. M., Jones, J. A., and Smith, L. J. (1999) Hydrodynamic radii of native and denatured proteins measured by pulse field gradient NMR techniques. *Biochemistry (Mosc)* **38**, 16424–16431.
90. Uversky, V. N. (1993) Use of fast protein size-exclusion liquid chromatography to study the unfolding of proteins which denature through the molten globule. *Biochemistry (Mosc)* **32**, 13288–13298.
91. Choy, W. Y., Mulder, F. A., Crowhurst, K. A., Muhandiram, D. R., Millett, I. S., Doniach, S., et al. (2002) Distribution of molecular size within an unfolded state ensemble using small-angle X-ray scattering and pulse field gradient NMR techniques. *J. Mol. Biol.* **316**, 101–112.
92. Damaschun, G., Damaschun, H., Gast, K., and Zirwer, D. (1998) Denatured states of yeast phosphoglycerate kinase. *Biochemistry (Mosc)* **63**, 259–275.
93. Marsh, J. A., and Forman-Kay, J. D. (2010) Sequence determinants of compaction in intrinsically disordered proteins. *Biophys. J.* **98**, 2383–2390.
94. Borg, M., Mittag, T., Pawson, T., Tyers, M., Forman-Kay, J. D., and Chan, H. S. (2007) Polyelectrostatic interactions of disordered ligands suggest a physical basis for ultrasensitivity. *Proc. Natl. Acad. Sci. USA* **104**, 9650–9655.
95. Iwahara, J., Schwieters, C. D., and Clore, G. M. (2004) Ensemble approach for NMR structure refinement against (1)H paramagnetic relaxation enhancement data arising from a flexible paramagnetic group attached

to a macromolecule. *J. Am. Chem. Soc.* **126**, 5879–5896.

96. Marsh, J. A., and Forman-Kay, J. D. (2009) Structure and disorder in an unfolded state under nondenaturing conditions from ensemble models consistent with a large number of experimental restraints. *J. Mol. Biol.* **391**, 359–374.
97. Hegedus, T., Serohijos, A. W., Dokholyan, N. V., He, L., and Riordan, J. R. (2008) Computational studies reveal phosphorylation-dependent changes in the unstructured R domain of CFTR. *J. Mol. Biol.* **378**, 1052–1063.
98. Mornon, J. P., Lehn, P., and Callebaut, I. (2009) Molecular models of the open and closed states of the whole human CFTR protein. *Cell. Mol. Life Sci.* **66**, 3469–3486.
99. Mittag, T., Marsh, J. A., Grishaev, A., Orlicky, S., Lin, H., Sicheri, F., et al. (2010) Structure/function implications in a dynamic complex of the intrinsically disordered Sic1 with the Cdc4 subunit of an SCF ubiquitin ligase. *Structure* **18**, 494–506.
100. Marsh, J. A., Dancheck, B., Ragusa, M. J., Allaire, M., Forman-Kay, J. D., and Peti, W. (2010) Structural diversity in free and bound states of intrinsically disordered protein phosphatase 1 regulators. *Structure* **18**, 1094–1103.
101. Bruschweiler, R., Liao, X., and Wright, P. E. (1995) Long-range motional restrictions in a multidomain zinc-finger protein from anisotropic tumbling. *Science* **268**, 886–889.
102. Macauley, M. S., Errington, W. J., Scharpf, M., Mackereth, C. D., Blaszczak, A. G., Graves, B. J., et al. (2006) Beads-on-a-string, characterization of ETS-1 sumoylated within its flexible N-terminal sequence. *J. Biol. Chem.* **281**, 4164–4172.
103. Marsh, J. A., Neale, C., Jack, F. E., Choy, W. Y., Lee, A. Y., Crowhurst, K. A., et al. (2007) Improved structural characterizations of the drkN SH3 domain unfolded state suggest a compact ensemble with native-like and non-native structure. *J. Mol. Biol.* **367**, 1494–1510.
104. Donaldson, L. W., Skrynnikov, N. R., Choy, W. Y., Muhandiram, D. R., Sarkar, B., Forman-Kay, J. D., et al. (2001) Structural characterization of proteins with an attached ATCUN motif by paramagnetic relaxation enhancement NMR spectroscopy. *J. Am. Chem. Soc.* **123**, 9843–9847.
105. Choy, W. Y., and Forman-Kay, J. D. (2001) Calculation of ensembles of structures representing the unfolded state of an SH3 domain. *J. Mol. Biol.* **308**, 1011–1032.
106. Lindorff-Larsen, K., Kristjansdottir, S., Teilum, K., Fieber, W., Dobson, C. M., Poulsen, F. M., et al. (2004) Determination of an ensemble of structures representing the denatured state of the bovine acyl-coenzyme a binding protein. *J. Am. Chem. Soc.* **126**, 3291–3299.
107. Jensen, M. R., Markwick, P. R., Meier, S., Griesinger, C., Zweckstetter, M., Grzesiek, S., et al. (2009) Quantitative determination of the conformational properties of partially folded and intrinsically disordered proteins using NMR dipolar couplings. *Structure* **17**, 1169–1185.
108. Naren, A. P., Cormet-Boyaka, E., Fu, J., Villain, M., Blalock, J. E., Quick, M. W., et al. (1999) CFTR chloride channel regulation by an interdomain interaction. *Science* **286**, 544–548.

Section V

CFTR Function

Chapter 26

Introduction to Section V: Assessment of CFTR Function

Karl Kunzelmann

Abstract

This chapter introduces the various techniques to asses the function of CFTR. The numerous functional interactions of CFTR and cellular properties affected by CFTR will be described initially. This will be followed by sections explaining the importance of patch clamping and double electrode voltage clamp experiments in *Xenopus* oocytes for expression analysis of CFTR, and the Ussing chamber technique to analyze CFTR in polarized epithelia. It is concluded that examining CFTR function should occur at different levels, starting with the intact epithelium and ending with isolated CFTR proteins.

Key words: CFTR, interactome, patch clamp, Ussing chamber, epithelial transport, double electrode voltage clamp, *Xenopus* oocytes, high-throughput analysis.

1. A Cellular Life with CFTR

Cells that express CFTR will certainly gain a cAMP-dependent Cl^- conductance of distinct properties. These properties are largely independent of the type of cell in which CFTR is expressed. This fact is taken as a proof of concept that CFTR itself is a Cl^- channel forming protein, rather than a regulator of endogenous Cl^- channels. However, as we have learned over the past 20 years or so, the functional consequences of CFTR expression are multifaceted, encompassing much more than simply supplying a cellular cAMP-regulated Cl^- conductance. To start, CFTR has been shown to influence properties and activity of other ion channels, such as the epithelial Na^+ channel ENaC (*see* **Chapter 3, Section I, Volume II**, by Berdiev et al.), K^+ channels, and Ca^{2+}-activated Cl^- channels, and it somehow controls cell swelling and concomitant volume regulatory decrease, partially by controlling Ca^{2+} influx through TRPV4 channels (**Fig. 26.1**)

M.D. Amaral, K. Kunzelmann (eds.), *Cystic Fibrosis*, Methods in Molecular Biology 741,
DOI 10.1007/978-1-61779-117-8_26,

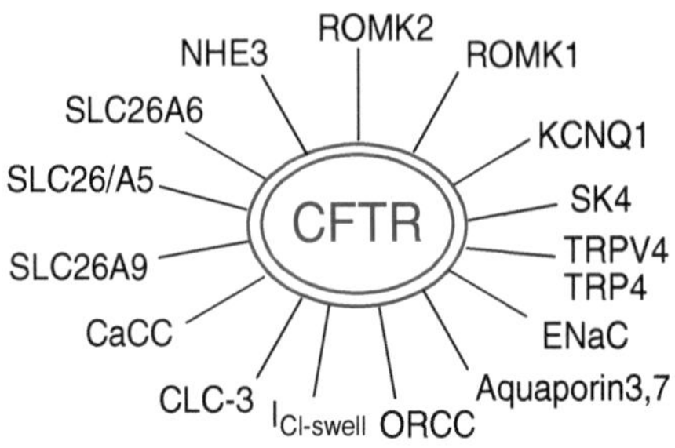

Fig. 26.1. Functional interaction of CFTR with membrane transport proteins.

(1–3). Moreover outwardly rectifying Cl^- channels, although not directly involved in the pathogenesis of cystic fibrosis (CF), are somehow regulated by CFTR (4, 5). Lately, it was discussed that CFTR activates another class of Cl^- channels, the SLC26A proteins. Since these currents have quite similar properties and pharmacology, it becomes rather difficult to discriminate the individual ion currents activated through expression of CFTR (6, 7).

Moreover, functional relationships exist between CFTR and carrier proteins such as the Cl^-/HCO_3^- exchanger SLC26A6 and the Na^+/H^+ exchanger NHE3 (8–10) (**Fig. 26.1**). Due to these properties and with the help of signal molecules such as PDZ-domain proteins (NHERF, CAL, CAP70, Shank-2) or IRBIT (**Fig. 26.2**), CFTR is essential for a coordinated transport of fluid and HCO_3^- and controls the cytosolic pH as outlined in **Chapter 30**, **Section V**, of this edition by Hug et al. (9, 11). PDZ-domain proteins play a major part in coordinating CFTR's function with that of other signaling molecules, kinases, transport proteins, and other elements of membrane trafficking (12) (**Fig. 26.2**). Although widely disputed, CFTR may also fulfill important intracellular/intravesicular functions and may control endosomal/lysosomal pH thereby controlling protein trafficking, renal protein absorption, and the function of immune cells (*see* **Chapter 19**, **Section III**, by Devuyst et al.) (13–17). Finally, CFTR has been shown to control transport of mucus and numerous substrates such as glutathione, ATP, glucose, and others (11).

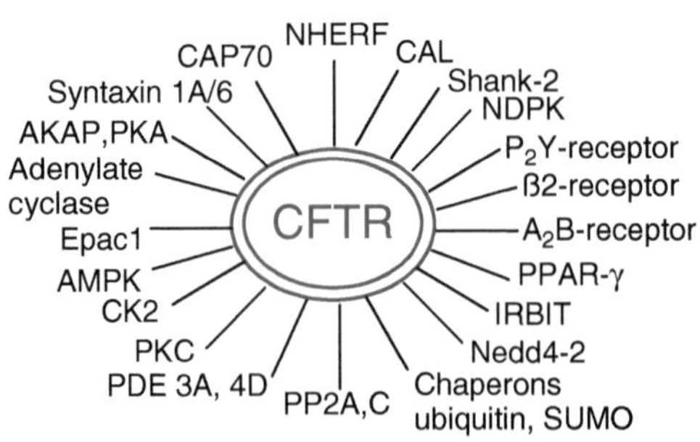

Fig. 26.2. Effects of CFTR on cellular signal transduction pathways.

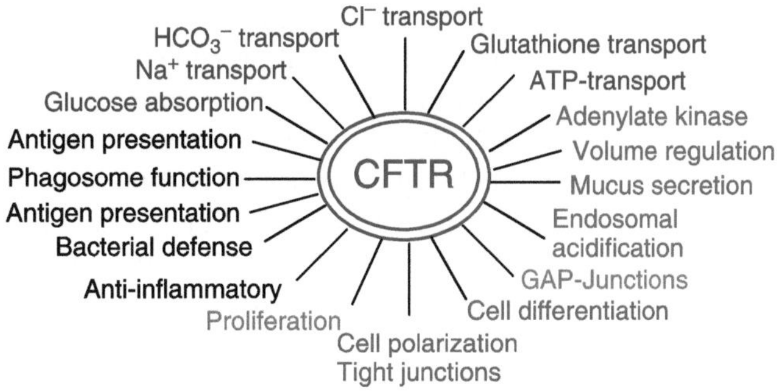

Fig. 26.3. Cellular effects of CFTR.

Thus CFTR interacts with a large number of transport proteins in the plasma membrane and thus affects a vast number of cellular transport processes (18) (**Fig. 26.3**).

Apart from these more or less direct effects on cellular transport, CFTR antagonizes pro-inflammatory pathways (*see* **Chapter 3** by Ziady and Davis, **Volume II, Section I**) and controls cytosolic Ca^{2+} signals (*see* **Chapter 7** by C. Ribeiro, **Volume II, Section I**) (19–24). More recent studies unmask the role of CFTR for cellular growth, differentiation, and polarization (*see* **Chapter 10** by M Chanson et al., **Volume II, Section I**) (25, 26), which has a major effect on cellular organization and asymmetric targeting of proteins to the luminal and basolateral membrane of polarized epithelial cells. When all these CFTR-related cellular effects are taken together, it becomes immediately clear that for a given cell, it makes quite a difference whether CFTR is expressed or not and thus assessment of CFTR's function suddenly becomes a major task. Thus, more comprehensive approaches are used recently to understand these multiple effects, using systems biology techniques as outlined in "Omic" section (**Section II** of **Volume II**). Despite this apparent complexity of CFTR-mediated effects, the primary read-out will be a cAMP/PKA-activated Cl^- current, which is analyzed in most detail by the patch clamp technique.

2. Single-Channel Patch Clamp Remains the Gold Standard to Examine CFTR Currents in Detail

CFTR's function as a Cl^- channel and its effects on other membrane ion conductances can be assessed by a number of methods outlined within this **Section V**. As every method has both strong and weak points, the most accurate analysis will make use of several techniques in parallel. Concerning the analysis of conductive and kinetic properties of CFTR, high-resolution single-channel patch clamp analysis still sets the gold standard. The analysis of ion currents in epithelial cells from CF patients and identification of CFTR coincided perfectly with establishment of the patch clamp technique, whose inventors, Sakmann and Neher, were later honored with the Nobel prize (27). In the past 20 years after cloning of the CFTR gene, the community of researchers analyzing CFTR made extensive use of patch clamping. Cai et al. describe in **Chapter 27** how this technique is applied to the analysis of both wt and mutant CFTR channels. They elucidate how the single-channel conductance and ion permeation, single-channel gating and the number of channels are determined. Dwell time analysis of open and closed channels gives a detailed insight into channel gating and how small molecule modulators affect current characteristics. In **Chapter 28**, Gadsby et al. demonstrate a detailed analysis of the regulation of CFTR channel gating.

After all patch clamping is still a very sophisticated and intellectually demanding method that requires proper biophysical knowledge and great experience and skills. Moreover, as with every other technique, there are limitations that may be overlooked by inexperienced researchers. Apart from the necessity to strictly control basic parameters throughout the experiments, such as temperature, pH, mechanical force, or ATP- and Ca^{2+} concentrations, it is indispensable that ion channel recordings are only accepted when there are proper pre-control and post-control phases. In this regard, short cutouts of only a few 100 ms of a channel "live" does appear inappropriate to assess detailed biophysical properties or pharmacological effects. Temperature-controlled bath perfusion is required as well as low noise setups to avoid heavy filtering of the current signal. Moreover, unless particular pharmacological tools are available to control gating of the channel, predictions regarding single-channel open probability and kinetic properties of single-channel currents are affected by some uncertainty. Thus, it comes to no surprise that the true open probability of the most common mutant, F508del–CFTR, is still a matter of debate (28). A comparison with data obtained from the analysis of CFTR currents by classical noise analysis might often be helpful (29, 30).

3. Protein Interaction Detected by Double Electrode Voltage Clamping

As outlined above, CFTR interacts with a number of other proteins and controls other membrane conductances. In order to be able to examine these interactions functionally, two or more proteins need to be coexpressed simultaneously in a particular stoichiometry. These interactions of CFTR with other ion channels or transporters, as well as analysis of a larger number of CFTR mutants are often done by double electrode voltage clamping (DEVC) in oocytes from *Xenopus laevis*, which is also described in **Chapter 3, Section I, Volume II**, by Berdiev et al. DEVC has many advantages since it is technically simple, and it produces large membrane currents and it offers a magnificent playground to examine all kinds of protein interactions. A larger number of different copy-RNAs can be injected in a stoichiometrically correct ratio and thus several proteins can be expressed simultaneously. As outlined in **Chapter 3, Section I, Volume II**, by Berdiev et al., this technique has been applied extensively to the question of how CFTR affects the function of the epithelial Na^+ channel ENaC, Ca^{2+}-activated Cl^- currents, and others. DEVC is sometimes used in combination with co-reconstitution of ion channels in planar lipid bilayers (31–34).

On a more critical notion, DEVC often provides results from unpaired experiments, i.e., from oocytes examined independently. As the quality of oocytes and injected cRNA may vary significantly from batch to batch and quantification of the injected cRNA is not always easy, it is indispensable to include multiple controls and to strictly perform a batch-wise comparison to avoid misinterpretation of the results (35). This is even more important when small changes are measured in the presence of large background conductances that are often observed in oocytes of low quality or when poorly impaled. Whenever possible absolute values rather than relative changes should be analyzed and continuous recordings with pre-and post-control traces should be presented. In contrast to mammalian epithelial cells, oocytes are kept at temperatures below 20°C and are non-polarized. Thus maturation and trafficking of proteins are different when compared to mammalian cells, e.g., allowing for substantial expression F508del–CFTR in the oocyte membrane. Thus F508del–CFTR currents are detected at magnitudes never observed in mammalian cells (36). Moreover, some regulatory features of CFTR are remarkably different in oocytes and may not reflect the situation in mammalian cells, such as the requirement of PDZ-binding proteins in mammalian cells or the contribution of exocytosis to the activation of CFTR (12, 37, 38).

4. CFTR Is Regulated by Phosphorylation

Protein phosphorylation is a key mechanism for regulation of ion channel activity and is also essential for controlling the activity of CFTR. As illustrated in **Fig. 26.2**, a number of kinases have been demonstrated meanwhile to phosphorylate CFTR, such as protein kinase A and C, CK2, and adenosine monophosphate-dependent kinase. The functional consequences of kinase regulation of CFTR have been demonstrated both in vitro and in vivo (36, 39–45). Phosphorylation sites have been identified and verified by biochemical methods including direct amino acid sequencing, site-directed mutagenesis combined with two-dimensional peptide mapping, and mass spectrometry. Kinase regulation has been examined by applying PKA, PKC, and other kinases to either full-length CFTR or recombinant CFTR domains such as R-domain or NBD1–R-domain peptides (45). In **Chapter 29**, Hallows et al. describe in detail the practical approaches to identify phosphorylation sites and explain the ups and downs of in vitro and in vivo phosphorylation. They focus specifically on the metabolic sensor AMP-activated protein kinase (AMPK) that has emerged as an important link between cellular metabolic status and ion transport activity. This appears to be of particular interest since specific serines in the R-domain of CFTR that have been considered to be inhibitory PKA sites have now been identified to be phosphorylated by AMPK and demonstrated to inhibit CFTR function (43, 46).

5. CFTR in a Polarized Cell: Ussing Chamber Recordings

Although established already in the late 1950s, Ussing chamber recordings remain the gold standard for electrical measurements in polarized cells and intact epithelia (47). Ussing chamber recordings are particularly relevant for CF-related research, since physiologically CFTR is expressed in a polarized epithelial environment. It turns out that, as recently proposed, CFTR may even control this environment by controlling tight junctions and cell polarity (26). Ussing chamber setups have been used extensively to measure expression and activity of CFTR currents in polarized grown epithelial cell lines (CFBE, H441, M1, Nuli, Cufi), primary airway epithelial cells, and native ex vivo mucosa from mouse and human airways and that of other species (48–50). Measurements can be performed in either short-circuit or open-circuit configuration and both methods have their advantages and their downsides. If required, luminal or basolateral membranes can be permeabilized selectively and made electrically silent, so that ion transport can be studied in an isolated luminal or basolateral epithelial monolayer membrane.

It is well established meanwhile that airway epithelial cells cultured on permeable supports for subsequent Ussing chamber recordings should be grown in the presence of an air–liquid interface (ALI), i.e., with no media on the apical side. ALI cultures increase formation of tight junctions and epithelial polarization and increase equivalent short-circuit currents (51, 52). ALI mimics the situation in vivo and allows to study fundamental aspects of airway epithelia, such as regulation of the air surface liquid (ASL) height/volume and mucociliary clearance. The mechanisms by which airways regulate their ASL volume are slowly emerging. It seems that apart from mechanical shear stress and purinergic agonists, the balance between proteases and protease inhibitors such as SPLUNC1 is crucial for the control of the ASL volume (53–56). Protease inhibitors are secreted onto the mucosal surface where they may work as soluble volume sensors, since they proteolytically cleave ENaC, which activates the channel and thus increases electrolyte absorption. In **Chapter 5, Section I, Volume II**, Worthington and Tarran outline the methods for ASL measurements and mucus transport rates in cell cultures.

Mucociliary transport can also be assessed more directly using particle tracking. The mucociliary particle transport of black polystyrene microspheres can be examined directly on either freshly isolated respiratory tissues or filter-grown epithelial cells in a humidified chamber and serves as direct measure for the mucociliary transport (57, 58). Direct measurements of the mucociliary transport and ASL volume may provide data that describe the pathophysiology of CF airways more reliably than data from Ussing chamber measurements, since Ussing chambers require a large volume on the apical side of the epithelium to allow immersion of the electrodes. However, due to expansion of the mucosal liquid, regulatory factors such as protease inhibitors and purinergic agonists are heavily diluted, thus generating an environment that is not present in vivo. What this means is that electrical read-outs such as large amiloride-sensitive short-circuit currents in Ussing chamber recordings may not necessarily indicate large Na^+ absorption in vivo, since all protease inhibitors have been washed away. This notion may actually challenge the established concepts of lung pathology in CF.

In a standard Ussing chamber recording with non-permeabilized membranes, it is important to keep in mind that the transport assessed, i.e., the short circuit current (I_{SC}) or equivalent short circuit current (Eq-I_{SC}), is always determined by the conductances of both membranes and the shunt conductance through tight junctions and leakage through edge damages. Thus, the quality of the preparations, the tightness of the cell monolayer and the geometry of the Ussing chamber, and positioning of the electrodes will have a major impact on the quality of the data. An Ussing chamber that can be perfused on both sides of the epithelium may supply excellent quality data, since such a setup provides pre- and post-control recordings that are essential to be able to evaluate the quality of the recordings. Short cutouts of I_{SC}-tracings put on a relative scale should be avoided as well as automatic computer-controlled corrections of the current tracings and are also unnecessary as long as the recordings are stable. Finally, CFTR function can also be assessed electrically in patients or under experimental conditions in animals as nasal potential difference (**Chapter 6**, **Section I**) or as rectal potential difference (44, 59, 60), which supplies valuable electrophysiological data to validate the outcome of therapeutic trials. However, it is often ignored that in contrast to short-circuit currents, potential measurements are not fully quantitative but only reflect relative changes, depending on the background conductance. A very useful and more quantitative alternative to PD measurements are ex vivo measurements on rectal biopsies (described in **Chapter 7**, **Section I** by Derichs et al.).

Ussing chamber measurements also become a very important tool in analyzing the contribution of CFTR to epithelial bicarbonate transport, as outlined in **Chapter 30**, this section by Hug, Clarke, and Gray. This chapter explains various techniques for measuring CFTR-dependent bicarbonate transport in single cells using fluorimetric techniques and patch clamping or analyzing transepithelial HCO_3^- secretion in monolayers and ex vivo tissues. Finally, the above-described noise analysis can also be applied to epithelial tissues. Similar to the data obtained through patch clamp experiments, transepithelial fluctuation analysis provides valuable information about the density and single-channel properties of ion channels in intact epithelia (61).

6. Large-Scale Analysis of CFTR Function by Fluorescence Quenching

The function of CFTR can be detected indirectly through quenching of a fluorescence dye by changes in the intracellular halide concentration (62). The use of fluorescence-based techniques for high-throughput screening of libraries of compounds to identify CFTR modulators is described in **Chapter 2**, **Section I**. Yellow fluorescence protein (YFP)-based assays have been proven to be particularly useful to identify small molecules as pharmacological CFTR modulators in large-scale high-throughput screenings of chemical libraries. Moreover, methods based on voltage-sensitive dyes are also effective in detecting cAMP-activated CFTR Cl^- conductance (63, 64). Naturally, changes in these fluorescence signals do not in any single case accurately and quantitatively reflect changes in CFTR conductance. These signals depend on a number of additional factors like membrane voltage, intracellular ion concentration, or additional factors such as intracellular Ca^{2+} concentration or pH. Thus, complementary methods are required in order to validate true changes in CFTR conductance.

Nevertheless, Galietta et al. describe in **Chapter 2, Section I** how large-scale screening has been very successfully used to identify CFTR inhibitors, correctors, and activators. Some of these compounds are now widely used as experimental tools, such as inhibitors CFTRinh-172 or GlyH101. Related compounds may be useful in the treatment of secretory diarrhea, which is caused by long-term activation of CFTR (65). More important, compounds that either correct the trafficking defects of mutant CFTR (correctors) or potentiate residual activity of membrane-localized mutant CFTR (potentiators) have been identified meanwhile and are already in clinical trials (66). This is described in more detail in **Chapter 15**, by Almaça et al. **Volume II, Section II**. More recently, fluorescence-based screening has been expanded to identify inhibitors of human intestinal calcium-activated chloride channels (67). It should also be noted that fluorescence-based assays are typically performed on non-polarized cells overexpressing CFTR, which does not take into account that CFTR is expressed in vivo in highly differentiated and polarized epithelial cells. Thus CFTR-interacting proteins (targets) or small chemical compounds affecting CFTR function (hits), which have been identified during screening assays, may not necessarily be valid in differentiated cells. Thus, additional methods based on large-scale Ussing chamber techniques, in which differentiated and polarized grown cells are used for the assays, may be helpful, if not for the primary screens themselves, at least to validate the above hits.

7. Concluding Remarks

Assessment of CFTR function is not simple. Expression of CFTR produces a large number of changes in a cell, which are not all detected by electrophysiological techniques. It is now well established that CFTR forms a membrane microdomain that organizes other ion channels and transporters; bundles receptors and signaling pathways; and exerts numerous effects on transport, cell polarization, and differentiation. Thereby, CFTR controls essential cellular functions including ion and substrate transport, mucus secretion, volume regulation, anti-inflammatory functions, and defense. Yet, the essential read-out has always been a cAMP-activated Cl^- conductance that is provided by CFTR. Electrophysiological analyses and transport studies related to CFTR should, whenever possible, occur at different levels. Results that have been obtained in a very isolated system, such as single channels in excised membrane patches, should be completed by analyzing whole-cell currents and by performing studies on highly differentiated and polarized epithelial cells and native epithelia to ensure that the results can be fully applied to CFTR in vivo.

References

1. Kunzelmann, K. (2001) CFTR: interacting with everything? *News Phys. Sci.* **17**, 167–170.
2. Valverde, M. A., O'Briens, J. A., Sepulveda, F. V., Ratcliff, R. A., Evans, M. J., and Colledge, W. H. (1995) Impaired cell volume regulation in intestinal crypt epithelia of cystic fibrosis. *Proc. Natl. Acad. Sci. USA* **92**, 9038–9041.
3. Arniges, M., Vazquez, E., Fernandez-Fernandez, J. M., and Valverde, M. A. (2004) Swelling-activated Ca^{2+} entry via TRPV4 channel is defective in cystic fibrosis airway epithelia. *J. Biol. Chem.* **279**, 54062–54068.
4. Kunzelmann, K., Pavenstädt, H., and Greger, R. (1989) Properties and regulation of chloride channels in cystic fibrosis and normal airway epithelial cells. *Pflügers Arch.* **415**, 172–182.
5. Gabriel, S. E., Clarke, L. L., Boucher, R. C., and Stutts, M. J. (1993) CFTR and outward rectifying chloride channels are distinct proteins with a regulatory relationship. *Nature* **363**, 263–268.
6. Bertrand, C. A., Zhang, R., Pilewski, J. M., and Frizzell, R. A. (2009) SLC26A9 is a constitutively active, CFTR-regulated anion conductance in human bronchial epithelia. *J. Gen. Physiol.* **133**, 421–438.
7. Chang, M. H., Plata, C., Sindic, A., Ranatunga, W. K., Chen, A. P., Zandi-Nejad, K., et al. (2009) Slc26a9 is inhibited by the R-region of CFTR via the STAS domain. *J. Biol. Chem.* **284**, 28306–28318.
8. Wang, Y., Soyombo, A. A., Shcheynikov, N., Zeng, W., Dorwart, M., Marino, C. R., et al. (2006) Slc26a6 regulates CFTR activity in vivo to determine pancreatic duct HCO(3)(−) secretion: relevance to cystic fibrosis. *EMBO J.* **25**, 5049–5057.
9. Ko, S. B., Zeng, W., Dorwart, M. R., Luo, X., Kim, K. H., Millen, L., et al. (2004) Gating of CFTR by the STAS domain of SLC26 transporters. *Nat. Cell Biol.* **6**, 343–350.
10. Seidler, U., Singh, A. K., Cinar, A., Chen, M., Hillesheim, J., Hogema, B., et al. (2009) The role of the NHERF family of PDZ scaffolding proteins in the regulation of salt and water transport. *Ann. NY Acad. Sci.* **1165**, 249–260.
11. Yang, D., Shcheynikov, N., Zeng, W., Ohana, E., So, I., Ando, H., et al. (2009) IRBIT coordinates epithelial fluid and HCO3-secretion by stimulating the transporters pNBC1 and CFTR in the murine pancreatic duct. *J. Clin. Invest.* **119**, 193–202.
12. Guggino, W. B., and Stanton, B. A. (2006) New insights into cystic fibrosis: molecular switches that regulate CFTR. *Nat. Rev. Mol. Cell Biol.* 7, 426–436.
13. Barasch, J., Kiss, B., Prince, A., Saiman, L., Gruenert, D. C., and Al-Awqati, Q. (1991) Defective acidification of intracellular organelles in cystic fibrosis. *Nature* **352**, 70–73.
14. Di, A., Brown, M. E., Deriy, L. V., Li, C., Szeto, F. L., Chen, Y., et al. (2006) CFTR regulates phagosome acidification in macrophages and alters bactericidal activity. *Nat. Cell Biol.* **8**, 933–944.
15. Haggie, P. M., and Verkman, A. S. (2009) Unimpaired lysosomal acidification in respiratory epithelial cells in cystic fibrosis. *J. Biol.Chem.* **284**, 7681–7686.
16. Jouret, F., Bernard, A., Hermans, C., Dom, G., Terryn, S., Leal, T., et al. (2007) Cystic fibrosis is associated with a defect in apical receptor-mediated endocytosis in mouse and human kidney. *J. Am. Soc. Nephrol.* **18**, 707–718.
17. Barriere, H., Bagdany, M., Bossard, F., Okiyoneda, T., Wojewodka, G., Gruenert, D., et al. (2009) Revisiting the role of cystic fibrosis transmembrane conductance regulator and counterion permeability in the pH regulation of endocytic organelles. *Mol. Biol. Cell* **20**, 3125–3141.
18. Kunzelmann, K. (1999) The Cystic Fibrosis Transmembrane Conductance Regulator and its function in epithelial transport. *Rev. Physiol. Biochem. Pharmacol.* **137**, 1–70.
19. Ribeiro, C. M., Paradiso, A. M., Schwab, U., Perez-Vilar, J., Jones, L., O'Neal, W., et al. (2005) Chronic airway infection/inflammation Induces a Ca^{2+}i-dependent hyperinflammatory response in human cystic fibrosis airway epithelia. *J. Biol. Chem.* **280**, 17798–17806.
20. Becker, M. N., Sauer, M. S., Muhlebach, M. S., Hirsh, A. J., Wu, Q., Verghese, M. W., et al. (2004) Cytokine secretion by cystic fibrosis airway epithelial cells. *Am. J. Respir. Crit. Care Med.* **169**, 645–653.
21. Hybiske, K., Fu, Z., Schwarzer, C., Tseng, J., Do, J., Huang, N., et al. (2007) Effects of cystic fibrosis transmembrane conductance regulator (CFTR) and delta F508-CFTR on inflammatory response, ER stress and Ca^{2+} of airway epithelia. *Am. J. Physiol. Lung Cell. Mol. Physiol.* **293**, L1250–L1260.
22. Perez, A., Issler, A. C., Cotton, C. U., Kelley, T. J., Verkman, A. S., and Davis, P. B. (2007) CFTR inhibition mimics the cystic

fibrosis inflammatory profile. *Am. J. Physiol. Lung Cell. Mol. Physiol.* **292**, L383–L395.
23. Antigny, F., Norez, C., Becq, F., and Vandebrouck, C. (2008) Calcium homeostasis is abnormal in cystic fibrosis airway epithelial cells but is normalized after rescue of F508del-CFTR. *Cell Calcium* **43**, 175–183.
24. Rottner, M., Kunzelmann, C., Mergey, M., Freyssinet, J. M., and Martinez, M. C. (2007) Exaggerated apoptosis and NF-κB activation in pancreatic and tracheal cystic fibrosis cells. *FASEB J.* **21**, 2939–2948.
25. Hajj, R., Lesimple, P., Nawrocki-Raby, B., Birembaut, P., Puchelle, E., and Coraux, C. (2007) Human airway surface epithelial regeneration is delayed and abnormal in cystic fibrosis. *J. Pathol.* **211**, 340–350.
26. Lesimple, P., Liao, J., Robert, R., Gruenert, D. C., and Hanrahan, J. W. (2010) CFTR trafficking modulates the barrier function of airway epithelial cell monolayers. *J. Physiol.* **588**, 1195–1209.
27. Hamill, O. P., Marty, A., Neher, E., Sakmann, B., and Sigworth, F. J. (1981) Improved patch-clamp techniques for high-resolution current recording from cells and cell-free membrane patches. *Pflügers Arch.* **391**, 85–100.
28. Dalemans, W., Barbry, P., Champigny, G., Jallat, S., Dott, K., Dreyer, D., et al. (1992) Altered chloride ion channel kinetics associated with the deltaF508 cystic fibrosis mutation. *Nature* **354**, 526–528.
29. Zhou, Z., Hu, S., and Hwang, T. C. (2001) Voltage-dependent flickery block of an open cystic fibrosis transmembrane conductance regulator (CFTR) channel pore. *J. Physiol.* **532**, 435–448.
30. Fischer, H., and Machen, T. E. (1994) CFTR displays voltage dependence and two gating modes during stimulation. *J. Gen. Physiol.* **104**, 541–566.
31. Bachhuber, T., König, J., Voelcker, T., Mürle, B., Schreiber, R., and Kunzelmann, K. (2005) Chloride interference with the epithelial Na^+ channel ENaC. *J. Biol. Chem.* **280**, 31587–31594.
32. Jiang, Q., Li, J., Dubroff, R., Ahn, Y. J., Foskett, J. K., Engelhardt, J. F., et al. (2000) Epithelial sodium channels regulate cystic fibrosis transmembrane conductance regulator chloride channels in *Xenopus oocytes. J. Biol. Chem.* **275**, 13266–13274.
33. Ismailov, I. I., Berdiev, B. K., Shlyonsky, V. G., Fuller, C. M., Prat, A. G., Jovov, B., et al. (1997) Role of actin in regulation of epithelial sodium channels by CFTR. *Am. J. Physiol.* **272**, C1077–C1086.
34. Kunzelmann, K., Mall, M., Briel, M., Hipper, A., Nitschke, R., Ricken, S., et al. (1997) The cystic fibrosis transmembrane conductance regulator attenuates the endogenous Ca^{2+} activated Cl^- conductance in *Xenopus* ooyctes. *Pflügers Arch.* **434**, 178–181.
35. Wagner, C. A., Friedrich, B., Setiawan, I., Lang, F., and Broer, S. (2000) The use of Xenopus laevis oocytes for the functional characterization of heterologously expressed membrane proteins. *Cell Physiol. Biochem.* **10**, 1–12.
36. Treharne, K. J., Xu, Z., Chen, J.-H., Best, O. G., Cassidy, D., Gruenert, D. C., et al. (2009) Inhibition of protein kinase CK2 closes the CFTR Cl^- channel, but has no effect on the cystic fibrosis mutant F508-CFTR. *Cell Physiol. Biochem.* **24**, 347–360.
37. Boucherot, A., Schreiber, R., and Kunzelmann, K. (2001) Role of CFTR's PDZ-binding domain, NBF1 and Cl^- conductance in inhibition of epithelial Na^+ channels in *Xenopus* oocytes. *Biochim. Biophys. Acta* **1515**, 64–71.
38. Kunzelmann, K., and Nitschke, R. (2000) Defects in processing and trafficking of CFTR. *Exp. Nephr.* **8**, 332–342.
39. Cheng, S. H., Rich, D. P., Marshall, J., Gregory, R. J., Welsh, M. J., and Smith, A. E. (1991) Phosphorylation of the R domain by cAMP-dependent protein kinase regulates the CFTR chloride channel. *Cell* **66**, 1027–1036.
40. Chappe, V., Hinkson, D. A., Zhu, T., Chang, X. B., Riordan, J. R., and Hanrahan, J. W. (2003) Phosphorylation of protein kinase C sites in NBD1 and the R domain control CFTR channel activation by PKA. *J. Physiol.* **548**, 39–52.
41. Hallows, K. R., Raghuram, V., Kemp, B. E., Witters, L. A., and Foskett, J. K. (2000) Inhibition of cystic fibrosis transmembrane conductance regulator by novel interaction with the metabolic sensor AMP-activated protein kinase. *J. Clin. Invest.* **105**, 1711–1721.
42. Chang, X.-B., Tabcharani, J. A., Hou, Y.-X., Jensen, T. J., Kartner, N., Alon, N., et al. (1993) Protein kinase A (PKA) still activates CFTR chloride channels after mutagenesis of all 10 PKA consensus phosphorylation sites. *J. Biol. Chem.* **268**, 11304–11311.
43. Kongsuphol, P., Cassidy, D., Hieke, B., Treharne, K. J., Schreiber, R., Mehta, A., et al. (2009) Mechanistic insight into control of CFTR by AMPK. *J. Biol. Chem.* **284**, 5645–5653.
44. Kongsuphol, P., Hieke, B., Ousingsawat, J., Almaça, J., Viollet, B., Schreiber, R., et al.

(2008) Regulation of Cl^- secretion by AMPK in vivo. *Pflügers Arch.* **457**, 1071–1078.
45. Gadsby, D. C., and Nairn, A. C. (1999) Control of CFTR channel gating by phosphorylation and nucleotide hydrolysis. *Physiol. Rev.* **79**, S77–S107.
46. King, J. D., Jr., Fitch, A. C., Lee, J. K., McCane, J. E., Mak, D. O., Foskett, J. K., et al. (2009) AMP-activated protein kinase phosphorylation of the R domain inhibits PKA stimulation of CFTR. *Am. J. Physiol. Cell Physiol.* **297**, C94–C101.
47. Koefoed-Johnsen, V., and Ussing, H. H. (1958) The nature of frog skin potential. *Acta Physiol. Scand.* **42**, 298–308.
48. Li, H., Sheppard, D. N., and Hug, M. J. (2004) Transepithelial electrical measurements with the Ussing chamber. *J. Cyst. Fibros.* **3**(Suppl 2), 123–126.
49. Mall, M., Hirtz, S., Gonska, T., and Kunzelmann, K. (2004) Assessment of CFTR function in rectal biopsies for the diagnosis of cystic fibrosis. *J. Cyst. Fibros.* **3**, 165–169.
50. Hirtz, S., Gonska, T., Seydewitz, H. H., Thomas, J., Greiner, P., Kuehr, J., et al. (2004) CFTR Cl^- channel function in native human colon correlates with the genotype and the phenotype in cystic fibrosis. *Gastroenterology* **127**, 1085–1095.
51. Robison, T. W., Dorio, R. J., and Kim, K. J. (1993) Formation of tight monolayers of guinea pig airway epithelial cells cultured in an air-interface: bioelectric properties. *Biotechniques* **15**, 468–473.
52. Johnson, L. G., Dickman, K. G., Moore, K. L., Mandel, L. J., and Boucher, R. C. (1993) Enhanced Na^+ transport in an air-liquid interface culture system. *Am. J. Physiol.* **264**, L560–L565.
53. Tarran, R., Trout, L., Donaldson, S. H., and Boucher, R. C. (2006) Soluble mediators, not cilia, determine airway surface liquid volume in normal and cystic fibrosis superficial airway epithelia. *J. Gen. Physiol.* **127**, 591–604.
54. Garcia-Caballero, A., Rasmussen, J. E., Gaillard, E., Watson, M. J., Olsen, J. C., Donaldson, S. H., et al. (2009) SPLUNC1 regulates airway surface liquid volume by protecting ENaC from proteolytic cleavage. *Proc. Natl. Acad. Sci. USA* **106**, 11412–11417.
55. Kleyman, T. R., Carattino, M. D., and Hughey, R. P. (2009) ENaC at the cutting edge: regulation of epithelial sodium channels by proteases. *J. Biol. Chem.* **284**, 20447–20451.
56. Kunzelmann, K., and Mall, M. (2003) Pharmacotherapy of the ion transport defect in cystic fibrosis: role of purinergic receptor agonists and other potential therapeutics. *Am. J. Resp. Med.* **2**, 299–309.
57. Ousingsawat, J., Martins, J. R., Schreiber, R., Rock, J. R., Harfe, B. D., and Kunzelmann, K. (2009) Loss of TMEM16A causes a defect in epithelial Ca^{2+} dependent chloride transport. *J. Biol. Chem.* **284**, 28698–28703.
58. Schreiber, R., Castrop, H., and Kunzelmann, K. (2008) Allergen induced airway hyperresponsiveness is absent in ecto-5′-nucleotidase (CD73) deficient mice. *Pflugers Arch.* **457**, 431–440.
59. Orlando, R. C., Powell, D. W., Croom, R. D., Berschneider, H. M., Boucher, R. C., and Knowles, M. R. (1989) Colonic and esophageal transepithelial potential difference in cystic fibrosis. *Gastroenterology* **96**, 1041–1048.
60. Wilschanski, M., Famini, H., Strauss-Liviatan, N., Rivlin, J., Blau, H., Bibi, H., et al. (2001) Nasal potential difference measurements in patients with atypical cystic fibrosis. *Eur. Respir. J.* **17**, 1208–1215.
61. Singh, A. K., Schultz, B. D., Van Driessche, W., and Bridges, R. J. (2004) Transepithelial fluctuation analysis of chloride secretion. *J. Cyst. Fibros.* **3**(Suppl 2), 127–132.
62. Galietta, L. J., Jayaraman, S., and Verkman, A. S. (2001) Cell-based assay for high-throughput quantitative screening of CFTR chloride transport agonists. *Am. J. Physiol. Cell Physiol.* **281**, C1734–C1742.
63. Galietta, L. J., Springsteel, M. F., Eda, M., Niedzinski, E. J., By, K., Haddadin, M. J., et al. (2001) Novel CFTR chloride channel activators identified by screening of combinatorial libraries based on flavone and benzoquinolizinium lead compounds. *J. Biol. Chem.* **276**, 19723–19728.
64. Miret, J. J., Zhang, J., Min, H., Lewis, K., Roth, M., Charlton, M., et al. (2005) Multiplexed G-protein-coupled receptor Ca^{2+} flux assays for high-throughput screening. *J. Biomol. Screen.* **10**, 780–787.
65. Thiagarajah, J. R., Broadbent, T., Hsieh, E., and Verkman, A. S. (2004) Prevention of toxin-induced intestinal ion and fluid secretion by a small-molecule CFTR inhibitor. *Gastroenterology* **126**, 511–519.
66. Pedemonte, N., Lukacs, G. L., Du, K., Caci, E., Zegarra-Moran, O., Galietta, L. J., et al. (2005) Small-molecule correctors of defective DeltaF508-CFTR cellular processing identified by high-throughput screening. *J. Clin. Invest.* **115**, 2564–2571.
67. de la Fuente, R., Namkung, W., Mills, A., and Verkman, A. S. (2007) Small molecule screen identifies inhibitors of a human intestinal calcium activated chloride channel. *Mol. Pharmacol.* **73**, 758–768.

Chapter 27

Application of High-Resolution Single-Channel Recording to Functional Studies of Cystic Fibrosis Mutants

Zhiwei Cai, Yoshiro Sohma, Silvia G. Bompadre,
David N. Sheppard, and Tzyh-Chang Hwang

Abstract

The patch-clamp technique is a powerful and versatile method to investigate the cystic fibrosis transmembrane conductance regulator (CFTR) Cl^- channel, its malfunction in disease and modulation by small molecules. Here, we discuss how the molecular behaviour of CFTR is investigated using high-resolution single-channel recording and kinetic analyses of channel gating. We review methods used to quantify how cystic fibrosis (CF) mutants perturb the biophysical properties and regulation of CFTR. By explaining the relationship between macroscopic and single-channel currents, we demonstrate how single-channel data provide molecular explanations for changes in CFTR-mediated transepithelial ion transport elicited by CF mutants.

Key words: ATP-binding cassette transporter, CFTR, chloride ion channel, patch-clamp technique, single-channel recording, channel gating.

1. Introduction

The patch-clamp technique (1, 2) is the method of choice to investigate the molecular and cellular behaviour of the cystic fibrosis transmembrane conductance regulator (CFTR) Cl^- channel. In combination with site-directed mutagenesis, this technique has provided invaluable insight into the relationship between CFTR structure and function, the malfunction of CFTR in disease and the use of small molecules to restore channel activity to cystic fibrosis (CF) mutants.

M.D. Amaral, K. Kunzelmann (eds.), *Cystic Fibrosis*, Methods in Molecular Biology 741,
DOI 10.1007/978-1-61779-117-8_27,

Because the CFTR Cl^- channel is regulated by cAMP-dependent phosphorylation and cycles of ATP binding and hydrolysis (3–5), CFTR is best studied using the excised inside-out configuration of the patch-clamp technique, which provides ready access to the intracellular side of the cell membrane. Here, we discuss how excised inside-out membrane patches are used to investigate the single-channel activity of wild-type CFTR and CF mutants. For information about the theory and operation of the patch-clamp technique, we refer the reader to *Single Channel Recording* (6), the reference book for this electrophysiological technique. Because the scope of this chapter is limited, we refer the reader to (7) and (8) for further information about how other configurations of the patch-clamp technique are used to investigate the CFTR Cl^- channel. For excellent reviews of the application of single-channel recording to the study of CFTR, *see* (9–12). For a review of strategies to investigate small molecules that modulate CFTR function, *see* (13).

2. Use of Excised Membrane Patches to Study the CFTR Cl^- Channel

Critical to the success of patch-clamp studies of CFTR are appropriate cells, solutions and reagents. These are required to optimize seal formation and ensure the detection of CFTR and not other ion channels.

2.1. Cells and CFTR Expression

For studies of CFTR structure and function, we prefer to heterologously express CFTR variants in mammalian cells that do not routinely express CFTR and possess no cAMP-stimulated Cl^- channels. Our cell lines of choice for single-channel recording are C127 (a mouse mammary epithelial cell line), CHO and NIH 3T3 cells (14–16). However, a wide variety of mammalian and non-mammalian cells have been used to heterologously express CFTR. Because of the difficulty of forming seals on epithelial cells, we do not routinely use native epithelial cells for structure–function studies. However, we recognize fully that it is important to use polarized epithelia to understand the physiological role of CFTR and its regulation.

The choice of cell lines is particularly pertinent for studies of CF mutants. Many CF mutants, including the most common F508del-CFTR, disrupt the processing of CFTR protein and its delivery to the cell surface (17). Because the trafficking defect of F508del-CFTR is attenuated in *Xenopus* oocytes (18), it is preferable to test the effects of CF mutants on CFTR function using mammalian cells (*see* below, **Section 6**).

In general, higher rates of seal formation can be achieved using stable cell lines rather than cells transiently expressing CFTR. Stable cell lines may provide more uniform levels of CFTR expression than transiently transfected cells. However, it is not practical to use stable cell lines to study CFTR variants especially when one has to study many mutants. When transient expression is necessary, we co-transfect CHO cells with plasmids encoding CFTR and green fluorescent protein (GFP) and then use a microscope equipped with epi-fluorescence to select fluorescent cells for study. In this way, data acquisition is efficient. For an example of this approach, *see* (19).

2.2. Experimental Solutions

To magnify the small single-channel current amplitude of CFTR, we routinely impose a large Cl^- concentration gradient across membrane patches by replacing most Cl^- in the pipette (extracellular) solution with the impermeant anion aspartate. However, it is important to ensure that there is a high concentration of electrolytes (~150 mM salt) in the bath (intracellular) solution to optimize channel gating (20). To prevent the activation of contaminating currents, we manipulate the composition of bath and pipette solutions. For example, we routinely use the large impermeant cation *N*-methyl-D-glucamine (NMDG) to preclude contaminating Na^+ and K^+ currents. To stop the activation of Ca^{2+}-activated Cl^- currents, we use CsEGTA to buffer $[Ca^{2+}]_{free}$ to ≤10 nM in the bath solution.

We routinely use the biological buffer TES or HEPES to buffer the pH of solutions. However, when present in the bath solution, many large anions such as biological buffers (e.g. MOPS and TES) cause a flickery block of CFTR that is most pronounced at strong negative voltages. Indeed, because tricine failed to block CFTR when present in the bath solution, Ishihara and Welsh (21) recommend the use of tricine-buffered bath solutions to study the conductance of CFTR (for discussion, *see* (21)).

Because CFTR Cl^- channels are regulated by cAMP-dependent phosphorylation and cycles of ATP binding and hydrolysis (3, 4), the bath solution must contain Mg^{2+}. To facilitate seal formation, the pipette solution contains millimolar Ca^{2+}. A sample of the composition of our bath and pipette solutions is listed below (mM):

Bath solution: 140 NMDG, 3 $MgCl_2$, 1 CsEGTA, 10 TES, pH 7.3 with 1 M HCl ($[Cl^-]_{Int}$, 147 mM; $[Ca^{2+}]_{free}$, ≤ 10 nM; osmolarity, 281 ± 0.5 mOsm ($n = 4$)).

Pipette solution: 140 NMDG, 5 $CaCl_2$, 2 $MgSO_4$, 140 aspartic acid, 10 TES, pH 7.3 with 1 M Tris ($[Cl^-]_{Ext}$, 10 mM; osmolarity, 279 ± 0.5 mOsm ($n = 7$)).

These bath and pipette solutions are not suitable for studies of the CFTR Cl^- channel using other configurations of the patch-clamp technique. For advice on the preparation of solutions for whole-cell and cell-attached recording, *see* (7) and (8).

We prepare bath and pipette solutions frequently (≤2 weeks) and store them at +4°C when not in use. To verify that solutions have been prepared correctly, we check their osmolarity.

2.3. Reagents

Phosphorylation of the R domain by protein kinase A (PKA) is critical for activation of the CFTR Cl^- channel (3, 22). In experiments using the excised inside-out configuration of the patch-clamp technique, the most effective way to phosphorylate CFTR at PKA consensus sites is to add the catalytic subunit of PKA (75–200 nM) to the intracellular solution in the presence of millimolar concentrations of ATP. Because of wide variation of the specific activity of commercial PKA and likely association of protein phophatases in the membrane patch, channel activation upon addition of PKA and ATP can vary greatly. Therefore, it is important to ensure the full activation of CFTR by continuously monitoring channel activity in real time. Even when CFTR is fully activated, phosphorylated CFTR is particularly susceptible to channel rundown. Rundown of CFTR is both phosphorylation-dependent and phosphorylation-independent. To prevent phosphorylation-dependent rundown, we add the catalytic subunit of PKA to all bath solutions. However, this does not guarantee the stability of channel activity. In our experience, PKA purified from bovine heart is more efficacious than recombinant PKA at stimulating CFTR and preventing rundown. However, batch-to-batch variation in the efficacy of PKA is not unknown. If rundown of CFTR becomes a problem, we recommend that the supply of PKA is checked first.

Once wild-type CFTR is phosphorylated, opening and closing (gating) are controlled by ATP. We store aliquots of ATP disodium salt desiccated at –20°C. For experiments, we prepare a stock of ATP (100–275 mM) dissolved in bath solution. Alternatively, the stock can be stored at –80°C for months. Other nucleotides are similarly stored and prepared. It is important to note that ATP acidifies the bath solution. We therefore add the required amount of NaOH to all bath solutions to readjust pH to 7.3. (Because CFTR channel gating is modulated by intracellular pH (23), we routinely test all agents added to the bath solution for their effects on pH).

CFTR modulators are prepared in their specified solvents, aliquoted into appropriate amounts and stored at –20°C in the dark. We test the effects of all solvents on the activity of CFTR in the absence of any modulator. Our preferred solvent is DMSO, which is without effect on the single-channel activity of CFTR

(14). We draw the readers' attention to the fact that tetrahydrofuran, a widely used solvent in chemistry, weakly potentiates CFTR channel gating (24).

Clean solutions are a prerequisite for successful seal formation. Therefore, we filter all bath and pipette solutions using 0.45 μm disposable filters prior to use.

3. Distinguishing CFTR Cl^- Channels and Currents

Using cells expressing recombinant CFTR and the recording conditions described above, CFTR will likely be the dominant channel observed. However, it is feasible that contaminating channels (e.g. large conductance anion channels or outwardly rectifying Cl^- channels) will be observed. For this reason, the experimenter must be able to identify with confidence the CFTR Cl^- channel.

CFTR Cl^- channels have a number of defining characteristics:

(i) They have a small single-channel conductance (6–10 pS).

(ii) The current–voltage (*I–V*) relationship is linear (but *see* (25)).

(iii) They are selective for anions over cations.

(iv) The anion permeability sequence is $Br^- \geq Cl^- > I^-$.

(v) They show time- and voltage-independent gating behaviour.

(vi) Channel activity is strictly dependent on cAMP-dependent phosphorylation and intracellular ATP (for discussion, *see* (3–5)).

(vii) CFTR channels open in bursts that typically last for hundreds of millisecond. Within each burst, one can easily discern short flickery closures with a lifetime <10 ms. These flickery closings show voltage dependence with fewer flickers observed at positive membrane voltages (25, 26).

The dependence of CFTR Cl^- currents on intracellular ATP is the simplest way to discriminate CFTR from other ion channels. Withdrawal of ATP from the bath solution rapidly decreases the activity of CFTR Cl^- channels (27). Although it was reported that this deactivation of CFTR can be irreversible (28), in most studies, one can readily reopen the closed channels. It is also important to note that a finite open probability is observed even in the absence of ATP (29).

4. Quantification of Single-Channel Conductance

Single-channel conductance is a measure of the ease with which ions flow through an ion channel. To determine single-channel conductance, the relationship between single-channel current amplitude (*i*) and voltage (*V*) is plotted over a range of voltages (e.g. –100 to +100 mV). If this relationship (termed a current–voltage (*I–V*) relationship) obeys Ohm's law, then the data can be fit with a first-order regression function and the slope of the line is a measure of single-channel conductance.

To measure single-channel current amplitude, a current amplitude histogram is created from a single-channel record (**Fig. 27.1**) and fitted with a two-component Gaussian function

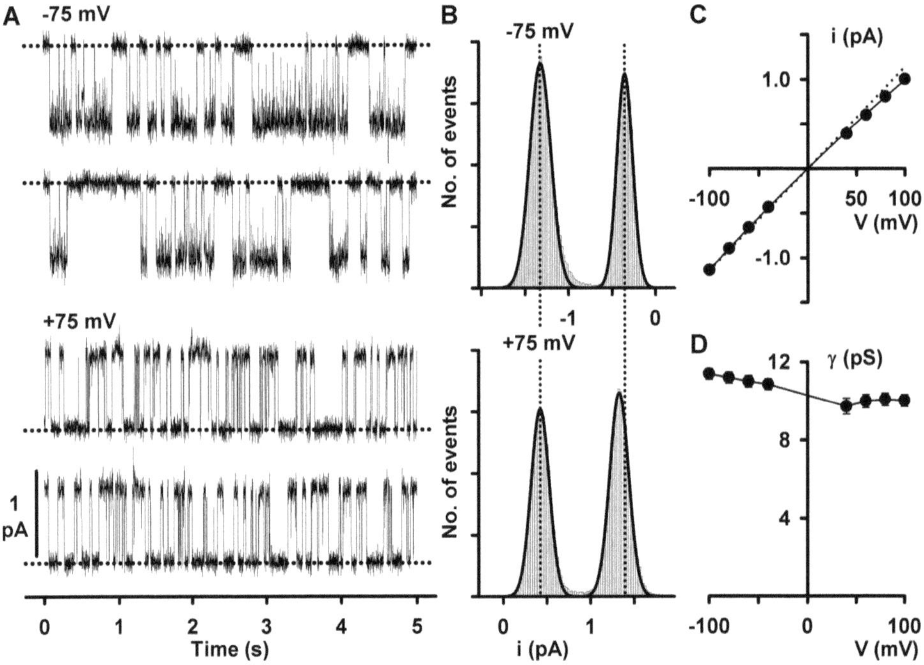

Fig. 27.1. **Effect of voltage on the single-channel activity of CFTR.** (**a**) Representative recordings of a single CFTR Cl^- channel at –75 mV (*top*) and +75 mV (*bottom*) in an excised inside-out membrane patch. The membrane patch was bathed in symmetrical 147 mM NMDGCl solutions, and ATP (1 mM) and PKA (75 nM) were continuously present in the intracellular solution. *Dotted lines* indicate the closed channel state. Downward and upward deflections correspond to channel openings at –75 and +75 mV, respectively. Each trace is 10 s long. (**b**) Single-channel current amplitude histograms of a single CFTR Cl^- channel at the indicated voltages. At –75 mV (*top*), the closed channel amplitude is shown on the *right*, whereas at +75 mV (*bottom*), the closed channel amplitude is shown on the *left*. The *continuous lines* represent the fit of Gaussian distributions to the data. The *vertical dotted lines* indicate the positions of the open and closed levels at –75 mV. (**c**) Single-channel *I–V* relationship of CFTR. Data are means ± SEM ($n = 10$); *error bars* are smaller than symbol size. The *dotted line* shows the *I–V* relationship of an ion channel with ohmic behaviour. (**d**) Relationship between chord conductance and voltage for the data shown in (**c**). For further information, *see* Cai et al. (25). Modified from The Journal of General Physiology 2003, 122:605–620. Copyright 2003 The Rockefeller University Press.

(assuming that the membrane patch contains just one active channel) to determine the mean closed and open levels. The difference between the closed and open levels in the current amplitude histogram provides a measure of single-channel current amplitude (**Fig. 27.1**). To avoid errors when measuring single-channel current amplitude, it is important to avoid baseline drift, current "glitches" and distorted channel openings.

Figure 27.1c demonstrates that the single-channel *I–V* relationship of wild-type CFTR weakly inwardly rectifies at positive voltages. To quantify this rectification, we measured chord conductance. Chord conductance is determined by dividing unitary current by the difference between the applied voltage and the reversal potential. **Figure 27.1d** demonstrates that the chord conductance of wild-type CFTR decreases from 11.4 $\pm$ 0.3 pS at –100 mV to 10.0 $\pm$ 0.3 pS at +100 mV ($n = 10$; $P < 0.01$).

As discussed further below in **Section 6**, measurement of single-channel conductance is used to identify CF mutations that disrupt Cl^- ion flow through the CFTR pore. An alternative method to generate an *I–V* relationship is to use a voltage ramp. This method for generating an *I–V* relationship can be used in an excised inside-out membrane patch containing large numbers of active channels (25, 30) or one single channel locked in an open state (31). Summation of single-channel currents generated by a voltage ramp protocol can also be used to demonstrate the relationship between single-channel and macroscopic currents (25).

Discussion of studies of CFTR permeation is beyond the scope of this chapter. We therefore refer the reader to (9) and (11) for excellent overviews of how to measure anion permeation through the CFTR pore.

5. Quantification of CFTR Channel Gating

The methods used to analyse CFTR channel gating are standard electrophysiological procedures. They involve a number of steps: (i) single-channel current amplitude is determined using a current amplitude histogram, as described above in **Section 4**; (ii) single-channel currents are idealized (e.g. **Fig. 27.2**); (iii) channel opening and closing events are detected and an events list is generated; (iv) open and closed times are plotted as either survivor functions or dwell-time histograms; and (v) exponential functions or probability density functions (pdfs) are fitted to estimate mean dwell times (e.g. **Fig. 27.2**). These procedures can be performed using standard data analysis software (e.g. IGOR Pro, WaveMetrics Inc., Lake Oswego, OR, USA), electrophysiological data analysis software (e.g. pCLAMP, Molecular Devices, Sunnyvale, CA,

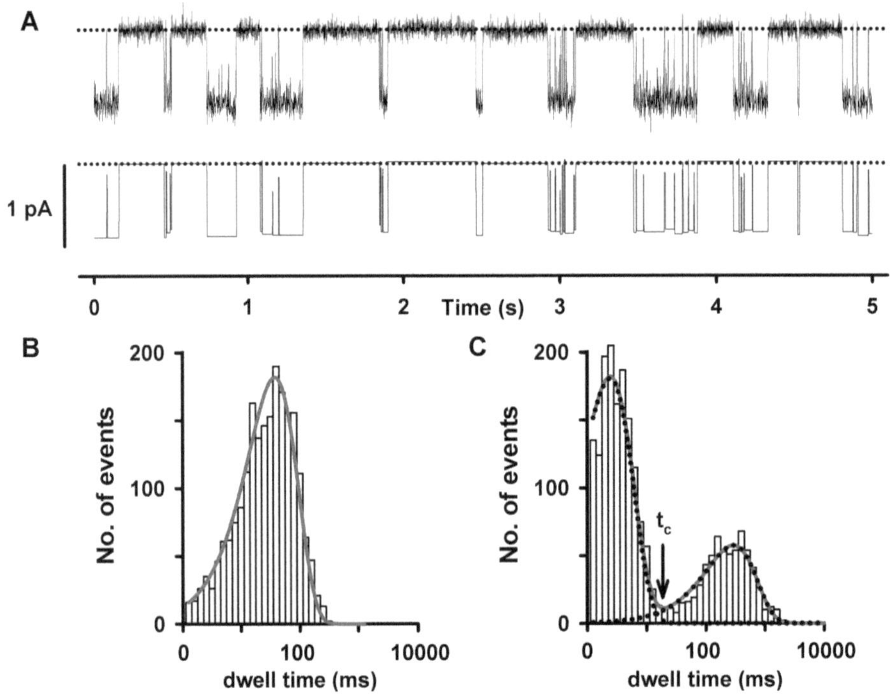

Fig. 27.2. **Dwell-time analysis of a single CFTR Cl⁻ channel.** (**a**) Representative recording of a single wild-type human CFTR Cl⁻ channel (*top*) and its corresponding idealized record (*bottom*). *Dotted lines* indicate where the channel is closed and downward deflections correspond to channel openings. For further information, *see* Cai et al. (37). (**b, c)** Representative open and closed dwell-time histograms, respectively. For the open-time histogram (**b**), the *continuous line* is the fit of a one-component exponential function. For the closed dwell-time histogram, the continuous line is the fit of a two-component exponential function. *Dotted lines* show the individual components of the exponential functions. The *vertical arrow* indicates the delimiter time (t_C) that separates interburst closures from intraburst closures.

USA) or data analysis software custom designed to analyse CFTR channel gating (32). The theory and operation of the different steps involved in the analysis of single-channel data are thoroughly explained in the book *Single Channel Recording* (6). Here, we provide specific guidance on the analysis of CFTR channel gating.

For accurate analysis of CFTR channel gating, it is important to acquire data that are kinetically stable over time. It is therefore critical to prevent the rundown of CFTR Cl⁻ channels in excised inside-out membrane patches (*see* above **Section 2.3**). Experimentalists therefore need to be vigilant when acquiring single-channel data to ensure that data are kinetically stable and suitable for gating analysis.

5.1. Determination of Number of Active Channels and Open Probability

The number (N) of active CFTR Cl⁻ channels in a membrane patch is determined from the maximum number of channels simultaneously observed using experimental conditions that maximally stimulate CFTR. For wild-type CFTR, we use enough PKA (i.e. 75 nM) to strongly phosphorylate CFTR and saturating concentrations of ATP (i.e. > 1 mM). However, for CF mutants, these conditions are not sufficient to maximally stimulate channel activity. We therefore use PKA (75 nM), ATP (1 mM) and a CFTR potentiator (e.g. phloxine B (5 μM)) (33) to maximally stimulate channel activity. Sometimes non-hydrolysable ATP analogues (e.g. AMP-PNP) (34) or the inorganic phosphate analogue (pyrophosphate) (35) are used to "lock open" channels to more easily detect the maximum number of active channels. For three reasons, these agents should be used with great care: (i) the effects of these agents are not completely reversible; (ii) AMP-PNP may not be effective at physiological temperatures; and (iii) pyrophosphate itself opens CFTR (36).

Open probability (P_o) is a measure of the average fraction of time that a channel is open. The open probability of CFTR can be calculated using the area under each peak in the current amplitude histogram and the number of active channels (N) as follows:

$$P_o = \frac{\sum(\text{current level} \times \text{area under peak})}{N \times \text{total area under all peaks}}. \quad [1]$$

The area under each peak is calculated using either the relevant macro in data analysis software or the parameters are obtained from the Gaussian function fitted to each peak.

Alternatively, P_o is calculated from open- and closed-times as follows:

$$P_o = (T_1 + T_2 + \cdots + T_N)/(NT_{tot}), \quad [2]$$

where N is the number of active channels, T_{tot} is the total time analysed, T_1 is the time that one or more channels are open, T_2 is the time two or more channels are open and so on. In practice, we prefer not to use membrane patches that contain more than five active channels to determine P_o. In the case of uncertainty about the number of active channels, apparent open probability (NP_o) is calculated as follows:

$$NP_o = (T_1 + T_2 + \cdots + T_N)/T_{tot}. \quad [3]$$

A major problem with using the maximum number of channel openings to determine the number of active channels in the membrane patch is that this method inevitably grossly overestimates P_o when P_o values are very low. Based on probability theorem, when a channel has a P_o of 0.01 in a membrane patch with two active channels, the probability that both channels are simultaneously open is 0.0001. Thus, for every 1,000 s recorded from this membrane patch, the two channels will be simultaneously open for only 1 s. If instead the membrane patch contained 100 channels each with a P_o of 0.01, it would be impossible to observe the simultaneous openings of all 100 channels. This technical issue is especially relevant when dealing with CF mutants that profoundly disrupt CFTR channel gating (e.g. G551D-CFTR (37, 38)).

To minimize errors when counting the number of active channels, we record channel activity for prolonged periods (i.e. >30 min including multiple interventions) and verify that recordings are of sufficient length to ascertain the correct number of active channels. To verify that recordings are of sufficient length, we use the method of Venglarik et al. (39). The time required to observe at least one single all-open event is $(3\tau_O/N)/(P_O)^N$ where τ_O is the open-time constant; N the number of active channels; and P_O the open probability.

5.2. Dwell-Time Analysis

Once CFTR is phosphorylated by PKA, channel gating is controlled by ATP (5). Thus, the main goal of kinetic analysis is to quantify ATP-dependent transitions to understand how ATP gates the channel, how CF mutants perturb gating and how small molecules rescue gating. However, not all gating transitions observed in single-channel records of CFTR are ATP dependent. It is therefore important to identify, with confidence, the ATP-dependent gating transitions of CFTR.

CFTR channel gating is characterized by bursts of channel openings that are separated by long closures in the range of hundreds of milliseconds to seconds (**Figs. 27.1a** and **27.2a**). As discussed above (**Section 4**), each individual open burst is interrupted by brief closures in the range of several to tens of milliseconds (**Figs. 27.1a** and **27.2a**). Because the ATP-independent brief flickery closures occur on a time scale much shorter than that of the ATP-dependent transitions, these fast events can be removed by filtering heavily the single-channel records prior to their analysis. For example, Zeltwanger et al. (40) demonstrated that filtering data at 25 Hz prior to digitization had little effect on ATP-dependent channel gating, but nearly completely eliminated brief, flickery closures. However, it should be recognized that heavy filtering causes a loss of information about the kinetics of channel gating. Researchers need to consider carefully the optimal settings for filtering and digitizing their data to address their particular research question. In general, we find that filtering and digitizing single-channel records of wild-type CFTR at 500 Hz and 5 kHz, respectively, provides good resolution of brief, flickery closures interrupting channel openings while still permitting clear separation of intraburst closures from interburst closures. Researchers also need to consider carefully the potential effects of their recording conditions on the single-channel activity of CFTR. Besides phosphorylation and ATP, the duration of CFTR channel openings and closings is influenced by temperature (41), voltage (25) and intracellular pH (23).

Temporal information about CFTR channel gating can be extracted from single-channel records by analysing the lifetimes (dwell times) of channel openings and closings. Because open and closed times are distributed exponentially, the time constant (τ) of the distribution can be derived from the exponential probability density function. We routinely plot dwell-time histograms using a logarithmic abscissa for dwell time and a linear ordinate for number of observations. With a logarithmic dwell-time scale, the exponential decay is transformed into a bell-shaped curve. As a result, the number of component exponential functions required to fit the data is readily determined from visual inspection of the dwell-time histogram. For example, in **Fig. 27.2b** the open-time histogram of wild-type CFTR is best described by a one-component exponential function, the open-time constant (τ_O). By contrast, the closed-time histogram is best described by a two-component exponential function (**Fig. 27.2c**). In **Fig. 27.2c**, the tall bell-shaped peak on the left, which represents the brief flickery closures interrupting bursts of channel openings, is described by a fast closed-time constant (τ_{cf}). The short bell-shaped peak on the right, which represents the long closures separating bursts, is described by a slow closed-time constant (τ_{cs}) (**Fig. 27.2c**).

An alternative approach to analyse the open- and closed-times of CFTR is to construct a "survivor plot" (42). The events list is sorted according to time interval from shortest to longest. Then, the events list is plotted against the upper cumulative probability that a particular opening or closing event will last at least time *t*. Note that the probability of an event being the shortest in the events list is 1. The resulting curve is fitted with one- or more-component exponential functions to determine the time constants that describe the open- and closed-times of CFTR.

The principal difficulty with dwell-time analysis of CFTR channel gating is the requirement of a large amount of data to generate histograms that convincingly describe open- and closed-times under specific experimental conditions. Because CFTR gates slowly, this is sometimes an almost insurmountable challenge particularly when studying CFTR inhibition by small molecules or CF mutants that perturb channel gating. Of note, using a dephosphorylation-resistant CFTR mutant, Bompadre et al. (29, 43) were able to acquire sufficient gating transitions to demonstrate the presence of multiple open- and closed-time components.

5.3. Burst Analysis

Burst analysis of CFTR channel gating depends critically on the choice of the burst delimiter (t_c, the time that separates interburst closures from intraburst closures). Theoretically, closures with a duration longer than t_c are classified as interburst closures, whereas closures shorter than t_c are classified as intraburst closures (**Fig. 27.2c**). We determine t_c by inspecting closed-time histograms to select the time value at the nadir separating the two closed-time populations, representing the brief, flickery closures interrupting bursts of channel openings and the prolonged closures separating bursts of channel openings, respectively (**Fig. 27.2c**). The large difference between the fast and slow time constants argues that errors caused by the misclassification of bursts should be rare. An alternative approach to inspecting experimental fits to closed-time distributions of CFTR constructs studied under the experimental conditions in question is to empirically choose t_c using the method of Sigurdson et al. (44). Using either method, the calculated mean open and closed times (or burst duration and interburst interval) for wild-type human CFTR are in the range of hundreds of milliseconds in the presence of saturating [ATP]. Based on the idea that the hydrolysis cycle of CFTR is coupled to the gating cycle of the channel, the data predict that the ATP hydrolysis rate of CFTR is ~1/s as indeed reported by Li et al. (45).

Because CFTR Cl^- channels seldom open in the absence of ATP, it is also possible to calculate burst duration by relaxation analysis of macroscopic currents. In excised inside-out membrane patches containing hundreds of CFTR Cl^- channels, the sudden withdrawal of ATP causes an exponential decay of the macroscopic current. The relaxation time constant determined by fitting the time course of current decay with a single exponential function is a measure of CFTR's burst duration (46). Relaxation analysis of macroscopic current can also be used to identify two populations of channel openings, when the exponential decay of macroscopic current is better fit by a double exponential function, resulting in two different relaxation time constants (e.g. (36); **Fig. 27.3b**). Furthermore, relaxation analysis of macroscopic currents is the method of choice to analyse the burst duration of CFTR constructs that open for tens of hundreds of seconds (e.g. E1371Q, (47)), because it can be very difficult to collect sufficient gating transitions for microscopic kinetic analysis of channel gating for these CFTR constructs.

5.4. Analysing Recordings from Multiple Channels to Obtain Kinetic Information

In **Sections 5.2** and **5.3**, we describe the analytical methods applicable to excised inside-out membrane patches containing a single active CFTR Cl^- channel. Unfortunately, such recordings are the exception, not the norm.

To circumvent this obstacle, Csanády (32) developed a suite of software programs to extract kinetic constants from membrane patches containing multiple active channels. Although this custom-designed software is powerful and rapid, it uses simple kinetic models to analyse CFTR channel gating and cannot accommodate cyclic gating schemes. Nevertheless, this methodology has been used successfully in several studies of CFTR channel gating (e.g. 38, 47–49).

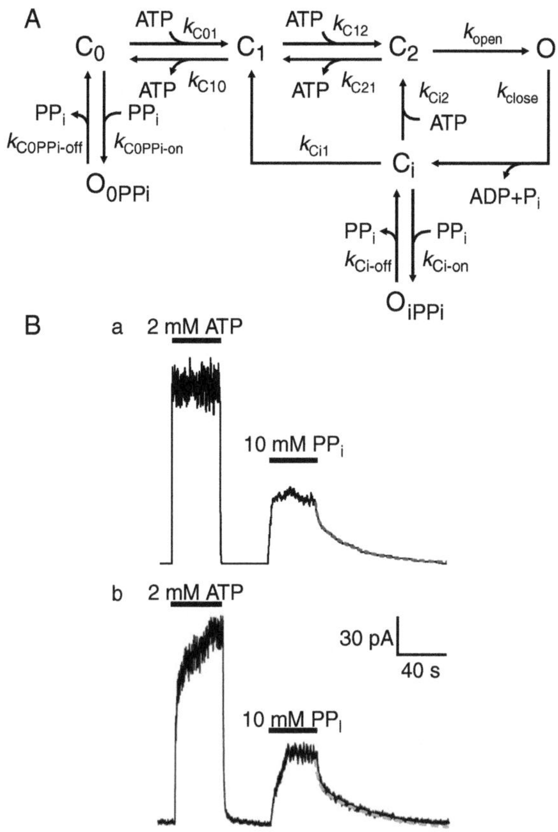

Fig. 27.3. **Monte Carlo simulation of the effects of pyrophosphate on macroscopic CFTR Cl⁻ currents.** (**a**) A kinetic model to simulate the reopening of macroscopic CFTR Cl⁻ currents induced by pyrophosphate (PP_i). In this model, C_0, C_1 and C_2 are closed states with zero, one and two ATP molecule bound, respectively, while C_i is an intermediate closed state sensitive to PP_i. 0, O_{iPPi} and O_{OPPi} are open states, with the latter two open states induced by PP_i binding from the C_i and C_0 states, respectively. The rate constants describing transitions between the different states are shown. (**b**) Comparison of (*a*) simulated and (*b*) experimental macroscopic current data for the PP_i-induced reopening of CFTR channels after removal of ATP. Double exponential fits to current relaxations after removal of PP_i are denoted by *continuous* and *dashed lines* in the simulated (*a*) and experimental (*b*) data, respectively. Time constants: (*a*) τ_{fast}: 1.7 s, τ_{slow}: 32.1 s; (*b*) τ_{fast}: 1.9 s, τ_{slow}: 32.4 s. For further information, *see* (36). Modified from The Journal of General Physiology 2009, 133:405–419. Copyright 2009 The Rockefeller University Press.

5.5. Data Interpretation and Mathematical Modelling

Dwell-time analysis of the ATP dependence of CFTR channel gating provides invaluable insight into the molecular mechanisms that control Cl⁻ flow through the CFTR pore. For example, Zeltwanger et al. (40) demonstrated that the closed-time histogram of CFTR contains a negative exponential component, suggesting that CFTR channel gating is not in equilibrium. Based on this result, the authors proposed a gating scheme with an irreversible step to describe CFTR channel gating (40). This gating scheme argues that ATP hydrolysis is strictly coupled to channel gating in the CFTR Cl^- channel.

Many studies have explored the relationship between ATP concentration and the kinetics of CFTR channel gating (e.g. 33, 40, 48). The data reveal that mean open time varies little with ATP concentration. By contrast, the relationship between mean closed time and ATP concentration is described by a simple Michaelis–Menten function. This result suggests that the rate-limiting step of channel opening occurs after ATP binding. Taken together, the data argue that CFTR channel gating is described by a cyclic scheme, which includes the irreversible step of ATP hydrolysis (47, 48, 50).

With these fundamental concepts of CFTR channel gating, it is possible to use Monte Carlo simulation to investigate whether kinetic models describe accurately CFTR channel gating. For this purpose, simulated single-channel currents based on a given kinetic model are analysed in an identical manner to real data. Then, the simulated and real data are compared to explore the underlying kinetic model. Importantly, Monte Carlo simulation can be used to model channel behaviour at steady state and during responses to channel modulators (**Fig. 27.3**). For examples of this type of approach, *see* (32, 38, 50).

In a given model, the mean lifetime of state i, MLT(i) is calculated using the equation:

$$\mathrm{MLT}(i) = \frac{1}{(\text{Sum of all rate constants away from state } i)}. \quad [4]$$

The actual lifetime of state i at each individual transition, LT(i) is calculated as follows:

$$\mathrm{LT}(i) = \mathrm{MLT}(i) \cdot (-\ln(\mathrm{Rnd})), \quad [5]$$

where MLT(i) is the mean lifetime of state i and Rnd is a random number between 0 and 1.

The probability that the channel moves from state i to one of the adjacent states (state j) is calculated using the equation:

$$P_{ij} = \frac{k_{ij}}{(\text{Sum of all rate constants away from state } i)}, \quad [6]$$

where k_{ij} is the rate constant from state i to state j (51).

To determine which state the channel moves to next after leaving state i, a computer-generated random number between 0 and 1 is used to calculate the cumulative distribution of the probabilities of leaving the state by the different possible pathways. To calculate the duration of individual open (or closed) events, the calculated lifetimes (durations) (LT(*i*)) of sequential states in the open (or closed) configurations are summed (52).

Next, the simulated current recordings are analysed in an identical way to the experimental data. Importantly, Monte Carlo simulation of CFTR channel gating provides values for the identical parameters used to analyse real data (e.g. relaxation time constants; **Fig. 27.3**). The results of this analysis of simulated data are then compared with the analysis of the real experimental data to statistically test the validity of a kinetic model of CFTR channel gating. Successful reproduction of multiple different experimental data by a single kinetic model would validate a particular model of CFTR channel gating.

6. Characterization of CF Mutants

To date, more than 1,600 mutations have been identified in the CFTR gene (www.genet.sickkids.on.ca/). Mutations associated with CF and CFTR-related disorders (e.g. congenital bilateral absence of the vas deferens and chronic pancreatitis) cause a loss of CFTR function by a number of different mechanisms: defective protein production (class I), defective protein processing (class II), defective regulation (class III), defective conductance (class IV) and reduced protein synthesis (class V) (53, 54). Electrophysiological techniques, including single-channel recording, play an important role in elucidating how CF mutants cause a loss of CFTR function and evaluating their severity.

The first step when characterizing a novel CF mutant is to learn whether the mutant generates functional CFTR Cl^- channels and quantify the magnitude of residual cAMP-stimulated Cl^- current relative to that of wild-type CFTR. For this purpose, either the Ussing chamber technique can be used to measure cAMP-stimulated apical membrane Cl^- currents (*see* below, **Section** 7) or the whole-cell configuration of the patch-clamp technique is used to measure macroscopic currents in mammalian cells heterologously expressing wild-type or mutant CFTR. Once the whole-cell configuration is achieved, the cAMP agonist forskolin (10 μM) and the membrane-permeant cAMP analogue 8-(4-chlorophenylthio)adenosine 3′:5′-cyclic monophosphate (CPT-cAMP; 100 μM) are used to stimulate CFTR Cl^- currents (55, 56). The mean current density is calculated using the mean current (maximal current minus leak current) and the membrane capacitance (obtained from the amplifier after compensation of the capacitance current). By averaging mean current density in many cells, it is possible to determine the average mean current density for the CF mutant.

Mean macroscopic CFTR Cl^- current (I) is the product of the number of CFTR Cl^- channels present in the cell membrane (N), the current flowing through an individual CFTR Cl^- channel (i) and the open probability of CFTR (P_o):

$$I = N \times i \times P_o. \quad [7]$$

Thus, a decrease in macroscopic CFTR Cl^- current might be caused by a decrease in N (classes I, II and V), i (class IV), P_o (class III) or a combination of several classes.

For CF mutants that only affect the number of functional channels in the plasma membrane (classes I, II and V), the comparison of whole-cell cAMP-stimulated current density between wild-type and mutant CFTR provides a quantitative assessment of the severity of the mutation. However, these mutations might be associated with other functional defects. For example, the most common CF mutation, F508del, not only disrupts the biosynthesis of CFTR protein (17), but also perturbs the gating behaviour of any mutant channels that reach the cell membrane (57). To identify and quantify these defects, single-channel recording using excised inside-out membrane patches is the method of choice.

The effect of a CF mutation on the cell surface expression of CFTR can be estimated from the magnitude of macroscopic whole-cell current. The ratio of the whole-cell CFTR Cl^- current of a CF mutant relative to that of wild-type CFTR (I_{mutant}/I_{WT}) is proportional to the ratio of the number of channels at the cells surface (N_{mutant}/N_{WT}). If single-channel conductance and P_o are unaltered by the CF mutant, then we can obtain the decrease in number of channels at the cell surface from the ratio of whole-cell CFTR Cl^- current (I_{mutant}/I_{WT}).

In **Section 5**, we emphasized the importance of kinetically stable recordings for kinetic analyses of CFTR channel gating and the need to guard against phosphorylation-dependent and -independent channel rundown. We find that phosphorylation-independent rundown is especially a problem when studying some CF mutants. For example, the F508del-CFTR Cl^- channel is structurally unstable, especially at elevated temperatures (58). At room temperature, F508del-CFTR is stable in excised inside-out membrane patches and amendable to study. By contrast, at 37°C, F508del-CFTR is thermally sensitive, leading to the rundown of many F508del-CFTR Cl^- channels within 10 min of patch excision. This rundown of F508del-CFTR at elevated temperatures constrains the design of experimental protocols to investigate the mechanism of dysfunction of F508del-CFTR and its rescue by small molecules.

The third most common CF mutation G551D is a classic example of a class III mutation because it completely abrogates the ATP-dependence of CFTR channel gating (38). Because of the extremely low P_O of G551D-CFTR, the methods used to study the single-channel behaviour of wild-type CFTR require some refinement before they can be applied to G551D-CFTR. As discussed above in **Section 5.1** it is very difficult to determine accurately the P_O of these channels. The issue resides in the difficulty of properly assessing the number of channels (N) present in the membrane patch given the very low P_O of G551D-CFTR. Although it is tempting to assume that N is equivalent to the number of simultaneous channel openings observed, in the case of G551D-CFTR, this can lead to a gross underestimation of N. Because G551D-CFTR Cl^- channels remain closed most of the time, different channel openings will likely originate from different channels present in the same membrane patch (for a discussion of this problem, *see* (51)). To have any possibility of estimating N for G551D-CFTR, the experimental conditions should be adjusted to maximize P_O. One manoeuvre that has been successfully employed with wild-type CFTR is to use either AMP-PNP or pyrophosphate, which locks open channels for many seconds. Unfortunately, these reagents do not always work with CF mutants. For example, AMP-PNP and pyrophosphate fail to lock-open the G551D-CFTR Cl^- channel (37, 38).

A compromise method used by Bompadre et al. (38) offers a rough estimation of the P_O of G551D-CFTR. When CHO cells are transfected with the same amount of cDNA encoding wild-type or G551D-CFTR, Western blot analysis demonstrates that the cells produce similar amounts of band C (mature protein) for the two constructs (38). This indicates that similar numbers of wild-type and G551D-CFTR Cl^- channels are present at the cell surface. In excised inside-out membrane patches, the mean current amplitude is measured after the channels are activated by PKA and ATP. Because neither the number of active channels nor the single-channel current amplitude is altered by the G551D mutation, the mean current amplitude directly reflects P_O. To obtain accurate results with this type of experiment, it is necessary to perform many experiments to overcome the variation observed between individual membrane patches.

One potential solution to the technical difficulty of measuring the P_O of CF mutants like G551D is to use CFTR potentiators or ATP analogues to augment robustly channel gating and hence P_O. However, so far in the literature, the most efficacious small molecules only increase the P_O of G551D-CFTR by $\sim$ 5-fold, far lower than the $\sim$100-fold decrease of P_O caused by this mutation. More efficacious CFTR potentiators are urgently required to address properly this issue.

Class IV mutations (defective conductance) attenuate the flow of Cl^- ions through the channel pore. As a result, these CF mutants (e.g. R334W and R347P; 59, 60) diminish single-channel current amplitude (i). To determine single-channel conductance, we measure single-channel current amplitude using current amplitude histograms, construct an *I–V* relationship and measure the slope of the line. In the case of some CF mutants, individual channel openings might not be easily resolvable. In this case, a large Cl^- concentration gradient and strong membrane hyperpolarization might be employed to magnify CFTR Cl^- currents. (Note that very tight seals are essential to successfully perform this type of experiment.) If individual channel openings remain unresolvable, non-stationary noise analysis might be applied to macroscopic CFTR Cl^- currents to calculate single-channel current amplitude. For this purpose, a low concentration of PKA (e.g. 20 nM) is used to slow the rate of channel activation (61).

It is important to note that if a CF mutation alters the single-channel conductance of CFTR, this does not necessarily mean that the affected amino acid residue lines the channel pore. A CF mutation might alter the packing of transmembrane segments and hence, the overall structure of the pore, causing a diminution of single-channel conductance. Consideration should also be given to the possibility that a CF mutation might reduce current flow through the CFTR pore by altering anion selectivity. For example, the CF mutant, P99L, in the first transmembrane segment attenuated the single-channel conductance (wild-type, 7.72 ± 0.22 pS (means ± SEM; $n = 4$); P99L, 4.97 ± 0.24 pS ($n = 5$, $p < 0.0001$)) and altered the anion selectivity sequence (wild-type, $Br^- \geq Cl^- > I^-$; P99L, $Br^- \geq Cl^- = I^-$) (62). However, Akabas et al. (63) concluded that P99 does not line the CFTR pore because the site-directed mutant P99C did not react with methanethiosulfonate reagents. This example illustrates the types of studies required to elucidate how an individual CF mutant disrupts CFTR function. As indicated earlier in this section, a single mutation might perturb CFTR function by multiple mechanisms. Experimentalists should be alert to this possibility.

7. Relationship Between Single-Channel and Macroscopic Behaviour

Studies of the biosynthesis and single-channel behaviour of CF mutants provide a molecular explanation for the greatly diminished cAMP-activated CFTR Cl^- current generated by CF mutants in the apical membrane of epithelia. Apical CFTR Cl^- current (I^{CFTR}(apical)) is determined by the product of the number of CFTR Cl^- channels in the apical membrane (*N*), the current amplitude (*i*) of an individual CFTR Cl^- channel and probability (P_o) that a single CFTR Cl^- channel is open: $I^{CFTR}(\text{apical}) = N \times i \times P_o$ (Eq. 7). Using biochemical (*N*) and functional

Table 27.1
Comparison of predicted apical membrane Cl⁻ current and measured cAMP-activated apical membrane Cl⁻ current for wild-type and mutant CFTRs

CFTR	*N* (%)	*i* (%)	P_o (%)	$N \times i \times P_o$ (%)	I^{CFTR} (apical) (%)
Wild-type	100	100	100	100	100
F508del	4	100	30	1.2	0
G551D	100	100	2.5	2.5	1.5
R117H	100	86	28	24	15
P574H	15	100	139	21.1	17

N, the number of Cl⁻ channels in the apical membrane; *i*, single-channel current amplitude; P_O, open probability; $N \times i \times P_O$, the predicted apical membrane Cl⁻ current; I^{CFTR} (apical), measured cAMP-activated apical membrane Cl⁻ current. Based on Cai & Sheppard (33), the P_O of F508del was set to 30% that of wild-type CFTR. Other details as in Sheppard and Ostedgaard (68). For G551D data, *N* and I^{CFTR} values are from Bompadre et al. (38) and Zegarra-Moran et al. (64), while *i* and P_O data are from Cai et al. (37). Modified, with permission, from Sheppard and Ostedgaard (68).

(*i* and P_O) data, the apical CFTR Cl⁻ current generated by F508del-CFTR and other CF-associated mutants can be predicted. For this purpose, *N*, *i* and P_O are set to 100% for wild-type CFTR. **Table 27.1** compares the predicted values of $N \times i \times P_O$ with the observed values of I^{CFTR}(apical) measured in FRT epithelia for F508del-CFTR and the CF mutants, R117H, G551D and P574H, which disrupt CFTR function by different mechanisms (33, 37, 59, 64, 65). Despite possible errors resulting from (i) the assumption that *N* is equivalent to the amount of fully glycosylated protein (band C) and (ii) the supposition that the P_O of CFTR Cl⁻ channels in the apical membrane of FRT epithelia is equivalent to values measured in excised membrane patches from non-polarized cells, the predicted values agree well with the measured data. The predicted values for F508del-CFTR also concur with values calculated by other investigators (e.g. Haws et al. (66), 2% and Wang et al. (67), 0.4%). Thus, the data demonstrate that biochemical and functional studies may be used to provide a molecular explanation for the quantitative decrease in cAMP-activated CFTR Cl⁻ current generated by CF-associated mutants.

8. Conclusions

The excised inside-out configuration of the patch-clamp technique is the premier method to investigate the CFTR Cl⁻ channel. The technique offers researchers the unique opportunity to observe in real-time conformational changes in a single membrane protein driven by cycles of ATP binding and hydrolysis.

The sheer excitement of such experiments more than compensates for the technical challenges of high-resolution recording of single CFTR Cl^- channels.

Acknowledgments

We thank our laboratory colleagues for valuable discussions. During the preparation of this chapter, DN Sheppard was supported by the Cystic Fibrosis Trust and EuroCareCF (LSHM-CT-2005-018932), Y Sohma by a Grant-in-Aid for Scientific Research (C) from the Japan Society for the Promotion of Science (JSPS) (19590215 and 22590212) and T-C Hwang by the National Institutes of Health (R01DK55835 and R01HL53445) and Cystic Fibrosis Foundation.

References

1. Neher, E., and Sakmann, B. (1976) Single-channel currents recorded from membrane of denervated frog muscle fibres. *Nature* **260**, 799–802.
2. Hamill, O. P., Marty, A., Neher, E., Sakmann, B., and Sigworth, F. J. (1981) Improved patch-clamp techniques for high-resolution current recording from cells and cell-free membrane patches. *Pflugers Arch.* **391**, 85–100.
3. Ostedgaard, L. S., Baldursson, O., and Welsh, M. J. (2001) Regulation of the cystic fibrosis transmembrane conductance regulator Cl^- channel by its R domain. *J. Biol. Chem.* **276**, 7689–7692.
4. Gadsby, D. C., Vergani, P., and Csanády, L. (2006) The ABC protein turned chloride channel whose failure causes cystic fibrosis. *Nature* **440**, 477–483.
5. Hwang, T. C., and Sheppard, D. N. (2009) Gating of the CFTR Cl^- channel by ATP-driven nucleotide-binding domain dimerisation. *J. Physiol.* **587**, 2151–2161.
6. Sakmann, B., and Neher, E. (1995) *Single-channel recording*, 2nd ed. Plenum, New York, NY.
7. Hug, M. J. (2002) The whole-cell patch-clamp technique – a powerful tool to approach CFTR function. Virtual Repository of Methods and Reagents for CFTR Expression and Functional Studies. http://central.igc.gulbenkian.pt/cftr/vr/physiology.html. Accessed 11 March 2010.
8. Gray, M. A. (2002) Investigating the properties of the CFTR channel using the cell-attached configuration of the patch clamp – monitoring single channel activity in a living cell. Virtual Repository of Methods and Reagents for CFTR Expression and Functional Studies. http://central.igc.gulbenkian.pt/cftr/vr/physiology.html. Accessed 11 March 2010.
9. Hanrahan, J. W., Kone, Z., Mathews, C. J., Luo, J., Jia, Y., and Linsdell, P. (1998) Patch-clamp studies of cystic fibrosis transmembrane conductance regulator chloride channel. *Methods Enzymol.* **293**, 169–194.
10. Scott-Ward, T. S., Chen, J. H., Li, H., Cai, Z., and Sheppard, D. N. (2002) Measurement of Cl^- flow through CFTR channels using the excised inside-out patch-clamp Virtual Repository of Methods and Reagents for CFTR Expression and Functional Studies. http://central.igc.gulbenkian.pt/cftr/vr/physiology.html. Accessed 11 March 2010.
11. Gong, X., Gupta, J., and Linsdell, P. (2002) Measurement of the permeation and conduction properties of the CFTR chloride channel using excised inside-out membrane. Virtual Repository of Methods and Reagents for CFTR Expression and Functional Studies. http://central.igc.gulbenkian.pt/cftr/vr/physiology.html. Accessed 11 March 2010.
12. Sohma, Y., and Hwang, T. C. (2002) Kinetic analysis of CFTR single-channel data. Virtual Repository of Methods and Reagents for

CFTR Expression and Functional Studies. http://central.igc.gulbenkian.pt/cftr/vr/physiology.html. Accessed 11 March 2010.

13. Cai, Z., Scott-Ward, T. S., Li, H., Schmidt, A., and Sheppard, D. N. (2002) Strategies to investigate the mechanism of action of CFTR modulators Virtual Repository of Methods and Reagents for CFTR Expression and Functional Studies. http://central.igc.gulbenkian.pt/cftr/vr/physiology.html. Accessed 11 March 2010.
14. Sheppard, D. N., and Robinson, K. A. (1997) Mechanism of glibenclamide inhibition of cystic fibrosis transmembrane conductance regulator Cl^- channels expressed in a murine cell line. *J. Physiol.* **503**, 333–346.
15. Lansdell, K. A., Delaney, S. J., Lunn, D. P., Thomson, S. A., Sheppard, D. N., and Wainwright, B. J. (1998) Comparison of the gating behaviour of human and murine cystic fibrosis transmembrane conductance regulator Cl^- channels expressed in mammalian cells. *J. Physiol.* **508**, 379–392.
16. Anderson, M. P., Gregory, R. J., Thompson, S., Souza, D. W., Paul, S., Mulligan, R. C., et al. (1991) Demonstration that CFTR is a chloride channel by alteration of its anion selectivity. *Science* **253**, 202–205.
17. Cheng, S. H., Gregory, R. J., Marshall, J., Paul, S., Souza, D. W., White, G. A., et al. (1990) Defective intracellular transport and processing of CFTR is the molecular basis of most cystic fibrosis. *Cell* **63**, 827–834.
18. Drumm, M. L., Wilkinson, D. J., Smit, L. S., Worrell, R. T., Strong, T. V., Frizzell, R. A., et al. (1991) Chloride conductance expressed by ΔF508 and other mutant CFTRs in Xenopus oocytes. *Science* **254**, 1797–1799.
19. Scott-Ward, T. S., Cai, Z., Dawson, E. S., Doherty, A., Da Paula, A. C., Davidson, H., et al. (2007) Chimeric constructs endow the human CFTR Cl^- channel with the gating behavior of murine CFTR. *Proc. Natl. Acad. Sci. USA* **104**, 16365–16370.
20. Wu, J. V., Joo, N. S., Krouse, M. E., and Wine, J. J. (2001) Cystic fibrosis transmembrane conductance regulator gating requires cytosolic electrolytes. *J. Biol. Chem.* **276**, 6473–6478.
21. Ishihara, H., and Welsh, M. J. (1997) Block by MOPS reveals a conformation change in the CFTR pore produced by ATP hydrolysis. *Am. J. Physiol.* **273**, C1278–C1289.
22. Tabcharani, J. A., Chang, X. B., Riordan, J. R., and Hanrahan, J. W. (1991) Phosphorylation-regulated Cl^- channel in CHO cells stably expressing the cystic fibrosis gene. *Nature* **352**, 628–631.
23. Chen, J. H., Cai, Z., and Sheppard, D. N. (2009) Direct sensing of intracellular pH by the cystic fibrosis transmembrane conductance regulator (CFTR) Cl^- channel. *J. Biol. Chem.* **284**, 35495–35506.
24. Hughes, L. K., Ju, M., and Sheppard, D. N. (2008) Potentiation of cystic fibrosis transmembrane conductance regulator (CFTR) Cl^- currents by the chemical solvent tetrahydrofuran. *Mol. Membr. Biol.* **25**, 528–538.
25. Cai, Z., Scott-Ward, T. S., and Sheppard, D. N. (2003) Voltage-dependent gating of the cystic fibrosis transmembrane conductance regulator Cl^- channel. *J. Gen. Physiol.* **122**, 605–620.
26. Zhou, Z., Hu, S., and Hwang, T. C. (2001) Voltage-dependent flickery block of an open cystic fibrosis transmembrane conductance regulator (CFTR) channel pore. *J. Physiol.* **532**, 435–448.
27. Anderson, M. P., Berger, H. A., Rich, D. P., Gregory, R. J., Smith, A. E., and Welsh, M. J. (1991) Nucleoside triphosphates are required to open the CFTR chloride channel. *Cell* **67**, 775–784.
28. Schultz, B. D., Frizzell, R. A., and Bridges, R. J. (1999) Rescue of dysfunctional ΔF508-CFTR chloride channel activity by IBMX. *J. Membr. Biol.* **170**, 51–66.
29. Bompadre, S. G., Cho, J. H., Wang, X., Zou, X., Sohma, Y., Li, M., et al. (2005) CFTR gating II: effects of nucleotide binding on the stability of open states. *J. Gen. Physiol.* **125**, 377–394.
30. Linsdell, P., and Hanrahan, J. W. (1996) Disulphonic stilbene block of cystic fibrosis transmembrane conductance regulator Cl^- channels expressed in a mammalian cell line and its regulation by a critical pore residue. *J. Physiol.* **496**, 687–693.
31. Zhou, Z., Hu, S., and Hwang, T. C. (2002) Probing an open CFTR pore with organic anion blockers. *J. Gen. Physiol.* **120**, 647–662.
32. Csanády, L., Chan, K. W., Seto-Young, D., Kopsco, D. C., Nairn, A. C., and Gadsby, D. C. (2000) Severed channels probe regulation of gating of cystic fibrosis transmembrane conductance regulator by its cytoplasmic domains. *J. Gen. Physiol.* **116**, 477–500.
33. Cai, Z., and Sheppard, D. N. (2002) Phloxine B interacts with the cystic fibrosis transmembrane conductance regulator at multiple sites to modulate channel activity. *J. Biol. Chem.* **277**, 19546–19553.
34. Hwang, T. C., Nagel, G., Nairn, A. C., and Gadsby, D. C. (1994) Regulation of the gating of cystic fibrosis transmembrane conductance regulator Cl channels by

phosphorylation and ATP hydrolysis. *Proc. Natl. Acad. Sci. USA* **91**, 4698–4702.
35. Carson, M. R., Winter, M. C., Travis, S. M., and Welsh, M. J. (1995) Pyrophosphate stimulates wild-type and mutant cystic fibrosis transmembrane conductance regulator Cl^- channels. *J. Biol. Chem.* **270**, 20466–20472.
36. Tsai, M. F., Shimizu, H., Sohma, Y., Li, M., and Hwang, T. C. (2009) State-dependent modulation of CFTR gating by pyrophosphate. *J. Gen. Physiol.* **133**, 405–419.
37. Cai, Z., Taddei, A., and Sheppard, D. N. (2006) Differential sensitivity of the cystic fibrosis (CF)-associated mutants G551D and G1349D to potentiators of the cystic fibrosis transmembrane conductance regulator (CFTR) Cl^- channel. *J. Biol. Chem.* **281**, 1970–1977.
38. Bompadre, S. G., Sohma, Y., Li, M., and Hwang, T. C. (2007) G551D and G1349D, two CF-associated mutations in the signature sequences of CFTR, exhibit distinct gating defects. *J. Gen. Physiol.* **129**, 285–298.
39. Venglarik, C. J., Schultz, B. D., Frizzell, R. A., and Bridges, R. J. (1994) ATP alters current fluctuations of cystic fibrosis transmembrane conductance regulator: evidence for a three-state activation mechanism. *J. Gen. Physiol.* **104**, 123–146.
40. Zeltwanger, S., Wang, F., Wang, G. T., Gillis, K. D., and Hwang, T. C. (1999) Gating of cystic fibrosis transmembrane conductance regulator chloride channels by adenosine triphosphate hydrolysis. Quantitative analysis of a cyclic gating scheme. *J. Gen. Physiol.* **113**, 541–554.
41. Aleksandrov, A. A., and Riordan, J. R. (1998) Regulation of CFTR ion channel gating by MgATP. *FEBS Lett.* **431**, 97–101.
42. Baukrowitz, T., Hwang, T. C., Nairn, A. C., and Gadsby, D. C. (1994) Coupling of CFTR Cl^- channel gating to an ATP hydrolysis cycle. *Neuron* **12**, 473–482.
43. Bompadre, S. G., Ai, T., Cho, J. H., Wang, X., Sohma, Y., Li, M., et al. (2005) CFTR gating I: characterization of the ATP-dependent gating of a phosphorylation-independent CFTR channel (ΔR-CFTR). *J. Gen. Physiol.* **125**, 361–375.
44. Sigurdson, W. J., Morris, C. E., Brezden, B. L., and Gardner, D. R. (1987) Stretch activation of a K^+ channel in molluscan heart cells. *J. Exp. Biol.* **127**, 191–209.
45. Li, C., Ramjeesingh, M., Wang, W., Garami, E., Hewryk, M., Lee, D., et al. (1996) ATPase activity of the cystic fibrosis transmembrane conductance regulator. *J. Biol. Chem.* **271**, 28463–28468.
46. Weinreich, F., Riordan, J. R., and Nagel, G. (1999) Dual effects of ADP and adenylylimidodiphosphate on CFTR channel kinetics show binding to two different nucleotide binding sites. *J. Gen. Physiol.* **114**, 55–70.
47. Vergani, P., Lockless, S. W., Nairn, A. C., and Gadsby, D. C. (2005) CFTR channel opening by ATP-driven tight dimerization of its nucleotide-binding domains. *Nature* **433**, 876–880.
48. Vergani, P., Nairn, A. C., and Gadsby, D. C. (2003) On the mechanism of MgATP-dependent gating of CFTR Cl^- channels. *J. Gen. Physiol.* **121**, 17–36.
49. Zhou, Z., Wang, X., Liu, H. Y., Zou, X., Li, M., and Hwang, T. C. (2006) The two ATP binding sites of cystic fibrosis transmembrane conductance regulator (CFTR) play distinct roles in gating kinetics and energetics. *J. Gen. Physiol.* **128**, 413–422.
50. Csanády, L., Vergani, P., and Gadsby, D. C. (2010) Strict coupling between CFTR's catalytic cycle and gating of its Cl^- ion pore revealed by distributions of open channel burst durations. *Proc. Natl. Acad. Sci. USA* **107**, 1241–1246.
51. Colquhoun, D., and Hawkes, A. G. (1995) The principles of stochastic interpretation of ion-channel mechanisms, in (Sakmann, B., Neher, E. eds.) *Single-channel recording*, 2nd ed. Plenum, New York, NY.
52. Blatz, A. L., and Magleby, K. L. (1986) Quantitative description of three modes of activity of fast chloride channels from rat skeletal muscle. *J. Physiol.* **378**, 141–174.
53. Welsh, M. J., and Smith, A. E. (1993) Molecular mechanisms of CFTR chloride channel dysfunction in cystic fibrosis. *Cell* **73**, 1251–1254.
54. Zielenski, J., and Tsui, L. C. (1995) Cystic fibrosis: genotypic and phenotypic variations. *Annu. Rev. Genet.* **29**, 777–807.
55. Hwang, T. C., Wang, F., Yang, I. C., and Reenstra, W. W. (1997) Genistein potentiates wild-type and F508-CFTR channel activity. *Am. J. Physiol.* **273**, C988–C998.
56. Al-Nakkash, L., and Hwang, T. C. (1999) Activation of wild-type and ΔF508-CFTR by phosphodiesterase inhibitors through cAMP-dependent and -independent mechanisms. *Pflugers Arch.* **437**, 553–561.
57. Dalemans, W., Barbry, P., Champigny, G., Jallat, S., Dott, K., Dreyer, D., et al. (1991) Altered chloride ion channel kinetics associated with the ΔF508 cystic fibrosis mutation. *Nature* **354**, 526–528.
58. Hegedus, T., Aleksandrov, A., Cui, L., Gentzsch, M., Chang, X. B., and Riordan, J. R. (2006) F508del CFTR with two

altered RXR motifs escapes from ER quality control but its channel activity is thermally sensitive. *Biochim. Biophys. Acta* **1758**, 565–572.
59. Sheppard, D. N., Rich, D. P., Ostedgaard, L. S., Gregory, R. J., Smith, A. E., and Welsh, M. J. (1993) Mutations in CFTR associated with mild-disease-form Cl^- channels with altered pore properties. *Nature* **362**, 160–164.
60. Gong, X., and Linsdell, P. (2004) Maximization of the rate of chloride conduction in the CFTR channel pore by ion-ion interactions. *Arch. Biochem. Biophys.* **426**, 78–82.
61. Linsdell, P. (2001) Relationship between anion binding and anion permeability revealed by mutagenesis within the cystic fibrosis transmembrane conductance regulator chloride channel pore. *J. Physiol.* **531**, 51–66.
62. Sheppard, D. N., Travis, S. M., Ishihara, H., and Welsh, M. J. (1996) Contribution of proline residues in the membrane-spanning domains of cystic fibrosis transmembrane conductance regulator to chloride channel function. *J. Biol. Chem.* **271**, 14995–15001.
63. Akabas, M. H., Kaufmann, C., Cook, T. A., and Archdeacon, P. (1994) Amino acid residues lining the chloride channel of the cystic fibrosis transmembrane conductance regulator. *J. Biol. Chem.* **269**, 14865–14868.
64. Zegarra-Moran, O., Romio, L., Folli, C., Caci, E., Becq, F., Vierfond, J. M., et al. (2002) Correction of G551D-CFTR transport defect in epithelial monolayers by genistein but not by CPX or MPB-07. *Br. J. Pharmacol.* **137**, 504–512.
65. Sheppard, D. N., Ostedgaard, L. S., Winter, M. C., and Welsh, M. J. (1995) Mechanism of dysfunction of two nucleotide binding domain mutations in cystic fibrosis transmembrane conductance regulator that are associated with pancreatic sufficiency. *EMBO J.* **14**, 876–883.
66. Haws, C. M., Nepomuceno, I. B., Krouse, M. E., Wakelee, H., Law, T., Xia, Y., et al. (1996) ΔF508-CFTR channels: kinetics, activation by forskolin, and potentiation by xanthines. *Am. J. Physiol.* **270**, C1544–C1555.
67. Wang, F., Zeltwanger, S., Hu, S., and Hwang, T. C. (2000) Deletion of phenylalanine 508 causes attenuated phosphorylation-dependent activation of CFTR chloride channels. *J. Physiol.* **524**, 637–648.
68. Sheppard, D. N., and Ostedgaard, L. S. (1996) Understanding how cystic fibrosis mutations cause a loss of Cl^- channel function. *Mol. Med. Today* **2**, 290–297.

Chapter 28

Electrophysiological, Biochemical, and Bioinformatic Methods for Studying CFTR Channel Gating and Its Regulation

László Csanády, Paola Vergani, Attila Gulyás-Kovács, and David C. Gadsby

Abstract

CFTR is the only member of the ABC (ATP-binding cassette) protein superfamily known to function as an ion channel. Most other ABC proteins are ATP-driven transporters, in which a cycle of ATP binding and hydrolysis, at intracellular nucleotide binding domains (NBDs), powers uphill substrate translocation across the membrane. In CFTR, this same ATP-driven cycle opens and closes a transmembrane pore through which chloride ions flow rapidly down their electrochemical gradient. Detailed analysis of the pattern of gating of CFTR channels thus offers the opportunity to learn about mechanisms of function not only of CFTR channels but also of their ABC transporter ancestors. In addition, CFTR channel gating is subject to complex regulation by kinase-mediated phosphorylation at multiple consensus sites in a cytoplasmic regulatory domain that is unique to CFTR. Here we offer a practical guide to extract useful information about the mechanisms that control opening and closing of CFTR channels: on how to plan (including information obtained from analysis of multiple sequence alignments), carry out, and analyze electrophysiological and biochemical experiments, as well as on how to circumvent potential pitfalls.

Key words: Single channels, multiple channels, kinetic analysis, energetic analysis, cysteine modification, coevolution.

1. Introduction

1.1. Present Understanding of Regulation of CFTR Channel Gating by Nucleotides

CFTR's pair of cytoplasmic NBDs (NBD1 and NBD2) are drawn together in head-to-tail orientation (1, 2), as in all other ABC proteins, by two ATP molecules bound within composite interfacial catalytic sites, between the Walker A and B motifs of one

M.D. Amaral, K. Kunzelmann (eds.), *Cystic Fibrosis*, Methods in Molecular Biology 741,
DOI 10.1007/978-1-61779-117-8_28, © Springer Science+Business Media, LLC 2011

NBD and the LSGGQ-like ABC signature sequence of the other (3–9). Hydrolysis of the ATP disrupts the interface, causing the NBDs to separate and allowing fresh ATP to bind. In CFTR, these cyclic, ATP-driven motions of the NBDs are transmitted to the transmembrane domains (TMDs) to alternately open and close the pore through which chloride ions flow rapidly across the membrane, down their electrochemical gradient. Dissimilarities between NBD1 and NBD2 in CFTR, mirrored in all members of the OAD (organic anion and drug; (10)) transporter subfamily of ABC proteins to which CFTR belongs, render only one of the composite interfacial ATP sites (the "NBD2 composite" site, incorporating the NBD2 Walker motifs) catalytically competent, while crippling the "NBD1 composite" site by substitutions on both sides of the interface. In the absence of ATP, phosphorylated (*see* **Section 1.2**) CFTR channels essentially remain closed (except for rare, brief, openings; e.g., (11, 12)). On exposure of the cytoplasmic surface of CFTR channels to millimolar ATP, its binding at the two interfacial sites causes NBD1–NBD2 heterodimerization and opening of the ion pore. The average channel opening rate is a saturable function of ATP concentration according to Michaelis–Menten kinetics and is half maximal near 50 μM ATP for wild-type (WT) CFTR (13). Because this apparent affinity for activation by ATP is diminished by mutations of either NBD that are expected to impair ATP binding, normal channel opening appears to require ATP binding in both composite sites (12).

The pore remains open until hydrolysis of the ATP in the competent "NBD2 site" triggers channel closure. That hydrolysis rate-limits closure is supported by prolongation of channel openings upon interference with hydrolysis by addition of inorganic phosphate analogues, such as orthovanadate or pyrophosphate (14–16), or of poorly hydrolyzable ATP analogs like AMP-PNP (15, 17) or by mutation of key catalytic residues (1, 11, 12, 15, 18). That the hydrolysis occurs only in the "NBD2 site," and not in the "NBD1 site," is demonstrated by the findings that only "NBD2 site" mutations prolong openings (11, 12, 15, 18), and that photocrosslinking with γ-^{32}P-8-azidoATP radio-labels only the "NBD1 site," since the ^{32}P is released from the "NBD2 site" too rapidly to be observed (19, 20). The photocrosslinking experiments also indicated that non-hydrolyzed ATP remained bound for minutes at the "NBD1 site" (19, 20), arguing that the seconds-long ATP binding and hydrolysis cycle that drives CFTR channel gating reflects events at the "NBD2 site" (12, 15, 20), a conclusion further supported by the much slower loss, after sudden ATP withdrawal, of the ability of brief exposures to pyrophosphate or AMP-PNP to elicit prolonged channel openings (21).

Because crystal structures of nucleotide-bound ABC transporters show the extracellular-side gate in the transmembrane domains open and the cytoplasmic-side gate closed (e.g., (7–9, 22)), whereas both gates must be open in an ATP-bound CFTR channel to allow the observed rapid chloride ion flow (millions of ions per second per channel), in CFTR the cytoplasmic-side gate would appear to have become atrophied or uncoupled from the outer gate (23). CFTR can therefore be considered to be a broken ABC transporter (e.g., (24–27)). Detailed analysis of the pattern of gating of CFTR channels thus offers the opportunity to learn about mechanisms of function not only of CFTR channels but also of their ABC transporter ancestors.

1.2. Present Understanding of Regulation of CFTR Channel Gating by Phosphorylation

Before a CFTR channel can be opened by ATP, cAMP-dependent protein kinase (PKA) must phosphorylate consensus-site serines in the ~200-residue cytoplasmic regulatory (R) domain that links CFTR's two homologous halves (28, 29), and phosphorylation of PKC sites in the R domain might be a prerequisite (30, 31). Because cells contain millimolar levels of ATP, enough to saturate binding at CFTR's NBDs, phosphorylation of the R domain by PKA may be presumed to be the principal physiological regulator of CFTR channel activity. The R domain is unique to CFTR, and its structure and mechanism remain controversial and incompletely understood (reviewed in (32)). Evidence of structural disorder of isolated R domain (33, 34) and of graded activation of CFTR channels with increasing phosphorylation (e.g., (28, 35, 36)) has been interpreted as indicating redundancy among up to nine R domain phosphoserines, with accumulated negative charge as the major factor. The positions of consensus serine-containing segments in crystal structures of CFTR NBD1 extended by an R domain fragment (37), and NMR measurements of NBD1-R domain interactions (34, 38), prompted the proposal that non-phosphorylated R domain binds to the NBDs and interferes with ATP-mediated formation of the NBD1–NBD2 heterodimer, and hence with CFTR channel opening; phosphorylation of the R domain is proposed to release it from the NBDs, relieving the inhibition of gating. Such a simple mechanism seems unlikely, as neither serine-containing segment is needed for channels to close in the absence of ATP, regardless of phosphorylation status, and their deletion or mutation does not alter the strict dependence of channel gating on phosphorylation by PKA (39). Moreover, deletion of the entire NBD2 (40, 41) or introduction of "constitutive" mutations (42), even the CF-causing mutation G551D (43), results in channels that gate regardless of the presence of ATP – but even this "spontaneous" activity remains strictly dependent on prior phosphorylation by PKA. Finally, two of the phosphoserines, including the one most readily generated by PKA (29, 36, 44, 45), seem to have an inhibitory, rather than stimulatory, influence on channel open probability (P_o, *see* **Section 3.4.2**) (36, 46). A region of density interpreted as R domain that extends between NBDs and TMDs in a cryo-EM low-resolution structure of CFTR (47) seems more consistent with an alternative proposal that the R domain somehow controls transmission of information from the NBDs to the channel gates (20).

2. Materials

2.1. Xenopus Oocyte Incubation Media

After injection with cRNA, oocytes are kept for 1–5 days at 18°C in solution containing (in mM) 83 NaCl, 2 KCl, 1 $MgCl_2$, 1.8 $CaCl_2$, 5 HEPES (pH 7.5), plus 50 μg/ml gentamycin (12, 13, 48).

2.2. Solutions Used for Electrophysiological Recordings

For recording in intact oocytes, the superfusion solution contains (in mM) 83 NaCl, 2 KCl, 1 $MgCl_2$, and 5 HEPES (pH 7.5). For excised patch recording, pipette solution contains (in mM) 138 NMDG-Cl, 2 $MgCl_2$, and 5 HEPES (pH 7.4); bath solution contains (in mM) 138 NMDG-Cl, 2 $MgCl_2$, 0.5 EGTA, 5 HEPES (pH 7.1); for chloride-free solutions, sulfamate or gluconate replace chloride (12, 13, 48).

3. Methods

3.1. Heterologous Expression of Human CFTR in Various Cell Types Including Xenopus Oocytes

3.1.1. Expression Plasmids

For expression in *Xenopus* oocytes, CFTR mutants are generated from pGEMHE-CFTR (48) by mutation with Quikchange, verified by automated DNA sequencing, and in vitro transcribed using mMessage T7 polymerase to yield cRNA. For expression in HEK293T cells, pIRES-CFTR constructs are generated by subcloning the corresponding CFTR into the *EcoRV* site of the pIRES vector (20).

3.1.2. Cell Preparation

Oocytes are isolated from anesthetized adult female *Xenopus laevis* and dispersed using collagenase, as described (13). HEK293T cells are maintained in DMEM medium supplemented with 10%fetal bovine serum, plated in 100 mm dishes, and transfected with pIRES-CFTR (20).

3.2. Biochemical Analysis of CFTR Regulation

3.2.1. Cysteine Modification as a Tool to Study Domain–Domain Interactions

To supplement the minimal structural information available for CFTR and to directly examine changes in conformation associated with gating, sulfhydryl-specific crosslinking can be used to probe proximity of pairs of target cysteines introduced into CFTR, provided that some or all of the 18 native Cys are first removed or shown not to interfere with the assay of target Cys reactivity. If the Cα atoms of residues approach each other to within 5–8 Å, then target Cys at those positions should form disulfide bonds upon oxidation with copper phenanthroline. Bifunctional sulfhydryl-specific reagents, e.g., based on maleimide (2) or methanethiosulfonate (MTS) (49, 50), with variable-length linkers can provide upper estimates for the minimum separation of Cys pairs under the conditions of the assay. These reagents can be applied to functioning CFTR channels in vivo. For example, crosslinking of several target Cys pairs across CFTR's head-to-tail NBD1–NBD2 heterodimer interface by BMOE (bismaleimidoethane; reactive groups ≤8 Å apart) in intact oocytes, assessed from large gel shifts of split CFTR channels with a target Cys in each half, has demonstrated that they must approach to within 8 Å of each other at some point during the gating cycle (2). In inside-out membrane patches excised from oocytes, formation of a disulfide bond across the NBD1–NBD2 interface, between Cys at position 1248 in the NBD2 Walker A motif and 549 in the NBD1 LSGGQ motif, prevented closure of the crosslinked CFTR channels after withdrawal of ATP; but the channels closed when the disulfide bonds were reduced by dithiothreitol (2), further supporting the association of dimerized NBDs with open channels. Similarly, bifunctional MTS reagents were found, in gel-shift assays, to crosslink NBD1 and NBD2 to cytoplasmic coupling helices that extend from the TMDs (50, 51) in a manner consistent with the "domain-swap" organization seen in the crystal structure of Sav1866, a prokaryotic multidrug transporter orthologue (7); when tested in inside-out patches, in contrast to the open-state stabilization caused by the NBD1–NBD2 crosslink (2), crosslinking either NBD to one of the coupling helices tended to impair channel opening (50, 51). These crosslinking experiments on CFTR have all used homology models to identify candidate target positions for Cys substitutions.

Modification of a single introduced target Cys, while assaying function as a monitor of reaction and its consequence, is an alternative way to probe CFTR channel structure and mechanism. Addition of *N*-ethylmaleimide (NEM) to the ATP-containing solution bathing inside-out patches irreversibly diminished the

P_O of CFTR channels with a single Cys introduced into Walker A or ABC signature motif of either composite interfacial site (52). Modification of the Walker A, but not the ABC signature, mutants became slower as ATP concentration was raised (52) and, at each [ATP], modification was much slower in the "NBD1" than in the "NBD2" composite site; these observations fit well with the present view of ATP-driven gating of CFTR channels (**Section 1.1**).

Further structural and mechanistic information may be obtained by determining the gating-state dependence of modification of single Cys or of crosslinking of Cys pairs (e.g., (53)).

3.2.2. Studying the Kinetics of CFTR Phosphorylation

Western blots of full-length (54) or split (2) CFTR, and Coomassie-stained gels or autoradiographs of isolated R domain peptide (29, 36), have all revealed mobility shifts induced by phosphorylation with PKA. By using low [ATP] to slow phosphorylation, taking samples at different times, and using SDS-PAGE followed by mass spectrometry of separated peptides, two-dimensional phosphopeptide mapping, and/or point mutation to identify individual phosphoserines, the kinetics of phosphorylation of individual Ser can be assessed. With this approach, Ser768 was found to be the first one phosphorylated and phosphorylation of Ser737 was found to cause the major mobility shift (36). Kinetic analysis of several small synthetic peptides (10–24 residues), each encompassing one (or two) of the R domain consensus PKA sites, showed that the peptide containing Ser768 was by far the preferred substrate for PKA (29), consistent with the results for isolated R domain and entire CFTR (36).

A difficulty in all biochemical studies of CFTR is availability of sufficient amounts of protein; expression and purification from Sf9 insect cells (55) and baby hamster kidney (BHK-21) fibroblast cells (56) have proven most successful so far. The large amplification of electrophysiological assays allows circumvention of this difficulty, as some biochemical studies can be done in real time on CFTR channels in voltage-clamped excised membrane patches or whole cells. For example, phosphorylation by PKA catalytic subunit or by PKC and dephosphorylation by specific phosphatases, of WT CFTR channels or mutants lacking one or more consensus phosphorylation sites, can be monitored by recording current in excised patches during direct application of exogenous kinases and/or phosphatases or inhibitors of endogenous phosphatases (e.g., (30, 31, 35, 36, 57–60)). The presence of active endogenous phosphatases in excised patches even permits determination of PKA concentration dependence of CFTR channel activation, assayed as P_O; enhanced sensitivity to PKA in Ser768Ala mutants compared to WT CFTR (36) confirmed the inhibitory influence of phosphoserine 768 concluded from measurements of sensitivity to the phosphodiesterase inhibitor IBMX in intact oocytes

(46). The enhanced sensitivity to phosphorylation resulted in substantial activation of Ser768Ala CFTR channels in resting oocytes, due to basal levels of PKA activity; phosphorylation of six Ser (including Ser768) in the R domains of WT CFTR channels in resting oocytes was confirmed by mass spectrometry (36).

3.3. Electrophysiological Recording of CFTR Currents

The possibility of following ion channel function using electrophysiological techniques makes CFTR uniquely suited for basic structure/function studies among ABC transporters. However, some of its gating characteristics – e.g., relatively slow and non-equilibrium gating – limit the usefulness of some techniques.

3.3.1. Recording CFTR Currents in Intact Cells by TEVC and Whole-Cell Patch Clamp

The two-microelectrode voltage-clamp (TEVC) method, and tight-seal current recording in the whole-cell configuration, allows little or no direct modification of the intracellular solution. However, as described above, the main factors regulating CFTR channel gating are phosphorylation and interaction with ATP, both acting on intracellular domains. In most intact cell studies CFTR is activated by extracellular application of membrane-penetrating forskolin, which activates adenylate cyclase, and hence PKA, eventually resulting in an increase in whole-cell conductance. For WT CFTR expressed in oocytes, held at –50 mV, the inward current peaks ~3 min after forskolin addition. For CFTR mutants with low P_{O}, conductance can increase more slowly, e.g., reaching a 10- to 100-fold lower maximal conductance in 10–20 min. The very indirect control of the channel gates somewhat limits the kinetic information that can be obtained with these techniques, yet they remain useful for screening (e.g., (2, 48)) or studying extreme alterations of gating kinetics (e.g., (61)). In addition, whole-cell current recordings can be valuable for studying endogenous CFTR in its physiological environment, with only minimal experimental modification (methods described in (62)).

3.3.2. Recording CFTR Currents in Inside-Out Patches

The experimenter has many more possibilities if, after sealing, the patch can be excised, so that the intracellular face of the patch is exposed. In *Xenopus* oocytes, this inside-out configuration is conveniently obtained by initially "cramming" the pipette toward the center of the cell, before extricating it with the excised membrane patch. Because of the characteristic slow gating of CFTR channels, relatively simple perfusion systems (e.g., available from ALA Scientific Instruments, www.alascience.com), which allow complete exchange of the solution bathing the intracellular (outside) face of the patch within a fraction of a second, are sufficient for most experiments. Most of the channels present in the patch will be activated within a few minutes after switching to a solution in which catalytic subunit of PKA (130 units/ml) and MgATP (concentrations 2–5 mM) is present. PKA extracted from bovine heart is commercially available (Sigma cat # P2645; note that recombinant PKA catalytic subunit, Promega cat # V5161, was found to be much less active even using up to 300 units/ml). Millimolar [ATP] are saturating for most mutants, the WT apparent dissociation constant being ~50 μM (e.g., (13)). Simple solutions with high Cl^-, *N*-methyl-D-glucamine as a counterion (to minimize cationic conductances), lightly buffered, and containing EGTA and millimolar Mg^{2+} are used as bath solutions, while pipettes (bathing the extracellular face) are filled with a similar solution but lacking EGTA (e.g., (27), *see* **Section 2.2**).

In some expression systems the level of channel expression can be modulated. This can be easily obtained when using *Xenopus* oocytes, by altering amounts of cRNA injected (typically from 0.1 to 10 ng/oocyte for WT CFTR), the time allowed for expression (~12 h to 1 week), and the position of the patch with respect to the injection site (when injecting within the animal pole, patches close to the injection site show higher expression). To a lesser extent, when using mammalian cell lines, variation in expression levels – among different cell lines and/or among clones obtained from different transfections – can be achieved (e.g., (63)). The experimenter can thus obtain two different, complementary, sets of kinetic information: either monitoring individual channels during steady-state gating (**Section 3.3.2.1**) or recording ensemble currents flowing through a high number of channels (**Section 3.3.2.2**).

3.3.2.1. Recording Individual CFTR Channel Currents in Inside-Out Patches

If the patch contains one or few (e.g., ≤8) channels the current "jumps" corresponding to the opening and closing of individual channel gates can be detected. Since the single-channel conductance of CFTR is small (~10 pS (64)), the main practical problem in performing these experiments is keeping electrical noise as low as possible to improve the signal-to-noise ratio. Practical considerations on this subject are discussed at length in excellent texts (65, 66). Most important, the electrical seal resistance between glass pipette tip and cell membrane needs to be very large (with *Xenopus* oocytes, seals >100 GΩ can be routinely obtained, using freshly stripped oocytes and 0.2 μm filtered solutions) and line-frequency interference needs to be minimized (by carefully grounding conducting objects close to the amplifier headstage, avoiding ground loops, and shielding in a Faraday cage). In addition, several parameters of the experimental setup can be optimized to obtain low-noise records (67). In our labs, the patches are excised in a large fluid-filled "patch-pulling chamber," and then transferred to a "flow chamber" for recording (**Fig. 28.1**). Here, to minimize the capacitance of the immersed pipette tip, the patch is immersed in a thin film of solution flowing down the walls of the flow chamber, along the Petri dish edge, and grounded (**Fig. 28.1**). Luckily, CFTR's slow gating character-

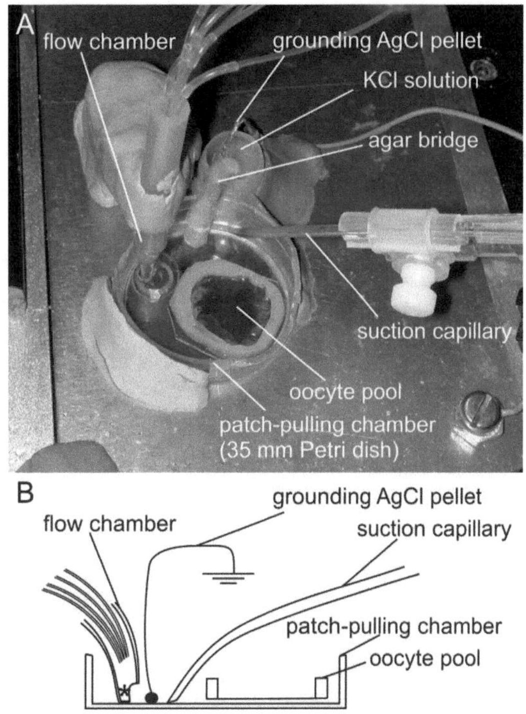

Fig. 28.1. **Photograph (a) and diagram (b) of a chamber for patch recording from oocytes.** The patch-pulling chamber (35 mm Petri dish) and oocyte pool are initially filled with bath solution. An oocyte stripped of its vitelline membrane is placed in the oocyte pool, which can be rotated to position it appropriately for pipette approach. After the patch is excised it is transferred to the flow chamber (to the position indicated by the *asterisk*) by moving the microscope stage, the perfusion flow is turned on, and most of the bath solution is removed using the suction capillary. The oocyte in the oocyte pool remains submerged by solution and can be used to provide further patches. The agar bridge (filled with 100 mM KCl + 4% agarose, providing an electrical connection to a small reservoir filled with KCl) is needed only when the bath solution does not contain Cl^- and is omitted from the diagram.

istics are here an advantage, since the recording bandwidth need not be wide and filtering at 50–200 Hz does not remove events of interest for ATP- and phosphorylation-dependent gating.

3.3.2.2. Recording Macroscopic, Multi-channel, CFTR Currents in Inside-Out Patches

When studying low probability events or mutants whose gating is very slow, accumulation of sufficient events cannot be achieved within the patch lifetime by recording from one or a few channels. In these cases, information on channel gating regulation is most simply obtained by recording ensemble current flow across patches containing a large number (typically hundreds or thousands) of CFTR channels ("macropatches"). Recording from macropatches allows relative steady-state parameters, e.g., relative P_o upon sudden change in [ATP] (13) or relative P_o in ATP vs. poorly hydrolyzable analogues (12), to be easily obtained. Alternatively, kinetic information can be extracted from measurements of the time course of current change following a maneuver that affects CFTR gating, e.g., burst duration upon washout of ATP (*see* **Section 3.5**).

3.4. Analysis of Steady-State CFTR Current Recordings

3.4.1. Idealization of Membrane Currents

The first step in the process of extracting information on channel gating kinetics from a raw current trace is to reconstruct the time series of channel opening/closing transitions. The output of this "idealization" procedure is an ordered list of events, each event described by a pair of numbers l_k, t_k; l_k denotes the number of channels open during the *k*th event and t_k its duration. This "events list" contains in a compact form all the information the raw data carry about gating.

The simplest idealization algorithm is the half-amplitude threshold crossing technique (68). In this procedure the baseline current and possible slow current drifts – not channel-related – are subtracted from the raw data. Ideal conductance levels are then set to integer multiples of the unitary current amplitude, and consecutive data points which fall within a half-amplitude distance of a given ideal conductance level are merged into an event. For reliable application of this simple procedure the signal-to-noise ratio must be sufficiently high to minimize half-amplitude threshold crossings caused by noise, while individual gating transitions should remain well resolved in time. In addition, the channels should open predominantly to a single, well-defined, conductance level. These criteria are typically met for WT CFTR under standard conditions (e.g., (11, 13, 18, 69)).

The half-amplitude procedure might present problems when using MOPS as an intracellular buffer (15), for certain pore mutants (70), or for murine CFTR channels, which open predominantly to subconductance levels (71). In such cases more elaborate algorithms are necessary for idealization. Time-course fitting (68) and hidden Markov modeling (72, 73) are procedures that allow for successful idealization of records with frequent subconductance openings and/or an insufficient signal-to-noise ratio; such algorithms are implemented by the free software packages HJCFIT (http://www.ucl.ac.uk/Pharmacology/dcpr95.html) and QuB (http://www.qub.buffalo.edu/), respectively.

3.4.2. Kinetic Analysis of Single-Channel Current Traces

Channel open probability (P_O), the fraction of time the pore is open, is simply obtained as the sum of all open-time durations in the events list divided by the total recording time. Although P_O can be viewed as the physiologically relevant readout of gating in terms of chloride transport, it provides essentially no information on mechanism. For instance, mutations might simultaneously alter the rates of both gating transitions by up to 1000-fold with no large effect on P_o (e.g., E1371Q; (1)), emphasizing the importance of kinetic analysis for mechanistic understanding.

WT CFTR channel gating is characterized by bursts of openings – groups of openings, interrupted by brief closures – that are flanked by long, interburst closures. Correspondingly, dwell-time analysis of single WT channels reveals a single open state and two distinct closed states (69). The three-state schemes $C_1—O—C_2$ and $C_1—C_2—O$ can equally well account for such a pattern of gating; assuming either scheme, the respective four rate constants can be estimated by maximum likelihood fitting. Two commonly used approaches for maximum likelihood fitting of single-channel event lists are fitting the open- and closed-time distributions (e.g., (74)) or fitting the entire series of closed- and open-time durations (75–77), implemented, e.g., by the MIL subprogram of the QuB package and by HJCFIT. In theory, the latter approach is more powerful because it exploits the information carried by correlations between the durations of adjacent closed and open events. However, for schemes with a single open state (or, in general, when a single "gateway" state connects the sets of open and closed states), like the two schemes above, open and closed events are uncorrelated and the two approaches therefore equivalent.

It is important to note that the schemes $C_1—O—C_2$ and $C_1—C_2—O$ cannot be distinguished in steady-state records. And, because of the short lifetime of state C_2 (~10 ms at 25°C) relative to C_1 (~1 s at 25°C), a distinction based on the time course of current change upon sudden addition/removal of the ligand ATP is technically not feasible. Thus, at present there is no strong evidence to support a choice between them. Correspondingly, both schemes have been used to interpret ATP dependence of CFTR gating, and fitting either scheme suggests [ATP] dependence of a single rate: rate $C_1 \rightarrow O$ (12) and rate $C_1 \rightarrow C_2$, respectively (69). Because these rates are meaningful only in the context of a particular scheme, it is customary to report only the mean durations of open burst and interburst closures, which are model-independent descriptive parameters, that can be calculated from the fitted rate constants regardless of the chosen scheme. Using this descriptive nomenclature it is generally agreed that increasing ATP concentrations shorten the mean interburst duration in a saturable fashion, while the mean burst duration, the mean intraburst closed time, and the mean number of intraburst closures per burst are little influenced by ATP concentration (12, 13, 69, 78).

An alternative approach for studying the kinetics of open burst and interburst closures is provided by conventional burst analysis. This method consists of ignoring brief intraburst closures by creating a new events list of bursts and interbursts in which closures shorter than a specified cutoff are suppressed. This cutoff is chosen based on the distribution of closed-time durations in the original events list and is ideally much larger than the mean duration of intraburst closures, but much smaller than that of interburst closures. Nevertheless, because the durations of both types of closures are exponentially distributed and therefore overlap, some fraction of closures will be necessarily misassigned regardless of the choice of the cutoff. This means that some fraction of intraburst closures will be erroneously kept and treated as interburst, and some fraction of interburst closures will be erroneously misclassified as intraburst and so eliminated. Two commonly used strategies for calculating the cutoff duration are to equalize the probabilities of the two types of error (79) or to minimize the total probability of committing any error (80). The merit of the first strategy is that the mean duration of reconstructed bursts provides an undistorted estimate of the true *mean* burst duration, whereas the second strategy was found to cause less distortion of the *shape* of the distribution of burst durations for a non-equilibrium cyclic gating mechanism like that of CFTR (27).

Because ATP concentration affects bursting, but not intraburst, kinetics, restricting kinetic analysis to a mere extraction of *mean* burst and interburst durations is equivalent to modeling ATP-dependent gating by a simple two-state process. Though more informative than just extracting P_O, such a simplification severely limits the amount of information that can be obtained about a complex process involving binding of ATP at two distinct sites, dynamic formation and disruption of an NBD1/NBD2 heterodimer, and hydrolysis of ATP in one of the composite binding sites. However, by reconstructing each burst, burst analysis offers the advantage of providing also the *distributions* of burst and interburst durations, not just their *mean values*. These distributions carry invaluable information on the mechanism of bursts and allow quantitative evaluation of alternative gating schemes by fitting them to the observed distributions using maximum likelihood. Although as a first approximation both interburst and burst durations are reasonably fit by single-exponential distributions (12, 13, 18), careful fitting of large sets of both interburst (11) and burst (27) durations has identified tell-tale deviations from single-exponential behavior that are indisputable signs of a highly non-equilibrium mechanism. Thus, the clear rising phases of these distributions (*see* histogram of burst durations in **Fig. 28.2b**) signal violation of microscopic reversibility (68). In addition, fitting these distributions by a cyclic mechanism (**Fig. 28.2a**; cf. **Section 1.1**) allows estimation of the rates of conformational transitions that are not associated with pore opening or closure (27).

3.4.3. Kinetic Analysis of Multi-channel Current Traces

Because CFTR gating is a slow process and gradual dephosphorylation by membrane-bound phosphatases limits the length of steady-state single-channel recordings, obtaining sufficient

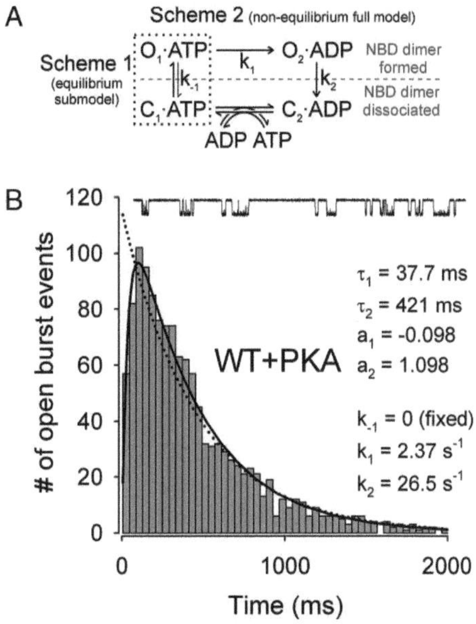

Fig. 28.2. **Distribution of open burst durations reports on mechanism of bursts.** (**a**) Cyclic scheme (*Scheme 2*) illustrating the proposed mechanism of CFTR gating in saturating ATP (*see* **Section 1.1**). The nucleotide specified for each state represents that bound at the "NBD2 site"; the "NBD1 site" is assumed to retain ATP bound in all four depicted states. *Scheme 1*, the subset of *Scheme 2* framed by the dotted line, is a simple equilibrium closed–open model. Note that extraction of just mean burst and interburst durations – using either the C_1—0—C_2 or C_1—C_2—0 scheme – is equivalent to simplifying the mechanism of bursts to *Scheme 1*. (**b**) Histogram of open burst durations, and 30 s segment of single-channel current recording, of WT CFTR gating in the presence of 2 mM ATP + 300 nM PKA. The *dotted* and *solid lines* are fits to Schemes 1 and 2, respectively; the fit parameters for *Scheme 2*, with predicted time constants and fractional amplitudes, are printed in the panel. The fit to *Scheme 2* is ranked significantly ($P = 4 \times 10^{-9}$) better by the log-likelihood ratio test (modified from (27)).

numbers of gating events from a patch containing only a single channel can become challenging. In contrast, from patches with multiple (e.g., two to eight) active channels comparable numbers of gating events are obtained in proportionately shorter duration recordings. An ensemble of several (N) channels gating via a common mechanism but independently of each other can be described by a single macro-system with N+1 conductance levels; transition rates between states of the macro-scheme are functions of the single-channel transition rates. Consequently, both maximum likelihood analysis approaches mentioned in **Section 3.4.2**, i.e., fitting of dwell-time distributions and fitting the entire time series, can be generalized to a multi-channel system. However, because the macro-system has many states, the computational burden for the latter approach becomes prohibitively large; even with improved present-day (2010) PC performances, fitting the entire time series for a record with more than three channels is still impractical. In contrast, maximum likelihood fitting of single-channel open- and closed-time distributions can be readily generalized to a simultaneous fitting of the ensemble of the dwell-time distributions of all conductance levels of a multi-channel patch. The computational burden of this approach is far smaller, because once the sequence in which the events follow each other is disregarded, the individual dwell-time distributions can be binned into histograms, resulting in a large reduction in the size of the data set to be fitted. Moreover, there is no disadvantage to losing correlation information between neighboring events for the simple C_1—O—C_2 and C_1—C_2—O schemes (as noted in **Section 3.4.2**). Finally, a first-order correction for missed events due to limited recording bandwidth is also readily incorporated into this approach (81). A program implementing these procedures has been used successfully by several groups and is freely available upon request (laszlo.csanady@eok.sote.hu).

3.5. Analysis of Macroscopic Current Relaxations

Information on gating kinetics of single ion channels can also be obtained from the time courses of macroscopic current relaxations in response to step changes in ligand concentration or voltage. These time courses can be fitted with sums of exponentials, whose time constants and fractional amplitudes are functions of the single-channel gating parameters. Non-linear least-squares fitting algorithms are included in most commercially available data acquisition software packages (e.g., PCLAMP and PulseFit).

Because, for CFTR, closing from a burst is little sensitive to ATP concentration and the rate of opening to a burst in the absence of ATP is vanishingly small, the time constant of macroscopic current relaxation upon sudden removal of ATP reflects the steady-state mean burst duration (13, 27, 82). This technique for estimating mean burst duration has been preferentially used for catalytic site mutants which abolish ATP hydrolysis at the composite NBD2 site (e.g., K1250A), or when non-hydrolyzable ATP analogs (e.g., AMP-PNP and pyrophosphate) are applied, because in either case burst durations are prolonged to several seconds or tens of seconds. While this makes it difficult to collect sufficient numbers of steady-state single-channel gating events, macroscopic ATP-removal experiments are easy to perform and require only moderately rapid solution exchange (e.g., (12, 13, 83, 84)).

One limitation of this approach is that for patches excised from certain cell types removal of PKA catalytic subunit results in a relatively abrupt shortening of mean burst durations, likely due to rapid partial dephosphorylation of CFTR channels by membrane-bound phosphatases (13, 17). In such systems the above approach can be used to study the mean burst duration of partially, but not of fully, phosphorylated channels. This is because sudden removal of ATP terminates not only channel opening but also activity of the co-applied PKA catalytic subunit, and so full phosphorylation of the channels throughout the time course of current relaxation cannot be guaranteed.

3.6. Thermodynamic Approaches to Studying the Energetics of Gating

3.6.1. Studying Temperature Dependence

Observing a chemical reaction at several different temperatures provides insight into the energetics of the process. For an equilibrium reaction A↔B the standard enthalpy change ΔH^{o} between states B and A can be calculated from the van't Hoff plot, which displays the natural logarithm of the equilibrium constant (ln K_{eq}) as a function of the inverse of absolute temperature ($1/T$). The slope of this linear plot is $-\Delta H^{o}/(R)$, where R is the gas constant (8.31 J/mol/K). If not only the equilibrium constant but also the rates of transition between states A and B can be measured, then temperature dependence of these rates can be used to calculate the activation enthalpies ($\Delta H^{\ddagger}$), i.e., the standard enthalpy differences between the transition state and the stable ground states A and B. With k_{AB} denoting transition rate A→B, plots of ln k_{AB} (Arrhenius plot) or ln (k_{AB}/T) (Eyring plot) as a function of $1/T$ yield linear graphs with slopes $-E_a/(R)$ or $-\Delta H^{\ddagger}/(R)$, respectively. Here, E_a denotes the activation energy and $\Delta H^{\ddagger}$ the enthalpy difference between the transition state and the ground state A; the two are related by the equation $E_a = \Delta H^{\ddagger} + RT$. The corresponding parameters for the reverse step B→A can be obtained analogously from Arrhenius or Eyring plots of the reverse rate k_{BA} (85).

Ion channels are especially well suited to such thermodynamic studies, because the average rates of opening (k_o) and closure (k_c) can be readily measured in single-channel recordings. If channel gating is an equilibrium process, then the open–closed equilibrium constant is given by $K_{eq}=P_o/(1-P_o)$; because $P_o=k_o/(k_o+k_c)$, an equivalent formulation is $K_{eq}= k_o/k_c$. Thus, measuring P_o of such a single channel at various temperatures allows construction of a van't Hoff plot (i.e., ln[$P_o/(1-P_o)$] versus $1/T$) for estimation of the standard enthalpy change between the open and the closed ground states. Similarly, measuring k_o and k_c at various temperatures allows estimation of the activation enthalpies for opening and closure by construction of Arrhenius or Eyring plots.

However, in the case of WT CFTR there is strong evidence that the gating involves irreversible steps and therefore follows a non-equilibrium cycle (11, 15, 27, 86), such that channels close from a burst predominantly through a pathway different from that by which they open (*see* **Section 1.2**). This circumstance has important implications for the interpretation of temperature dependence of WT CFTR bursting kinetics. First, if the process is not at equilibrium, then the apparent equilibrium constant $K_{app} = P_o/(1-P_o)$ is not a true equilibrium constant. Thus, construction of a van't Hoff plot is meaningless, as the slope of a plot of ln K_{app} versus $1/T$ does not report $\Delta H^{o}_{open-closed}$. (Note that if ΔH^{o} for the process closed→open→closed is non-zero, then the quantity $\Delta H^{o}_{open-closed}$ cannot even be defined in general; statements must be limited to comparing an open state to either the *preceding* or the *subsequent* closed state (84).) It is also important to note that a linear van't Hoff plot does not *imply* an equilibrium mechanism, as has been argued (87). Because the apparent equilibrium constant $K_{app}= P_{o}/(1-P_{o})$ is always equal to k_{o}/k_{c}, the relationship $\ln K_{app}=\ln k_{o}-\ln k_{c}$ also holds regardless of the mechanism. Therefore, if the Arrhenius (or Eyring) plots for opening and closure are linear – as observed for CFTR (84, 87, 88) – then the plot of ln K_{app} versus $1/T$ will also be linear, regardless of the mechanism. Similarly, caution must be applied to the interpretation of energetic barriers. If WT CFTR indeed exits the open burst state through a pathway which involves ATP hydrolysis, then $\Delta H^{\ddagger}$ for opening and closure characterize single sides of two distinct energy barriers, rather than the two sides of a single barrier. In this case the barrier height for the reversal of the opening step must be obtained from the temperature dependence of closing rate under conditions that prevent ATP hydrolysis (e.g., using NBD2 composite catalytic site mutations or non-hydrolyzable ATP analogs). Together the three $\Delta H^{\ddagger}$ values for opening, non-hydrolytic closure, and normal hydrolytic closure then allow reconstruction of the ΔH^{o} profile for a partial gating cycle which involves transition from an ATP-bound closed state through a transition state to the open state, and then from the open state to a second, distinct, transition state for closure (84).

By transition-state theory (e.g., (85, 89)) the absolute value of a transition rate k, measured at a given temperature, provides at least an upper estimate of the activation free energy ($\Delta G^{\ddagger}$) in the form $\Delta G^{\ddagger} \leq RT\ln(k_{B}T/(kh))$, where k_{B} is Boltzmann's constant (1.38×10^{-23} J/K) and h is Planck's constant (6.63×10^{-34} J s). This upper estimate of $\Delta G^{\ddagger}$ ($\Delta G^{\ddagger}_{max}$) together with the estimate of $\Delta H^{\ddagger}$ yields a lower estimate of the activation entropy $\Delta S^{\ddagger}$: $\Delta S^{\ddagger}_{min}=(\Delta H^{\ddagger}-\Delta G^{\ddagger}_{max})/T$ (cf. (84)) which provides additional information about the mechanisms underlying CFTR channel gating.

3.6.2. Mutant Cycle Analysis

The thermodynamic mutant cycle formalism (89) can be used to detect energetic coupling between two amino acid positions in a protein. In a generalized double mutant cycle, the WT, two single-site mutants, and the double mutant form the vertices of a thermodynamic cycle. From patch recordings of CFTR channel currents, several kinetic parameters can be measured that can be used to characterize WT and single and double mutants in terms of the ΔG between two states. If the two residues do not interact, the effects of mutating one site will not depend on whether that mutation was done in a WT or mutant (at the other site) background, i.e., mutation-linked changes in ΔG on parallel sides of the cycle are equal ($\Delta\Delta G_{int} = 0$). Any difference ($\Delta\Delta G_{int} \neq 0$) signifies, and (to some extent) quantifies, energetic coupling between the two residues. Effective dissociation constants for ATP activation of channel gating, opening rates, and equilibrium constant between closed and open states in a nonhydrolytic background[1] can all be used to estimate a mutation-induced change in free energy, in each case probing a different step of the gating cycle. Several energetic coupling values can therefore be determined for each pair of target sites, allowing inferences to be made about how coupling between two positions changes as the NBDs bind ATP, and the channel opens, and transits between open and closed states, i.e., as the channel progresses through its gating cycle (1).

Unfortunately, interpretation of data obtained using the mutant cycle formalism is rarely straightforward. A first complicating factor relates to the large statistical variability observed in CFTR gating measurements. Because coupling energies are obtained as sums (of mutation-linked changes in ΔG on parallel sides of the cycle), the errors on the individual sets of measurements are summed too, resulting in coupling energies, $\Delta\Delta G_{int}$, which are not significantly different from zero unless the mutation effects are large. A second problem arises from the oversimplifying assumptions required to reduce kinetic data to free energy differences between two states. Thus, it is likely that the "equilibrium constants" estimated from measurements reflect the steady-state distribution of channels among more than two underlying states; and states with low occupancy in WT might become important in certain mutants with severe phenotypes. A third problem can arise from the quantitative interpretation of $\Delta\Delta G_{int}$ as interaction energy in the WT when the target site residues still form significant interactions in the single and double mutants (89). Such interactions can usually be avoided by using alanine substitutions (90). However, mutant cycles in which the substitutions form a novel interaction in the double mutant only result in a stronger deviation from simple additivity, and this might help reveal energetic coupling when the single mutation effects are small.

3.6.3. REFER Analysis

Rate-equilibrium free energy relationship (REFER) analysis provides information on transition-state structures and has been used to study the temporal sequence in which various regions of an

[1] After reducing the cyclic gating scheme to a closed-to-open equilibrium by impairing hydrolysis, this equilibrium constant can be obtained from P_o, as $K_{eq} = P_o/(1-P_o)$

ion channel protein move during a closed–open conformational transition. REFER theory uses transition-state formalism and was developed for equilibrium reactions. The method assumes that structural perturbations introduced into a given region of an ion channel protein affect the free energy of the transition state for opening in proportion to their effects on the free energy of the open ground state (both free energies measured relative to the closed ground state), i.e., $\delta\Delta G^{o}_{\text{transition–closed}}=\Phi\cdot\delta\Delta G^{o}_{\text{open–closed}}$ $(0 \leq \Phi \leq 1)$. Because the logarithm of the opening rate (k_o) and of the closed–open equilibrium constant (K_{eq}) are identically sensitive to $\Delta G^{o}_{\text{transition–closed}}$ and $\Delta G^{o}_{\text{open–closed}}$, respectively, the slope of a plot of ln k_o as a function of ln K_{eq} for a series of structural perturbations to a particular region of a protein (Brønsted or REFER plot) provides the proportionality coefficient Φ. (Because $\delta\Delta G^{o}_{\text{transition–closed}}=\Phi\cdot\delta\Delta G^{o}_{\text{open–closed}}$ implies $\delta\Delta G^{o}_{\text{transition–open}}=(\Phi-1)\cdot\delta\Delta G^{o}_{\text{open–closed}}$, the slope of the Brønsted plot for channel closure is $\Phi-1$.) Large Φ values (close to 1) indicate that in the transition state the perturbed region is already near its open-state conformation, while a Φ value close to 0 is an indication that the region is still closed-like in the transition state. Therefore, high Φ values are generally interpreted to signal early, and low Φ values late, movement of the target region during the closed-to-open transition (91).

The success of REFER analysis for ligand-gated ion channels (e.g., (92, 93)) has encouraged its application to CFTR gating (94, 95). Unfortunately, however, interpretation of REFER plots depends strictly on the assumption of an underlying equilibrium process. For this reason, although the observed linearity of the REFER plots and the complementarity of the slopes of such plots for opening and closure of CFTR channels have been argued to support an equilibrium mechanism (95), such inferences have no theoretical foundation. Indeed, it has been shown that both equilibrium and non-equilibrium mechanisms can result in either linear or non-linear REFER plots and that the complementary REFER slopes for opening and closure are a trivial feature of all ion channels regardless of their gating mechanism; moreover, for non-equilibrium mechanisms REFER analysis provides no information on the transition-state structures (96). These limitations should be considered before applying REFER analysis to CFTR.

3.7. Bioinformatic Approaches to Identify Coevolving Amino Acid Positions

3.7.1. Coevolution Reports on Functional Residue–Residue Interactions

Information about gating of CFTR channels can also be gleaned from the evolutionary record in the form of correlated amino acid substitutions. The conformational changes associated with gating are controlled by residue interactions, and interacting residues exert evolutionary pressure on each other, such that substitutions at one position are coupled to substitutions at another. In terms of multiple sequence alignments, this means that the variation of residues found in one column will correlate with the variation in some other column(s). This is illustrated schematically in **Fig. 28.3** for evolution of positions *x* and *y* in a hypothetical protein family. In **Fig. 28.3a**, because of strong interaction between positions *x* and *y*, their substitutions are correlated, leading to their coevolution, whereas in **Fig. 28.3b** the positions

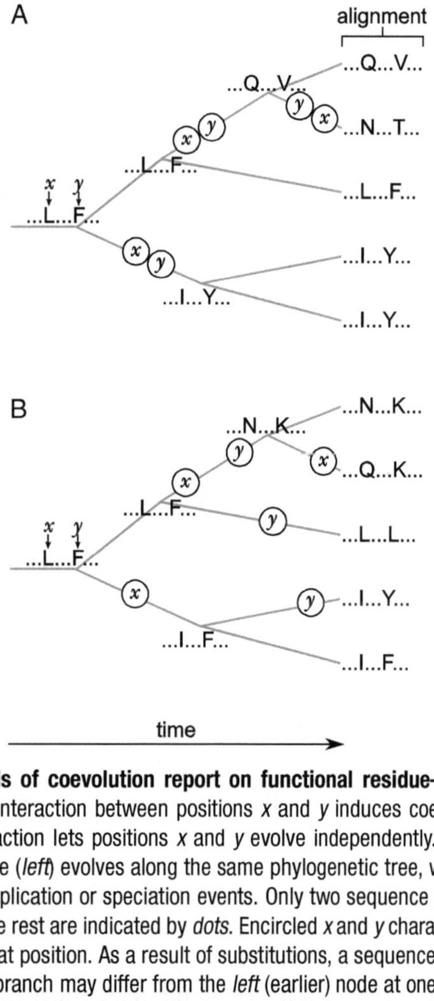

Fig. 28.3. **Signals of coevolution report on functional residue–residue interactions.** (**a**) Strong interaction between positions *x* and *y* induces coevolution. (**b**) Negligibly weak interaction lets positions *x* and *y* evolve independently. In both cases an ancestral sequence (*left*) evolves along the same phylogenetic tree, whose bifurcations represent gene duplication or speciation events. Only two sequence positions, *x* and *y*, are considered; the rest are indicated by *dots*. Encircled *x* and *y* characters mark substitution events at that position. As a result of substitutions, a sequence at the *right* (more recent) node of a branch may differ from the *left* (earlier) node at one or both positions. The process results in the set of contemporary sequences on the *right*, organized into a multiple alignment. Though substitutions occur stochastically in both cases, only in case (**a**) do they correlate temporally between the two positions. Since the protracted timescale of evolution precludes direct observation of substitution events, the challenge is to distinguish between the two cases (**a**) and (**b**) indirectly, using the alignment as the only available input data.

do not interact strongly, and so they evolve independently, and hence substitutions at those positions are uncorrelated ((97, 98) cf. (99)).

Because CFTR belongs to the ABC protein superfamily, the large quantity of sequence data available make such coevolution analysis attractive. Depending on which ABC subfamily sequences are included in the alignment, the analysis may illuminate general mechanisms shared by the whole ABC superfamily (e.g., interactions across the NBD dimer interface (1)) or may relate specifically to a particular subfamily. An alignment restricted to OAD family sequences, for instance, may be expected to yield information about mechanism applicable not only to CFTR but also to paralogs such as the SUR and MRP proteins.

3.7.2. Statistical Approaches for Coevolution Prediction

In practice, given the protracted timescale of evolution, inferences about past substitution events made from alignments of contemporary sequences are used to generate a statistic that relates to the probability that two positions coevolved. A number of methods have been developed for these analyses, and they use one of two basic approaches (for recent reviews, *see* (97, 100)). In one, the coevolution statistic is derived from correlated patterns in the alignment; methods using this approach include McBASC (101), SCA (102), ELSC (103), OMES (104), CAPS (105), and MIp (106). In the other, an assumed evolutionary mechanism is used to reconstruct the history of amino acid mutations, from which correlations in the substitution process can be extracted; this approach is used by CoMap (107, 108), BMM (109), CorrMut (110), and methods based on explicit coevolution models (111, 112). This latter approach adheres closely to the above (**Section 3.7.1**) definition of coevolution as temporally correlated substitutions, but is subject to the uncertainty inherent in inferring past substitution and branching events from present sequences.

3.7.3. Input Data and Practical Aspects

A multiple sequence alignment comprises the input data for coevolution prediction. As misalignments increase with sequence divergence, filtering out distant sequences improves alignment quality but at the expense of discarding useful information. Calculation of BLAST E-values (113) or HMMER log-odds likelihood scores (114), combined with estimates of local (115) or global (116) alignment quality, can help guide this tradeoff between sequence number and divergence. Once sequences are aligned, gaps need to be removed by deleting entire columns and/or sequences. Ideally, the resulting multiple sequence alignment will retain hundreds of homologs each containing hundreds of positions.

3.7.4. Validation of Methods with Structural Contact Prediction

Benchmarking, to validate the predictive performance of a method on a test set of data under particular conditions, would ideally require a protein family for which all coevolving, and independently evolving, position pairs are known. As no such family exists, a data set can be simulated, which offers precise control over phylogenetic tree parameters and rates of evolution, and allows clear distinction between coevolving and independently evolving pairs. Applicability of the assumptions about mechanisms of (co)evolution used in the model, however, remains uncertain. An alternative approach is to use a known physical quantity, such as spatial proximity, to characterize position pairs. The ability of a method to predict coevolution that arose from structural contact can then be assessed for protein conformations for which a high-resolution 3D structure exists. In the absence of an X-ray crystal structure for CFTR, homology models (e.g., (51, 117, 118)) based on the structure of Sav1866 (7, 8) provide a reasonable alternative (118).

Coevolution analysis has been shown to predict structural contact between amino acids in proteins significantly (108, 119, 120) better than random choice. Limits to the performance of coevolution analysis assessed by contact prediction include incomplete overlap between functional and structural interactions, in part due to functional interactions between spatially distant positions (connected by chains of direct, structural, interactions) that nevertheless induce coevolution (121). In general, correction for phylogenetic relatedness of sequences (122), instead of assuming sequence independence, improves performance (106, 109, 123–125). In addition, coevolution analysis methods show different sensitivities to the heterogeneity of substitution rates across positions, i.e., conserved, slowly evolving positions versus rapidly evolving, variable positions (126, 127), and the accuracy of coevolution prediction may be improved by taking this into account.

In the case of CFTR, comparison of the results obtained from different methods of coevolution analysis, followed by structural contact tests, can exploit the strengths and overcome the weaknesses of individual methods, and so yield useful functional information.

References

1. Vergani, P., Lockless, S. W., Nairn, A. C., and Gadsby, D. C. (2005) CFTR channel opening by ATP-driven tight dimerization of its nucleotide-binding domains. *Nature* **433**, 876–880.
2. Mense, M., Vergani, P., White, D. M., Altberg, G., Nairn, A. C., and Gadsby, D. C. (2006) In vivo phosphorylation of CFTR promotes formation of a nucleotide-binding domain heterodimer. *EMBO J.* **25**, 4728–4740.
3. Hopfner, K. P., Karcher, A., Shin, D. S., Craig, L., Arthur, L. M., Carney, J. P., et al. (2000) Structural biology of Rad50 ATPase: ATP-driven conformational control in DNA double-strand break repair and the ABC-ATPase superfamily. *Cell* **101**, 789–800.
4. Locher, K. P., Lee, A. T., and Rees, D. C. (2002) The E. coli BtuCD structure: a framework for ABC transporter architecture and mechanism. *Science* **296**, 1038–1040.

5. Smith, P. C., Karpowich, N., Millen, L., Moody, J. E., Rosen, J., Thomas, P. J., et al. (2002) ATP binding to the motor domain from an ABC transporter drives formation of a nucleotide sandwich dimer. *Mol. Cell* **10**, 139–149.
6. Chen, T. Y., Chen, M. F., and Lin, C. W. (2003) Electrostatic control and chloride regulation of the fast gating of ClC-0 chloride. *J. Gen. Physiol.* **122**, 641–651.
7. Dawson, R. J., and Locher, K. P. (2006) Structure of a bacterial multidrug ABC transporter. *Nature* **443**, 180–185.
8. Dawson, R. J., and Locher, K. P. (2007) Structure of the multidrug ABC transporter Sav1866 from Staphylococcus aureus in complex with AMP-PNP. *FEBS Lett.* **581**, 935–938.
9. Oldham, M. L., Khare, D., Quiocho, F. A., Davidson, A. L., and Chen, J. (2007) Crystal structure of a catalytic intermediate of the maltose transporter. *Nature* **450**, 515–521.
10. Dassa, E. B. P. (2001) The ABC of ABCS: a phylogenetic and functional classification of ABC systems in living organisms. *Res. Microbiol.* **152**, 211–229.
11. Zeltwanger, S., Wang, F., Wang, G. T., Gillis, K. D., and Hwang, T. C. (1999) Gating of cystic fibrosis transmembrane conductance regulator chloride channels by adenosine triphosphate hydrolysis. Quantitative analysis of a cyclic gating scheme. *J. Gen. Physiol.* **113**, 541–554.
12. Vergani, P., Nairn, A. C., and Gadsby, D. C. (2003) On the mechanism of MgATP-dependent gating of CFTR Cl- channels. *J. Gen. Physiol.* **121**, 17–36.
13. Csanády, L., Chan, K. W., Seto-Young, D., Kopsco, D. C., Nairn, A. C., and Gadsby, D. C. (2000) Severed channels probe regulation of gating of cystic fibrosis transmembrane conductance regulator by its cytoplasmic domains. *J. Gen. Physiol.* **116**, 477–500.
14. Baukrowitz, T., Hwang, T. C., Nairn, A. C., and Gadsby, D. C. (1994) Coupling of CFTR Cl- channel gating to an ATP hydrolysis cycle. *Neuron* **12**, 473–482.
15. Gunderson, K. L., and Kopito, R. R. (1995) Conformational states of CFTR associated with channel gating: the role ATP binding and hydrolysis. *Cell* **82**, 231–239.
16. Carson, M. R., Winter, M. C., Travis, S. M., and Welsh, M. J. (1995b) Pyrophosphate stimulates wild-type and mutant cystic fibrosis transmembrane conductance regulator Cl- channels. *J. Biol. Chem.* **270**, 20466–20472.
17. Hwang, T. C., Nagel, G., Nairn, A. C., and Gadsby, D. C. (1994) Regulation of the gating of cystic fibrosis transmembrane conductance regulator Cl channels by phosphorylation and ATP hydrolysis. *Proc. Natl. Acad. Sci. USA* **91**, 4698–4702.
18. Carson, M. R., Travis, S. M., and Welsh, M. J. (1995a) The two nucleotide-binding domains of cystic fibrosis transmembrane conductance regulator (CFTR) have distinct functions in controlling channel activity. *J. Biol. Chem.* **270**, 1711–1717.
19. Aleksandrov, L., Aleksandrov, A. A., Chang, X. B., and Riordan, J. R. (2002) The first nucleotide binding domain of cystic fibrosis transmembrane conductance regulator is a site of stable nucleotide interaction, whereas the second is a site of rapid turnover. *J. Biol. Chem.* **277**, 15419–15425.
20. Basso, C., Vergani, P., Nairn, A. C., and Gadsby, D. C. (2003) Prolonged nonhydrolytic interaction of nucleotide with CFTR's NH2-terminal nucleotide binding domain and its role in channel gating. *J. Gen. Physiol.* **122**, 333–348.
21. Tsai, M. F., Shimizu, H., Sohma, Y., Li, M., and Hwang, T. C. (2009) State-dependent modulation of CFTR gating by pyrophosphate. *J. Gen. Physiol.* **133**, 405–419.
22. Ward, A., Reyes, C. L., Yu, J., Roth, C. B., and Chang, G. (2007) Flexibility in the ABC transporter MsbA: alternating access with a twist. *Proc. Natl. Acad. Sci. USA* **104**, 19005–19010.
23. Gadsby, D. C. (2009) Ion channels versus ion pumps: the principal difference, in principle. *Nat. Rev. Mol. Cell. Biol.* **10**, 344–352.
24. Jordan, I. K., Kota, K. C., Cui, G., Thompson, C. H., and McCarty, N. A. (2008) Evolutionary and functional divergence between the cystic fibrosis transmembrane conductance regulator and related ATP-binding cassette transporter. *Proc. Natl. Acad. Sci. USA* **105**, 18865–18870.
25. Chen, T. Y., and Hwang, T. C. (2008) CLC-0 and CFTR: chloride channels evolved from transporters. *Physiol. Rev.* **88**, 351–387.
26. Muallem, D., and Vergani, P. (2009) ATP hydrolysis-driven gating in cystic fibrosis transmembrane conductance regulator. *Philos. Trans. R. Soc. Lond. B Biol. Sci.* **364**, 247–255.
27. Csanády, L., Vergani, P., and Gadsby, D. C. (2010) Strict coupling between CFTR's catalytic cycle and gating of its Cl- ion pore revealed by distributions of open channel burst durations. *Proc. Natl. Acad. Sci. USA* **107**, 1241–1246.
28. Cheng, S. H., Rich, D. P., Marshall, J., Gregory, R. J., Welsh, M. J., and Smith, A. E. (1991) Phosphorylation of the R domain

by camp-dependent protein kinase regulates the CFTR chloride channel. *Cell* **66**, 1027–1036.
29. Picciotto, M. R., Cohn, J. A., Bertuzzi, G., Greengard, P., and Nairn, A. C. (1992) Phosphorylation of the cystic fibrosis transmembrane conductance. *J. Biol. Chem.* **267**, 12742–12752.
30. Jia, Y., Mathews, C. J., and Hanrahan, J. W. (1997) Phosphorylation by protein kinase C is required for acute activation of cystic fibrosis transmembrane conductance regulator by protein kinase A. *J. Biol. Chem.* **272**, 4978–4984.
31. Chappe, V., Hinkson, D. A., Zhu, T., Chang, X. B., Riordan, J. R., and Hanrahan, J. W. (2003) Phosphorylation of protein kinase C sites in NBD1 and the R domain control CFTR channel activation by PKA. *J. Physiol.* **548**, 39–52.
32. Gadsby, D. C., Vergani, P., and Csanady, L. (2006) The ABC protein turned chloride channel whose failure causes cystic fibrosis. *Nature* **440**, 477–483.
33. Ostedgaard, L. S., Baldursson, O., Vermeer, D. W., Welsh, M. J., and Robertson, A. D. (2000) A functional R domain from cystic fibrosis transmembrane conductance regulator is predominantly unstructured in solution. *Proc. Natl. Acad. Sci. USA* **97**, 5657–5662.
34. Baker, J. M., Hudson, R. P., Kanelis, V., Choy, W. H., Thibodeau, P. H., Thomas, P. J., et al. (2007) CFTR regulatory region interacts with NBD1 predominantly via multiple transient helices. *Nat. Struct. Mol. Biol.* **14**, 738–745.
35. Chang, X. B., Tabcharani, J. A., Hou, Y. X., Jenson, T. J., Kartner, N., Alon, N., et al. (1993) Protein kinase A (PKA) still activates CFTR chloride channel after mutagenesis of all 10 PKA consensus phosphorylation sites. *J. Biol. Chem.* **268**, 11304–11311.
36. Csanady, L., Seto-Young, D., Chan, K. W., Cenciarelli, C., Angel, B. B., Qin, J., et al. (2005) Preferential phosphorylation of R-domain serine 768 dampens activation of CFTR channels by PKA. *J. Gen. Physiol.* **125**, 171–181.
37. Lewis, H. A., Buchanan, S. G., Burley, S. K., Conners, K., Dickey, M., Dorwart, M., et al. (2004) Structure of nucleotide-binding domain 1 of the cystic fibrosis transmembrane conductance regulator. *EMBO J.* **23**, 282–293.
38. Kanelis, V., Hudson, R. P., Thibodeau, P. H., Thomas, P. J., and Forman-Kay, J. D. (2010) NMR evidence for differential phosphorylation-dependent interactions in WT and DeltaF508 CFTR. *EMBO J.* **29**, 263–277, PMCID: PMC2808376.
39. Csanady, L., Chan, K. W., Nairn, A. C., and Gadsby, D. C. (2005) Functional roles of non conserved structural segments in CFTR's NH2-terminal nucleotide binding domain. *J. Gen. Physiol.* **125**, 43–55.
40. Zerhusen, B., and Ma, J. (1999) Function of the second nucleotide-binding fold in the CFTR chloride channel. *FEBS Lett.* **459**, 177–185.
41. Chan, K. W., Csanády, L., Nairn, A. C., and Gadsby, D. C. (1999) Deletion analysis of CFTR channel R domain using severed molecules. *Biophys. J.* **76**, A405.
42. Wang, W., Wu, J., Bernard, K., Li, G., Wang, G., Bevensee, M. O., et al. (2010) ATP-independent CFTR channel gating and allosteric modulation by phosphorylation. *Proc. Natl. Acad. Sci. USA* **107**, 3888–3893.
43. Bompadre, S. G., Sohma, Y., Li, M., and Hwang, T. C. (2007) G551D and G1349D, two CF-associated mutations in the signature sequences of CFTR, exhibit distinct gating defects. *J. Gen. Physiol.* **129**, 285–298.
44. King, J. D., Jr., Fitch, A. C., Lee, J. K., McCane, J. E., Mak, D. O., Foskett, J. K., et al. (2009) AMP-activated protein kinase phosphorylation of the R domain inhibits PKA stimulation of CFTR. *Am. J. Physiol. Cell Physiol.* **297**, C94–C101.
45. Kongsuphol, P., Cassidy, D., Hieke, B., Treharne, K. J., Schreiber, R., Mehta, A., et al. (2009) Mechanistic insight into control of CFTR by AMPK. *J. Biol. Chem.* **284**, 5645–5653.
46. Wilkinson, D. J., Strong, T. V., Mansoura, M. K., Wood, D. L., Smith, S. S., Collins, F. S., et al. (1997) CFTR activation: additive effects of stimulatory and inhibitory phosphorylation sites in the R domain. *Am. J. Physiol.* **273**, L127–L133.
47. Zhang, L., Aleksandrov, L. A., Zhao, Z., Birtley, J. R., Riordan, J. R., et al. (2009) Architecture of the cystic fibrosis transmembrane conductance regulator protein and structural changes associated with phosphorylation and nucleotide binding. *J. Struct. Biol.* **167**, 242–251.
48. Chan, K. W., Csanády, L., Seto-Young, D., Nairn, A. C., and Gadsby, D. C. (2000) Severed molecules functionally define the boundaries of the cystic fibrosis transmembrane conductance regulator's NH_2-terminal nucleotide binding domain. *J. Gen. Physiol.* **116**, 163–180.
49. Loo, T. W., and Clarke, D. M. (2001) Defining the drug-binding site in the human

multidrug resistance P-glycoprotein using a methanethiosulfonate analog of verapamil, MTS-verapamil. *J. Biol. Chem.* **276**, 14972–14979.
50. He, L., Aleksandrov, A. A., Serohijos, A. W., Hegedus, T., Aleksandrov, L. A., Cui, L., et al. (2008) Multiple membrane-cytoplasmic domain contacts in the cystic fibrosis transmembrane conductance regulator (CFTR) mediate regulation of channel gating. *J. Biol. Chem.* **283**, 26383–26390.
51. Serohijos, A. W., Hegedus, T., Aleksandrov, A. A., He, L., Cui, L., Dokholyan, N. V., et al. (2008) Phenylalanine-508 mediates a cytoplasmic-membrane domain contact in the CFTR 3D structure crucial to assembly and channel function. *Proc. Natl. Acad. Sci. USA* **105**, 3256–3261.
52. Cotten, J. F., and Welsh, M. J. (1998) Covalent modification of the nucleotide binding domains of cystic fibrosis transmembrane conductance regulator. *J. Biol. Chem.* **273**, 31873–31879.
53. Zhang, Z.-R., Song, B., and McCarty, N. A. (2005b) State-dependent chemical reactivity of an engineered cysteine reveals conformational changes in the outer vestibule of the cystic fibrosis transmembrane conductance regulator. *J. Biol. Chem.* **280**, 41997–42003.
54. Seibert, F. S., Chang, X. B., Aleksandrov, A. A., Clarke, D. M., Hanrahan, J. W., and Riordan, J. R. (1999) Influence of phosphorylation by protein kinase A on CFTR at the cell surface and endoplasmic reticulum. *Biochim. Biophys. Acta* **1461**, 275–283.
55. Ramjeesingh, M., Li, C., Garami, E., Huan, L. J., Hewryk, M., Wang, Y., Galley, K., et al. (1997) A novel procedure for the efficient purification of the cystic fibrosis transmembrane conductance regulator (CFTR). *Biochem. J.* **327**, 17–21.
56. Aleksandrov, L., Mengos, A., Chang, X., Aleksandrov, A., and Riordan, J. R. (2001) Differential interactions of nucleotides at the nucleotide binding domains of the cystic fibrosis transmembrane conductance regulator. *J. Biol. Chem.* **276**, 12918–12923.
57. Berger, H. A., Travis, S. M., and Welsh, M. J. (1993) Regulation of the cystic fibrosis transmembrane conductance regulator Cl- channel by specific protein kinases and protein phosphatases. *J. Biol. Chem.* **268**, 2037–2047.
58. Travis, S. M., Berger, H. A., and Welsh, M. J. (1997) Protein phosphate 2C dephosphorylates and inactivates cystic fibrosis transmembrane conductance regulator. *Proc. Natl. Acad. Sci. USA* **94**, 11055–11060.
59. Luo, J., Pato, M. D., Riordan, J. R., and Hanrahan, J. W. (1998) Differential regulation of single CFTR channels by PP2C, PP2A, and other phosphatases. *Am. J. Physiol.* **274**, C1397–C1410.
60. Chappe, V., Hinkson, D. A., Howell, L. D., Evagelidis, A., Liao, J., Chang, X. B., et al. (2004) Stimulatory and inhibitory protein kinase C consensus sequences regulate the cystic fibrosis transmembrane conductance regulator. *Proc. Natl. Acad. Sci. USA* **101**, 390–395.
61. Wilkinson, D. J., Mansoura, M. K., Watson, P. Y., Smit, L. S., Collins, F. S., and Dawson, D. C. (1996) CFTR: the nucleotide binding folds regulate the accessibility and stability of the activated state. *J. Gen. Physiol.* **107**, 103–119.
62. Sheppard, D. N., Gray, M. A., Gong, X., Sohma, Y., Kogan, I., Benos, D. J., et al. (2004) The patch-clamp and planar lipid bilayer techniques: powerful and versatile tools to investigate the CFTR Cl- channel. *J. Cyst. Fibros.* **3**, 101–108.
63. Thomas, P., and Smart, T. G. (2005) HEK293 cell line: a vehicle for the expression of recombinant proteins. *J. Pharmacol. Toxicol. Methods* **51**, 187–200.
64. Bear, C., Li, C., Kartner, N., Bridges, R., Jensen, T., Ramjeesingh, M., et al. (1992) Purification and functional reconstitution of the cystic fibrosis transmembrane conductance regulator (CFTR). *Cell* **68**, 809–818.
65. Sakmann, B., Neher, E. (eds.) (1995) *Single-Channel Recording*, Plenum Press, New York, NY, p. 700.
66. Ashley, R. H. (ed.) (1995) *Ion Channels: A Practical Approach.* Practical Approach Series, Oxford University Press, Oxford, p. 328.
67. Benndorf, K. (1995) Low-noise recording, in (Sakmann, B., Neher, E. eds.) *Single-Channel Recording.* Plenum Press, New York, NY, pp. 129–145.
68. Kijima, S., and Kijima, H. (1987) Statistical analysis of channel current from a membrane patch I. Some stochastic properties of ion channels or molecular systems in equilibrium. *J. Theor. Biol.* **128**, 423–434.
69. Winter, M. C., Sheppard, D. N., Carson, M. R., and Welsh, M. J. (1994) Effect of ATP concentration on CFTR Cl- channels: a kinetic analysis of channel regulation. *Biophys. J.* **66**, 1398–1403.
70. Zhang, Z. R., Cui, G., Liu, X., Song, B., Dawson, D. C., and McCarty, N. A. (2005a) Determination of the functional unit of the cystic fibrosis transmembrane conductance

regulator chloride channel. One polypeptide forms one pore. *J. Biol. Chem.* **280**, 458–468.
71. Lansdell, K. A., Kidd, J. F., Delaney, S. J., Wainwright, B. J., and Sheppard, D. N. (1998) Regulation of murine cystic fibrosis transmembrane conductance regulator Cl- channels expressed in Chinese hamster ovary cells. *J. Physiol.* **512**(Pt 3), 751–764.
72. Venkataramanan, L., and Sigworth, F. J. (2002) Applying hidden Markov models to the analysis of single ion channel activity. *Biophys. J.* **82**, 1930–1942.
73. Qin, F. (2004) Restoration of single-channel currents using the segmental k-means method based on hidden Markov modeling. *Biophys. J.* **86**, 1488–1501.
74. Sigworth, F. J., and Sine, S. M. (1987) Data transformations for improved display and fitting of single-channel dwell time histograms. *Biophys. J.* **52**, 1047–1054.
75. Horn, R., and Lange, K. (1983) Estimating kinetic constants from single channel data. *Biophys. J.* **43**, 207–223.
76. Ball, F. G., and Sansom, M. S. (1989) Ion-channel gating mechanisms: model identification and parameter estimation from single channel recordings. *Proc. R. Soc. Lond. B Biol. Sci.* **236**, 385–416.
77. Qin, F., Auerbach, A., and Sachs, F. (1996) Estimating single-channel kinetic parameters from idealized patch-clamp data containing missed events. *Biophys. J.* **70**, 264–280.
78. Bompadre, S. G., Ai, T., Cho, J. H., Wang, X., Sohma, Y., Li, M., et al. (2005a) CFTR gating I: characterization of the ATP-dependent gating of a phosphorylation-independent CFTR channel (DeltaR-CFTR). *J. Gen. Physiol.* **125**, 361–375.
79. Magleby, K. L., and Pallotta, B. S. (1983) Burst kinetics of single calcium-activated potassium channels in cultured rat muscle. *J. Physiol.* **344**, 605–623.
80. Jackson, M. B., Wong, B. S., Morris, C. E., Lecar, H., and Christian, C. N. (1983) Successive openings of the same acetylcholine receptor channel are correlated in open time. *Biophys. J.* **42**, 109–114.
81. Csanády, L. (2000) Rapid kinetic analysis of multichannel records by a simultaneous fit to all dwell-time histograms. *Biophys. J.* **78**, 785–799.
82. Weinreich, F., Riordan, J. R., and Nagel, G. (1999) Dual effects of ADP and adenylylimidodiphosphate on CFTR channel kinetics show binding to two different nucleotide binding sites. *J. Gen. Physiol.* **114**, 55–70.
83. Bompadre, S. G., Cho, J. H., Wang, X., Zou, X., Sohma, Y., Li, M., et al. (2005) CFTR gating II: effects of nucleotide binding on the stability of open states. *J. Gen. Physiol.* **125**, 377–394.
84. Csanády, L., Nairn, A. C., and Gadsby, D. C. (2006) Thermodynamics of CFTR channel gating: a spreading conformational change initiates an irreversible gating cycle. *J. Gen. Physiol.* **128**, 523–533.
85. Segel, I. H. (1993) *Enzyme Kinetics. Behavior and Analysis of Rapid Equilibrium and Steady-State Enzyme Systems*, Wiley, New York, NY.
86. Ishihara, H., and Welsh, M. J. (1997) Block by MOPS reveals a conformation change in the CFTR pore produced by ATP hydrolysis. *Am. J. Physiol.* **273**, C1278–C1289.
87. Aleksandrov, A. A., and Riordan, J. R. (1998) Regulation of CFTR ion channel gating by MgATP. *FEBS Lett.* **431**, 97–101.
88. Mathews, C. J., Tabcharani, J. A., and Hanrahan, J. W. (1998) The CFTR chloride channel: nucleotide interactions and temperature-dependent gating. *J. Membr. Biol.* **163**, 55–66.
89. Fersht, A. (2002) *Structure and Mechanism in Protein Science*, 4th ed. W.H. Freeman and Company, New York, NY.
90. Faiman, G. A., and Horovitz, A. (1996) On the choice of reference mutant states in the application of the double-mutant cycle method. *Protein Eng.* **9**, 315–316.
91. Auerbach, A. (2007) How to turn the reaction coordinate into time. *J. Gen. Physiol.* **130**, 543–546.
92. Chakrapani, S., Bailey, T. D., and Auerbach, A. (2004) Gating dynamics of the acetylcholine receptor extracellular domain. *J. Gen. Physiol.* **123**, 341–356.
93. Purohit, P., Mitra, A., and Auerbach, A. (2007) A stepwise mechanism for acetylcholine receptor channel gating. *Nature* **446**, 930–933.
94. Scott-Ward, T. S., Cai, Z., Dawson, E. S., Doherty, A., Da Paula, A. C., Davidson, H., et al. (2007) Chimeric constructs endow the human CFTR Cl- channel with the gating behavior of murine CFTR. *Proc. Natl. Acad. Sci. USA* **104**, 16365–16370.
95. Aleksandrov, A. A., Cui, L., and Riordan, J. R. (2009) Relationship between nucleotide binding and ion channel gating in cystic fibrosis transmembrane conductance regulator. *J. Physiol.* **587**, 2875–2886.
96. Csanády, L. (2009) Application of rate-equilibrium free energy relationship analysis to nonequilibrium ion channel gating mechanisms. *J. Gen. Physiol.* **134**, 129–136.

97. Galtier, N., and Dutheil, J. (2007) Coevolution within and between genes. *Genome Dyn.* **3**, 1–12.
98. Fitch, W. M., and Markowitz, E. (1970) An improved method for determining codon variability in a gene and its application to the rate of fixation of mutations in evolution. *Biochem. Genet.* **4**, 579–593.
99. Gutell, R. R., Larsen, N., and Woese, C. R. (1994) Lessons from an evolving rRNA: 16S and 23S rRNA structures from a comparative perspective. *Micro. Biol.* **58**, 10–26.
100. Codoñer, F. M., O'Dea, S., and Fares, M. A. (2008) Reducing the false positive rate in the non-parametric analysis of molecular coevolution. *BMC Evol. Biol.* **8**, 106.
101. Olmea, O., and Valencia, A. (1997) Improving contact predictions by the combination of correlated mutations and other sources of sequence information. *Fold Des.* **2**, S25–S32.
102. Lockless, S. W., and Ranganathan, R. (1999) Evolutionarily conserved pathways of energetic connectivity in protein families. *Science* **286**, 295–299.
103. Dekker, J. P., Fodor, A., Aldrich, R. W., and Yellen, G. (2004) A perturbation-based method for calculating explicit likelihood of evolutionary co-variance in multiple sequence alignments. *Bioinformatics* **20**, 1565–1572.
104. Kass, I., and Horovitz, A. (2002) Mapping pathways of allosteric communication in GroEL by analysis of correlated mutations. *Proteins* **48**, 611–617.
105. Fares, M. A., and Travers, S. A. A. (2006) A novel method for detecting intramolecular coevolution: adding a further dimension to selective constraints analyses. *Genetics* **173**, 9–23.
106. Dunn, S. D., Wahl, L. M., and Gloor, G. B. (2008) Mutual information without the influence of phylogeny or entropy dramatically improves residue contact prediction. *Bioinformatics* **24**, 333–340.
107. Dutheil, J., Pupko, T., Jean-Marie, A., and Galtier, N. (2005) A model-based approach for detecting coevolving positions in a molecule. *Mol. Biol. Evol.* **22**, 1919–1928.
108. Dutheil, J., and Galtier, N. (2007) Detecting groups of coevolving positions in a molecule: a clustering approach. *BMC Evol. Biol.* **7**, 242.
109. Dimmic, M. W., Hubisz, M. J., Bustamante, C. D., and Nielsen, R. (2005) Detecting coevolving amino acid sites using Bayesian mutational mapping. *Bioinformatics* **21**(Suppl 1), i126–i135.
110. Fleishman, S. J., Yifrach, O., and Ben-Tal, N. (2004) An evolutionarily conserved network of amino acids mediates gating in voltage-dependent potassium channels. *J. Mol. Biol.* **340**, 307–318.
111. Pollock, D. D., Taylor, W. R., and Goldman, N. (1999) Coevolving protein residues: maximum likelihood identification and relationship to structure. *J. Mol. Biol.* **287**, 187–198.
112. Yeang, C.-H., and Haussler, D. (2007) Detecting coevolution in and among protein domains. *PLoS Comput. Biol.* **3**, e211.
113. Altschul, S. F., Gish, W., Miller, W., Myers, E. W., and Lipman, D. J. (1990) Basic local alignment search tool. *J. Mol. Biol.* **215**, 403–410.
114. Eddy, S. R. (2009) A new generation of homology search tools based on probabilistic inference. *Genome Inform.* **23**, 205–211.
115. Notredame, C., and Abergel, C. (2003) Using multiple alignment methods to assess the quality of genomic data analysis, in *Bioinformatics and Genomes: Current Perspectives.* Horizon Scientific Press, Wymondham, Norfolk, pp. 30–55.
116. Lassmann, T., and Sonnhammer, E. L. L. (2005) Automatic assessment of alignment quality. *Nucleic Acids Res.* **33**, 7120–7128. doi:10.1093/nar/gki1020.
117. Mornon, J. P., Lehn, P., and Callebaut, I. (2009) Molecular models of the open and closed states of the whole human CFTR protein. *Cell. Mol. Life Sci.* **66**, 3469–3486.
118. Alexander, C., Ivetac, A., Liu, X., Norimatsu, Y., Serrano, J. R., Landstrom, A., et al. (2009) Cystic fibrosis transmembrane conductance regulator: using differential reactivity toward channel-permeant and channel-impermeant thiol-reactive probes to test a molecular model for the pore. *Biochemistry* **48**, 10078–10088.
119. Fodor, A. A., and Aldrich, R. W. (2004b) On evolutionary conservation of thermodynamic coupling in proteins. *J. Biol. Chem.* **279**, 19046–19050.
120. Fuchs, A., Martin-Galiano, A. J., Kalman, M., Fleishman, S., Ben-Tal, N., and Frishman, D. (2007) Co-evolving residues in membrane proteins. *Bioinformatics* **23**, 3312–3319.
121. Burger, L., and van Nimwegen, E. (2010) Disentangling direct from indirect co-evolution of residues in protein alignments. *PLoS Comput. Biol.* **6**, e1000633.
122. Felsenstein, J. (1985) Phylogenies and the comparative method. *Am. Nat.* **125**, 1.
123. Wollenberg, K. R., and Atchley, W. R. (2000) Separation of phylogenetic and functional associations in biological sequences by using the parametric bootstrap. *Proc. Natl. Acad. Sci. USA* **97**, 3288–3291.

124. Tillier, E. R. M., and Lui, T. W. H. (2003) Using multiple interdependency to separate functional from phylogenetic correlations in protein alignments. *Bioinformatics* **19**, 750–755.
125. Noivirt, O., Eisenstein, M., and Horovitz, A. (2005) Detection and reduction of evolutionary noise in correlated mutation analysis. *Protein Eng. Des. Sel.* **18**, 247–253.
126. Fodor, A. A., and Aldrich, R. W. (2004) Influence of conservation on calculations of amino acid covariance in multiple sequence alignments. *Proteins* **56**, 211–221.
127. Martin, L. C., Gloor, G. B., Dunn, S. D., and Wahl, L. M. (2005) Using information theory to search for co-evolving residues in proteins. *Bioinformatics* **21**, 4116–4124.

Chapter 29

CFTR Regulation by Phosphorylation

Rodrigo Alzamora, J Darwin King, and Kenneth R. Hallows

Abstract

The cystic fibrosis transmembrane conductance regulator (CFTR) is the gene product mutated in cystic fibrosis, a common lethal genetic disease characterized by abnormal electrolyte transport across epithelia. CFTR functions as an ATP-gated, phosphorylation-regulated Cl^- channel that mediates agonist-stimulated apical membrane epithelial Cl^- and bicarbonate secretion and also regulates a variety of other transport proteins and cellular processes. CFTR belongs to the ATP-binding cassette (ABC) transporter superfamily. Its presumed architecture consists of two transmembrane domain regions that form the channel pore, two nucleotide-binding domains that bind and hydrolyze ATP, and a unique regulatory (R) domain that contains numerous protein kinase A (PKA) and protein kinase C (PKC) phosphorylation sites. Other kinases have also been shown more recently to phosphorylate and regulate CFTR activity. This chapter describes strategies and methods for studying the phosphorylation of CFTR both in vitro and whole-cell systems.

Key words: Kinases, PKA, PKC, AMPK, mass spectrometry, immunoprecipitation, immunoblotting, autoradiography, phosphoproteins.

1. Introduction

Protein phosphorylation is a critical post-translational modification that plays a key regulatory role for many biological functions. There are a growing number of signaling cascades and kinases that mediate phosphorylation. These processes regulate diverse cellular functions such as signal transduction, gene expression, cell division and differentiation, and membrane transport protein activity and localization. Phosphorylation can also serve as a means of transducing extracellular events to intracellular processes. The identification of protein phosphorylation sites and

M.D. Amaral, K. Kunzelmann (eds.), *Cystic Fibrosis*, Methods in Molecular Biology 741,
DOI 10.1007/978-1-61779-117-8_29, © Springer Science+Business Media, LLC 2011

cellular signaling cascades represents technical challenges that can be partially addressed through the use of both in vitro and in vivo phosphorylation techniques.

1.1. CFTR as a Phosphoprotein

The cystic fibrosis transmembrane conductance regulator (CFTR) channel, defective in cystic fibrosis, is a chloride channel containing 12 predicted transmembrane helices and 5 cytoplasmic domains with 2 nucleotide-binding domains (NBDs), a regulatory R domain with multiple PKA and PKC phosphorylation sites, and NH_2- and COOH-terminal cytoplasmic tails (1, 2). The gating of CFTR requires both PKA-dependent phosphorylation of the R domain and ATP binding and subsequent hydrolysis at the NBDs (3, 4). PKC-dependent phosphorylation at multiple sites is necessary for full PKA-dependent activation of CFTR (5, 6). Conversely, the metabolic sensor AMP-activated protein kinase (AMPK) binds to the COOH-terminal tail and phosphorylates CFTR, which inhibits PKA-stimulated CFTR channel gating (7–10). An inhibitory PKA site on the R domain of CFTR, Ser768, appears to be the dominant site of AMPK phosphorylation in vitro (10, 11). Other kinases have also been reported to phosphorylate and regulate CFTR, including the p60Src tyrosine kinase and CK2 (12, 13).

1.2. Characterization of Protein Phosphorylation

Protein phosphorylation may be characterized in two stages. First, the protein of interest should be shown to be phosphorylated by a particular kinase. To demonstrate phosphorylation of a protein by a particular kinase, one can use both in vitro and in vivo phosphorylation approaches. For in vitro phosphorylation assays, the target protein is first immunoprecipitated from cell lysates or over-expressed recombinantly. Then, purified kinase and [γ-^{32}P]-ATP are added to the purified target protein in a kinase reaction buffer to allow phosphorylation to occur in vitro. Phosphorylation of the protein is detected as a labeled band either on a gel by autoradiography or on a phosphorimaging screen after SDS-PAGE. To detect whether a protein may be a target for a particular kinase in an intact cellular milieu, an in vivo phosphorylation technique is employed, which involves [^{32}P]-orthophosphate labeling of cells for a period of time under conditions where the kinase to be tested is either activated or inhibited using either over-expression or RNAi knockdown approaches or by pharmacological modulators of kinase activity. The target protein is then immunoprecipitated from cell lysates and subjected to SDS-PAGE followed by either autoradiography or phospho-screen imaging.

The second stage of protein phosphorylation characterization involves determining which amino acids in the protein are the phosphorylation targets by the particular kinase. One approach to do this is through mass spectrometry, which can detect various post-translational modifications on proteins, including the addition of phosphate groups on particular residues (*see* **Section 1.4.1** for more details). Another approach is to mutate candidate phosphorylation sites and compare the extent of in vitro or in vivo ^{32}P labeling of the mutant protein with that of wild-type protein (*see* **Section 1.4.3**). This candidate site mutagenesis approach is more feasible for kinases that have well-defined and predictable target phosphorylation motifs. Indeed, there are various available algorithms that may be useful for screening a protein of interest for potential phosphorylation sites by various kinases (*see* **Section 1.4.2**). Once specific phosphorylation sites have been identified, phosphorylation-deficient (e.g., Ser/Thr to Ala) or phospho-mimic (e.g., Ser/Thr to Asp) site mutants can be generated to test the functional consequences of phosphorylation by a kinase at the particular site(s) identified. In addition, phosphorylation site-specific antibodies that recognize the phosphorylated residue (e.g., Ser, Thr, or Tyr) within the context of the target phosphorylation sequence can be generated and used in experiments to detect changes in phosphorylation at a particular site in the protein under various relevant cellular conditions (14). Indeed, antibodies have been recently developed to detect changes in the phosphorylation status of various PKA sites in the CFTR R domain (15). This powerful approach enables the simultaneous investigation of multiple PKA phosphorylation sites in the CFTR R domain without the need for radioactive labeling.

1.3. Advantages and Disadvantages of In Vitro and In Vivo Phosphorylation Approaches

In vitro phosphorylation assays are useful to demonstrate direct phosphorylation of a purified target protein by a particular kinase. Because the phosphorylation of the target protein occurs in vitro (i.e., outside a normal cellular environment) with the target protein potentially in a non-native conformation, the physiological significance of any phosphorylation observed in this setting is unclear by itself. One major advantage of using the in vivo phosphorylation approach is that phosphorylation events are detected in the intact cellular milieu where the particular kinase of interest is either activated or inhibited. Thus, any kinase-dependent phosphorylation observed is more likely to be physiologically relevant. However, a disadvantage of the in vivo phosphorylation assay is that this approach by itself cannot be used to discern whether a particular kinase directly or indirectly (e.g., through modulation of another intermediate kinase or signaling cascade) phosphorylates the target protein of interest. Therefore, the use of in vitro and in vivo phosphorylation assays is complementary in the information that they yield when analyzing whether a particular kinase phosphorylates a protein of interest. For example, if a purified kinase phosphorylates a target protein in vitro and if enhanced kinase-dependent in vivo phosphorylation of the protein is found in cells, then it is highly likely that the kinase directly phosphorylates the target protein in intact cells. Moreover, if mutation of the candidate phosphorylation site(s) causes a change in the function of the target protein, then it is very likely that the phosphorylation event(s) are physiologically relevant in regulating the function of the target protein.

1.4. Identification and Validation of Phosphorylation Sites

An important step in studying phosphorylation of a protein like CFTR is to determine which residues are the sites of phosphorylation. There are several approaches to determine the identity of a phosphorylated residue, including phosphopeptide mapping, mass spectrometry, and site-directed mutagenesis. This section briefly describes the advantages and disadvantages of these techniques in determining the identity of phosphorylated residues.

1.4.1. Direct Identification by Mass Spectrometry

Several analytical methods are available for the identification of phosphorylated peptides within proteins. Mass spectrometry is becoming a commonly used method for identifying these sites (16). The peptide may be directly isolated from a two-dimensional phosphopeptide map, although the yield from this approach is often low. Alternatively, the complete tryptic digest can be first fractionated by high-performance liquid chromatography (HPLC) and then the eluted radioactive peptides can be used for Edman degradation sequencing and/or mass spectrometry. Tandem mass spectrometry is an additional step that not only gives the mass of a peptide, but then by further analysis of the peptide can help identify phosphorylated residues (17). One caveat of all of these techniques is the relatively low amount of phosphorylated peptides compared to non-phosphorylated peptides. Thus, even after two-dimensional analysis or high-performance liquid chromatography, the peptide is usually not pure or even a major constituent of the sample for mass spectrometry.

1.4.2. Bio-informatic Approaches to Identify Potential Phosphorylation Sites

An alternative approach to identify phosphorylation sites is to analyze the protein sequence to determine the presence of phosphorylation consensus sequences using bio-informatic approaches. Approximately 10 different software programs have been created and are available online to search for phosphorylation consensus motifs for a variety of protein kinases. Many of them are freely available on the Internet. The search algorithms of each differ slightly, but most of them are based on locating specific motifs within the peptide sequence. One of the most used programs is NetPhosK (http://www.cbs.dtu.dk/services/NetPhosK) (18). This software analyzes the sequence using an integrated database of motifs for several kinases and assigns a score depending on the probability that a particular site will be phosphorylated by one or more protein kinases. However, NetPhosK has the limitation that it will only search for phosphorylation sites for the kinases in its database. Another popular search engine is Phosida (http://www.phosida.com). This program also allows one to search for phosphorylation sites using a predetermined database of kinases, although it is not as comprehensive as that of NetPhosK. However, it does offer the advantage of searching for the specific consensus sequence for any kinase where the consensus sequence can be specified by the investigator. This tool is particularly advantageous for more recently discovered protein kinases that are yet to be included in these programs or for protein kinases that have variable consensus motifs such as AMPK. Determining candidate phosphorylation sites using these bio-informatic tools is extremely helpful to narrow down the number of potential sites. However, one important caveat of this approach is that it does not consider whether the candidate sites are accessible to the protein kinases. Additional software available online for phosphorylation site prediction includes ScanSite (http://scansite.mit.edu) and PhoScan (http://bioinfo.au.tsinghua.edu.cn/phoscan).

1.4.3. Candidate Site Mutagenesis

The usual next step in determining phosphopeptide identity is to test a mutation of CFTR where the putative site identified above has been mutated to an Ala. If there are multiple phosphorylation sites, mutation of any one site may not be detected as a loss of phosphate incorporation. Depending on the reproducibility of the in vitro kinase assay, it may be difficult to observe less than a 50% reduction in incorporation. The loss of phosphate labeling is a good evidence (but not conclusive) that a site has been determined. A caveat of this test is that the Ser/Thr to Ala mutation could alter the conformation of the protein and thus reduce phosphorylation without it actually being a site of phosphorylation. **Figure 29.1** illustrates a typical experiment in which site-directed mutagenesis of one candidate site results in the inhibition of in vitro phosphorylation of CFTR by AMPK.

2. Materials

2.1. In Vitro Phosphorylation Measurements

2.1.1. Cell Maintenance

1. HEK-293, COS-7, or NIH 3T3 cells (American Type Culture Collection).
2. Fetal bovine serum (FBS; Atlanta Biologicals).
3. Dulbecco's modified Eagle medium (DMEM; Sigma-Aldrich).
4. Trypsin/ethylenediaminetetraacetic acid (EDTA) solution (Sigma-Aldrich).

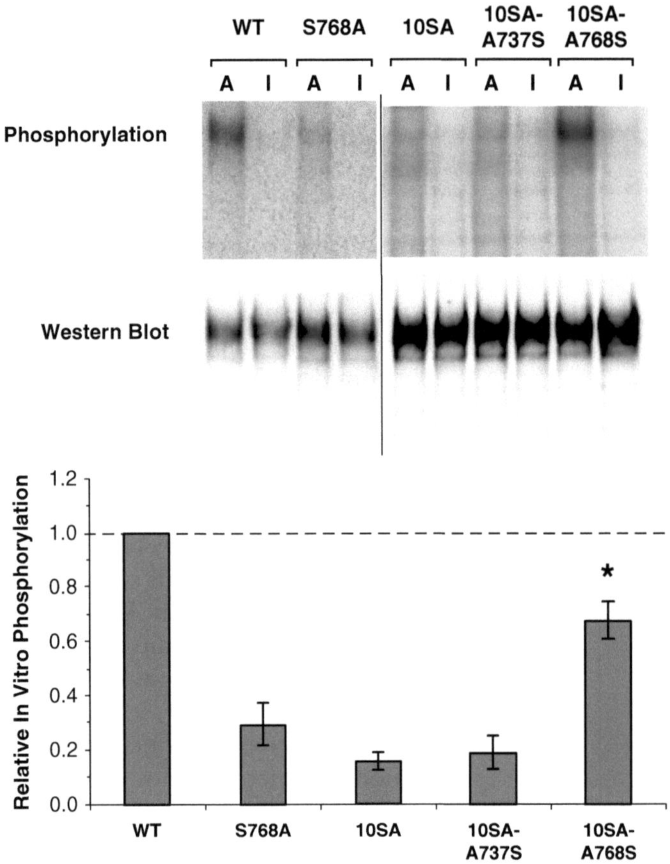

Fig. 29.1. In vitro phosphorylation of CFTR wild type (WT) and various mutants by purified active (A) versus inactive (I) AMPK holoenzyme. HEK-293 cells were transiently transfected with CFTR for 48 h. Cell lysates were immunoprecipitated with M24-1 anti-CFTR antibody. In vitro phosphorylation assay was carried out in the presence of γ-^{32}P-ATP. The amount of CFTR protein was detected by immunoblotting using the M3A7 anti-CFTR antibody. Phosphorylation of CFTR was detected by exposing the nitrocellulose membrane to a phosphoscreen and the signals were recorded and quantified using a Phosphorimager system. *Top panel:* representative phospho-screen images and corresponding western blots of the various CFTR mutants. The WT and S768A images shown are from a different membrane than the rest of the mutants shown. *Bottom panel*: in vitro phosphorylation corrected for CFTR protein expression and normalized to that of CFTR-WT. The results suggest that the Ser-768 site is the only relevant one among the candidate sites for AMPK phosphorylation in vitro. Adapted from (10) (used with permission).

5. Penicillin/streptomycin 100X solution (Lonza).
6. Sterile phosphate-buffered saline (PBS).
7. 37°C humidified CO_2 incubator.
8. Tissue culture 75 cm^2 flasks.
9. Sterile Pasteur pipettes.
10. Sterile disposable 5, 10, and 25 ml pipettes.

2.1.2. Cell Transfection

1. Tissue culture dishes, 60 or 100 mm.
2. Sterile 15 ml polystyrene tubes.
3. Transfection reagent (Lipofectamine 2000, Invitrogen; Superfect, Qiagen).
4. Transfection medium (Opti-MEM, Invitrogen Life Technologies).
5. Purified CFTR cDNA in mammalian expression vector (human CFTR in pAd.CMV.Link.1 vector, American Type Culture Collection, Cat# 75468).

2.1.3. Cell Lysis

1. Ice-cold PBS.
2. RIPA lysis buffer (100 mM NaCl, 50 mM NaF, 5 mM EDTA, 5 mM Na-pyrophosphate, 1% Na-deoxycholate, 1% Triton X-100, 0.1% SDS, 50 mM Tris–HCl, pH 7.5; before use add 1 mM EGTA, 0.1 mg/ml aprotinin, 0.1 mM PMSF, 1 mM sodium orthovanadate, and protein and phosphate inhibitor cocktails).
3. Complete protease inhibitor cocktail (Roche).
4. Phosphatase inhibitor cocktail (PhosSTOP, Roche).
5. Cell scrapers.

2.1.4. Immunoprecipitation

1. Protein Sepharose A/G beads (Pierce; Santa Cruz Biotechnology).
2. Mouse anti-CFTR antibody clone M24-1 (R&D Systems, *see* **Note 1**).
3. Epitope tag antibodies (*see* **Table 29.1** for epitope sequences and suggested sources of antibodies).

Table 29.1
Epitope tag antibodies

Epitope	Sequence	Antibody	Company	Species
HA	MYPYDVPDYA	3F10	Roche	Rat
		16B12	Covance	Mouse
FLAG	MDYKDDDDK	M2	Sigma-Aldrich	Mouse
Myc	MEQKLISEEDL	9E10	Roche	Mouse
			Invitrogen	Mouse
V5	GKPIPNPLLGLDST	V5-10	Invitrogen	Mouse

This table should be used only as a guide when selecting epitope tag antibodies. Several other companies also make these antibodies. The manufacturer's instructions should be followed when evaluating the suitability of each antibody for immunoprecipitation and/or immunoblotting.

4. Rocking platform.
5. Vacuum aspirator.
6. RIPA lysis buffer plus 0.5% SDS.
7. Laemmli SDS sample buffer 2X.

2.1.5. In Vitro Kinase Assay

1. Immunoprecipitated CFTR.
2. Recombinant purified protein kinase (Promega; Millipore/Upstate; Cell Signaling Technology).
3. Kinase buffer and cofactors (*see* **Note 2**).
4. [γ-^{32}P]-Adenosine triphosphate (ATP) in buffered solution (100 μl, 10 mCi/ml; MP Biomedicals).
5. Laemmli SDS sample buffer (2X).

2.1.6. Western Blotting

1. SDS polyacrylamide gel electrophoresis apparatus (Bio-Rad; Invitrogen).
2. Nitrocellulose membrane (GE Healthcare).
3. Tris-buffered saline (TBS); 10 mM Tris–HCl pH 8.0, 150 mM NaCl.
4. Tween-20 (Sigma-Aldrich).
5. Bovine serum albumin (BSA, EMD Chemicals).
6. CFTR-specific antibodies (e.g., M3A7, Millipore/Upstate) or epitope tag antibodies.
7. Secondary horseradish peroxidase-coupled antibodies (anti-mouse, anti-rabbit, anti-goat; GE Healthcare).
8. Chemiluminescence reagents: ECL Plus (GE Healthcare) or Supersignal West PICO (Pierce Biotechnology).
9. Chemiluminescence detection system (Molecular Imager VersaDoc MP System, Bio-Rad).
10. Phosphorimager system (Personal Molecular Imager PMI System, Bio-Rad).

2.2. In Vivo Phosphorylation Measurements

2.2.1. Cell Culture

See **Section 2.1.1**.

2.2.2. Cell Transfection

See **Section 2.1.2**.

2.2.3. Cell Stimulation and Orthophosphate Labeling

1. Agonists such as growth factors (insulin-like growth factor-1 (IGF-1), epidermal growth factor (EGF)), hormones (insulin, vasopressin, angiotensin), or specific protein kinase activators or inhibitors.

2. ^{32}P-Orthophosphate sodium salt in buffered solution (1 ml, 5 mCi/ml; MP Biomedicals).
3. Orthophosphate efflux buffer: 140 mM NaCl, 3 mM KCl, 1 mM $MgSO_4$, 1 mM $CaCl_2$, 10 mM D-glucose, 10 mM HEPES pH 7.4 (adjust pH with 1 M Tris base).

3. Methods

3.1. Cell Culture

The procedures described below have been developed for detecting CFTR phosphorylation purified from transiently transfected human embryonic kidney (HEK-293) cells, mouse fibroblasts (NIH 3T3), or African green monkey kidney cells (COS-7, SV40 transformed). All of these cell lines are easily transfected and produce high yields of protein. Numerous studies addressing the regulation of CFTR by phosphorylation have used these cells. However, the methodologies described can also be applied to other cell lines with minor modifications to the growth conditions and media requirements depending on the cell type. Cells are grown in a humidified CO_2 (5%) incubator at 37°C in DMEM supplemented with 10% FBS. We routinely also supplement with an antibiotic/antimycotic. Standard sterile tissue culture techniques should be used at all times. Cells are typically seeded in 75 cm^2 flasks. Cells are serially passaged prior to confluence, typically at 50–70% confluence. To reduce basal phosphorylation of CFTR, cells can be serum starved before treatment. The conditions for serum starvation vary greatly depending on the cell type, but as a general guide a minimum of 10–14 h starvation in DMEM in the absence of FBS should be used. One percent BSA can be used as a supplement and some researchers also use 0.1% FBS.

3.2. Transient Transfection of Cells with CFTR cDNA

Although the phosphorylation of CFTR can be monitored using endogenous protein, it is often useful and advantageous to monitor the phosphorylation of CFTR expressed heterologously in a naïve cell line, which can be achieved by transient transfection. There are a number of reasons for this such as the phosphorylation of CFTR is more readily detected when present in larger quantities as compared to endogenous levels; the CFTR cDNA can be tagged with a variety of epitopes and highly specific antibodies are available to such tags (thereby circumventing the low specificity or affinity of some CFTR antibodies and potentially reducing costs); and point-specific mutations can be readily introduced into the cDNA used for heterologous CFTR expression. The use of epitope tags also eliminates the risk of the anti-CFTR antibody binding to a phosphorylation site or a domain required for protein kinase interaction with CFTR.

Transient transfection with CFTR cDNA has been widely used and numerous mammalian expression vectors are available. The most commonly used vectors contain the cytomegalovirus (CMV) promoter to achieve high expression in transient transfections. Examples of such vectors are the pcDNA3 series (Invitrogen Life Technologies). We recommend the subcloning of CFTR cDNA into a CMV promoter-based vector, along with in-frame addition of an epitope tag to the amino or carboxyl terminus of the CFTR open reading frame. We routinely use the epitope tags shown in **Table 29.1**.

Epitope tags may be added to the CFTR cDNA by PCR using oligonucleotide primers under standard PCR conditions. The CFTR cDNA plasmids are then purified using conventional plasmid isolation techniques from bacterial cultures. The procedure below describes a transient transfection protocol for HEK 293 cells using Lipofectamine 2000, adapted from the manufacturer's protocol (Invitrogen). There are numerous other transfection reagents and procedures. In each case the transfection efficiency of a given CFTR cDNA should be determined empirically for each procedure and cell line:

1. Seed cells into 60 mm dishes at a density of 1×10^6 in DMEM + 10% FBS. Allow cells to reach a density of 70–80% confluence.
2. Wash cells twice with serum-free DMEM media and then replace with 4 ml of DMEM media.
3. In one sterile, 15 ml polystyrene tube add 500 μl Opti-MEM media and 12 μl Lipofectamine 2000 reagent for each dish to be transfected. Mix by gently tapping the tube.
4. In a separate tube, add 500 μl Opti-MEM media and 5 μg of CFTR plasmid DNA for each dish to be transfected. Mix by gently tapping the tube.
5. Add Opti-MEM/Lipofectamine 2000 mixture to tube containing Opti-MEM/DNA mixture. Mix by tapping gently. Do not vortex. Incubate for 20 min at room temperature.
6. Gently overlay 1 ml of transfection mixture to each dish.
7. Return cells to incubator and allow transfection to proceed for 4–6 h.
8. Aspirate transfection mixture from cells and add 5 ml of complete media.
9. Cells are typically harvested 24–48 h after transfection, although the optimal time for maximal protein expression has to be determined for each DNA and cell line.

3.3. Cell Lysis and Immunoprecipitation

1. Wash cells twice with 2 ml of ice-cold PBS.
2. Add 150 μl of RIPA buffer to which fresh protease inhibitor and phosphatase inhibitor cocktails have been added to a final concentration recommended by the manufacturer.
3. Incubate cells for 15 min on ice.
4. Scrape cells into a 0.5 ml centrifuge tube.
5. Centrifuge lysate for 30 min at 4°C and 14,000×*g*.
6. Decant supernatant into a new centrifuge tube and discard pellet.
7. Measure protein concentrations of the lysate supernatants for each condition (e.g., using the Bradford assay or bicinchoninic acid assay).
8. Make lysate supernatants for all conditions the same volume and protein concentration by adding extra RIPA buffer as needed.
9. Pre-clear the lysate supernatants by adding 30 μl of a 50% slurry of protein Sepharose A/G beads (previously washed and equilibrated in RIPA buffer).
10. Incubate for 1 h with rocking at 4°C.
11. Pellet beads by centrifugation at 5,000×*g* for 2 min at 4°C (*see* **Note 3**).
12. Transfer the supernatant to a clean 1.5 ml centrifuge tube and discard beads.
13. Add either CFTR-specific antibody (M24-1) or epitope tag antibody to the lysate. Typically, concentrations of 1–5 μg/ml for each antibody are sufficient or follow manufacturer's suggestions. Supplement the RIPA buffer with 10% SDS to achieve a final SDS concentration of 0.5%.
14. Incubate for 1 h with rocking at 4°C.
15. Add 30 μl of a 50% slurry of protein Sepharose A/G beads.
16. Incubate for a minimum of 3 h with rocking at 4°C. For convenience overnight incubations at 4°C can be performed.
17. Pellet beads by centrifugation at 5,000×*g* for 2 min at 4°C.
18. Aspirate supernatant and wash three times with 0.5% SDS-RIPA buffer. Centrifuge at 5,000×*g* for 2 min at 4°C after each wash.

3.4. In Vitro Phosphorylation of CFTR

The procedure described below is a general guideline for detecting phosphorylation of immunoprecipitated CFTR by most kinases. Active recombinant protein kinases can be obtained from several companies with high specific activities.

1. Pellet beads by centrifugation at 5,000×*g* for 2 min at 4°C.
2. Aspirate supernatant and wash three times with the appropriate kinase reaction buffer. Centrifuge at 5,000×*g* for 2 min at 4°C after each wash.
3. Resuspend beads in 40 μl of kinase reaction buffer supplemented with the appropriate cofactors if required.
4. Add the desired protein kinase. One microgram of purified recombinant protein kinase is usually recommended (*see* **Note 4**).
5. Start the reaction by adding 20 μCi (2 μl) of ^{32}P-γ-ATP using a 10 μl pipette filter tip to prevent pipette contamination.
6. Incubate the reaction for 30–60 min at room temperature (*see* **Note 4**).
7. Pellet beads by centrifugation at 5,000×*g* for 2 min at 4°C.
8. Aspirate supernatant and wash three times with 1 ml of ice-cold PBS. Centrifuge at 5,000×*g* for 2 min at 4°C after each wash.
9. Pellet beads by centrifugation at 5,000×*g* for 2 min at 4°C and remove any supernatant left using a fine pipette tip such as a gel loading tip.
10. Add 20 μl of Laemmli SDS sample buffer 2X. Mix thoroughly and incubate at 37°C for 30 min. Do not boil samples as this may significantly reduce the immunoblotting signal.

3.5. Western Immunoblotting

1. Using a standard sodium dodecyl sulfate polyacrylamide gel electrophoresis (SDS-PAGE) apparatus and reagents, prepare a 7.5% SDS polyacrylamide gel. Alternatively, precast 7.5 or 4–10% gels can be used.
2. Pellet beads at 14,000×*g* for 2 min at room temperature and carefully load supernatant into stacking gel avoiding any carryover of beads. Load appropriate pre-stained molecular mass standard proteins in separate lanes.
3. Separate proteins using constant current.
4. Transfer proteins to a nitrocellulose membrane in a semidry or wet-transfer apparatus.
5. Rinse membrane with TBS for 5 min with rocking.
6. Block membrane with 5% BSA in TBS with rocking for 1–2 h at room temperature (*see* **Note 5**).
7. Rinse in TBST (TBS + 0.1% Tween-20) for 5 min with rocking.

8. Incubate with primary anti-CFTR antibody (e.g., M3A7) at appropriate dilution (typically 1:500–1:10,000) in TBST + 1% BSA overnight at 4°C with gently rocking. Alternatively, if the CFTR protein is epitope tagged, use an anti-epitope tag primary antibody with overnight incubation at 4°C or an HRP-linked anti-epitope tag antibody for 1 h at room temperature.
9. Rinse four times in TBST for 10 min each time.
10. Incubate with secondary antibody at an appropriate dilution (typically 1:5000) in TBST + 1% BSA for 1 h at room temperature, with rocking. If an HRP-linked anti-epitope tag antibody was used as the primary antibody, proceed to step 12 directly.
11. Rinse four times in TBST for 10 min each time.
12. Expose to chemiluminescence reagents as recommended by the manufacturer, typically 1–5 min.
13. Detect CFTR protein using an image acquisition system such as Molecular Imager VersaDoc MP system with Quantity One software (Bio-Rad) (*see* **Note 6**).
14. Expose membrane to a phosphoscreen to detect protein phosphorylation. Exposure time must be determined empirically depending on protein amount and kinase activity. Detect radiolabeled CFTR using a Phosphorimager (Bio-Rad) (*see* **Note 6**).
15. The intensity of each band in the immunoblot and phosphoimage must be corrected by subtracting out the local background in the same lane. The ratio of the phosphorylation signal to the immunoblot signal in each lane is then compared across conditions to derive relative phosphorylation levels.

3.6. In Vivo Phosphorylation of CFTR

The protocols described below have been developed for detecting CFTR phosphorylation in a cell system (in vivo) in transiently transfected human embryonic kidney cells (HEK-293), mouse fibroblasts (NIH 3T3), or African green monkey kidney cells (COS-7, SV40 transformed). Alternatively, cell lines expressing high amounts of endogenous CFTR, such as human colonic epithelial (T84) cells or human bronchial epithelial (Calu-3) cells, could be used. These cells offer the advantage of being a more physiologically relevant model for the study of growth factor-, hormone-, or osmotic-dependent phosphorylation of CFTR in cells. Cells may be grown non-polarized in tissue culture dishes or polarized in permeable supports. The methodologies described may also be applied to other cell lines with minor modifications to the growth conditions and media requirements depending on the cell type. To determine stimulation-dependent phosphorylation of CFTR, cells should be serum starved before stimulation; the conditions for serum starvation should be determined empirically depending on cell type and growing conditions. Modulation of kinase activity can be achieved by different means; the simplest of them is a pharmacological approach if specific activators and inhibitors are available. However, many protein kinase inhibitors are not very specific, especially when it comes to isoforms of one kinase in particular (e.g., PKC; 12 isoforms) and specific activators are often rare and poorly described. Alternatively, protein kinase activity can be suppressed using specific siRNA or shRNA probes against a particular protein kinase. This approach is particularly helpful in inhibiting specific isoforms of a protein kinase. Coexpression of an active or a kinase-dead mutant is also an efficient means for modulating kinase activity in a more specific manner.

1. For cell culture refer to protocol in **Section 3.1**.
2. For transient transfection refer to protocol in **Section 3.2**.
3. After CFTR transfection allow 36–48 h for expression.
4. Serum starve cells for a period of 4–12 h before experimentation.
5. Wash cells twice with 3 ml of orthophosphate efflux buffer.
6. Add 2 ml of orthophosphate efflux buffer.
7. Add ^{32}P-orthophosphate (300 μCi per dish) and gently tilt and swirl the dish to distribute radioactivity.
8. Place cells in radioactivity shielding container and place in incubator for 2 h.
9. Remove dishes from incubator and carefully remove the radioactive orthophosphate efflux buffer. Discard buffer in appropriate radioactivity-shielded liquid waste container.
10. Wash cells twice with 3 ml of ice-cold TBS. Place cells on ice behind a radioactivity shielding screen.
11. Add 150 μl of RIPA buffer + phosphatase and protease inhibitors and allow lysis for 15 min on ice. Tilt and swirl the dishes twice during the 15-min period to ensure good lysis.
12. Scrape cells/dish with a plastic cell scraper. Place lysate in 0.5 ml centrifuge tube. Repeat for each condition.
13. Centrifuge lysates at 14,000×*g* at 4°C in a microcentrifuge for 30 min. Remove and keep supernatant (place in a 1.5 ml microcentrifuge tube) discard pellet in radioactive waste.
14. Measure protein concentrations of the lysate supernatants for each condition.

15. Make lysate supernatants for all conditions the same volume (1 ml) and protein concentration (1 mg) by adding extra RIPA buffer as needed.
16. Proceed with immunoprecipitation as described in **Section 3.3**.
17. Pellet beads by centrifugation at 5,000×*g* for 2 min at 4°C and remove any supernatant left using a fine pipette tip such as a gel loading tip.
18. Add 20 μl of Laemmli SDS sample buffer 2X. Mix thoughtfully and incubate at 37°C for 30 min.
19. Perform SDS-PAGE, immunoblotting, and radiolabeled CFTR quantification as described in **Section 3.5**.

3.7. Confirmation of Kinase Activity Modulation in Cells

When performing in vivo phosphorylation assays, it is critical to control for modulation of protein kinase activity. To implicate the activation of a particular protein kinase in response to an agonist, one typically should demonstrate that (1) the agonist or stimulus (e.g., growth factors, hormones, and osmolality change) activates the protein kinase; (2) specific protein kinase activators replicate the effect; and (3) specific protein kinase inhibitors block it. Observing consistent effects with down-regulation or knockout of the protein kinase versus overexpression of a catalytically active kinase would strengthen the argument. Stimulation of protein kinase activity in cells can be evaluated by several means such as immunoblotting using an antibody against the activated form of the protein kinase (e.g., antibodies against phospho-PKC isoforms or phospho-Thr172-AMPKα1). If specific antibodies for activated forms of a particular kinase are not available, then direct measurement of protein kinase activity in whole-cell lysates should be performed using a specific peptide substrate for each kinase. Alternatively, activation of a protein kinase can be measured by immunoblotting against a protein known to be a specific substrate for that kinase using specific anti-phosphopeptide antibodies (e.g., phospho-CREB for PKA).

4. Notes

1. The mouse monoclonal anti-CFTR antibody is derived from the mouse hybridoma M24-1 and is available from the American Type Culture Collection (Cat# HB-11947). The hybridoma can be cultured and the supernatant can be collected for direct use in immunoblotting. Alternatively, the supernatant can be purified using HiTRAP protein

G columns (GE Healthcare). The resulting antibody can be used for immunoprecipitation, immunoblotting, and immunohistochemistry.

2. The composition of the reaction buffer must be determined for each specific kinase. As a general rule one should use the kinase buffer recommended by the manufacturer and supplement the buffer with all cofactors that are required to achieve maximal kinase activity (e.g., phospholipids, phosphate nucleotides, and magnesium).
3. Perform all bead centrifugation steps for 2 min at low speed. Centrifuging at speeds greater than $5,000 \times g$ may cause the resin to clump and make resuspension and washes difficult. However, after incubation with Laemmli SDS loading buffer a high centrifugation speed is recommended to produce a compact pellet that facilitates sample collection, preventing the carryover of beads.
4. The amount of protein kinase and the incubation time required for in vitro phosphorylation assays must be determined empirically. In general, high amounts of kinase require shorter incubation times but increase the probability of nonspecific phosphorylation. In contrast, low amounts of kinase may reduce this problem but may require longer incubation times.
5. Although lower backgrounds are often obtained on autoradiographs of immunoblots when using non-fat milk (5% in TBS) as the blocking agent, this is known to contain active phosphatases which can effectively strip the phosphate groups off many proteins. Although this is particularly troublesome when evaluating tyrosine phosphorylation, we favor the use of BSA as the blocking agent to circumvent this issue.
6. To detect CFTR protein amounts and phosphorylation we routinely use the same nitrocellulose membrane. This approach has the advantage that the phosphorylation signal for each sample is then normalized by the amount of CFTR in each lane without requiring running a parallel gel for loading control. However, if an imaging system and/or Phosphorimager system are not available to the investigator we recommend staining the SDS-polyacrylamide gel with Coomassie Blue or a silver stain and then drying the gel. Once dry, take a picture or scan of the stained gel for quantification of CFTR protein. Normally, three prominent bands should be observed after staining corresponding to CFTR (170 kDa), the IgG heavy (50 kDa), and IgG light (25 kDa) chains of the antibody. The dry gel is then exposed to a photographic film for quantification of CFTR phosphorylation by autoradiography.

Acknowledgments

The authors wish to thank Dr. William Reenstra for the past sharing of his laboratory protocols for CFTR in vitro and in vivo phosphorylation. This work was supported by an American Heart Association Postdoctoral Fellowship (AHA 0825540D) to R.A., by the National Institutes of Health (T32 HL007563 to J.D.K. and R01 DK075048 to K.R.H.) and by the Cystic Fibrosis Foundation (HALLOW06P0 to K.R.H.)

References

1. Riordan, J. R., Rommens, J. M., Kerem, B., Alon, N., Rozmahel, R., Grzelczak, Z., et al. (1989) Identification of the cystic fibrosis gene: cloning and characterization of complementary DNA. *Science* **245**, 1066–1073.
2. Rommens, J. M., Iannuzzi, M. C., Kerem, B., Drumm, M. L., Melmer, G., Dean, M., et al. (1989) Identification of the cystic fibrosis gene: chromosome walking and jumping. *Science* **245**, 1059–1065.
3. Carson, M. R., Travis, S. M., and Welsh, M. J. (1995) The two nucleotide-binding domains of cystic fibrosis transmembrane conductance regulator (CFTR) have distinct functions in controlling channel activity. *J. Biol. Chem.* **270**, 1711–1717.
4. Cheng, S. H., Rich, D. P., Marshall, J., Gregory, R. J., Welsh, M. J., and Smith, A. E. (1991) Phosphorylation of the R domain by cAMP-dependent protein kinase regulates the CFTR chloride channel. *Cell* **66**, 1027–1036.
5. Chappe, V., Hinkson, D. A., Zhu, T., Chang, X. B., Riordan, J. R., and Hanrahan, J. W. (2003) Phosphorylation of protein kinase C sites in NBD1 and the R domain control CFTR channel activation by PKA. *J. Physiol.* **548**, 39–52.
6. Jia, Y., Mathews, C. J., and Hanrahan, J. W. (1997) Phosphorylation by protein kinase C is required for acute activation of cystic fibrosis transmembrane conductance regulator by protein kinase A. *J. Biol. Chem.* **272**, 4978–4984.
7. Hallows, K. R., Raghuram, V., Kemp, B. E., Witters, L. A., and Foskett, J. K. (2000) Inhibition of cystic fibrosis transmembrane conductance regulator by novel interaction with the metabolic sensor AMP-activated protein kinase. *J. Clin. Invest.* **105**, 1711–1721.
8. Hallows, K. R., McCane, J. E., Kemp, B. E., Witters, L. A., and Foskett, J. K. (2003) Regulation of channel gating by AMP-activated protein kinase modulates cystic fibrosis transmembrane conductance regulator activity in lung submucosal cells. *J. Biol. Chem.* **278**, 998–1004.
9. Hallows, K. R., Kobinger, G. P., Wilson, J. M., Witters, L. A., and Foskett, J. K. (2003) Physiological modulation of CFTR activity by AMP-activated protein kinase in polarized T84 cells. *Am. J. Physiol. Cell Physiol.* **284**, C1297–C1308.
10. King, J. D., Jr., Fitch, A. C., Lee, J. K., McCane, J. E., Mak, D. O., Foskett, J. K., et al. (2009) AMP-activated protein kinase phosphorylation of the R domain inhibits PKA stimulation of CFTR. *Am. J. Physiol. Cell Physiol.* **297**, C94–C101.
11. Kongsuphol, P., Cassidy, D., Hieke, B., Treharne, K. J., Schreiber, R., Mehta, A., et al. (2009) Mechanistic insight into control of CFTR by AMPK. *J. Biol. Chem.* **284**, 5645–5653.
12. Fischer, H., and Machen, T. E. (1996) The tyrosine kinase p60c-src regulates the fast gate of the cystic fibrosis transmembrane conductance regulator chloride channel. *Biophys. J.* **71**, 3073–3082.
13. Treharne, K. J., Xu, Z., Chen, J. H., Best, O. G., Cassidy, D. M., Gruenert, D. C., et al. (2009) Inhibition of protein kinase CK2 closes the CFTR Cl channel, but has no effect on the cystic fibrosis mutant deltaF508-CFTR. *Cell Physiol. Biochem.* **24**, 347–360.
14. Blaydes, J. P., Vojtesek, B., Bloomberg, G. B., and Hupp, T. R. (2000) The development and use of phospho-specific antibodies to study protein phosphorylation. *Methods Mol. Biol.* **99**, 177–189.
15. Hegedus, T., Aleksandrov, A., Mengos, A., Cui, L., Jensen, T. J., and Riordan, J. R. (2009) Role of individual R domain phos-

phorylation sites in CFTR regulation by protein kinase A. *Biochim. Biophys. Acta* **1788**, 1341–1349.
16. Zhou, H., Watts, J. D., and Aebersold, R. (2001) A systematic approach to the analysis of protein phosphorylation. *Nat. Biotechnol.* **19**, 375–378.
17. Carr, S. A., Huddleston, M. J., and Annan, R. S. (1996) Selective detection and sequencing of phosphopeptides at the femtomole level by mass spectrometry. *Anal. Biochem.* **239**, 180–192.
18. Bloom, N., Sicheritz-Ponten, T., Gupta, R., Gammeltoft, S., and Brunak, S. (2004) Prediction of post-translational glycosylation and phosphorylation of proteins from the amino acid sequence. *Proteomics* **4**, 1633–1649.

Chapter 30

How to Measure CFTR-Dependent Bicarbonate Transport: From Single Channels to the Intact Epithelium

Martin J. Hug, Lane L. Clarke, and Michael A. Gray

Abstract

Bicarbonate serves many functions in our body. It is the predominant buffer maintaining a physiological pH in the blood and within our cells. It is also essential for proper digestion of nutrients and solubilization of complex protein mixtures, such as digestive enzymes and mucins, in epithelial secretions. Transepithelial HCO_3^- transport also drives net fluid secretion in many epithelial tissues including those in the gastrointestinal and reproductive tracts as well as the airways. Indeed, defective bicarbonate secretion is a hallmark of the pathophysiology in the pancreas of most patients suffering from cystic fibrosis. Some, but not all, disease-causing mutations in the CF gene lead to impaired bicarbonate transport when expressed in heterologous systems. Recently developed pharmacological modulators of mutant CFTR have demonstrated an ability to activate chloride transport but little is known about whether they also increase the secretion of bicarbonate. It is therefore essential to assay bicarbonate transport when studying the effect of small molecules on CFTR function. However, due to the chaotropic nature of the ion, the measurement of the absolute bicarbonate concentration and its permeability through CFTR is far from trivial. In this chapter we will review some of the techniques available to measure bicarbonate transport through single ion channels, individual cells, and intact epithelial layers.

Key words: Bicarbonate transport, epithelial cells, cystic fibrosis, CFTR, patch clamp technique, pH stat, Ussing chambers, intracellular pH, fluorescent dyes.

1. Introduction

1.1. Chemistry of HCO_3^-

One problem faced by researchers working with HCO_3^--based salt solutions is the fact that HCO_3^- is a volatile buffer and without careful control of experimental conditions large variations in both pH and concentration can occur. When CO_2 dissolves in water it

M.D. Amaral, K. Kunzelmann (eds.), *Cystic Fibrosis*, Methods in Molecular Biology 741,
DOI 10.1007/978-1-61779-117-8_30,

forms carbonic acid (H_2CO_3), which in turn may dissociate into HCO_3^- and H^+ ions (Equation **1**).

$$CO_2 + H_2O \leftrightarrow H_2CO_3 \leftrightarrow HCO_3^- + H^+ \qquad [1]$$

Due to the reversible nature of this reaction, it is easily appreciated that the HCO_3^- ion is very volatile and not easily accessible to direct measurement. HCO_3^- is the most important buffer in our body fluids and disturbances in our buffering systems can result in severe metabolic disorders. In order to estimate HCO_3^- concentrations, several approaches have been developed, but the most widely used is to directly measure the actual CO_2 concentration (pCO_2) and the respective pH using ion-sensitive electrodes.

From these two parameters, the Henderson–Hasselbalch equation (Equation **2**) best describes the relation between HCO_3^-, pCO_2, and pH, respectively:

$$\mathrm{pH} = \mathrm{p}K_\mathrm{a} + \log_{10}\frac{\mathrm{A}^-}{\mathrm{HA}} \qquad [2]$$

For the HCO_3^-/CO_2 system a pK_a of 6.1 can be assumed; 'A^-' corresponds to the actual HCO_3^- and 'HA' to the CO_2 concentration that can be derived from the partial pressure for CO_2 multiplied by the solubility constant (0.03 mmHg^{-1}).

If we fill in these parameters the equation reads

$$\mathrm{pH} = 6.1 + \log_{10}\frac{[HCO_3^-]}{0.03pCO_2(\mathrm{mmHg})} \qquad [3]$$

Now we can solve for the concentration of HCO_3^-:

$$[HCO_3^-] = 0.03pCO_2(\mathrm{mmHg})10^{\mathrm{pH}-6.1} \qquad [4]$$

Clearly, this equation cannot fully account for the several buffer systems present in a physiological environment. For most purposes, however, Equation **4** is sufficient enough to make assumptions about changes occurring in the acid/base system of a cell or its environment once pH and pCO_2 can be determined. One important outcome of the above is that any experimental solution that contains HCO_3^- will have to be gassed with CO_2 in order to stabilize pH. If this is not done then pH will vary during the course of the experiment and this will have to be taken into account. In addition, if pH is required to be kept constant but [HCO_3^-] varied then different concentrations of CO_2 will be required (*see* **Note 1**).

2. Materials

2.1. Patch Clamp

2.1.1. Introduction to the Patch Clamp Technique

The patch clamp (PC) technique is the gold-standard method to directly determine the transport of any ion of interest through CFTR. An excellent introduction to the equipment required and theory of the PC technique can be found in the book by Molleman (1). The PC technique measures the electric current, which equals the number of ions flowing per second, as they flow through the CFTR pore. Measuring ion flow through either a single CFTR channel or multiple channels requires that a high-resistance seal be obtained between a glass microelectrode (patch pipette) and the plasma membrane of the cell. After the patch pipette is carefully attached to the surface of the cell (bathed in a saline solution) a high-resistance (GΩ) seal is then formed between the glass pipette and membrane by applying slight negative pressure to the back of the pipette. The high resistance of this seal makes it possible to electronically clamp the voltage across the patch of membrane enclosed by the glass pipette (hence the name patch clamp) as well as measure the electrical current that flows across the membrane patch. The GΩ seal also provides mechanical stability to the recording. A high-gain operational amplifier is connected to the patch pipette via a Ag/$AgCl_2$ electrode, which is inserted into the patch pipette filling solution. An additional electrode is also placed in the bath solution to act as a ground electrode which completes the simple equivalent circuit as depicted in **Fig. 30.1a**. The current flowing through the ion channel when it opens is measured as a voltage drop across a feedback resistor (FR). The FR has a resistance of 50 GΩ allowing very small

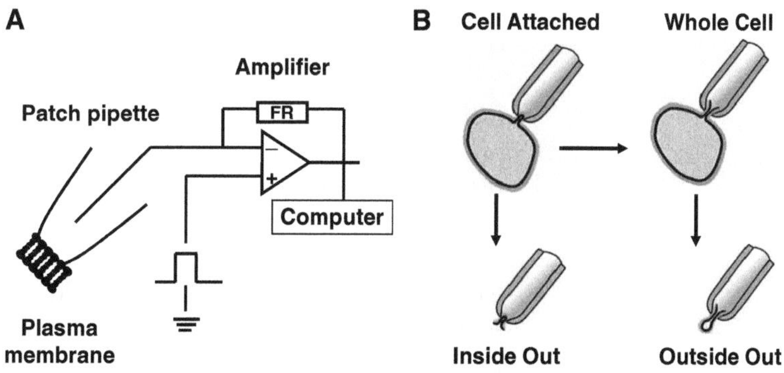

Fig. 30.1. (**a**) Schematic of the patch clamp recording circuit. (**b**) Schematic of the four possible recording configurations of the patch clamp technique after formation of a high-resistance seal between the patch pipette and the cell.

currents ($\sim 10^{-12}$ A) to be resolved. For measurement of a large number of channels then a lower FR is normally used.

There are four different recording configurations of the PC technique (**Fig. 30.1b**). Formation of a high-resistance seal between the patch pipette and the cell produces the cell-attached configuration. From here two other configurations can then be obtained. Excision of the patch of membrane from the cell creates the inside-out configuration, where the cytoplasmic face of the plasma membrane is exposed to the bath solution. Alternatively, disruption of the small patch of membrane enclosed by the patch pipette by hard suction or high membrane voltage (zapping) creates the whole-cell recording configuration. In this case the contents of the pipette filling solution diffuse into the cell and exchange with the normal cell constituents. In this configuration the whole cell is voltage clamped and resulting whole-cell currents reflect the contribution from all the channels in the cell. Finally, after obtaining the whole-cell configuration the outside-out configuration can be created by slowly excising the patch pipette from the cell. Here the extracellular face of the plasma membrane is exposed to the bathing solution. The cell-attached and whole-cell configurations therefore study the behaviour of CFTR Cl^- channels in the intact cell, whereas the excised inside- and outside-out configurations monitor CFTR in isolated membrane patches. Apart from whole cell, the other configurations are generally used to make single-channel recordings. However, in cell expressing very high numbers of CFTR channels large macroscopic currents from a small patch of membrane can be obtained. In principle, all four configurations permit direct measurements of HCO_3^- transport through CFTR. For a more detailed discussion of the different configurations, refer to (1).

Patch clamp amplifiers: Patch clamp amplifiers are built by a number of manufacturers, i.e. Alembic, Axon Instruments, Dagan, and HEKA to name a few. Their products differ not only in price but also in the mode of operation. Some patch clamp amplifiers are completely computer controlled (i.e. HEKA EPC-10), the majority are not.

Patch pipettes: These are prepared from borosilicate glass using a patch pipette puller. One of the most reliable pipette pullers is manufactured by Sutter Instruments. For single-channel recordings pipette resistances should be between 4 and 10 MΩ when filled with a normal saline solution. For whole-cell recording or for macroscopic current recordings, lower resistances need to be employed (2–5 MΩ). Generally patch pipettes do not need to be coated with an insulating material such as Sylgard. After pulling, the tip of pipette generally needs to be firepolished to smooth the tip which improves sealing to cell membranes. Pipette polishers can be bought from a number of companies such as Narishge and Digitimer.

Micromanipulators: These are essential in order to finely position the patch pipette onto the surface of the cell to obtain a seal onto the plasma membrane. Manipulators need to be mechanically stable and not drift with time. Again a variety of manufacturers provide suitable manipulators including Scientifica, Sutter, and Narishige. Some are motorized while others use piezoelectric devices to function.

Microscope: Inverted microscopes are required since access to the cells from above is needed in order to attach the patch pipette to the cells. Optically, phase-contrast microscopes are generally used as they produce the best image of the cell plasma membrane for seal formation, but other microscopes such as DIC are also suitable. A minimum of ×200, but preferably ×400 magnification is needed. Most major manufacturers produce suitable microscopes (Nikon, Olympus, Zeiss).

Anti-vibration table: The microscope plus cell perfusion chamber and micromanipulator, all need to be isolated from mechanical disturbances caused by vibrations from external sources. Isolation (anti-vibration) tables suitable for this purpose are sold by Narishige, Heka, TMC, and Digitimer.

2.1.2. Solutions

In order to measure ionic currents that flow through CFTR, cells are bathed in an extracellular or bath solution (pH 7.2–7.4) while the patch pipette is also filled with a saline solution (pH 7.0–7.2). However, the composition of these solutions for a typical patch clamp experiment involving CFTR varies considerably and depends on the cell type and the endogenous complement of ion channels. In a 'typical' experiment (*see* **Fig. 30.3**) a quasi-physiological NaCl-rich bath solution of the following composition can be used; in mM: 145 NaCl, 4.5 KCl, 2 $CaCl_2$, 1 $MgCl_2$, 10 HEPES, and 5 glucose (pH 7.4 with NaOH). The osmolarity of the external solution should be adjusted to 300 mOsm/L. For HCO_3^- containing solutions, NaCl can be replaced with equimolar $NaHCO_3$. However, as indicated in **Section 1.1**, pH will vary unless the solution is gassed with an appropriate CO_2/O_2 mixture. Having HEPES present will stabilize pH to some extent but can be removed (*see* **Note 2**). A standard pipette solution containing (in mM): 110 CsCl, 2 $MgCl_2$, 5.0 ethylene glycol-bis(*b*-aminoethyl ether)-*N*,*N*,*N'*,*N'*-tetraacetic acid (EGTA), 10 HEPES, and 1 Na_2ATP (pH 7.2 with CsOH). MgATP is required in order for CFTR to open. The osmolarity of the pipette solution should be ~20–40 mOsm/L less than the bath solution to avoid cell swelling, but again depends on cell type. Agents to replace large cations are listed under **Note 3**.

2.2. pH Stat

2.2.1. Introduction to pH Stat

The pH stat technique is used to measure the serosal-to-mucosal flux of HCO_3^- $\left(J_{sm}^{HCO_3^-}\right)$ across an epithelium. Application of the pH stat method for this purpose was largely advanced using the Ussing chamber technique for studies of ex vivo mucosal preparations and cultured epithelial monolayers that retain tight junction integrity. The Ussing chamber technique including tissue preparation, equipment, and theory has been recently reviewed in detail (2). As depicted schematically in **Fig. 30.2a**, the mucosa (or an epithelial monolayer) is secured between two halves of an Ussing

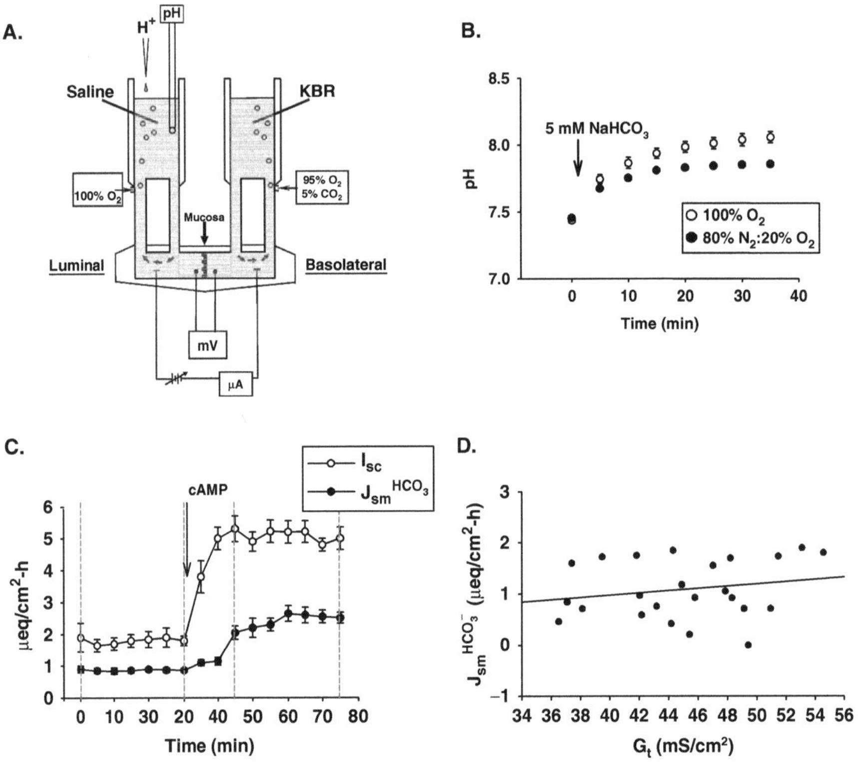

Fig. 30.2. (**a**) Schematic diagram of an Ussing chamber apparatus adapted for pH stat measurement. The mucosa (*arrow*) separates two halves of the Ussing chamber. In this case, the solution bathing the basolateral side is Kreb's bicarbonate Ringers (KBR) solution which is gassed with 95% O_2:5% CO_2. The luminal side is bathed with an unbuffered solution that is similar in composition to KBR and gassed with 100% O_2. The pH of the luminal bath is measured and continuously titrated to a target pH (7.0–7.4) by acid addition, e.g. 5 mM HCl. The rate of acid addition is considered equivalent to the rate of HCO_3^- secretion. The spontaneous V_t of the mucosa is clamped to 0 mV to allow the measurement of G_t and I_{SC}. (**b**) Time course of the pH change resulting from the addition of 5 mM $NaHCO_3$ to an unbuffered luminal solution gassed with either 100% O_2 or 80% N_2:20% O_2 ($n = 3$). (**c**) Time course of $J_{sm}^{HCO_3^-}$ and I_{SC} of wild-type murine duodena before and after cAMP stimulation (10 μM forskolin) of electrogenic HCO_3^- secretion ($n = 6$). *Vertical dashed lines* indicate the beginning and end of 30-min flux periods (basal and cAMP stimulation). (**d**) Relationship between the basal $J_{sm}^{HCO_3^-}$ and the G_t of wild-type mouse duodenum.

chamber, so that the epithelium separates the luminal (mucosal) and basolateral (serosal) solutions. Gas lift circulates and mixes the solution on each side of the mucosa and water-jacketed reservoirs adjust the temperature of the solution (e.g. to 37°C).

The application of pH stat requires the removal of buffers (HCO_3^-, PO_4^-) from the luminal bath and maintenance of a target pH (typically pH 7.0 or 7.4) by titration of the net HCO_3^- equivalents appearing in the luminal bath. The rate of acid equivalent addition necessary to maintain the target pH is assumed equivalent to $J_{sm}^{HCO_3^-}$. Kreb's bicarbonate Ringer's (KBR) is typically used for the basolateral solution and contains physiological levels of CO_2 and HCO_3^- serving as the source for HCO_3^- uptake via basolateral $NaHCO_3^-$ cotransporters or through the hydration of CO_2 (*see* **Section 2.2.2**). A significant advantage of the Ussing chamber technique for pH stat is that the spontaneous electrical potential (V_t) of the mucosa can be clamped to zero (i.e. short circuited) allowing measurement of the short-circuit current I_{sc}, which is equivalent to the algebraic sum of all electrogenic transport processes, and the transepithelial conductance (G_t), which provides a measure of the paracellular conductance. In a leaky mucosa like the small intestine, greater than 90% of G_t is due to paracellular conductance (3). Constant monitoring of the G_t is necessary because most pH stat experiments have a standing mucosal-to-serosal HCO_3^- gradient across the epithelium which will introduce a passive contribution to $J_{sm}^{HCO_3^-}$ if G_t increases significantly (*see* **Section 3.2**). The Ussing chamber pH stat technique is useful for $J_{sm}^{HCO_3^-}$ measurement in native mucosa, but two-dimensional monolayers of cultured cells have about one-tenth the number of cells/cm^2. Therefore, special effort is required to grow confluent polarized monolayers over greater surface areas, increase epithelial differentiation, or reduce perfusate volume to improve detection of pH changes.

2.2.2. Solutions

The unbuffered solution of the luminal bath in pH stat experiments is typically saline solution similar in composition and identical in osmolarity to the basolateral solution. The ideal replacement for HCO_3^- and H_2PO_4/HPO_4 in the luminal solution is a Na^+ salt (to avoid a transepithelial Na^+ gradient) that does not have buffering capacity or alter transport function. These characteristics are uncommon for most non-toxic Na^+ salts. NaCl can be used to replace HCO_3^- and PO_4 but this introduces a mucosal-to-serosal Cl^- concentration gradient (~20 mM) that must be considered if voltage clamping is used. Another alternative is using the Na^+ salt of a membrane-impermeable anion such as gluconate$^-$ or isethionate$^-$. Gluconate has a low p*K*a (3.86) and demonstrates significant buffering capacity at target pH of 7.0 or 7.4. In contrast, Na^+ isethionate is an alkali salt that at

Table 30.1
Example of solution composition for pH stat experiments

Chemical	Luminal unbuffered solution (mM)	Basolateral KBR solution (mM)
NaCl	109.8	115.0
$NaHCO_3$	–	25.0
Na isethionate	34.0	–
KCl	5.2	–
K_2HPO_4	–	2.4
KH_2PO_4	–	0.4
$CaCl_2$	1.2	1.2
$MgCl_2$	1.2	1.2
Glucose	–	10.0

low concentrations has a pH of ~8 and little buffering capacity at pH 7.0–7.4. The composition of an unbuffered luminal solution in which Na^+ isethionate is used to replace HCO_3^- and $HPO_4^{2-}/H_2PO_4^-$ in KBR is given in **Table 30.1**.

2.2.3. Gasses

The titration of HCO_3^- in an unbuffered saline solution for pH stat requires constant displacement of CO_2 (solubility ~1.1 g/kg water, at 37°C) with a less soluble gas to minimize the pH effects due to spontaneous hydration of CO_2. This is accomplished by vigorous gassing of the luminal solution with either 100% O_2 or an 80% N_2:20% O_2 mixture (simulates air) to minimize the partial pressure of CO_2 in solution. Oxygen has aqueous solubility of ~0.03 g/kg water at 37°C, whereas nitrogen gas has aqueous solubility of ~0.01 g/kg water, at 37°C. Physically, an 80% N_2:20% O_2 mixture has lower solubility and is more efficient than 100% O_2 at displacing CO_2. As shown in **Fig. 30.2b**, a faster return to steady-state pH can be demonstrated after addition of a small amount of $NaHCO_3$ to an unbuffered solution that is gassed with 80% N_2:20% O_2. However, this small difference cannot be appreciated in a pH stat experiment during a 20- to 30-min steady-state flux period. In a comparison of the two different luminal gases, differences in the cAMP-stimulated $J_{sm}^{HCO_3^-}$ of murine duodenum were not apparent over a 30-min flux period (100% O_2 $\Delta J_{sm}^{HCO_3^-} = 0.6 \pm 0.1$ vs. 80% N_2:20% O_2 $\Delta J_{sm}^{HCO_3^-} = 0.7 \pm 0.3$ μeq/cm^2·h; $n = 4$). Standard Ussing chambers are relatively inefficient for gas dissolution due to the small surface area of large gas bubbles for gas lift but this can be improved by modifying the gas ports to produce smaller bubbles, e.g. using small diameter polyethylene tubing.

2.2.4. Titration

$J_{sm}^{HCO_3^-}$ is measured by the rate of acid equivalent addition that is necessary to maintain the target pH of the luminal bath during a timed flux period. For intestinal preparations with an exposed surface area of 0.25 cm^2, a titrant concentration of 5 mM HCl is appropriate. The HCl titrant is freshly formulated in a saline solution to approximate the osmolarity of the luminal bath and degassed under vacuum before use to minimize dissolved CO_2. Titration of the bath to target pH is accomplished with either an automatic titration burette system (e.g. Radiometer America PHM290 pH stat controller/ABU900 autoburette, 2 ml volume) or by manual pipetting using an extended pipette tip. Both methods yield similar results in a 20- to 30-min steady-state flux period. Measurement of the luminal solution pH during the experiment involves the introduction of a pH electrode into the luminal reservoir about 1 cm below the fluid surface. A small diameter glass pH electrode (EW-05990-30, Cole-Parmer, Vernon Hills, IL, USA) provides rapid measurement, minimizes the mucosal-to-serosal hydrostatic pressure due to volume displacement in the luminal reservoir, and allows sufficient room for the placement of acid titrant delivery tube or pipettor.

2.2.5. Mucus Removal

Mucus production continues for >1 h in ex vivo preparations and accumulation on the mucosal surface can affect drug access to the epithelium (4) and pH changes in the luminal solution. Chemical agents such as *N*-acetylcysteine and dithiothreitol (DTT, 1 10 mM, 15 min exposure) facilitate physical removal of mucus, although mucus will continue to accumulate, especially in the crypts (5). DTT pretreatment does not appreciably affect basal $J_{sm}^{HCO_3^-}$ or I_{sc} of the intestine, but introduces the problem of non-specific reduction of disulfide bonds in membrane proteins. Other methods include pretreatment with papain, a cysteine protease (0.1 U/ml, 30 min), and maximal stimulation of mucus secretion using muscarinic agonists (e.g. carbachol 250 μg/kg, i.p.) prior to killing of the animal (4–6).

To avoid the non-specific effects of chemical or pharmacological agents, physical removal of accumulated mucus is an acceptable practice. Approximately 15 min after an intestinal preparation is mounted in the Ussing chamber, the luminal solution reservoir is disconnected to allow access to the luminal surface of the mucosa. The mucosal surface is rinsed with a gentle stream of warmed unbuffered solution applied through large bore tubing (1.5 mm, I.D.) until the mucus is visibly detached (approximately 5 s). The experiment is resumed with fresh luminal unbuffered solution after flushing the chamber and reservoir. In a direct comparison, this method was found to be superior to DTT or carbachol pretreatment by yielding larger cAMP-stimulated $J_{sm}^{HCO_3^-}$

responses and glucose-stimulated I_{sc} responses in murine intestine (unpublished observations).

2.3. Fluorimetric Techniques

The measurement of intracellular pH (pH_i) has been revolutionized by the introduction of fluorescent indicators such as the fluorescein derivative 2′,7′-bis(carboxyethyl)-5(6)-carboxyfluorescein (BCECF) (7). BCECF can be injected into cells as the free acid or added to the incubation medium as the acetoxymethyl (AM) ester (8), a method by which the molecule permeates the cell membrane and remains trapped in the cytosol. The dye has an emission maximum at 526 nm when excited at 490 nm. Closer inspection of the spectral properties of BCECF reveals that the pH dependence of the dye can be observed when excited at 490 nm. At 430 nm, however, the emission intensity is largely pH independent.

In addition to the dye, microfluorimetry of pH_i requires three more components: a source for the excitation light, a means to immobilize the cells or tissue, respectively, and a detection device to collect the emitted fluorescence. In order to yield sufficient spatial resolution a microscope is often used as central part of this machinery.

Excitation pathway: high-intensity xenon or mercury lamps can be utilized as illumination source. These lamps provide a light which is broad and evenly distributed. The desired wavelength can be selected using bandpass filters or by a variable wavelength monochromator. For a ratiometric measurement fast switching of the spectrum in the illumination pathway is necessary. This can be achieved using a rotating wheel that holds at least two filters. A computer that also monitors the intensity in the emission pathway usually controls the position of the respective filter. When using a monochromator, the latter is set to alternating positions of the internal gate that selects the individual wavelength. More recently confocal imaging has been introduced into physiological experiments. However, an extensive description of the use of optically tuned lasers to record changes in pH_i is beyond the scope of this chapter.

It is apparent that due to the inherent properties of the fluorophore the emission has to be separated from the excitation pathway. This is most challenging when a technique is chosen that is called epifluorescence. In this configuration both the excitation and the emission light travel through the same objective. The key to the optics in an epifluorescence apparatus is the separation of the illumination light from the fluorescence emission emanating from the sample. In order to obtain either an image of the emission without excessive background illumination or a measurement of the fluorescence emission without background ‘contamination’, the optical elements used to separate these two light components must be very efficient. For this purpose a dichroic mirror is used to separate the excitation and emission light paths. The dichroic mirror's special reflective properties allow it to separate the two light paths. Each dichroic mirror has a set wavelength value – called the transition wavelength value – which is the wavelength of 50% transmission. The mirror reflects wavelengths of light below the transition wavelength value and transmits wavelengths above this value. This property accounts for the name given to this mirror (*dichroic*, two colour). Ideally, the wavelength of the dichroic mirror is chosen to be between the wavelengths used for excitation and emission. For BCECF a dichroic mirror with a cut-off wavelength of 510–520 nm is typically chosen.

Emission pathway: In order to more specifically select the emission wavelength of the light emitted from the sample and to remove traces of excitation light, emission filters can be placed beneath the dichroic mirror or in front of the detection device. When measuring BCECF epifluorescence a 530–540 nm emission filter can be recommended.

Detection: Even though a fluorescence signal emitted at 530 nm can be picked up by the naked eye, a researcher will hardly judge pH changes by simply looking through the ocular of his microscope. To monitor emission intensity several approaches can be chosen.

Photomultiplier (PMT): a PMT is an extremely sensitive detector of even the least traces of light. It uses a cathode inside an evacuated tube and converts photons into electrical signals. The voltage generated by the PMT is proportional to the intensity of the detected light. PMTs have a high temporal but hardly any spatial resolution. The latter can be improved by placing a pinhole or slit in front of the PMT by which a region of interest can be defined.

Photodiode array (PDA): PDA consists of multiple discrete photodiode elements, formed in a linear or matrix arrangement and usually placed on an integrated circuit chip. Diode arrays having numbers of elements ranging from 128 to 1024 and even up to 4,096 are nowadays available. Due to the inherent properties of the photodiode PDA require a relative high light level.

Charge-coupled device (CCD) camera: a CCD is designed to convert optical brightness into electrical amplitude signals similar to the PMT or the PDA and requires less of an electrical charge than PDA. CCDs are ideal for low-light-level detection.

The signal generated by either device can be converted into digital values using an analogue–digital converter connected to a computer. Custom-made or commercially available software (i.e. Metafluor®, Molecular Devices, Sunnyvale, CA, USA) can be used for analysis and documentation of the results.

3. Methods

3.1. Direct Measurement of HCO_3^- Transport by CFTR Using the Patch Clamp Technique

3.1.1. Introduction to Ion Channel Terminology and Practice

For studies of CFTR HCO_3^- permeability the patch clamp amplifier is normally used in the voltage-clamp mode. Here the amount of electric current (in amp), denoted 'i' for a single channel or capital 'I' for measurements from many (N) channels, is measured at a fixed membrane voltage (V). By convention all voltages are referenced to the outside of the cell and are measured in millivolts. In addition, by convention positive charge leaving the cell (equivalent electrically to negative charge entering the cell) equates to positive or *outward* current. *Inward* current represents negative charge leaving the cell. From these measurements a current–voltage relationship (i/I–V) can be constructed. For both single-channel and multi-channel recordings, the i/I–V plot for CFTR is linear when Cl^- gradients are equal on both sides of the membrane. From the i/I–V plot two different parameters can be obtained. The first is conductance which is a direct measure of the number of ions flowing through the channel. Conductance is the reciprocal of resistance and has units of siemens. From Ohm's law $R = V/I$ and therefore conductance ($1/R$) is obtained from the slope of the I–V plot (or for single-channel recordings, the i–V plot). However, this is only valid when there is a linear relationship between current and voltage (in other words conductance is voltage independent and the channel is ohmic). In practice, especially with mixed solutions of anions, the i/I–V plot may not be linear. In these cases chord conductances are generally calculated which is obtained from the following relationship:

$$G = \frac{\Delta i/I}{\Delta V} \qquad [5]$$

where G = conductance.

The second parameter is the membrane potential at which there is zero current flow (E_{rev}). Both these parameters give important information about absolute rates of ion transport (electrodiffusion) through CFTR as well as the relative selectivity of CFTR to different ions (*see* below).

3.1.2. How to Measure HCO_3^- Permeability and Conductance Selectivity of CFTR from a Whole-Cell Recording Experiment

Anion selectivity is often determined by exposing channels to different anions and measuring the E_{rev} and conductance from the $i/I–V$ relationship. In most cases selectivity is usually determined under biioinic conditions where Cl^- is present on one side of the channel and anion X^- on the other. This can be done using three of the four PC recording configurations but cannot be achieved for cell-attached patches, since the concentration inside the cell cannot (easily) be controlled. With identical Cl^- on both sides of the channel E_{rev} will be 0 mV. If all the Cl^- on one side is then changed for X^-, then the relative permeability (P) of X to Cl is given by the Goldman–Hodgkin–Katz voltage equation:

$$\frac{P_X}{P_{Cl}} = e^{\frac{\Delta E_{rev} F}{RT}} \qquad [6]$$

where ΔE_{rev} is the change in reversal potential following replacement of Cl^- with X^-, F is the Faraday's constant, R is the gas constant, and T is the temperature in kelvin.

In practice PC experiments usually require some Cl^- to be present in both patch pipette and bath solutions in order to achieve stable recordings. Under these conditions the concentration of all anion species needs to be considered. In this case,

$$\frac{P_X}{P_{Cl}} = \frac{[Cl]_{in} - e^{\frac{E_{rev} F}{RT}} [Cl]_{out}}{e^{\frac{E_{rev} F}{RT}} [X]_{out} - [X]_{in}} \qquad [7]$$

where 'out' and 'in' represent the concentrations of Cl^- or anion X^- in the extracellular and intracellular solutions. Note that electrical recordings made under conditions with two different anions may result in a liquid junction potential being generated between the two different solutions. These potentials can be quite large depending on the anions used, and need to be corrected for (*see* (9), for further discussion), or serious errors in relative permeability values can arise.

As described above, CFTR conductance is obtained from $i/I–V$ plots. In the case where Cl^- is present in one solution and anion X^- in the other solution then conductance can be obtained for each ion by focussing on the part of the $i/I–V$ plot that corresponds to current carried by that ion.

An example of this type of experiment is illustrated in **Fig. 30.3**. These data are taken from a whole-cell recording made from a single pancreatic duct cell containing thousands of CFTR channels. The bath solution initially contained an NaCl-rich solution (total [Cl] of 155 mM) and the pipette (filling) solution a CsCl-rich solution (total [Cl] of 114 mM) as depicted in the cartoon (**Fig. 30.3a**). Whole-cell currents (**Fig. 30.3b**) were recorded in the absence of stimulants (control) and then

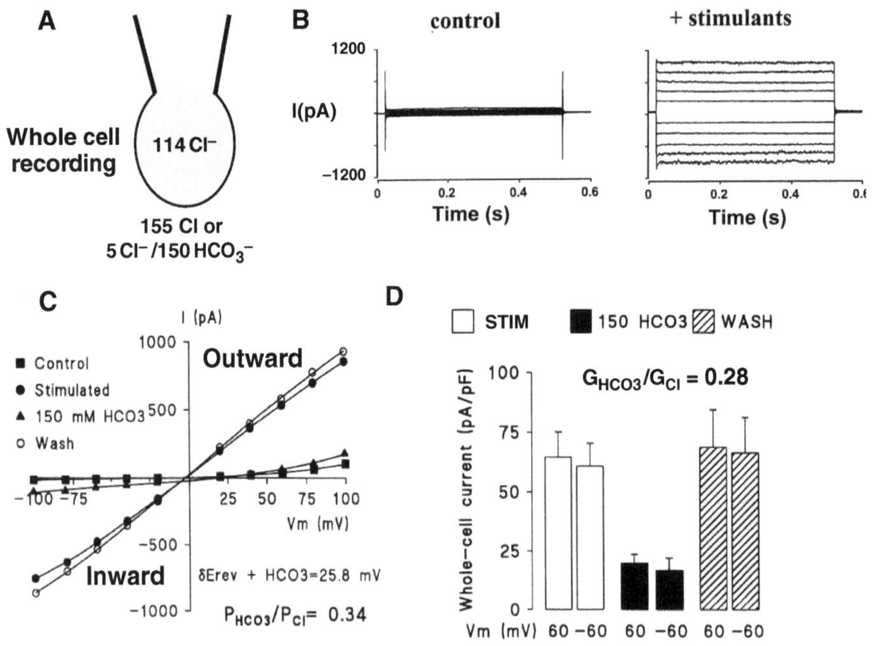

Fig. 30.3. (**a**) shows a schematic of the whole-cell recording configuration. Bath solution was (in mM) NaCl (145), KCl (4.5), $CaCl_2$ (2.0), $MgCl_2$ (1.0), HEPES (10.0), and glucose (5) (pH 7.4) with NaOH. For the high HCO_3^- solution NaCl and $CaCl_2$ were replaced with 150 $NaHCO_3$. Pipette solution: CsCl (110), $MgCl_2$ (2.0), HEPES (10.0), EGTA (5.0), Na_2ATP (1.0) (pH 7.2) with CsOH. (**b**) shows currents in the absence of stimulants (control) and then after forskolin exposure (stimulants). Whole-cell currents were measured between ±100 mV in steps of 20 mV, with each step lasting 0.5 s. Between the voltage steps the membrane potential was held at 0 mV. (**c**) shows *I–V* relationships for control (*solid squares*), stimulated (*solid circles*), after Cl^- was replaced by HCO_3^- (*solid triangles*), and washout (*open circles*). (**d**) plots the current density (pA/pF). For further details, *see* (11).

after forskolin exposure to raise cAMP levels and activate CFTR (stimulants). The whole-cell currents were measured between ±100 mV in steps of 20 mV, with each step lasting 0.5 s. Between the voltage steps the membrane potential was held at 0 mV. The resulting currents were then overlaid for illustration purposes. **Figure 30.3c** shows the resulting *I–V* relationships for the control data (solid squares) and the stimulated data (solid circles). The bath solution was then changed, so that most of the Cl^- was replaced by HCO_3^- (plus forskolin) and an *I–V* again obtained (**Fig. 30.3c**, solid triangles). Under these conditions E_{rev} shifted by a total of 26 mV in the positive direction giving a P_{HCO_3}/P_{Cl} of 0.34, calculated using Equation 7, which is similar to published values (10–17). The HCO_3^- was then washed out and replaced with the original Cl^--rich solution (open circles). In terms of conductance it is also very clear from the *I–V* plots that outward HCO_3^- currents (i.e. inward flow of HCO_3^- ions from the bath into the cell) are markedly lower than outward Cl^- currents. In order to compare the relative outward conductance for the two anions, the size of the current at E_{rev} to ±60 mV was measured, in order to compare conductance at the same electrochemical driving force (10, 11). **Figure 30.3d** plots the current density, where currents have been normalized to cell size (using capacitance which is measured in farads) and expressed in pA/pF, using the above method. It can be seen that when most of the Cl^- is replaced with HCO_3^- outward current density decreases. The calculated conductance (I/V) is reduced by ~70% compared to Cl^- ($G_{HCO_3^-}/G_{Cl^-}$ 0.28).

An additional effect is also quite clearly observed in these experiments; inward currents carried by Cl^- ions leaving the cell are reduced by a similar extent. This result is not predicted for a channel in which ion movement (flow) is independent of the presence of other ions and particularly where $[Cl^-]$ is constant (inside the cell). Although there is evidence that CFTR displays multi-ion pore behaviour (12, 18, but *see* 19) and thus interactions can occur within the pore between different permeant ions, the reason for this large drop in conductance when Cl^- is reduced is not likely to be for this reason. Indeed it appears that the drop in conductance is due to a substantial alteration in the gating (or open probability) of CFTR channels when external Cl^- is reduced and not because of a major decrease in transport of Cl^- ions through the channel (11, 13). Furthermore, this reduction in the open-state probability of CFTR is specific to changes in *extracellular* Cl^- concentration. For this reason measurements of relative permselectivity and/or conductance selectivity of CFTR for different anions need to be aware of this confounding effect of external $[Cl^-]$ (11, 13).

3.2. Measurement of Transepithelial HCO_3^- Secretion in Tissues and Monolayers Using the pH Stat Technique

After an epithelium has been mounted in the Ussing chamber for a pH stat experiment, an equilibration period is necessary for the system to attain the proper temperature and allow time for drug action, e.g. 20 min for tetrodotoxin neural blockade. At this point, mucus can be removed manually and the luminal solution is refreshed before positioning the pH electrode and titrant delivery tube. Whether titrating by hand or using an automatic titrator, it is important to position the delivery of the acid titrant below the pH electrode and near the reservoir bottom, so that the titrant is immediately circulated and mixed with the luminal solution. Patience becomes a key element when allowing the epithelium to attain a steady-state rate of net HCO_3^- secretion or, under some conditions, net H^+ secretion. Typically, the initial pH of the freshened luminal bath is slightly below the target pH, possibly due to ambient CO_2 absorption. Rather than adjusting the pH to its target value with NaOH, the reproducibility of the $J_{sm}^{HCO_3^-}$ measurement is improved by allowing time for the preparation to attain the target pH by endogenous HCO_3^- secretion. Although this practice may require ~30 min, rapid titration with

NaOH often results in a prolonged cessation of HCO_3^- secretion in intestinal preparations. After attaining target pH, $J_{sm}^{HCO_3^-}$ is measured over a 20- or 30-min time period with the starting point determined retrospectively. The total length of the experiment is limited by the viability of the tissue and the magnitude of mucus accumulation. Thus, it may be more acceptable in practice to restrict comparisons to single 30-min $J_{sm}^{HCO_3^-}$ flux periods. If two or more flux periods are warranted, then mucus removal may be necessary between flux periods.

It should be recognized that changes in the measured $J_{sm}^{HCO_3^-}$ are artificially delayed by the time necessary for each acid addition to mix within the luminal solution and attain a steady-state pH. The error is illustrated by the experiment shown in **Fig. 30.2c** where measurement of cAMP-stimulated electrogenic $J_{sm}^{HCO_3^-}$ is delayed by ~5–10 min relative to the instantaneous measurement of I_{sc}. Each titrant addition also causes a pH excursion about the target pH as mixing occurs (2). Therefore, $J_{sm}^{HCO_3^-}$ measurement is best performed over a 20- to 30-min flux period once a steady rate of titrant addition has been achieved. Reporting single time points (e.g. 'peak' $J_{sm}^{HCO_3^-}$) may misrepresent the data because titration error is greater during rapid changes in HCO_3^- secretion.

Comparing steady-state periods of $J_{sm}^{HCO_3^-}$ also simplifies the interpretation of a pH stat experiment. For studies where CFTR provides electrogenic HCO_3^- secretion (for example, **Fig. 30.2c**), the magnitude of the I_{sc} averaged over the flux period can be directly compared to $J_{sm}^{HCO_3^-}$ by expressing the I_{sc} ($\mu A/cm^2$) as C/cm^2 h and dividing by the Faraday constant (C/eq) to calculate univalent ion flux units. This reduces to $I_{sc} = \mu A/cm^2 \times 0.0373 = \mu eq/cm^2$ h (2). However, the accuracy of equating I_{sc} and $J_{sm}^{HCO_3^-}$ for the purpose of demonstrating electrogenic HCO_3^- secretion may be compromised by the contribution of other acid–base transporters (e.g. Cl^-/HCO_3^-, Na^+/H^+ exchangers) or the activity of other electrogenic ion transport proteins at the luminal membrane. Thus, the simplicity inherent in measuring transepithelial HCO_3^- secretion by pH stat can belie the complexity of its underlying molecular determinants.

Since a standing HCO_3^- concentration gradient exists across the mucosa (~25 mM HCO_3^- serosal to mucosal) in a pH stat experiment, differences in G_t confound interpretation of the $J_{sm}^{HCO_3^-}$ because passive movement of HCO_3^- through the paracellular pathway would be expected to change proportionally. Fortunately, as compared to most univalent ions, HCO_3^- has a lower diffusivity in solution and does not show a steep relationship with changes in G_t (20). Nonetheless, the contribution of paracellular HCO_3^- movement can be appreciated empirically. As shown in **Fig. 30.2d**, a positive relationship between basal $J_{sm}^{HCO_3^-}$ and G_t yields an increase in $J_{sm}^{HCO_3^-}$ of +0.2 μeq/cm^2 h per decade in G_t (e.g. 40–50 mS/cm^2). The magnitude of this change is near the resolution of the assay, so paracellular HCO_3^- movement is not likely appreciated in a single experiment but should be considered when experimental groups show differences in mean G_t or individual preparations exceed the range of G_t normally expected. Continuous short circuiting of V_t is used to prevent paracellular ion movement in response to the electrical gradient but the serosal-to-mucosal HCO_3^- diffusion potential will introduce a small error in the I_{sc}. The error is acceptable if large changes in electrogenic transport are expected during an experiment. Alternatively, the experiment can be performed in open circuit where V_t is monitored and intermittently clamped to 0 mV to enable calculation of G_t from Ohm's law.

3.3. Indirect Measurement of Bicarbonate Transport Using Fluorimetric Dyes

As discussed earlier in this chapter the measurement of HCO_3^- concentration inside cells (or in extracellular fluid) is not trivial and requires a value for pCO_2 and pH. Simultaneous recording of pCO_2 and pH in living cells using ion-selective electrodes has been limited to body fluids and the interstitial space. An approach to circumvent this problem is to use pH-sensitive dyes such as BCECF.

3.3.1. Basic Principle of Ratiometric Analysis

As with any other fluorophore the apparent concentration of BCECF decreases over time due to photolytic destruction and compartmentalization (to decrease the amount of compartmentalization, *see* **Note 4**). To make changes in pH comparable throughout the entire time course of an experiment, ratio metric techniques have been applied to recordings with BCECF. For this purpose the emission intensity of the fluorescence is sequentially monitored at two different excitation wavelengths. In most experimental protocols the intensity at the pH-sensitive spectrum of the dye (490 nm) is divided by the intensity at the pH-insensitive end of the spectrum (430 nm) resulting in a ratio value.

Figure 30.4 shows a representative recording where the pH of rat pancreatic duct cells has been experimentally altered using a protocol that has generally been referred to as ammonium pulse technique. Panel A shows the raw data (photon counts) as fluorescence intensity measured after excitation with either 488 or 436 nm, respectively. Addition of NH_4Cl to the perfusate results in a transient shift in the emission intensity after excitation at 488 nm while the fluorescence at 436 nm remains largely unaffected by this manoeuvre. Upon washout of NH_4Cl a

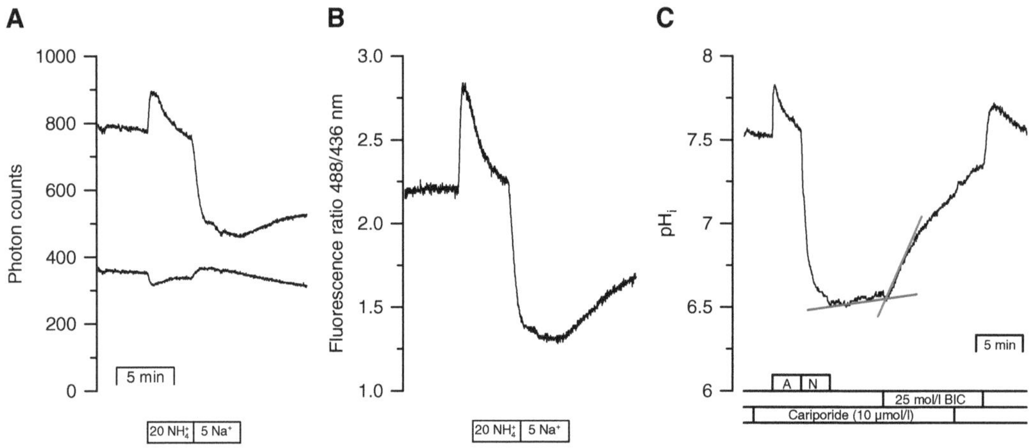

Fig. 30.4. Conversion of the raw signal of fluorescence intensity into a ratio. (**a**) shows the fluorescence of Calu-3 human airway cells loaded with BCECF during exposure to 20 mmol/l NH_4Cl. Addition of NH_4 results in a transient increase in the fluorescence measured after excitation at 488 nm while the fluorescence signal at 436 nm remains unaffected. (**b**) shows the ratio calculated from the raw data. After calibration the ratio can be converted into absolute values for pH_i. (**c**) Recovery of pH_i of porcine SMG after acid load in the presence of HCO_3^-. Cells were exposed to 20 mmol/l NH_4Cl (*A*) followed by a brief washout in a sodium-free solution (*N*). pH_i recovery after re-admission of Na^+ is prevented in the presence of the NHE 1-specific inhibitor cariporide. After addition of HCO_3^-/CO_2 (25 mmol/l BIC) pH_i starts to recover to a neutral value. Removal of HCO_3^-/CO_2 leads to subsequent alkalinization.

sharp decrease in the intensity after excitation at 488 nm can be observed. Panel B shows the ratio calculated from the raw data. After proper calibration the ratio values can be converted into the actual pH.

3.3.2. Calibration of the Fluorimetric Signal

It can be easily anticipated that the absolute intensity, the ratio, and the total range thereof will depend on several factors such as the dye concentration, the optical properties of the excitation–emission pathway, and last but not least the tissue or cell type chosen for the measurement. Using merely the fluorescence ratio between a pH_i-sensitive and a pH_i-insensitive signal may be sufficient to compare the effects of different manoeuvres within one single experiment or – if the conditions are well chosen – even between several experiments using the same set-up and cell type. However, when summarizing a larger number of experiments or when putting the results obtained with a certain cell type in the context of an entire tissue one needs to present the data in a standardized format. It is therefore recommended to calibrate the ratio values to absolute values of pH_i.

An established technique to calibrate the signal of pH-sensitive dyes is to equilibrate pH_i and external pH (pH_e) with the K^+/H^+ exchanger nigericin dissolved in a medium with a cytoplasmic-like (145 mmol/l) K^+ concentration (21). Stepwise changes in the pH_e will lead to consecutive changes in pH_i. The values obtained by this procedure can be fitted to a linear equation that serves as calibration curve for further experiments.

3.3.3. Mechanisms That Regulate pH_i

When HCO_3^- is transported into or out of a cell it will have an impact on the cytosolic buffering capacity and thus on pH_i. Most if not all cells have mechanisms to counterbalance changes in pH_i, which are dependent on or independent of the presence of HCO_3^-. Proper understanding of the complex interaction between these pathways is mandatory when using pH_i changes as a read-out of HCO_3^- transport.

3.3.4. Experimental Approach to Study HCO_3^- Transport

Several experimental approaches have been developed to study the movement of HCO_3^-. The major hurdle to overcome is to separate the activity of the HCO_3^- transporters from that of the H^+ transporters. Due to the fact that most if not all cells express the isoform 1 of the Na^+/H^+ exchanger family, the activity of that protein has to be eliminated or at least greatly reduced to study other transport pathways. In the past decade highly specific inhibitors of NHE1 have been developed. All these compounds are derived from the blocker of the epithelial Na^+ channel (ENaC), amiloride, but in contrast to the latter have no inhibitory action on electrogenic Na^+ transport (22–24). When cells are incubated with any of these NHE1 blockers, a concentration-dependent inhibition of pH_i after acidification can be observed. Now how does this approach help to study HCO_3^- transport? When cells are acidic and H^+ elimination is inhibited either by a pharmacologic blocker or by eliminating Na^+ as the key substrate for secondary active H^+ transport, HCO_3^- influx may be a possibility to restore neutral pH. **Figure 30.4c** shows a recording where HCO_3^- has been added to the bath while pH_i recovery was inhibited by the compound cariporide. It is apparent that immediately after the addition of HCO_3^- pH_i starts to recover to neutral values. The rate of pH_i recovery can then be used as a measure of HCO_3^- influx. Experimentally elicited changes in the recovery rate reflect modulation of HCO_3^- transport. It is possible though to study the influence of CFTR on HCO_3^- transport using specific modulators of CFTR activity. Changes in the pH_i recovery rate upon stimulation of CFTR might be indicative for its involvement in the regulation of HCO_3^- transport.

A major caveat of this approach is that it does not allow for discrimination of the several proteins involved in HCO_3^- transport. To this end at least four different classes of HCO_3^- transporters are described, which, for some, no specific inhibitors are known. It is therefore mandatory to supplement pH_i recordings with molecular and/or biochemical techniques to identify the transporters present in the cell membrane.

4. Notes

1. As an example if we choose two different [HCO_3^-] of 25 and 150 mM and we wish to set pH to 7.4, then from Equation **3**, pCO_2 will need to be 40 mmHg (or 5% CO_2) and 250 mmHg (or 35% CO_2), respectively. Since 5% CO_2/95% O_2 gas cylinders are readily available this is not a problem, but 35% CO_2 gas cylinders are generally more difficult to obtain and far more expensive. A very useful alternative is to use a gas mixer that allows for individual adjustment of pCO_2/pO_2.
2. When preparing HCO_3^--based solutions containing greater than 50 mM HCO_3^- care has to be taken to avoid precipitation of $CaCO_3$. One way to prevent this is to completely remove $CaCl_2$ from the solution.
3. Many researchers studying CFTR replace all permeant cations with larger, non-permeant, cations such as *N*-methyl-D-glucosamine, Tris, or choline.
4. Fluorescent dyes such as BCECF tend to compartmentalize. In most experiments it is desirable to keep this phenomenon at a minimum to avoid contamination of the signal due to a high proportion of organelles with a pH different from the cytosol. The degree of compartmentalization correlates with both time and temperature of incubation. In our hands incubation at room temperature for not longer than 30 min gave the best results.

Acknowledgements

MJH acknowledges generous support from Mukoviszidose e.V. (N03/07), Innovative Medizinische Förderung Münster (HU 1 1 01 03), and EuroCare CF (LSHM-CT-2005-018932). LLC acknowledges the technical assistance of Erin E. Hoover and support from the National Institutes of Health (DK48816). MAG gratefully acknowledges support from the Welcome Trust (079673), the Cystic Fibrosis Trust (PJ540), and the Royal Society (2006R1/JP).

References

1. Molleman, A. (2003) *Patch clamping: an introductory guide to patch clamp electrophysiology*, Wiley, Chichester, ISBN 047148685X.
2. Clarke, L. L. (2009) A guide to Ussing chamber studies of mouse intestine. *Am. J. Physiol.* **296**, G1151–G1166.

3. Frizzell, R. A., and Schultz, S. G. (1972) Ionic conductances of extracellular shunt pathway in rabbit ileum: influence of shunt on transmural sodium transport and electrical potential differences. *J. Gen. Physiol.* **59**, 318–337.
4. Flemstrom, G., Hallgren, A., Nylander, O., Engstrand, L., Wilander, E., and Allen, A. (1999) Adherent surface mucus gel restricts diffusion of macromolecules in rat duodenum in vivo. *Am. J. Physiol.* **277**, G375–G382.
5. Sandberg, J. W., Lau, C., Jacomino, M., Finegold, M., and Henning, S. J. (1994) Improving access to intestinal stem cells as a step toward intestinal gene transfer. *Hum. Gene Ther.* **5**, 323–329.
6. Phillips, T. E. (1992) Both crypt and villus intestinal goblet cells secrete mucin in response to cholinergic stimulation. *Am. J. Physiol.* **262**, G327–G331.
7. Rink, T. J., Tsien, R. Y., and Pozzan, T. (1982) Cytoplasmic pH and free Mg^{2+} in lymphocytes. *J. Cell Biol.* **95**, 189–196.
8. Paradiso, A. M., Tsien, R. Y., and Machen, T. E. (1984) Na^{+}-H^{+} exchange in gastric glands as measured with a cytoplasmic-trapped, fluorescent pH indicator. *Proc. Natl. Acad. Sci. USA* **81**, 7436–7440.
9. Barry, P. H., and Lynch, J. W. (1991) Liquid junction potentials and small cell effects in patch clamp analysis. *J. Membr. Biol.* **121**, 101 117.
10. Gray, M. A., Plant, S., and Argent, B. E. (1993) cAMP regulated whole cell chloride currents in pancreatic duct cells. *Am. J. Physiol.* **264**, C591–C602.
11. O'Reilly, C. M., Winpenny, J. P., Argent, B. E., and Gray, M. A. (2000) Cystic fibrosis transmembrane conductance regulator currents in guinea pig pancreatic duct cells: inhibition by bicarbonate ions. *Gastroenterology* **118**, 1187–1196.
12. Tabcharani, J. A., Rommens, J. M., Hou, Y. X., Chang, X. B., Tsui, L. C., Riordan, J. R., et al. (1993) Multi-ion pore behaviour in the CFTR chloride channel. *Nature* **366**, 79–82.
13. Wright, A. M., Gong, X., Verdon, B., Linsdell, P., Mehta, A., Riordan, J. R., et al. (2004) Novel regulation of the cystic fibrosis transmembrane conductance regulator(CFTR) channel gating by external chloride. *J. Biol. Chem.* **279**, 41658–41663.
14. Gray, M. A., Pollard, C. E., Harris, A., Coleman, L., Greenwell, J. R., and Argent, B. E. (1990) Anion selectivity and block of the small conductance chloride channel on pancreatic duct cells. *Am. J. Physiol.* **259**, C752–C761.
15. Poulsen, J. H., Fisher, H., Illek, B., and Machen, T. E. (1994) Bicarbonate conductance and pH regulatory capability of cystic fibrosis transmembrane conductance regulator. *Proc. Natl. Acad. Sci. USA* **91**, 5340–5344.
16. Linsdell, P., Tabcharani, J. A., Rommens, J. M., Hou, Y. X., Chang, X. B., Tsui, L. C., et al. (1997) Permeability of wild type and mutant cystic fibrosis transmembrane conductance regulator chloride channels to polyatomic anions. *J. Gen. Physiol.* **110**, 355–364.
17. Tang, L., Fatehi, M., and Linsdell, P. (2009) Mechanism of direct bicarbonate transport by the CFTR anion channel. *J. Cyst. Fibros.* **8**, 115–121.
18. Linsdell, P., Tabcharani, J. A., and Hanrahan, J. W. (1997) Multi-ion mechanism for ion permeation and block in the cystic fibrosis transmembrane conductance regulator chloride channel. *J. Gen. Physiol.* **110**, 365–377.
19. Linsdell, P. (2001) Thiocyanate as a probe of the cystic fibrosis transmembrane conductance regulator chloride channel pore. *Can. J. Physiol. Pharmacol.* **79**, 573–579.
20. Walker, N. M., Flagella, M., Gawenis, L. R., Shull, G. E., and Clarke, L. L. (2002) An alternate pathway of cAMP-stimulated Cl^{-} secretion across the NKCC1-null murine duodenum. *Gastroenterology* **123**, 531–541.
21. Chaillet, J. R., and Boron, W. F. (1985) Intracellular calibration of a pH-sensitive dye in isolated, perfused salamander proximal tubules. *J. Gen. Physiol.* **86**, 765–794.
22. Vigne, P., Frelin, C., Cragoe, E. J., and Lazdunski, M. (1983) Ethylisopropyl-amiloride: a new and highly potent derivative of amiloride for the inhibition of the Na^{+}/H^{+} exchange system in various cell types. *Biochem. Biophys. Res. Commun.* **116**, 86–90.
23. Schmid, A., Scholz, W., Lang, H. J., and Popp, R. (1992) Na^{+}/H^{+} exchange in porcine cerebral capillary endothelial cells is inhibited by a benzoylguanidine derivative. *Biochem. Biophys. Res. Commun.* **184**, 112–117.
24. Scholz, W., Albus, U., Counillon, L., Gögelein, H., Lang, H. J., and Linz, W. (1995) Protective effects of HOE642, a selective sodium-hydrogen exchange subtype 1 inhibitor, on cardiac ischaemia and reperfusion. *Cardiovasc. Res.* **29**, 260–268.

INDEX

Note: The letters 'f' and 't' following the locators refer to figures and tables respectively.

M.D. Amaral, K. Kunzelmann (eds.), *Cystic Fibrosis*, Methods in Molecular Biology 741,
DOI 10.1007/978-1-61779-117-8, © Springer Science+Business Media, LLC 2011

T

MIX
Papier aus verantwortungsvollen Quellen
Paper from responsible sources
FSC® C105338

If you have any concerns about our products,
you can contact us on
ProductSafety@springernature.com

In case Publisher is established outside the EU,
the EU authorized representative is:
Springer Nature Customer Service Center GmbH
Europaplatz 3, 69115 Heidelberg, Germany

Printed by Libri Plureos GmbH
in Hamburg, Germany